ATLAS OF ORTHOPAEDIC SURGERY:
A MULTIMEDIA REFERENCE

ATLAS OF ORTHOPAEDIC SURGERY: A MULTIMEDIA REFERENCE

Editors

KENNETH J. KOVAL, M.D.

Professor of Orthopaedic Surgery
New York University School of Medicine
Director, Trauma Service
New York University—Hospital for Joint Diseases Department of Orthopaedic Surgery
New York, New York

JOSEPH D. ZUCKERMAN, M.D.

Chairman, New York University—Hospital for Joint Diseases Department of Orthopaedic Surgery
Walter A.L. Thompson Professor of Orthopaedic Surgery
New York University School of Medicine
Surgeon-in-Chief
Hospital for Joint Diseases
New York, New York

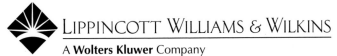

LIPPINCOTT WILLIAMS & WILKINS
A **Wolters Kluwer** Company
Philadelphia · Baltimore · New York · London
Buenos Aires · Hong Kong · Sydney · Tokyo

Acquisitions Editor: Robert Hurley
Developmental Editor: Keith Donnellan
Production Editor: Robin E. Cook
Manufacturing Manager: Colin Warnock
Cover Designer: Christine Jenny
Compositor: Maryland Composition
Printer: Walsworth

© 2004 by LIPPINCOTT WILLIAMS & WILKINS
530 Walnut St.
Philadelphia, PA 19106 USA
LWW.com

Printed in the USA

Library of Congress Cataloging-in-Publication Data
Atlas of orthopaedic surgery : a multimedia reference / editors, Joseph D. Zuckerman, Kenneth J. Koval
    p. ; cm.
  Includes bibliographical references and index.
  ISBN 0-7817-1788-4
  1. Orthopedic surgery—Atlases. I. Koval, Kenneth J. II. Zuckerman, Joseph D. (Joseph David), 1952-
  [DNLM: 1. Orthopedic Procedures—Atlases. WE 17 A8806325 2004]
  RD 731.A886 2004
  617.4′7—dc22
                                                        2003060621

Care has been taken to confirm the accuracy of the information presented and to describe generally accepted practices. However, the authors, editors, and publisher are not responsible for errors or omissions or for any consequences from application of the information in this book and make no warranty, expressed or implied, with respect to the currency, completeness, or accuracy of the contents of the publication. Application of this information in a particular situation remains the professional responsibility of the practitioner.

The authors, editors, and publisher have exerted every effort to ensure that drug selection and dosage set forth in this text are in accordance with current recommendations and practice at the time of publication. However, in view of ongoing research, changes in government regulations, and the constant flow of information relating to drug therapy and drug reactions, the reader is urged to check the package insert for each drug for any change in indications and dosage and for added warnings and precautions. This is particularly important when the recommended agent is a new or infrequently employed drug.

Some drugs and medical devices presented in this publication have Food and Drug Administration (FDA) clearance for limited use in restricted research settings. It is the responsibility of the health care provider to ascertain the FDA status of each drug or device planned for use in their clinical practice.

10 9 8 7 6 5 4 3 2 1

For my loving and understanding wife, Mary, and my fantastic children, Courtney, Michael, and Lauren.

KJK

To my esteemed colleagues in the NYU-Hospital for Joint Diseases Department of Orthopaedic Surgery for their outstanding contributions to this multimedia reference and for their dedication to our academic mission.
And, as always, to the joys of my life—my wife, Janet, and my sons, Scott and Matthew.

JDZ

CONTENTS

CONTRIBUTING AUTHORS

Arash Araghi, D.O., Former Shoulder and Elbow Fellow, NYU–Hospital for Joint Diseases Department of Orthopaedic Surgery, New York, New York, and Attending Physician, Department of Orthpaedic Surgery, Del E. Webb Memorial Hospital, Sun City West, Arizona

Donna J. Astion, M.D., Former Attending Physician, Foot and Ankle Service, NYU–Hospital for Joint Diseases Department of Orthopaedic Surgery, New York, New York, and Attending Physician, Department of Orthopaedic Surgery, St. Luke's Roosevelt Hospital Center, New York, New York

John A. Bendo, M.D., Clinical Assistant Professor of Orthopaedic Surgery, New York University School of Medicine, New York, New York, and Associate Director, Hospital for Joint Diseases Spine Center, New York, New York

Peter Bono, D.O., Former Spine Fellow, NYU–Hospital for Joint Diseases Department of Orthopaedic Surgery, New York, New York, and Clinical Assistant Professor of Osteopathic Surgical Specialties, Michigan State University College of Osteopathic Medicine, East Lansing, Michigan

Biren V. Chokshi, M.D., M.S., Former Sports Medicine Fellow, NYU–Hospital for Joint Diseases Department of Orthopaedic Surgery, New York, New York, and Orthopedic Associates of Windham County, Putnam, Connecticut

Gail S. Chorney, M.D., Assistant Professor of Orthopaedic Surgery, New York University School of Medicine, New York, New York, and Attending Physician, NYU–Hospital for Joint Diseases Department of Orthopaedic Surgery, New York, New York

Brian S. DeLay, M.D., Former Sports Medicine Fellow, NYU–Hospital for Joint Diseases Department of Orthopaedic Surgery, New York, New York, and Charlotte Orthopaedic Specialists, Lake Norman Office, Moorsville, North Carolina

Craig J. Della Valle, M.D., Former Chief Resident, NYU–Hospital for Joint Diseases Department of Orthopaedic Surgery, New York, New York, and Assistant Professor of Orthopaedic Surgery, Rush Medical College, Chicago, Illinois

Paul E. Di Cesare, M.D., F.A.C.S., Associate Professor of Orthopaedic Surgery and Cell Biology, New York University School of Medicine, New York, New York, and Director, Musculoskeletal Research Center, NYU–Hospital for Joint Diseases Department of Orthopaedic Surgery, New York, New York

Kenneth A. Egol, M.D., Assistant Professor of Orthopaedic Surgery, New York University School of Medicine, New York, New York, and Attending Physician, Trauma Service, NYU–Hospital for Joint Diseases, Department of Orthopaedic Surgery, New York, New York

Thomas J. Errico, M.D., Associate Professor of Orthopaedic Surgery and Neurosurgery, New York University School of Medicine, New York, New York, and Chief, Spine Service, NYU–Hospital for Joint Diseases, Department of Orthopaedic Surgery, New York, New York

David S. Feldman, M.D., Assistant Professor of Orthopaedic Surgery, New York University School of Medicine, New York, New York, and Chief, Pediatric Service, NYU–Hospital for Joint Diseases Department of Orthopaedic Surgery, New York, New York

Steven M. Green, M.D., Clinical Associate Professor of Orthopaedic Surgery, New York University of School of Medicine, New York, New York, and Associate Chief, Hand Service, NYU–Hospital for Joint Diseases Department of Orthopaedic Surgery, New York, New York

Amir Hasharoni, M.D., Ph.D., Former Spine Fellow, NYU–Hospital for Joint Diseases Department of Orthopaedic Surgery, New York, New York, and Attending Spine Surgeon, Hadassah Hebrew University Medical Center, Jerusalem, Israel

William L. Jaffe, M.D., Clinical Professor of Orthopaedic Surgery, New York University School of Medicine, New York, New York, and Vice-Chairman, NYU–Hospital for Joint Diseases Department of Orthopaedic Surgery, New York, New York

Kenneth J. Koval, M.D., Professor of Orthopaedic Surgery, New York University School of Medicine, New York, New York, and Director, Trauma Service, NYU–Hospital for Joint Diseases Department of Orthopaedic Surgery, New York, New York

Mark I. Loebenberg, M.D., Former Attending Physician, Shoulder and Elbow Service, NYU–Hospital for Joint Diseases Department of Orthopaedic Surgery, New York, New York, and Senior Consultant Surgeon, Department of Orthopaedic Surgery, Assaf HaRofeh Medical Center, Tel Aviv University School of Medicine, Tzrifin, Israel

Patrick A. Meere, M.D., Clinical Assistant Professor of Orthopaedic Surgery, New York University School of Medicine, New York, New York, and Attending Physician, Adult Reconstructive Service, NYU–Hospital for Joint Diseases Department of Orthopaedic Surgery, New York, New York

Young Ho Oh, M.D., Former Sports Medicine Fellow, NYU–Hospital for Joint Diseases Department of Orthopaedic Surgery, New York, New York, and Attending Physician, Department of Surgery, MetroWest Medical Center, Framingham, Massachusetts

J. Serge Parisien, M.D., Clinical Professor of Orthopaedic Surgery, New York University School of Medicine, New York, New York, and Attending Physician, Sports Medicine Service, NYU–Hospital for Joint Diseases Department of Orthopaedic Surgery, New York, New York

Mark I. Pitman, M.D., Clinical Associate Professor of Orthopaedic Surgery, New York University School of Medicine, New York, New York, and Chief Emeritus, Sports Medicine Service, NYU–Hospital for Joint Diseases Department of Orthopaedic Surgery, New York, New York

Ann-Marie R. Plate, M.D., Assistant Professor of Orthopaedic Surgery, New York University School of Medicine, New York, New York, and Attending Physician, Hand Service, NYU–Hospital for Joint Diseases Department of Orthopaedic Surgery, New York, New York

Martin A. Posner, M.D., Clinical Professor of Orthopaedic Surgery, New York University School of Medicine, New York, New York, and Chief, Hand Service, NYU–Hospital for Joint Diseases Department of Orthopaedic Surgery, New York, New York

Keith B. Raskin, M.D., Clinical Associate Professor of Orthopaedic Surgery, New York University School of Medicine, New York, New York, and Attending Physician, Hand Service, NYU–Hospital for Joint Diseases Department of Orthopaedic Surgery, New York, New York

Ponnavolu D. Reddy, M.D., Former Foot and Ankle Fellow, NYU–Hospital for Joint Diseases Department of Orthopaedic Surgery, New York, New York, and Attending Orthopaedic Surgeon, Winter Haven Hospital, Winter Haven, Florida

Michael E. Rettig, M.D., Assistant Professor of Orthopaedic Surgery, New York University School of Medicine, New York, New York, and Attending Physician, Hand Service, NYU–Hospital for Joint Diseases Department of Orthopaedic Surgery, New York, New York

Andrew S. Rokito, M.D., Assistant Professor of Orthopaedic Surgery, New York University School of Medicine, New York, New York, and Chief, Shoulder and Elbow Service, NYU–Hospital for Joint Diseases Department of Orthopaedic Surgery, New York, New York

Jeffrey E. Rosen, M.D., Assistant Professor of Orthopaedic Surgery, New York University School of Medicine, New York, New York, and Attending Physician, Sports Medicine Service, NYU–Hospital for Joint Diseases Department of Orthopaedic Surgery, New York, New York

Steven C. Sheskier, M.D., Clinical Assistant Professor of Orthopaedic Surgery, New York University School of Medicine, New York, New York, and Attending Physician, Foot and Ankle Service, NYU–Hospital for Joint Diseases Department of Orthopaedic Surgery, New York, New York

Jeffrey M. Spivak, M.D., Assistant Professor of Orthopaedic Surgery, New York University School of Medicine, New York, New York, and Director, Hospital for Joint Diseases Spine Center, New York, New York

Richard A. Zell, M.D., Former Foot and Ankle Fellow, NYU–Hospital for Joint Diseases Department of Orthopaedic Surgery, New York, New York, and Staff Orthopaedic Surgeon, Department of Orthopaedics, Yale-New Haven Hospital and Hospital of Saint Raphael, New Haven, Connecticut

Joseph D. Zuckerman, M.D., Walter A.L. Thompson Professor of Orthopaedic Surgery, New York University School of Medicine, New York, New York, and Chairman, NYU–Hospital for Joint Diseases Department of Orthopaedic Surgery, New York, New York

PREFACE

Atlas of Orthopaedic Surgery: A Multimedia Reference represents the effort of many members of the NYU-Hospital for Joint Diseases Department of Orthopaedic Surgery. The creation of an interactive video guide for use by practicing orthopaedists, residents, and fellows in training is the culmination of our many years of commitment to graduate medical education. The chapters and procedures included for presentation are based on a consensus of the most common procedures performed by orthopaedists and represent the subspecialty areas of adult reconstruction; shoulder and elbow; sports medicine; hand, spine, foot, and ankle pediatrics; and trauma. Chapters were prepared by contributors with special expertise and extensive experience in the operative case illustrated. Each chapter follows an outline consisting of: pertinent surgical anatomy; surgical indications; classification, when appropriate; preoperative planning, including equipment, patient positioning, a step-by-step approach to the operative procedure; and postoperative care. "Pearls" and "pitfalls" are provided throughout the text to help the clinician achieve successful outcomes; pearls are <u>underlined</u> and pitfalls appear in **bold**.

It is our hope that this reference will provide orthopaedic surgeons with important and useful information on commonly performed surgical procedures in our specialty, with the ultimate goal of enhancing the care we provide our patients.

Kenneth J. Koval, M.D.
Joseph D. Zuckerman, M.D.

ACKNOWLEDGMENTS

We would like to acknowledge: 1) the efforts made by all of the outstanding contributors—they provided their expertise, time and effort to produce the chapters comprising this book; 2) the faculty and residents of the NYU–Hospital for Joint Diseases Department of Orthopaedic Surgery who provided the academic environment for this project; 3) David Ruchelsman, B.S., New York University School of Medicine, for his excellent assistance in preparation of Chapter 12, "Supracondylar Fractures: Operative Management"; 4) Baynon McDowell, our editorial assistant, who was essential in the completion and coordination of the entire work and without whose tremendous effort, this work would not have been possible; 5) Frank Martucci, medical photographer *par excellence,* who was responsible for the photographic and video work; and 6) all of the staff at Lippincott Williams & Wilkins responsible for shepherding this project, most particularly Keith Donnellan, Developmental Editor, and Robin Cook, Production Editor, for their expertise, patience, and understanding during the many hours and days required for the completion of what we believe is a distinctive contribution to the roster of orthopaedic publications.

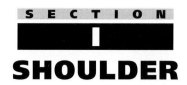
CHAPTER 1

SHOULDER ARTHROSCOPY: DIAGNOSTIC

MARK I. LOEBENBERG

The therapeutic use of arthroscopy in shoulder surgery has expanded rapidly in the last decade. Arthroscopic subacromial decompressions, instability procedures, and rotator cuff repairs are now all common interventions. However, diagnostic arthroscopy remains the foundation on which all of these procedures are built. The competent surgeon must be familiar with normal arthroscopic anatomy before pathology can be identified. The surgeon should be able to visualize all of the structures within the glenohumeral joint and subacromial before undertaking any reconstructive procedures. This chapter describes the steps necessary to perform a complete diagnostic arthroscopy of the glenohumeral joint, including positioning, setup, instruments, and technical advice to assist with full visualization.

ANATOMY

A full understanding of both the surface and intraarticular anatomy of the glenohumeral joint and the subacromial space are prerequisites for successful arthroscopic surgery of the shoulder. Proper portal placement can allow the surgeon to routinely visualize the entire glenohumeral joint and subacromial space. A complete understanding of normal anatomy, including its normal variants allows the surgeon to quickly recognize the presence of pathologic conditions.

Biceps Tendon

The proximal or long head tendon of the biceps brachii is the first major structure that should be identified within the glenohumeral joint, because it acts as a major landmark for orientation within the joint. When the patient is in the lateral decubitus position the biceps tendon is seen approximately 10 degrees to 15 degrees from an imaginary vertical line. In the beachchair position, the tendon runs quite parallel to floor before it enters the bicipital groove. The tendon originates from the supraglenoid tubercle at the superior rim of the glenoid and from the superior, usually posterior,

glenoid labrum (Fig. 1-1). However, it is important to note that the sites of origin are variable. Studies have documented that 20% of normal biceps tendons attach only to the supraglenoid tubercle; 48% only to the superior, posterior glenoid labrum; and 28% originating from both points. To facilitate visualization of the tendon as it courses anterolaterally through the joint, the arm should be externally rotated. The tendon can be observed as it exits into the bicipital groove, between the tendons of the subscapularis and supraspinatus muscles. In the anatomic position, the intraarticular portion of the biceps tendon courses below the coracohumeral ligament, which strengthens the rotator interval, a space between the tendons of the subscapularis and supraspinatus muscles. The coracohumeral ligament and superior glenohumeral ligament aid in the support of the biceps tendon in the rotator interval.

The surface of a healthy biceps tendon appears smooth; glistening; and free of any adhesions, fraying, or partial tears. The arthroscope can be used to diagnose any dislocation or subluxation of the tendon out of the bicipital groove in addition to partial tears or detachment of the biceps anchor. Superior labrum anterior and posterior (SLAP) lesions of the biceps origin can also be identified and treated.

Articular Surfaces

The appearance and integrity of the articular surfaces of the glenoid and the humeral head must be fully evaluated during arthroscopy. The glenoid is an ovoid or pear-shaped cavity that is approximately one fourth the size of the humeral head. Its surface is covered by articular cartilage. However, there is a normal central area with little or no cartilage present. At the anterior glenoid margin a notch or indentation is present, which should not be mistaken for an anterior lip or Bankart lesion related to anterior instability. The humeral head is typically round and covered with smooth articular cartilage. Posteriorly, it has a normal "bare area" or sulcus, which is a region of bare bone present between the edge of the articular surface and the insertion of the poste-

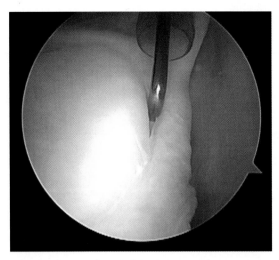

FIGURE 1-1. The long head of the biceps tendon acts as a major landmark for orientation within the joint. When the patient is in the lateral decubitus position the biceps tendon is seen approximately 10 to 15 degrees from an imaginary vertical line. In the beachchair position, the tendon runs quite parallel to floor before it enters the bicipital groove. The tendon originates from the supraglenoid tubercle at the superior rim of the glenoid and from the superior, usually posterior, glenoid labrum. Variable sites of origin include the supraglenoid tubercle and either or both of the anterior and posterior labrum.

rior capsule (Fig. 1-2). This bare area should not be confused with a Hill Sachs lesion, a posterior humeral head compression fracture associated with anterior dislocations of the glenohumeral joint. A Hill Sachs lesion typically is found posterosuperiorly on the humeral head and has no vascular channels, whereas the bare area has normally ap-

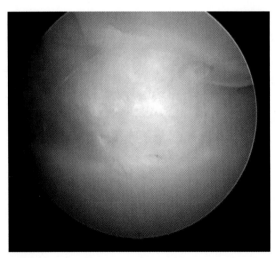

FIGURE 1-2. The humeral head is typically round and covered with smooth articular cartilage. A normal "bare area" of bare bone is present between the edge of the articular surface and the insertion of the posterior capsule. This bare area should not be confused with a traumatic Hill Sachs lesion. A Hill Sachs lesion typically is found posterosuperiorly on the humeral head and has no vascular channels, whereas the bare area has normally appearing vascular channels.

pearing vascular channels. A reverse Hill Sachs lesion, associated with posterior dislocations is an extremely rare pathologic finding during arthroscopy. It appears as a wedge-shaped defect toward the lateral insertion of the subscapularis tendon on the lesser tuberosity. In all cases, the cartilage should be scanned for any traumatic lesions, inflammatory or degenerative conditions, or chondromalacia. In osteoarthritis, significant osteophyte formation tends to occur along the edges of the articular surface, particularly along the anteroinferior surface of the joint. In the presence of full-thickness rotator cuff tears, the edge of the articular surface near the cuff insertion often becomes roughened with small spurs and osteophytes.

Glenoid Labrum

By deepening the glenoid fossa, the wedge-shaped glenoid labrum serves to provide substantial stability to the glenohumeral joint and extends its arc of stable rotation. The labrum consists of hyaline cartilage, fibrocartilage, and fibrous tissue. Its capsular surface blends with the joint capsule, whereas the glenoid surface is directly continuous with the hyaline cartilage of the glenoid fossa. The labrum varies greatly in its anatomy, ranging in width from 1 to 5 mm and in shape from ovoid to meniscoid. Five normal labral anatomic variations have been described. A wedge labrum located only at the superior glenoid margin, a wedge labrum at the posterior glenoid margin, a wedge labrum at the anterior glenoid margin, a wedge labrum extending from the superior to the anterior glenoid margin, and a meniscoid labrum extending around the circumference of the glenoid margin. In addition, a subcoracoid labral sulcus or foramen, present superoanteriorly on the glenoid margin and characterized by smooth borders, is a normal anatomic variant. This sulcus is far more superior than the pathologic "Bankart" lesion described later. The "Buford complex" described by Snyder is a normal anatomic variant in which the cordlike middle glenohumeral ligament inserts directly into the biceps tendon, creating an area on the glenoid with no labrum superiorly, appearing as a sublabral hole. These normal variations need to be recognized and differentiated from pathologic conditions.

The entire glenoid labrum should be visualized during the procedure and should appear smooth, without fraying or partial tearing and should not be hypermobile (see Fig. 4-1).

Capsule/Ligaments

With close intraarticular arthroscopic examination, three distinct thickenings of the anterior capsule can be recognized as the superior, middle, and inferior glenohumeral ligaments. They are named for their origins on the humeral head rather than for their scapular attachments and function to stabilize the anterior and inferior portions of the joint capsule. When viewed arthroscopically, the insertions may appear to be labral rather than the more typical capsular or glenoid insertions.

The superior glenohumeral ligament is the smallest of the three glenohumeral ligaments. It combines with the coracohumeral ligament and rotator interval to form the superior glenohumeral ligamentous complex. This functions to stabilize the shoulder joint when the arm is in the adducted dependent position and to prevent inferior instability. The superior glenohumeral ligament courses laterally across the joint from its points of origin to insert into the anterior aspect of the anatomic neck of the humerus, just superior to the lesser tuberosity. Arthroscopically it may be difficult to find because its position may be hidden by the biceps tendon. Insufflation of the joint also blurs the margins of the ligament when the entire capsule is placed under tension.

The middle glenohumeral ligament stabilizes the glenohumeral joint when the shoulder is abducted to 45 degrees. It attaches to the superior aspect of the labrum, just caudal to the superior glenohumeral ligament, and to the scapular neck. Running laterally, it crosses just posterior to the subscapularis tendon at an approximate angle of 60 degrees and inserts on the anterior anatomic humeral neck just medial to the lesser tuberosity. A cordlike or very thin appearance of the ligament are both normal variants.

Viewed arthroscopically, the triangular inferior glenohumeral ligament is typically the most conspicuous of the capsular ligaments. The sling-like ligament consists of anterior and posterior band and an intervening "axillary pouch." When the arm is abducted to approximately 90 degrees, the inferior glenohumeral ligament acts to stabilize the glenohumeral joint. The ligament originates from the medial aspect of the surgical neck of the humerus and attaches to the anteroinferior and posteroinferior aspects of the glenoid labrum.

Rotator Interval and Rotator Cuff

Arthroscopy of the glenohumeral joint allows for full visualization of the rotator interval, the intraarticular portion of the subscapularis tendon, and the insertion of the rotator cuff on the humeral head.

The rotator interval is a triangular space between supraspinatus and subscapularis tendons (Fig. 1-3). It contains both the superior glenohumeral and the coracohumeral ligaments, the latter overlying the biceps tendon. The rotator interval serves as an important landmark for anterior portal placement. The tissue appears less dense than the tendons that border it. A healthy, normal interval should appear almost empty. Copious amounts of scar can present in this area when significant preoperative restrictions in range of motion, particularly external rotation, are present.

The most superior aspects of the subscapularis tendon can be examined during glenohumeral arthroscopy. This region of the tendon, commonly referred to as the "rolled edge" of the tendon because of its thickness in this region can be ob-

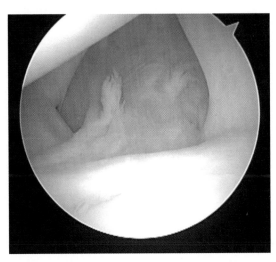

FIGURE 1-3. The rotator interval is a triangular space between supraspinatus and subscapularis tendons. It contains both the superior glenohumeral and the coracohumeral ligaments, the latter overlying the biceps tendon. The anterior portal is placed through the rotator interval. The tissue appears less dense than the tendons that border it. A healthy, normal interval should appear almost empty.

served in the anterior aspect of the shoulder (Fig. 1-4). The tendon can be seen entering the glenohumeral joint through the subscapular recess or bursa. The bursa lies between the superior and middle glenohumeral ligaments. Occasionally, the middle glenohumeral ligament may obscure vision of the subscapularis tendon or even appear to blend with it, because the ligament lies posterior to the tendon. Differentiation is based on the tendon's fibers running perpendicular to the

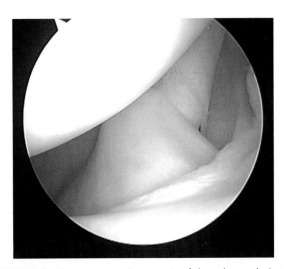

FIGURE 1-4. The most superior aspects of the subscapularis tendon can be examined during glenohumeral arthroscopy. This "rolled edge" of the tendon can be observed in the anterior aspect of the shoulder. The tendon's lateral margin can be seen entering the glenohumeral joint through the subscapular recess or bursa. Occasionally, the middle glenohumeral ligament may obscure vision of the subscapularis tendon. A healthy tendon should be free of any fraying or adhesions to surrounding capsular tissues and translate freely with internal and external rotation of the humeral head.

long axis of the glenoid, and the ligament runs more obliquely. A healthy tendon should be free of any fraying or adhesions to surrounding capsular tissues and translate freely with internal and external rotation of the humeral head.

Intraarticular arthroscopic observation of the rotator cuff allows for examination of the tendons of the supraspinatus, infraspinatus, and most of the teres minor as they course together toward their insertion on the greater tuberosity of the humerus. The anterior edge of the supraspinatus tendon can be observed just superior to the biceps tendon as it enters the bicipital groove. The supraspinatus originates from the supraspinatus fossa on the posterior scapula and inserts on the superior aspect of the greater tuberosity of the humerus. The infraspinatus inserts on the posterolateral aspect of the greater tuberosity, whereas the teres minor inserts on its lower portion. Closer to the insertion points the three tendons appear to fuse. A thin layer of synovium and joint capsule, with a smooth appearance, should cover the surface of these tendons.

Subacromial Space

Arthroscopy of the subacromial space allows for examination of the superior surface of the rotator cuff, the undersurface of the coracoacromial arch including the coracoacromial ligament, the acromioclavicular joint, and the subacromial bursa. The superior surface of the rotator cuff should be smooth and homogenous, without any tears, fraying, or calcifications. A layer of periosteum covers the undersurface of the acromion and should also appear smooth without spurring. Acromial shape may be characterized according to the curvature of their undersurface, ranging from flat to hooked. The superior aspect of the coracoacromial ligament should be visualized as it courses obliquely from its origin on the anterior undersurface and tip of the acromion toward its insertion on the lateral aspect of the coracoid process. Medially, the acromioclavicular joint can be seen and any spurs or prominences noted. Finally, the bursa itself should be evaluated. It extends from the deltoid muscle laterally to the coracoacromial ligament medially. Anteriorly, the bursa stretches from the coracoacromial ligament and the deltoid to approximately one third of the way back under the acromion. The roof of the bursa is limited by the undersurface of the coracoacromial ligament and acromion and the floor by the rotator cuff.

CLASSIFICATION

A number of anatomic and pathologic conditions exist that characterize structures observed during diagnostic arthroscopy and allow for determination of proper treatment. Snyder and his coauthors have described and classified tears of the superior labrum and biceps anchor (Fig. 1-5). SLAP lesions are categorized into four types. In type I lesions there is fraying and degeneration of the superior labrum but there

is no tearing present. The biceps tendon is healthy and intact. A type II lesion also exhibits fraying of the superior labrum, but there is pathologic detachment of the labrum and biceps anchor from the underlying superior glenoid. A type III SLAP lesion is a bucket-handle type tear strictly of the superior labrum, with no involvement of the biceps tendon. Type IV lesions involve a bucket handle tear of the superior labrum that extends up into the biceps tendon, with both displaced into the joint. Most SLAP lesions are type II (55%) or type I (21%).

The morphology of the acromion has been classified by Bigliani and Morrison into three types. The shape of the acromion seems to correlate with the risk of impingement pathologies. Type I acromions, with the least associated with rotator cuff pathology, are characterized by a flat undersurface. The undersurfaces of type II acromions are curved. Finally, a type III acromion has a hooked or beak shaped undersurface, which narrows the outlet pathway of the supraspinatus muscle and tendon. Patients with type III acromions are most at risk for impingement syndrome and its resulting complications.

Rotator cuff tears should be characterized by history as acute, subacute, or chronic. Imaging and arthroscopy allow for characterization based on size, shape, and tendon quality. Cuff tears can be described as either partial- or full-thickness tears. Partial-thickness tears are characterized by fraying of the cuff and may be located on either the intraarticular or bursal side of the rotator cuff. Grade I partial thickness tears are less than one fourth of the thickness of the tendon, Grade II are less than $^1/_2$ of the thickness, and Grade III are greater than $^1/_2$ of the thickness of the tendon. Full-thickness tears can be characterized as small ($<$1cm) medium (1 to 3 cm), large ($>$3 to 5 cm), or massive ($>$5 cm). In some cases of massive, retracted full-thickness tears the rotator cuff may appear to be completely absent. The shape of the tear should also be characterized. A transverse linear tear exists at the insertion. L-shaped tears extend from the transverse linear in between the supraspinatus and infraspinatus tendons. A reverse L-shaped tear extends into the rotator interval. Massive tears include all of the supraspinatus and infraspinatus tendons and extend into the teres minor as well.

SPECIAL EQUIPMENT/INSTRUMENTS

Diagnostic arthroscopy of the shoulder requires basic arthroscopic equipment. Typically, a 30-degree arthroscope, between 4 to 5 mm, allows for observation of the entire joint. The size and degree of visualization of the arthroscope are more significant than its specific designer. To allow for easy and clear visualization of the joint a video camera and monitor are necessary. A set of spinal needles should be present to allow for an accurate assessment of portal position before their placement. Basic arthroscopic in-

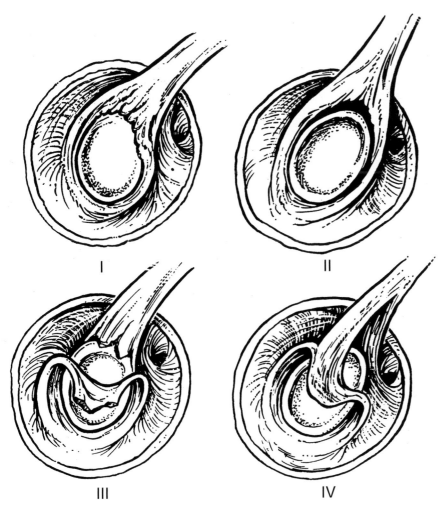

I

II

III

IV

FIGURE 1-5. The classification of superior labrum anterior and posterior (SLAP) lesions. Type I lesions have fraying and degeneration of the superior labrum, but there is no tearing present. A type II lesion also exhibits fraying of the superior labrum, but there is pathologic detachment of the labrum and biceps anchor from the underlying superior glenoid. A type III SLAP lesion is a bucket-handle type tear strictly of the superior labrum, with no involvement of the biceps tendon. Type IV lesions involve a bucket handle tear of the superior labrum that extends up into the biceps tendon, with both easily displaced into the joint. (From Park SS, Loebenberg MI, Rokito AS, Zuckerman JD: The shoulder in baseball pitching: biomechanics and related injuries-Part 2. Bull Hosp Jt Dis 2002-2003;61 (1-2):80-8, with permission.)

struments, including probes, hooks, and grabbers (Fig. 1-6) should be present and are often critical for a complete diagnostic assessment of intraarticular structures.

A cannula system (Fig. 1-7) should be used to act both as a conduit for the arthroscope and other instruments and as an irrigation tool. Diaphragm inserts for the cannulas are helpful in maintaining joint distension. An arthroscopy pump, with a pressure sensor, and tubing should be used to create joint distension and introduce a constant flow of clear fluid (Fig. 1-8). In addition, a suction-equipped system of shavers of various sizes and shapes should be available (Fig. 1-9). Radiofrequency ablation devices can be a great assis-

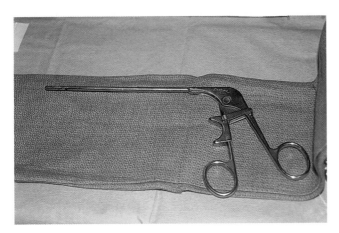

FIGURE 1-6. Arthroscopic graspers.

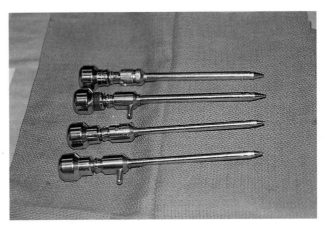

FIGURE 1-7. Arthroscopic cannulas.

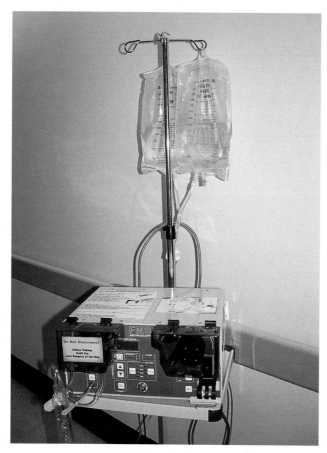

FIGURE 1-8. Infusion pump.

tance for intraoperative hemostasis and the removal of soft tissues when appropriate.

INDICATIONS

Diagnostic arthroscopy can be used for the confirmation of pathology before operative intervention. Most patients who undergo diagnostic arthroscopy should have had a definitive

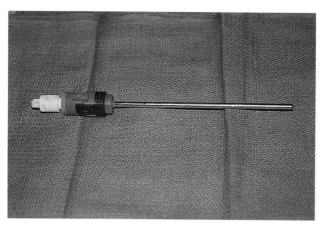

FIGURE 1-9. Arthroscopic shaver.

diagnosis made through a complete history, physical examination, and the appropriate radiographic imaging. In addition to a proper examination under anesthesia, diagnostic arthroscopy should confirm the diagnosis for which surgery was scheduled, assist in the discovery of secondary diagnoses, and allow for proper planning with regard to the placement of additional operative arthroscopy portals or open incisions.

PREOPERATIVE PLANNING

The proper preoperative plan will vary depending on the diagnosis that resulted in a surgical indication. Plain radiographs should be obtained before any surgical procedure. Anteroposterior views in both external and internal rotation, supraspinatus outlet views, and an axillary view should be obtained to allow for proper orthogonal assessment of the glenohumeral and acromioclavicular joints in addition to the subacromial space. Advanced imaging studies such as arthrography, ultrasonography, and magnetic resonance imaging should be obtained when appropriate. These studies can provide valuable preoperative assessment of the integrity and quality of the rotator cuff and the presence and absence of Bankart or SLAP lesions. A full preoperative understanding of the extent of the pathology not only allows for adequate planning on the part of the surgeon but also allows the patient to be fully cognizant of the extent of his or her pathology. This information can serve as a valuable aid in the establishment of reasonable outcome expectations.

PATIENT POSITIONING AND PREPARATION

For proper patient positioning, additional equipment may be necessary. If the beachchair sitting position is used, it is valuable to use a special operative table addition that allows the patient to be placed in a seated upright position without the table resting against the posterior aspect of the operative shoulder. **It is critical to have access to almost the entire scapula when positioning the patient. If the table rests too close to the posterior portal site, visualization of the lateral aspect of the glenohumeral joint, including the rotator cuff insertion may be significantly restricted** (Fig. 1-10). A disposable cervical collar can be used to stabilize the neck during the procedure. The head is placed in a stable head rest and gently secured in place with an elastic bandage, taking care to protect the patients' eyes. The bed should be flexed slightly and the legs elevated on several pillows to prevent the patient from sliding into a more supine position during the procedure. Surgical preparation of the entire operative extremity should be undertaken to allow for full access to the surface anatomy of the entire shoulder (Fig. 1-11). The monitor should be positioned in such a manner to allow the surgeon to stand behind the shoulder and look easily toward both the shoulder and the monitor (Fig. 1-12).

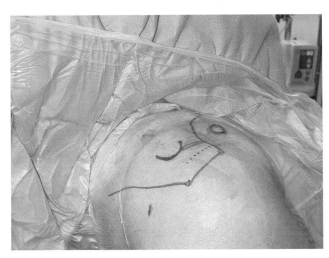

FIGURE 1-10. The beach chair position after the extremity has been prepped and draped. It is critical to have access to almost the entire scapula when positioning the patient. If the table rests too close to the posterior portal site, visualization of the lateral aspect of the glenohumeral joint, including the rotator cuff insertion may be significantly restricted.

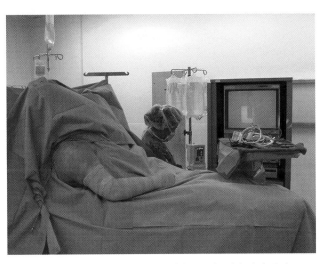

FIGURE 1-11. The beach chair position. It is critical that the entire arm is draped free to allow the surgeon to move the limb at will. The patient should be in a semireclined position to allow the surgeon access to both the anterior and posterior surfaces of the shoulder.

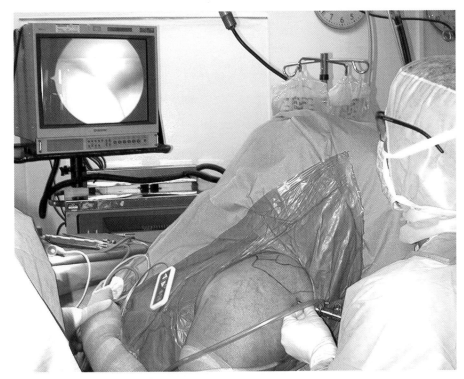

FIGURE 1-12. The beach chair position. The monitor should be positioned in such a manner to allow the surgeon to stand behind the shoulder and look easily toward both the shoulder and the monitor. An elevated Mayo stand can serve as a convenient shelf for arthroscopic instruments when placed above the patients midportion.

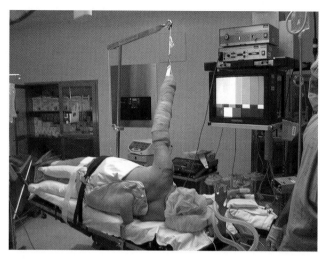

FIGURE 1-13. The lateral position. This position requires that the patient be secured in a direct lateral position with the operative extremity placed in a traction apparatus with the arm elevated roughly 45 degrees in the plane of the scapular. Lateral positioning affords the option of easier glenohumeral joint distraction when desired.

A lateral position may also be used for shoulder arthroscopy. This position requires that the patient be secured in a direct lateral position with the operative extremity placed in a traction apparatus with the arm elevated roughly 45 degrees in the plane of the scapular. An inflatable bean bag and kidney rest attachments help secure the patient in a stable position. An axillary roll should be placed to protect the dependent extremity and all bony prominences should be carefully padded. The operative extremity can then be prepared and draped up to the edge of the forearm traction device (Fig. 1-13).

LANDMARKS/PORTALS

After the shoulder is properly prepared and draped with sterile towels and adhesive drapes, the major bony anatomic landmarks are identified and marked with a skin marking pen. The demarcation of these structures allows for the site of the primary portals to be reproducibly located (Fig. 1-14). The landmarks are the anterior, lateral, and posterior borders of the acromion, the distal clavicle and the acromioclavicular joint, the scapular spine, and the coracoid process. ◖▶

For diagnostic arthroscopy two primary portals are used. The posterior portal is the first portal to be established. This approach is preferred because the posterior portal allows for almost complete observation of the glenohumeral joint and aids in placing subsequent portals. The posterior portal is located approximately 2 to 3 cm inferior and 1 to 2 cm medial to the posterolateral tip of the acromion. This allows the portal to pass through the "soft spot" of the posterior shoulder, representing the interval between the infraspinatus and the teres minor muscle. By placing an index finger on the coracoid process, the thumb can be used to feel for the direction of the glenohumeral joint. Neither the posterior circumflex arteries nor the axillary nerve, the nearest neurovas-

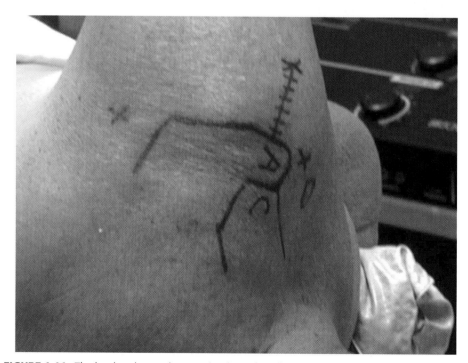

FIGURE 1-14. The landmarks are the anterior, lateral, and posterior borders of the acromion (A), the distal clavicle (C) and the acromioclavicular joint, the scapular spine, and the coracoid. The three most common portals are marked with an X as well as the incision necessary for a mini-open type rotator cuff repair.

cular structures, are at risk with proper portal placement. **It is important that this portal is established directly in line with the glenohumeral joint. A portal that is too lateral or too medial may allow for entry into the joint but prevent full visualization of the joint, particularly of the anteroinferior joint and the insertions of the rotator cuff muscles.**

The anterior portal is used to visualize the posterior capsule and the anterior aspects of the glenohumeral ligaments and the subscapularis tendon. It is placed approximately 2 cm inferior and 1 cm medial to the anterior edge of the acromion, that is one half of the distance between the anterolateral margin of the acromion and the coracoid process. With accurate placement, the anterior portal should pass through the rotator interval. ◉ By establishing the portal lateral to the coracoid process the risk to the musculocutaneous nerve is minimized. This portal should be established with the camera already placed through the posterior portal and in the glenohumeral joint. The anterior portal can then be accurately placed with either an inside out or outside in technique depending on the surgeon's preference. An inside-out technique involves placing the camera itself in the rotator interval and then replacing the arthroscope with its trocar sheath and then advancing the instrument until the skin is tented anteriorly. A skin incision is then made over the palpable instrument that is advanced to allow the anterior cannula to be placed over the trocar. The entire construct is then retracted back into the glenohumeral joint and disassembled under direct visualization (Fig. 1-15).

A lateral portal can be placed 2 cm distal to the lateral border of the acromion and 1 cm posterior to its anterior margin. This portal is not necessary usually necessary for di-

agnostic arthroscopy but is used during acromioplasty and rotator cuff repair. During diagnostic arthroscopy, this portal may be helpful to aid in the palpation of the rotator cuff insertion, to assess the mobility and quality of the rotator cuff in the presence of complete tears. **It is important that this portal not be placed too close to the lateral edge of the acromion. A portal that is too superior can result in significant interference between the instruments and the edge of cannula when working in the lateral aspects of the subacromial space.** Other accessory portals are not used in diagnostic arthroscopy.

PROCEDURE

All patients who are indicated for surgery of the shoulder should have a complete examination under anesthesia before any incision. ◉ If general anesthesia is used, this examination can be undertaken immediately after intubation. If regional anesthesia is used, it is critical that the block is allowed to set in with a complete motor and sensory block so that the examination and any indicated manipulation can be performed with complete relaxation and without pain. With the patient in the supine position, the operative extremity is taken through a complete gentle passive range of motion that is compared with the uninvolved extremity. If a passive deficit remains, a closed, gentle manipulation can be performed. Closed manipulations should also be avoided in those patients with questionable bone quality. The patient with marked osteopenia is at considerable risk for a fracture during manipulation. The intraarticular and subacromial adhesions may provide a greater resistance to manipulation than the bone itself. In these patients, this step should be skipped, and a gentle complete arthroscopic or open release undertaken if indicated.

The technique for closed manipulation is standard in all patients and is performed in the supine position before the patient is placed in the "beach chair" or lateral positions for the operative procedure. A short lever arm is used for all stages of the manipulation to prevent injury to the collateral ligaments of the elbow or fractures within the humerus. The scapula is stabilized. Bringing the arm slowly into full forward elevation, with flexion and traction in the plane of the scapula first stretches the inferior capsule. A clear audible lysis of adhesions is often heard along with an accompanying loss of resistance. The arm is then stretched across the patient's chest into adduction to stretch the posterior capsule. In 90 degrees of scapular plane abduction, external rotation is performed to stretch the anteroinferior capsule. Any remaining anterior capsular adhesions are released by slowly adducting the externally rotated arm toward the patient's side. With arm held in scapular plane abduction, internal rotation is performed, further releasing the posterior capsular release.

Once the patient has been properly prepared and draped

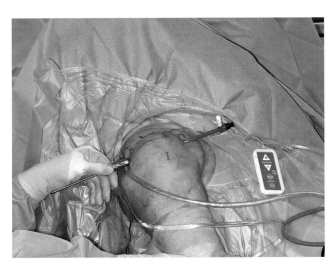

FIGURE 1-15. Placement of the rotator interval portal. An inside-out technique involves placing the camera itself in the rotator interval and then replacing the arthroscope with its trocar sheath and then advancing the instrument until the skin is tented anteriorly. A skin incision is then made over the palpable instrument, which is advanced to allow the anterior cannula to be placed over the trocar. The entire construct is then retracted back into the glenohumeral joint and disassembled under direct visualization.

and all the arthroscopic equipment assembled and accessible, the portals can be established. The glenohumeral joint is cannulated with a spinal needle through the proposed posterior portal directed toward the coracoid. The glenohumeral joint is then insufflated with 30 to 50 cc of arthroscopy fluid. Epinephrine 1:100,000 dilution in the arthroscopy fluid can aid in hemostasis. Hypotensive anesthesia, when appropriate, can also help to diminish hemorrhage within the glenohumeral joint or subacromial space. The position of the spinal needle, when lying freely in the glenohumeral joint can be used to adjust the placement of the proposed portal. If the needle appears to be directed to medial or lateral to enter the glenohumeral joint, the portal position can be adjusted appropriately. The arthroscope can then be placed through the posterior portal and into the glenohumeral joint. A semiblunt trocar tip should be used to allow the arthroscope to penetrate the capsule without inflicting iatrogenic trauma to the structures within the joint. The trocar should be advanced gently until the space between the edge of the glenoid and the humeral head can be felt (Fig. 1-16). The trocar can then be safely advanced into the joint with gentle pressure, if one is assured that the arthroscope is properly placed. 🎥 As the trocar is removed, a return of the arthroscopy fluid will confirm proper placement. The camera is then attached to the arthroscope and the flow of fluid opened into the joint (Fig. 1-17). At this point a routine diagnostic assessment of the glenohumeral joint is undertaken.

If visualization of the joint is adequate, examination can occur before placement of an anterior portal. If hemorrhage from manipulation is present, placement of the anterior portal for outflow may aid in visualization.

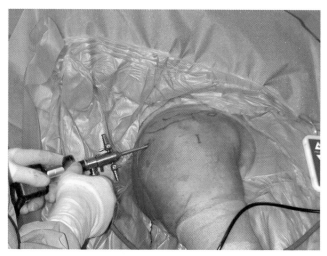

FIGURE 1-17. Placement of posterior portal. As the trocar is removed, a return of the arthroscopy fluid will confirm proper placement. The camera is then attached to the arthroscope and the flow of fluid opened into the joint. At this point a routine diagnostic assessment of the glenohumeral joint is undertaken.

A consistent step-wise assessment of the glenohumeral will ensure that all necessary structures are visualized. The biceps tendon is identified initially and the joint oriented appropriately on the monitor (Fig. 1-18). The biceps origin is carefully inspected for the presence of a SLAP lesion and should be palpated with a nerve hook through the anterior portal to document its integrity and stability. 🎥 A probe can be used to place tension on the biceps tendon and assess whether any origin lesions result in instability of the tendon. The biceps tendon should be followed along its course to

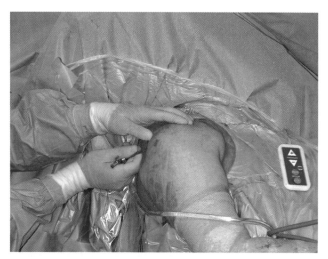

FIGURE 1-16. Placement of posterior portal. A semiblunt trocar tip should be used to allow the arthroscope to penetrate the capsule without inflicting iatrogenic trauma to the structures within the joint. The trocar should be advanced gently until the space between the edge of the glenoid and the humeral head can be felt. The trocar can then be safely advanced into the joint with gentle pressure, if one is assured that the arthroscope is properly placed.

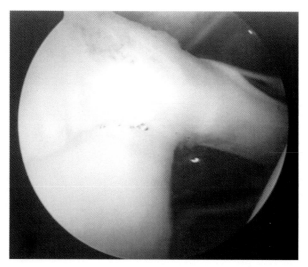

FIGURE 1-18. View from the posterior portal. The biceps tendon is identified initially and the joint oriented appropriately on the monitor. The biceps origin must be carefully inspected for the presence of a superior labrum anterior and posterior (SLAP) lesion and should be palpated with a nerve hook through the anterior portal to document its integrity and stability.

document any fraying or instability. Abduction of the arm, accompanied by rotation of the arthroscope should allow for visualization of the tendon into the bicipital groove (Fig. 1-19). The arm can be further abducted allowing the arthroscope to visualize the tendon as it exits from the shoulder into the arm through the bicipital groove (Fig. 1-20). The arthroscope is then rotated anteriorly and the subscapularis tendon is examined (Fig. 1-21). The arm can be rotated to gain further visualization of the lateral subscapularis tendon. ◘ The rotator interval should be examined for the presence of adhesions or insufficiencies.

The arthroscope is then directed in an anterior and inferior direction to assess the size of the inferior capsular pouch and the anterior inferior glenohumeral ligament. This ligament can be seen as a distinct band within the anterior capsule that merges into the glenoid position at the anterior inferior edge of the glenoid (Fig. 1-22) ◘ This ligament should tighten with external rotation of the arm. The arthroscope should be directed further inferior to visualize in the inferior capsular recess and then directed superiorly to follow the margin of the posterior glenoid to allow circumferential visualization of the labrum until the arthroscope is returned to its position just posterior to the origin of the long head of the biceps. It is important to remember to keep the posterior aspect of the glenoid in view at all times when inspecting the posterior aspect of the glenohumeral joint. This will minimize inadvertent loss of the portal and minimize soft tissue swelling which can occur after multiple cannulations of the joint.

At this point the articular surfaces of the humeral head and glenoid should be examined for any signs of degeneration or injury. The camera should then be directed just pos-

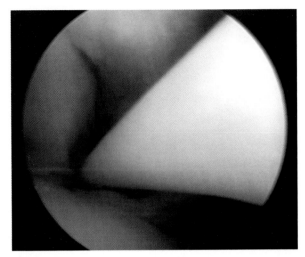

FIGURE 1-20. View of the long head of the biceps from the posterior portal. The arm can be further abducted allowing the arthroscope to visualize the tendon as it exits from the shoulder into the arm through the bicipital groove. This is a common site for loose bodies to lodge.

terior to the biceps tendon at its entry into the bicipital groove. This is a good starting position to visualize the insertion of the rotator cuff. ◘ The supraspinatus insertion can be identified just posterior to the bicipital groove and followed posteriorly by abducting the arm while rotating the arthroscope posteriorly (Fig. 1-23). This can allow for complete visualization of the insertions of the infraspinatus and teres minor (Fig. 1-24). The posterosuperior aspect of the humeral head should be examined in this position to document the presence or absence of a Hill Sachs lesion.

Once the entire joint has been inspected and arthro-

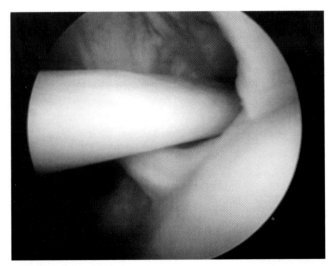

FIGURE 1-19. View of the biceps tendon from the posterior portal. The long head of the biceps tendon should be followed along its course to document any fraying or instability. Abduction of the arm, accompanied by rotation of the arthroscope should allow for visualization of the tendon as it enters into the bicipital groove.

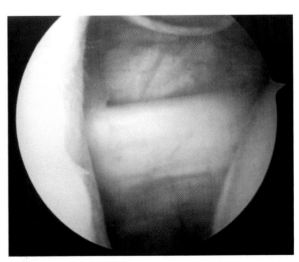

FIGURE 1-21. View from the posterior portal. The superior rolled edge of the subscapularis tendon can be clearly visualized in the anterior portion of the joint. Abduction and external rotation aid in the visualization of the superior insertion of the tendon at the bicipital groove.

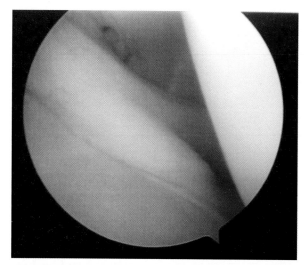

FIGURE 1-22. View from the posterior portal. The arthroscope can be directed in an anterior and inferior direction to assess the size of the inferior capsular pouch and the integrity of the anterior inferior glenohumeral ligament. This ligament can be seen as a distinct band within the anterior capsule, which merges into the glenoid at the anterior inferior edge of the glenoid. This ligament should tighten with external rotation of the arm.

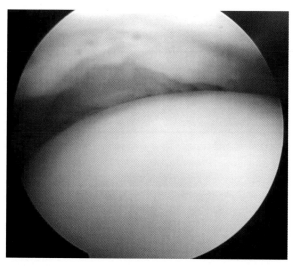

FIGURE 1-24. View from the posterior portal. Abduction and internal rotation of the arm while the camera is directed posteriorly can allow for full visualization of the insertions of all of the rotator cuff tendons. It is important to be able to visualize the entire insertion to adequately assess the extent of any evident tears.

scopic photographs taken to document the findings, the anterior rotator interval portal should be established as necessary to allow for proper palpation and assessment of any noted pathology (Fig. 1-25). Rotator cuff tears can be marked with the placement of a suture through a spinal needle to allow for its easier localization in the subacromial space. Arthroscopic grabbers can be used to assess tendon quality and mobility.

Following arthroscopy of the glenohumeral joint, the subacromial space should be visualized. The arthroscope cannula is removed from the glenohumeral and the camera replaced with the semiblunt trocar. The cannula is then placed in the subacromial space through the posterior portal by sliding directly under the posterior edge of the acromion. Use a sliding-type motion to direct the cannula off the lateral edge of the acromion, sweeping the bursa off the undersurface of the acromion. It can be an effective way to quickly improve visualization in the subacromial space.

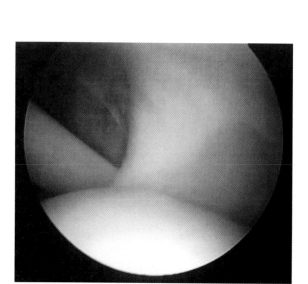

FIGURE 1-23. View from the posterior portal. The anterior insertion of the supraspinatus tendon can be seen here as it begins just posterior to bicipital groove. The rotator cuff insertion should appear as a continuous tendinous veil as it meets the lateral articular margin of the humerus along the greater tuberosity.

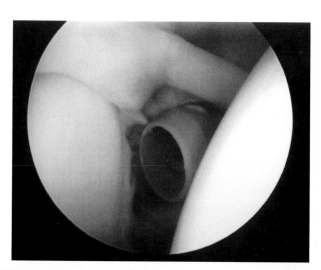

FIGURE 1-25. View from posterior portal. Placement of a cannula in the rotator interval portal. Cannulae should be used in all open portals to ease exchange of instruments and to prevent the leakage of excess arthroscopy fluid into the surrounding soft tissue. The rotator interval portal should be used during every diagnostic arthroscopy to allow for palpation of intraarticular structures.

The camera is then placed within the subacromial space. Assessment of the thickness of the bursa, the degree of inflammation, and the presence of fraying or erythema on the bursal surface of the rotator cuff should be undertaken. ◼︎◄ This often requires the establishment of the lateral portal and débridement of bursal tissue with a shaver or radiofrequency ablater to enhance visualization. It is important that the insertion of the rotator cuff is thoroughly inspected in the subacromial space. Significant bursal sided tears that mandate repair can often appear quite benign from the articular surface. Arthroscopic photographs should be taken to document the condition of the subacromial space both before and after any operative procedures.

Once the diagnostic arthroscopy has been completed and documented, operative interventions can be undertaken to address specific pathology. Additional portals may be necessary for further arthroscopic interventions and are detailed in the appropriate chapters. After adequate hemostasis is obtained within the joint and subacromial space, the portals are closed with interrupted skin sutures that can be removed in the office 7 to 10 days after the procedure. A sterile waterproof dressing is applied to the portal sites and a sling is usually provided for comfort.

POSTOPERATIVE PROTOCOL/FOLLOW-UP

The postoperative protocol will vary with the pathology encountered and the treatment rendered. If only a diagnostic arthroscopy is undertaken, a sling may only be necessary for comfort for a couple of days after the surgery. It should be moved early to enhance the recovery of postoperative ranges of motion. The procedure usually occurs on an outpatient basis and the patient should follow-up for routine examination and suture removal within 7 to 10 days.

SUGGESTED READINGS

Baechler MF, Kim DH. Patient positioning for shoulder arthroscopy based on variability in lateral acromion morphology. *Arthroscopy* 2002; 18: 547–549.

Bennett WF. Visualization of the anatomy of the rotator interval and bicipital sheath. *Arthroscopy* 2001; 17: 107–1011.

Cofield RH. Arthroscopy of the shoulder. *Mayo Clin Proc* 1983; 58: 501–508.

Favorito PJ, Harding WG 3rd, Heidt RS Jr. Complete arthroscopic examination of the long head of the biceps tendon. *Arthroscopy* 2001; 17: 430–432.

Hulstyn MJ, Fadale PD. Arthroscopic anatomy of the shoulder. *Orthop Clin North Am* 1995; 26: 597–612.

Mohammed KD, Hayes MG, Saies AD. Unusual complications of shoulder arthroscopy. *J Shoulder Elbow Surg* 2000; 9: 350–353.

Nottage WM. Arthroscopic anatomy of the glenohumeral joint and subacromial bursa. *Orthop Clin North Am* 1993; 24: 27–32.

Nottage WM. Arthroscopic portals: anatomy at risk. *Orthop Clin North Am* 1993; 24: 19–26.

Ruotolo C, Nottage WM, Flatow EL, et al. Controversial topics in shoulder arthroscopy. *Arthroscopy* 2002; 18[2 Suppl 1]: 65–75.

Scoggin JF 3rd, Mayfield G, Awaya DJ, et al. Subacromial and intra-articular morphine versus bupivacaine after shoulder arthroscopy. *Arthroscopy* 2002; 18: 464–468.

Weber SC, Abrams JS, Nottage WM. Complications associated with arthroscopic shoulder surgery. *Arthroscopy* 2002; 18[2 Suppl 1]: 88–95.

Wright JM, Heavrin B, Hawkins RJ, et al. Arthroscopic visualization of the subscapularis tendon. *Arthroscopy* 2001; 17: 677–684

CHAPTER 2

ARTHROSCOPIC ACROMIOPLASTY AND MINI-OPEN ROTATOR CUFF REPAIR

ANDREW S. ROKITO
BRIAN S. DELAY

Impingement syndrome is one of the most common causes of shoulder pain and dysfunction. This condition is typically caused by mechanical encroachment of the bursal surface of the rotator cuff resulting from a narrowed coracoacromial arch. This disorder has been classified into three progressive stages based on the degree of rotator cuff disease: inflammation and edema, fibrosis and tendinitis, and finally partial- or full-thickness tears. Arthroscopic acromioplasty has become the procedure of choice for the treatment of impingement syndrome in those cases refractory to nonoperative care. This procedure allows for a thorough inspection of the glenohumeral joint; complete decompression of the subacromial space; and early, aggressive rehabilitation. When a tear is present it can be combined with a mini-open rotator cuff repair through a deltoid-splitting approach. This approach allows for adequate tendon mobilization and secure repair, while preserving the anterior deltoid attachment.

ANATOMY

The rotator cuff is composed of the supraspinatus, infraspinatus, teres minor, and subscapularis muscles (Fig. 2-1). These insert onto the lesser and greater tuberosities as a conjoined tendon. The interval between the supraspinatus and subscapularis is occupied by the biceps tendon and coracohumeral ligament. The latter structure functions as a suspensory ligament for the humeral head and may require release during mobilization of a rotator cuff tear. The biceps tendon is an intraarticular, intrasynovial structure, which originates on the supraglenoid tubercle and is intimately related to the rotator cuff. It exits the joint through the rotator interval before entering the intertubercular groove.

The major portion of the blood supply to the rotator cuff and biceps tendon arises from branches of the axillary artery, with the most important contribution coming from the suprascapular and anterior and posterior humeral circumflex vessels (Fig. 2-2). An anastomotic area known as the "critical zone" is found in the region of the supraspinatus tendon just proximal to its insertion. It is in this region that most rotator cuff tears occur.

The coracoacromial arch is formed by the acromion and coracoacromial ligament (Fig. 2-3). The acromion forms the osseous roof of the arch. The coracoacromial ligament, which extends from the lateral edge of the coracoid and inserts onto the undersurface of the acromion, forms the anterior extent of the arch. The subacromial bursa is a filmy synovium-lined sac that separates the rotator cuff tendons from the overlying coracoacromial arch and thus serves to enhance the biomechanics of the shoulder by allowing for relatively frictionless motion. Recent studies suggest that acromial morphology may be related to rotator cuff disease. Individuals with a downward sloping or hooked acromion may be more likely to develop subacromial impingement and rotator cuff tears. These studies, however, are based primarily on cadaveric specimens and the impact of acromion slope and shape on cuff degeneration remains unclear.

CLASSIFICATION, DIAGNOSIS, AND INDICATIONS

Classic outlet or primary impingement refers to compression of the rotator cuff against the undersurface of the anterior one third of the acromion, the coracoacromial ligament, and, in some instances, the inferior aspect of the acromioclavicular joint. Three progressive stages of subacromial impingement have been described: stage I, edema and hemorrhage in patients younger than 25 years; stage II, fibrosis and tendinitis in patients 25 to 40 years old; stage III, osteophytes and tendon ruptures typically in patients older than 40 years.

More recently nonoutlet or secondary impingement has been described. This refers to impingement or injury of the rotator cuff by factors other than a narrowed or compromised coracoacromial arch. Such pathology includes glenohumeral instability, neurologic injury such as axillary or suprascapular nerve palsy, overuse or fatigue of the scapular stabilizers, eccentric overload of the rotator cuff tendons, or acute trauma to the rotator cuff. Successful treatment of secondary impingement depends on recognition and correction of the underlying cause.

The diagnosis of impingement is based primarily on a careful history and physical examination. Patients with impingement typically present with pain, difficulty with over-

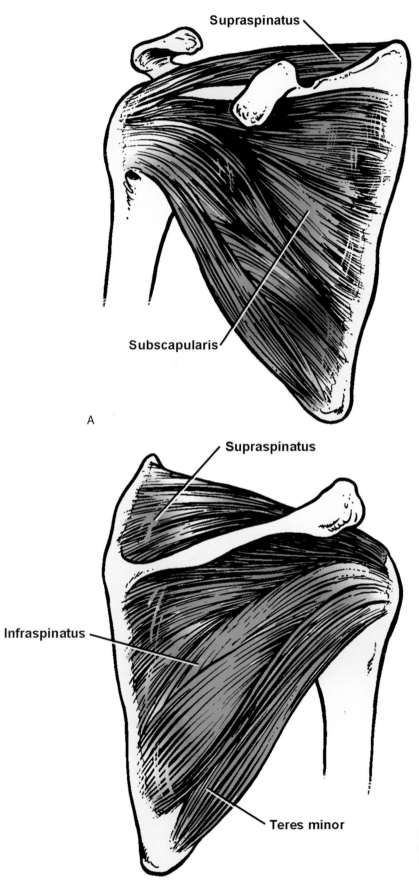

Supraspinatus

Subscapularis

A

Supraspinatus

Infraspinatus

Teres minor

B

FIGURE 2-1. The rotator cuff is composed of the suprasinatus, infraspinatus, teres minor, and subscapularis muscles. **A:** Anterior view. **B:** Posterior view.

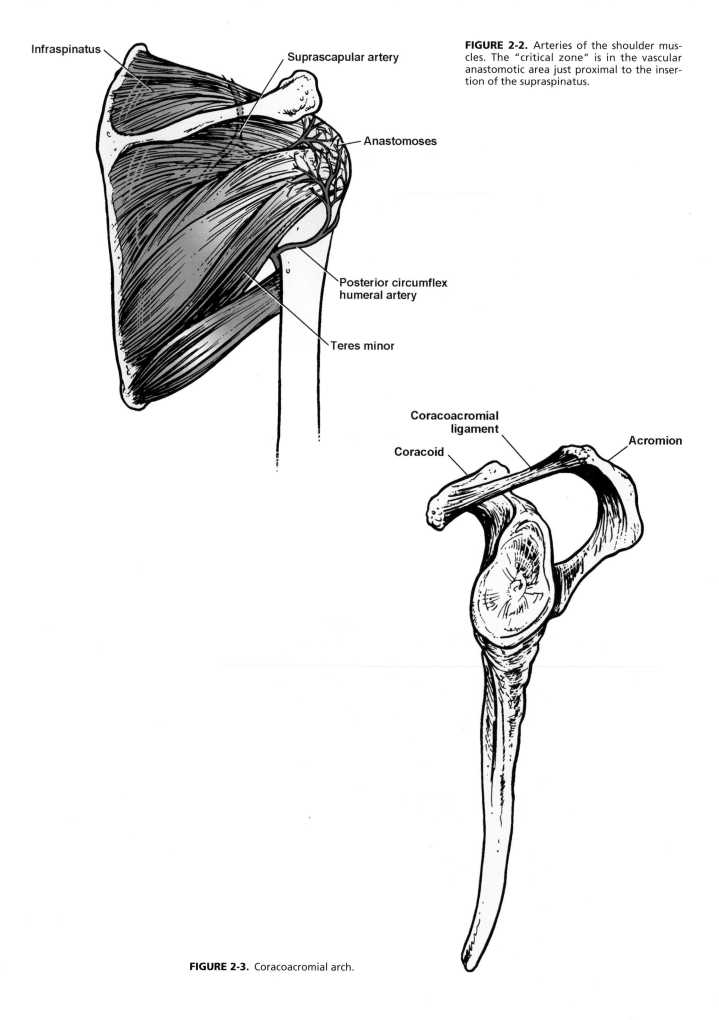

Infraspinatus

Suprascapular artery

Anastomoses

Posterior circumflex humeral artery

Teres minor

FIGURE 2-2. Arteries of the shoulder muscles. The "critical zone" is in the vascular anastomotic area just proximal to the insertion of the supraspinatus.

Coracoacromial ligament

Coracoid

Acromion

FIGURE 2-3. Coracoacromial arch.

head activities, stiffness, and weakness. Night pain, particularly when rolling onto the affected side is commonly found in patients with rotator cuff disease. From a functional standpoint patients often report having difficulty with those activities that require reaching overhead or behind the back. Women for example often describe an inability to fasten their brassiere. Physical examination findings may include tenderness along the anterior acromion or supraspinatus insertion, a painful arc of shoulder motion, and pain with provocative impingement maneuvers (Fig. 2-4). A selective lidocaine injection into the subacromial space followed by reassessment of the patient's response to these impingement maneuvers provides valuable diagnostic information. A standard radiographic assessment includes anteroposterior,

axillary, supraspinatus outlet (Fig. 2-5), and acromioclavicular joint views. The presence of a rotator cuff tear is confirmed by magnetic resonance imaging or arthrography.

Most patients with primary impingement can be successfully treated without surgery. Nonoperative treatment involves rest from those activities that exacerbate the symptoms, stretching and strengthening exercises, nonsteroidal antiinflammatory medications, and the judicious use of cortisone injections. Indications for surgery include chronic stage II impingement and acute or chronic, symptomatic full-thickness or large partial-thickness (>50%) tears. The mini-open deltoid-splitting approach can be used successfully to treat most tears, regardless of size provided that adequate tendon mobilization can be achieved.

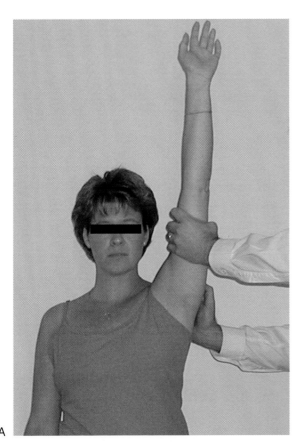

A

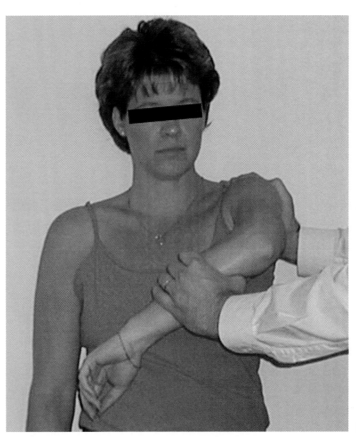

B

FIGURE 2-4. A: The classic impingement sign occurs as the shoulder is placed in the position of maximum forward elevation, reproducing the patient's pain. **B:** Impingement of the greater tuberosity on the coracoacromial ligament occurs when the shoulder is forward-flexed to 90 degrees and internally rotated, reproducing the patient's pain.

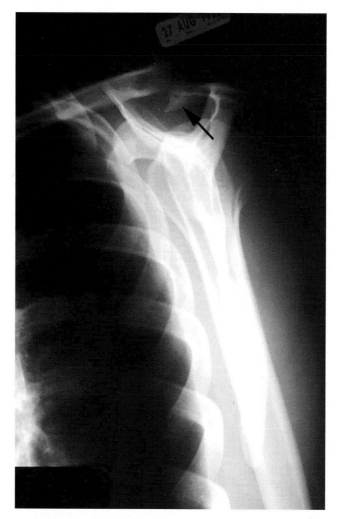

FIGURE 2-5. A supraspinatus outlet view demonstrating large subacromial spur (*arrow*).

SPECIAL EQUIPMENT/INSTRUMENTATION

The basic instruments necessary for arthroscopic acromioplasty and mini-open rotator cuff repair includes the following (Fig. 2-6):

- Arthroscopic video camera/monitor
- 4.5-mm, 30-degree angled arthroscope/sheath/trocar
- Arthroscopic instrument cannulas of various sizes
- Wissinger rod and switching sticks
- Motorized arthroscopic shaver system/shaver and burr blades
- Arthroscopic electrocautery or radiofrequency system
- Arthroscopic infusion pump
- Several 3-L bags of normal saline with 1 to 3 ampules of epinephrine per bag
- Angled/offset awls
- Suture anchors
- Self-retaining retractor

- No. 2 nonabsorbable braided sutures
- Shoulder traction system with weights and bean bag or beach chair table attachment

ANESTHESIA AND POSITIONING

The procedure can be performed under general, regional, or a combination of general and regional anesthesia. The advantages of regional anesthesia include better postoperative pain control, the ability to immediately begin range of motion exercises, and the tendency for greater patient acceptance. Ideally, shoulder arthroscopy should be performed under controlled hypotensive anesthesia. The systolic blood pressure should be kept less than 100 mm Hg whenever possible to control bleeding. This is especially critical during the subacromial decompression portion of the procedure when visualization can be compromised when bleeding is encountered.

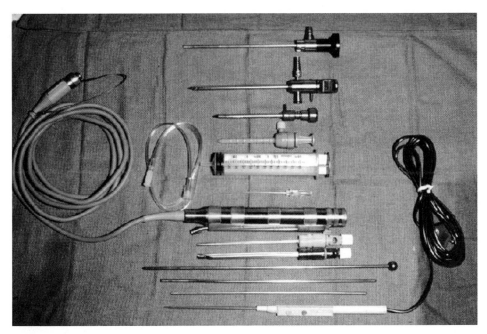

FIGURE 2-6. Instruments (from *top to bottom*): 4.5-mm 30-degree angled arthroscope, arthroscope sheath/trocar, arthroscopic cannulas, 60-cc syringe and tubing, spinal needle, motorized arthroscopic shaver system, 4.5-mm shaver, 5.0-mm acromionizer, Wissinger rod and switching sticks, and electrofrequency device.

The procedure is performed in either the beach chair or lateral decubitus position (Fig. 2-7). Advantages of the beach chair position are relative ease of patient positioning, normal anatomic orientation of the shoulder, the ability to manipulate the arm during the procedure, and a lower risk of neuropraxia that is associated with excessive traction used with the lateral decubitus position. Many surgeons, however, prefer the lateral decubitus position, because it is more familiar to them and allows for distraction, which facilitates work in the subacromial space. **With the patient in the lat-**

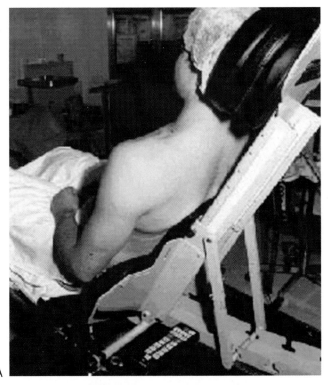

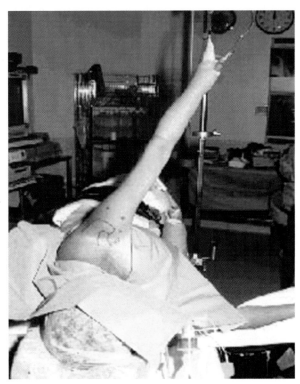

A

B

FIGURE 2-7. The arthroscopic procedure may be performed in the beach chair **(A)** or lateral decubitus **(B)** position.

eral decubitus position, careful attention must be paid to protecting the dependant bony prominences as well as the brachial plexus, ulnar, and peroneal nerves with appropriate padding.

EXAMINATION UNDER ANESTHESIA AND PORTAL PLACEMENT

The procedure begins with a thorough, systematic examination under anesthesia (Fig. 2-8). Range of motion in all planes is assessed first. Stability is then tested in the anterior, posterior, and inferior directions. If a manipulation under anesthesia is required to address any preoperative stiffness, this should be performed in a controlled, systematic fashion, always maintaining a short lever arm by grasping the humerus close to the axilla to avoid iatrogenic fracture. The shoulder is then gently manipulated in a slow, gradual fashion assessing for audible, and/or palpable lysis of adhesions. Manipulation is performed in all planes—elevation, abduction, adduction, internal, and external rotation—with the goal of achieving range of motion that is symmetrical with the contralateral side.

The bony landmarks, arthroscopic portals, and planned skin incision are carefully identified before beginning the procedure, because this becomes difficult once fluid extravasation occurs (Fig. 2-9). Three basic arthroscopic portals are used for this procedure. The posterior portal is located approximately 2 cm inferior and 1 cm medial to the posterolateral corner of the acromion. This portal allows adequate visualization of most of the glenohumeral joint and facilitates placement of other portals. When establishing this portal, one hand is placed on top of the shoulder with the thumb palpating the "soft spot." The index finger of that same hand is used to palpate the coracoid process. Using a number 11 scalpel blade, a puncture is made through the skin only. The arthroscopic sheath and blunt tipped trocar are then passed through the posterior deltoid and directed

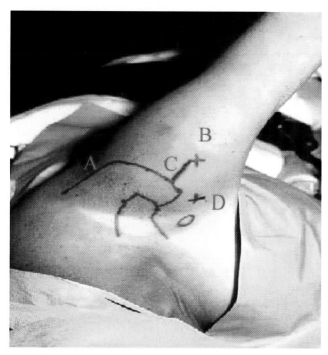

FIGURE 2-9. Bony landmarks, portal placement, and planned incision. *A:* Posterior portal. *B:* Lateral portal. *C:* Mini-open incision. *D:* Anterosuperior portal.

toward the coracoid process. The tip of the trocar is then used to palpate the "step-off" between the posterior glenoid rim and capsule. The sheath and trocar are then advanced between the humeral head and glenoid through the capsule. **Precise placement of this portal is critical because if it is too medial or inferior the suprascapular and axillary nerves, respectively, are at risk for injury.**

The anterosuperior portal is used mainly for instrumentation. It is also used for better visualization of the posterior and anteroinferior portions of the joint when this is necessary. It is located approximately 1 cm inferior and medial to the anterolateral corner of the acromion, lateral to the coracoid process. When a distal clavicle excision is planned, it is helpful to place this portal more medial in line with the acromioclavicular joint. The portal can be created either with an "inside-out" technique using a Wissinger rod or with an "outside-in" technique in which an 18-gauge spinal needle is used to confirm portal placement and direction.

The posterior portal established initially for glenohumeral inspection can also be used for initial visualization of the subacromial space. The arthroscopic sheath and trocar are simply redirected beneath the acromion. A lateral portal located 2 to 3 cm distal and parallel to the anterior margin of the acromion is used initially for instrumentation and then for visualization because it provides an "outlet" view of the subacromial space. **Excessive distal placement of this portal risks injury to the axillary nerve which lies approximately 5 cm distal to the acromion.**

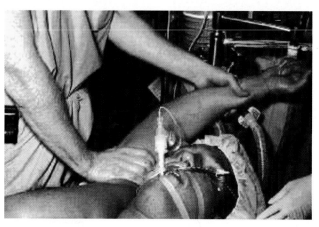

FIGURE 2-8. Examination under anesthesia.

SURGICAL APPROACH AND PROCEDURE

The procedure begins with a thorough, systematic arthroscopic evaluation of the glenohumeral joint. The articular surface of the rotator cuff is carefully inspected and partial- or full-thickness tears are identified (Fig. 2-10). A suture marker can be used to better assess the extent of a tear. A monofilament suture is placed through a spinal needle passed percutaneously across the area in question (Fig. 2-11). The end of the suture is then brought out through the anterosuperior portal using an arthroscopic grasping device. The suture is subsequently identified on the bursal surface of the rotator cuff and the questionable region is closely inspected (Fig. 2-12). ▣

Once the glenohumeral examination is completed and any associated intraarticular pathology is addressed, attention is directed toward the subacromial space. The angle of traction is adjusted so as to maximize the acromiohumeral interval. Typically, 10 lb of traction is sufficient. The arthroscopic sheath and trocar are directed beneath the acromion and swept laterally to clear bursal tissue and lyse adhesions. **To prevent excessive bleeding, the fat pad located medially beneath the acromioclavicular joint should be avoided.**

The subacromial space is distended and the lateral portal is created. This portal is typically placed 2 to 3 cm distal and parallel to the anterior margin of the acromion (Fig. 2-9). Placement of this portal slightly more posterior may allow for better access to larger size tears. A self-sealing arthroscopic cannula is used through this portal and a motorized shaver or radiofrequency soft tissue ablation device is introduced to perform a partial bursectomy and to remove periosteum from the undersurface of the acromion.

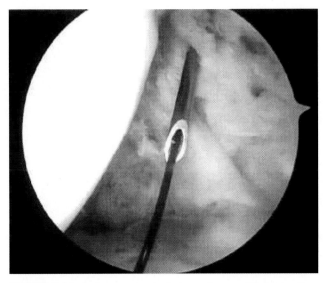

FIGURE 2-11. Suture marker technique. A monofilament suture is passed through spinal needle placed through area of suspected rotator cuff tear. The end of the suture is then brought out through the anterior portal. The suture is subsequently identified on the bursal surface of the rotator cuff.

The medial and lateral extents of the acromion are identified along with the coracoacromial ligament. The ligament is then released from medial to lateral using either an electrocautery or radiofrequency device (Fig. 2-13). The ligament is released from the undersurface of the acromion until the subdeltoid fascia is seen, avoiding injury to the overlying muscle. If the acromial branch of the thoracoacromial artery, which is located along the superomedial aspect of the coracoacromial ligament, is encountered, it should be cauterized to avoid excessive bleeding.

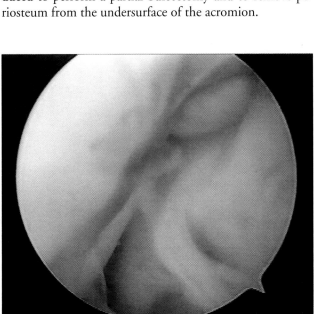

FIGURE 2-10. Arthroscopic view of the rotator cuff tear. This tear is located just posterior to the biceps tendon at the insertion of the supraspinatus.

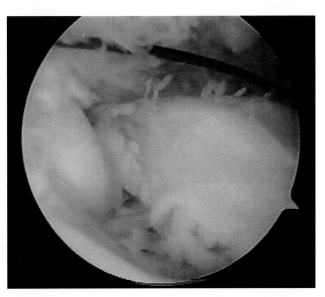

FIGURE 2-12. Rotator cuff tear with the PDS suture marker as viewed arthroscopically on the bursal side of the tear.

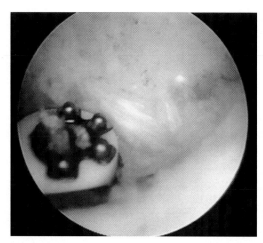

FIGURE 2-13. Release of the coracoacromial ligament using a radiofrequency device.

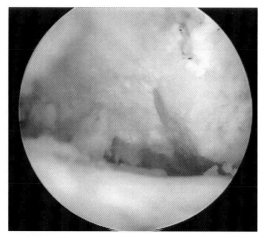

FIGURE 2-15. Appearance after the anterior acromial spur is resected as viewed from the lateral portal before using the "cutting block technique" to smooth off the posterior acromion.

The acromioplasty is then performed using an arthroscopic burr. The anterior inferior acromion is approached first. While viewing from the posterior portal, the burr is used to remove 5 to 8 mm of the inferior surface of the acromion, beginning at the anterolateral corner and proceeding medially. In addition the acromial osteophyte projecting anterior to the leading edge of the clavicle is removed (Fig. 2-14). ▮◀

The arthroscope and burr are then interchanged to perform the posterior acromion resection. While viewing from the lateral portal, the resection of the anterior spur (Fig. 2-15) and the thickness and shape of the acromial arch are assessed. It is important to place the burr just underneath and parallel to the undersurface of the acromion. The spine of the scapula is then used as a cutting block, as the burr is used to plane the undersurface of the acromion. Beginning at the low point of the acromion posteriorly, the burr is swept from medial to lateral proceeding to the anterior resection (Fig. 2-16). This technique allows for the reproducible creation of a smooth, flat acromion. The final resection should be assessed by viewing from both the lateral and posterior portals. Final smoothing can be performed with an arthroscopic rasp if desired. The final resection should be checked from the posterior and lateral portals (Fig. 2-17). ▮◀

The acromioclavicular joint is left undisturbed unless there is pathology that warrants correction. This includes

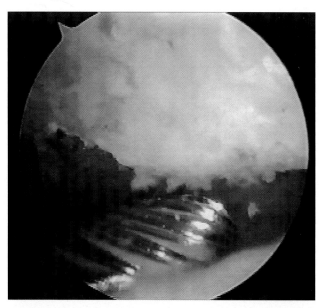

FIGURE 2-14. Anterior acromion resection. While viewing from the posterior portal, the burr is used to resect the anteroinferior aspect of the acromion.

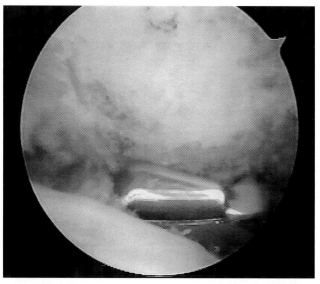

FIGURE 2-16. Posterior acromion resection. While viewing from the lateral portal, the burr is used to plane the undersurface of the acromion, using the spine of the scapula as a cutting block.

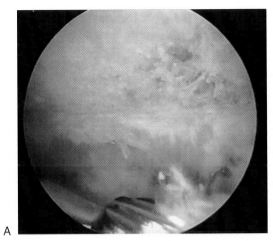 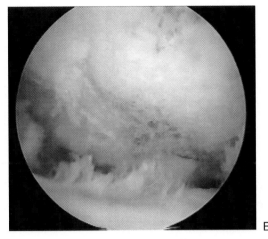

A   B

FIGURE 2-17. Final resection viewed from **(A)** posterior and **(B)** lateral portals.

symptomatic acromioclavicular joint arthritis and inferior projecting osteophytes that contribute to impingement. Resecting the inferior capsule exposes the acromioclavicular joint. The burr is then used to resect osteophytes emanating from the distal clavicle and medial acromion. The distal 7 to 10 mm of distal clavicle can then be resected if clinically indicated. This is best accomplished with the arthroscope laterally and the burr anterior through an ancillary portal created in line with the acromioclavicular joint.

Once the acromioclavicular joint has been addressed, the rotator cuff tear is inspected. Tear size, morphology, and mobility is assessed through both the posterior and anterior portals. A traction suture or arthroscopic grasper can be used to assess the mobility of the tear (Fig. 2-18). If desired, a soft tissue elevator can be used to release articular and bursal-sided adhesions.

If a mini-open repair is indicated, the arm is left in trac-

tion and a 4 cm incision is made from the anterolateral corner of the acromion and extended distally, incorporating the lateral subacromial portal (Fig. 2-19). Generous subcutaneous flaps are raised in all directions and the deltoid is split from the acromion proximally and extended distally for the length of the incision (Fig. 2-20). <u>A suture can be placed at the distal aspect of the deltoid split to prevent inadvertent extension and possible injury to the axillary nerve.</u> Subdeltoid adhesions are released manually. There should be no detachment of the deltoid from the acromion with this muscle-splitting approach. The adequacy of the subacromial decompression can be assessed by palpating the undersurface of the acromion. A rasp may be used to address any rough areas or remaining osteophytes if necessary.

A self-retaining retractor is now placed for retraction of the deltoid. Additional bursectomy is performed as needed to completely expose the rotator cuff tear (Fig. 2-21). Soft

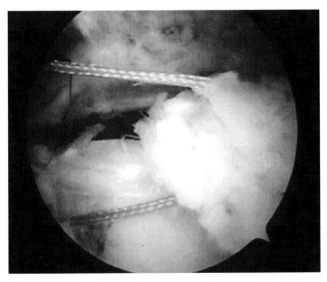

FIGURE 2-18. Arthroscopic assessment of tear mobility using a traction suture.

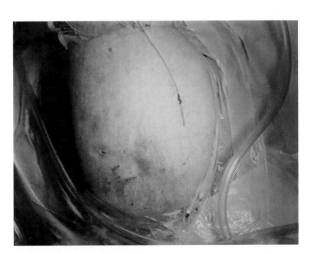

FIGURE 2-19. Skin incision for the mini-open approach incorporates the lateral subacromial portal.

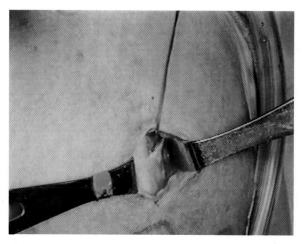

FIGURE 2-20. Deltoid split is made after raising subcutaneous flaps. Care is taken not to extend distally more than 5 cm from the edge of the acromion.

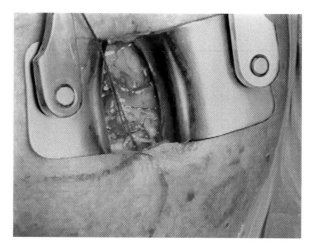

FIGURE 2-22. Exposure of rotator cuff tear. Traction sutures are placed through the torn edge of the tear and a rongeur is used to create a bleeding bone bed adjacent to the articular surface of the humeral head.

tissue elevators and dissecting scissors are then used to release any remaining adhesions that may restrict cuff mobility. <u>If additional mobilization is required this may be accomplished through releasing the coracohumeral ligament; dissecting the articular side of the cuff from the superior margin of the glenoid; or, in cases of very large, retracted tears, performing a rotator interval release and advancement.</u> ◖▉◗

The arthroscopic burr or a rongeur is then used to create a bone bed adjacent to the articular surface (Fig. 2-22). A bleeding bed, not a trough, is established. **Excessive decortication should be avoided, because this will diminish the pull-out strength of suture anchors if they are used.** The tendon is then repaired to bone using no. 2 nonabsorbable sutures either through transosseous tunnels or with suture anchors (Fig. 2-23). In cases of poor bone quality, tran-

sosseous tunnels are preferred over suture anchors. Several commercially available angled awls and suture passing devices are available to assist in the transosseous tunnel technique. Often, however, the sutures can be passed directly through the bone bed and out through the lateral cortex using a trocar-tipped needle.

Sutures are evenly spaced through the torn edge of the rotator cuff in a simple, horizontal mattress, or modified Mason-Allen configuration. For U-shaped tears, side-to-side sutures are placed beginning at the apex proceeding laterally. The converged margins are then repaired to bone. <u>If suture anchors are used, these are placed adjacent to the articular surface into the prepared bone bed at a 45-degree angle with respect to the pull of the rotator cuff. Insertion of the anchor at this angle has been shown to re-</u>

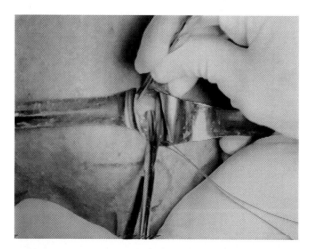

FIGURE 2-21. Bursectomy is performed to expose the rotator cuff tear.

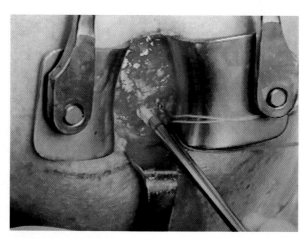

FIGURE 2-23. Suture anchors are placed to allow distribution of forces across the repair.

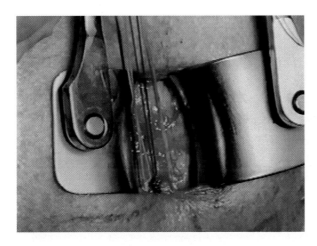

FIGURE 2-24. Simple sutures are spaced evenly throughout the tear.

duce tension within the suture and increase anchor pullout strength. Each anchor is tested for security after being placed by pulling on the sutures. Either simple or horizontal mattress sutures are then used to establish a stable rotator cuff margin (Fig. 2-24). Regardless of the technique used, the rotator cuff should be repaired with traction released without excessive tension. With large U-shaped tears it is often impossible to reapproximate the central portion to bone. In such cases it is preferable to repair the anterior and posterior leaflets while leaving the central portion of the cuff open rather than overtightening the repair, which would be prone to failure. ◖▪◗

The deltoid split is closed by reapproximating the fascia with interrupted absorbable sutures. The subcutaneous tissue and skin are then closed in routine fashion, and an arm sling is applied. Most patients are discharged from the hospital on the day of surgery.

POSTOPERATIVE PROTOCOL

Physical therapy initially consists of passive range of motion exercises (Fig. 2-25), attempting to achieve full range of motion within the first 6 to 8 weeks following surgery. Active range of motion exercises are begun once the rotator cuff is presumed healed at 6 weeks. Rotator cuff strengthening exercises are delayed until approximately 12 weeks (Fig. 2-26). Stretching exercises are continued throughout the strengthening phase of rehabilitation (Fig. 2-27). Patients are usually able to resume heavy manual labor and sports at approximately 9 to 12 months following surgery.

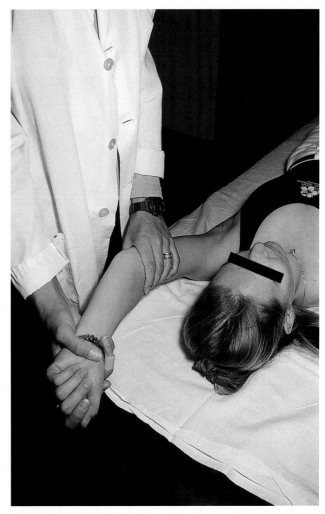

FIGURE 2-25. Passive range of motion exercises.

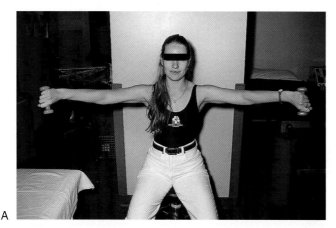

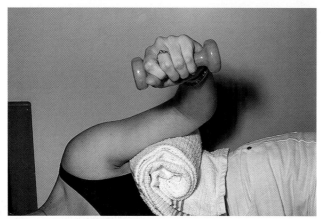

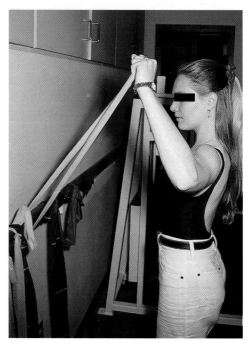

FIGURE 2-26. Rotator cuff strengthening exercises. **A:** Supraspinatus strengthening exercises. **B:** External rotator strengthening exercises. **C:** Tubing exercises.

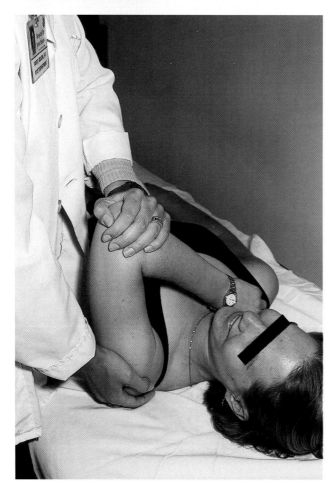

FIGURE 2-27. Posterior capsule stretching exercises.

SUGGESTED READING

Baker CL, Liu SH. Comparison of open and arthroscopically assisted rotator cuff repairs. *Am J Sports Med* 1995; 23: 99–104.

Blevins FT, Warren RF, Cavo C, et al. Arthroscopic assisted rotator cuff repair: results using a mini-open deltoid splitting approach. *Arthroscopy* 1996; 12: 50–59.

Hersch JC, Sgaglione NA. Arthroscopically assisted mini-open rotator cuff repairs. Functional outcome at 2- to 7-year follow-up. *Am J Sports Med* 2000; 28: 301–311.

Liu SH. Arthroscopically-assisted rotator cuff repair. *J Bone Joint Surg (Br)* 1994; 76-B: 592–595.

Park JY, Levine WN, Marro G, et al. Portal-extension approach for the repair of small and medium rotator cuff tears. *Am J Sports Med* 2000; 28: 312–316.

Paulos LE, Kody MH. Arthroscopically enhanced "Miniapproach" to rotator cuff repair. *Am J Sports Med* 1994; 22: 19–25.

Pollock RG, Flatow EL. The rotator cuff. Full-thickness tears. Mini-open repair. *Orthop Clin North Am* 1997; 28: 169–177.

Weber SC, Schaefer R: "Mini-open" versus traditional open repair in the management of small and moderate size tears of the rotator cuff. *Arthroscopy* 1993; 9: 365–366.

CHAPTER 3

ACROMIOPLASTY AND ROTATOR CUFF REPAIR

JOSEPH D. ZUCKERMAN
ARASH ARAGHI

The repair of full-thickness rotator cuff tears is a common procedure in orthopaedic surgery. Up until the early 1990s, it was performed primarily as an open procedure consisting of anterior acromioplasty and repair of the full-thickness tear. Today, there are alternative procedures including arthroscopic subacromial decompression and mini-open repair or arthroscopic subacromial decompression combined with arthroscopic rotator cuff repair. The outcomes of these arthroscopic procedures have been promising when compared with the results of open procedures. However, the role of open acromioplasty and rotator cuff repair continues to be important in the treatment of these injuries. In our practice, this approach is used primarily for large, retracted full-thickness tears that require extensive mobilization techniques to obtain closure and as an option when arthroscopic or mini-open techniques are not possible or have been unsuccessful. In these latter situations, an open approach will continue to have an important role in the treatment of full-thickness rotator cuff tears. In this chapter we describe the technique that we have found successful.

ANATOMY

To understand the relevant anatomy for acromioplasty and rotator cuff repair, it is important to understand the anatomy of the coracoacromial arch and the supraspinatus outlet (Fig. 3-1). The coracoacromial arch is formed by the anterior one third of the acromion and the coracoacromial ligament with its insertion into the coracoid process. The humeral head is located within the coracoacromial arch and the rotator cuff tendons pass underneath the arch to insert into the proximal humerus. The passage through this coracoacromial arch has been described as the "supraspinatus outlet." Any anatomic variant that decreases the size of the outlet can result in impingement on the rotator cuff. The supraspinatus outlet can be decreased by several mechanisms: osteophytes from the anterior inferior acromion, a downward sloping acromion, an acromion with significant concavity, and osteophytes about the inferior aspect of the acromioclavicular (AC) joint. Neer has introduced the concept of impingement as a critical factor in the etiology of rotator cuff tears. He postulated that with forward elevation of the arm, the supraspinatus tendon was impinged by structures of the coracoacromial arch. Repetitive overhead activities have the potential to cause repetitive impingement that leads to wear of the tendons. Over time, this can result in disruption of tendon fibers, partial tearing, and eventually full-thickness tears. When injury is superimposed on an already weakened rotator cuff, a full-thickness tear can result or a previously existing small full-thickness tear can be extended into a larger tear.

The rotator cuff consists of the tendons of the supraspinatus, infraspinatus, and teres minor (which insert on the great tuberosity superiorly and posteriorly) and the subscapularis (which inserts on the lesser tuberosity anteriorly) (Fig. 3-2). The rotator interval is the area of capsular tissue that joins the anterior edge of the supraspinatus tendon with the superior edge of the subscapularis tendon. The most important function of the rotator cuff is to stabilize the humeral head against the glenoid as the arm is elevated. The rotator cuff tendons form half of the "force couple" with the deltoid and together they allow elevation of the arm overhead. If the stabilizing function of the rotator cuff is compromised (as in a full-thickness rotator cuff tear) there will be an unopposed pull of the deltoid, which displaces the humeral head upward toward the acromion. Elevation is generally limited to 30 or 40 degrees. This is a classical finding in some patients with large full-thickness rotator cuff tears. Most rotator cuff tears—particularly those secondary to impingement—involve the supraspinatus tendon near its insertion into the greater tuberosity. As a tear enlarges, more of the supraspinatus insertion becomes involved, often with an intratendinous extension into the infraspinatus. When a traumatic event is superimposed onto a rotator cuff with chronic degeneration, there may be a more significant avulsion component that includes the infraspinatus tendon. As rotator cuff degeneration progresses, there can also be involvement of the subscapularis tendon, particularly its superior one-third. Traumatic, complete subscapularis ruptures can also occur. These often represent an isolated injury and are not included in this chapter.

CLASSIFICATION

There is no uniformity accepted classification of full-thickness rotator cuff tears. However, evaluation of each tear in

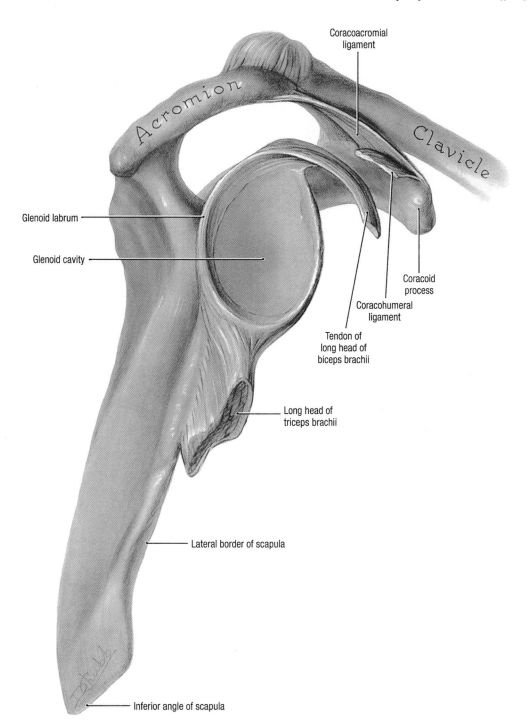

Coracoacromial
ligament

Acromion

Clavicle

Glenoid labrum

Glenoid cavity

Coracoid
process

Coracohumeral
ligament

Tendon of
long head of
biceps brachii

Long head of
triceps brachii

Lateral border of scapula

Inferior angle of scapula

FIGURE 3-1. Glenoid cavity, lateral view. The coracoacromial arch is formed by the acromion, coracoacromial ligament, and the tip of the coracoid process. The supraspinatus passes under it and inserts onto the greater tuberosity. Compromise of the space within the coracoacromial arch results in "outlet impingement."

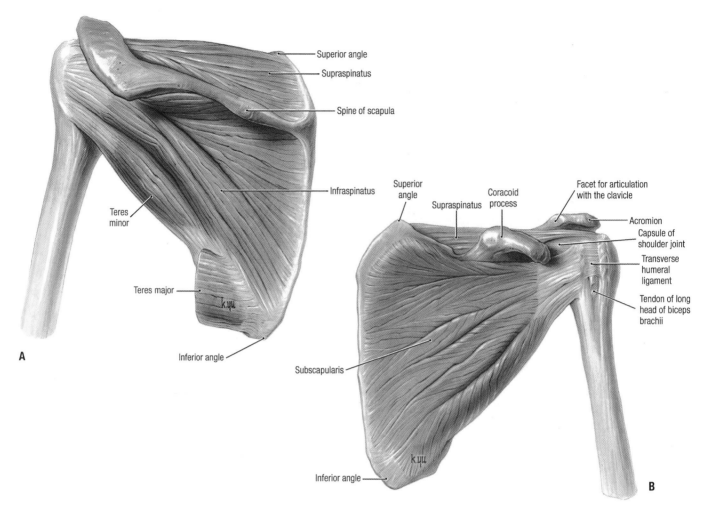

FIGURE 3-2. Rotator cuff. **A:** Posterior view. **B:** Anterior view. The rotator cuff consists of the supraspinatus, infraspinatus, and teres minor muscles inserting on the greater tuberosity and the subscapularis inserting on the lesser tuberosity.

relation to its etiology and size are important considerations. Most full-thickness rotator cuff tears are associated with an underlying impingement syndrome. Exceptions include full-thickness tears that occur in younger patients as a result of significant trauma. Most rotator cuff tears that occur in older patients represent acute extensions in areas of preexisting rotator cuff degeneration. This "acute-on-chronic" category is applicable to most full-thickness tears in older patients.

When a full-thickness tear is present, size is an important consideration and is determined by direct observation of the rotator cuff at the time of surgery. As such, full-thickness tears can be grouped by and are often classified on the basis of the largest linear dimension of the tear: less than 1 cm is a small tear, 1 to 3 cm is medium, 3 to 5 cm is large, and greater than 5 cm is a massive tear. Although this is a gener-

ally accepted classification system, it has significant limitations when attempting to compare tears within the same size category. Although the "resting" size of the tear is an important consideration, its significance has to be considered in the context of mobility of the tissues and tissue quality. A 5-cm tear that occurs in mobile tissue of good quality may be much easier to repair than a 2-cm tear in immobile, degenerative tissue that does not hold suture material. The most important consideration relating to the size of the tear is whether there is a tissue defect present after all mobilization techniques have been performed. The goal of surgery is to obtain a secure repair that brings the tendon tissue back to its insertion onto the tuberosity and restores the integrity of the cuff. The ease or difficulty in achieving this result is certainly affected by the size of the tear but is also significantly impacted by tissue mobility and tissue quality.

INDICATIONS

Patients with full-thickness rotator cuff tears present with a wide range of symptoms and findings. Symptoms can range from constant pain that interferes with sleep to little or no pain. The effect of the rotator cuff tear on active range of motion of the shoulder is quite variable. Some patients will be able to maintain full range of motion, although it will be painful, particularly through the midrange of elevation and at the extremes of motion. Other patients will have significant loss of active motion that can be representative of a "true" loss of active motion resulting from the disruption of the musculotendinous unit or, for many patients, a loss of active motion secondary to pain. In these latter patients, a subacromial lidocaine injection test can be helpful in determining the true active range of motion. There are also some patients who have a limitation of passive range of motion. This probably develops over time as a result of decreased use of the painful shoulder and inflammation associated with the tendon tear. When significant limitation of passive range of motion is present preoperatively, a therapy program directed at regaining range of motion is important. In patients who cannot regain range of motion, manipulation and possibly arthroscopic releases at the time of rotator cuff repair should be performed.

The primary indication for rotator cuff repair is shoulder pain. The secondary indication is immobility and dysfunction in patients with significant loss of active range of motion. Although these indications are described as primary and secondary, clinically it is important to integrate them to identify patients who are candidates for surgery. Successful resolution of pain following rotator cuff repair can be achieved in more than 90% of patients. The ability to restore active range of motion is more variable and depends on many factors including the size of the tear, the ability to achieve a secure repair, the degree of preoperative stiffness and muscular atrophy, and compliance with the postoperative rehabilitation program. Although most patients who undergo rotator cuff repair have significant associated symptoms, there is a small group of patients in whom rotator cuff repair is indicated primarily because of the loss of active motion and the loss of function. These patients have generally sustained an acute injury resulting in a large or massive rotator cuff tear. Although the degree of pain and discomfort may not be substantial, the precipitous loss of active range of motion and function in the context of an acute injury is a clear indication for surgical repair. We emphasize that this latter group represents a very small percentage of patients undergoing surgery for rotator cuff repair.

PREOPERATIVE PLANNING

An accurate assessment of rotator cuff function is an important part of preoperative planning. In addition to the history and physical examination, appropriate imaging studies are necessary: standard radiographs of the right shoulder consisting of anteroposterior (AP) views with internal and external rotation, scapular lateral outlet view, and an axillary view. These views provide important information about the bony architecture of the coracoacromial arch, particularly with respect to the presence of significant anterior and inferior acromial spurs and osteophytes about the inferior aspect of the AC joint, as well as the presence of an os acromiale. The presence of degenerative arthritis of the AC and glenohumeral joints is an important consideration in ascertaining that the source of pain is indeed the rotator cuff tear and not degenerative arthritis. A preoperative magnetic resonance imaging (MRI) provides important information about the size and location of the tear. It also provides information about the amount of retraction of the tear and which tendons are involved. An estimation of the chronicity of the tear can also be obtained, based on the presence of atrophic changes in the rotator cuff muscles that may make tissue mobilization and repair more difficult. An MRI also provides additional information about acromial morphology. One of the most important aspects of the preoperative evaluation is to confirm that all other potential causes of shoulder pain other than rotator cuff tear have been excluded. The coexistence of rotator cuff tears with other conditions that can cause shoulder pain—including cervical spondylosis, cervical radiculopathy, scapulothoracic bursitis, AC arthritis, glenohumeral arthritis, and pulmonary tumors—is well-recognized.

EQUIPMENT

Although there is considerable individual variation and personal choice involved in equipment and instruments, there are specific retractors and instruments that make it easier to perform the procedure (Fig. 3-3). Specific retractors that can be beneficial include (a) angled self-retaining retractors used to retract the skin edges, (b) right-angled Richardson

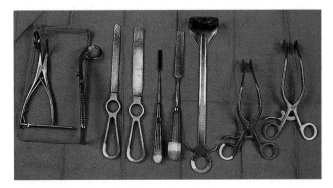

FIGURE 3-3. Instruments used to facilitate open rotator cuff tear include (*left* to *right*): angled self-retaining retractors, deltoid retractor, large rasp, small rasp, flat Darrach elevators (two), and humeral head "ring" retractors (two).

retractors to facilitate retraction of the deltoid muscle, (c) a "deltoid retractor" specifically designed to retract the lateral and posterior deltoid and to expose the humeral head, and (d) specific humeral head "ring" retractors to enhance exposure of the retracted rotator cuff by displacing the humeral head downward as counterforce is placed on the underside of the acromion.

We prefer to use a microsagittal saw with blades of varying width to perform the acromioplasty. The final contouring of the acromioplasty can be accomplished easily with small rasps to smooth the undersurface of the acromion.

The most important aspect of the rotator cuff repair is the reattachment to the insertion at the greater tuberosity. There are different techniques that can be used for this approach. We describe the technique that uses bone tunnels and the passing and placement of horizontal mattress sutures. We accomplish this using an awl to prepare the bone tunnels and a large cutting needle to pass the sutures through the tunnels. There are a variety of bone anchors currently available that can also be used for the tendon-to-bone reattachment. Bone tunnels have a long track record of use and an established record of success. Anchors have been used more recently and early results indicate that they can be used successfully. The choice of bone tunnels versus anchors is based on surgeon preference. We perform the tendon-to-bone reattachment with no. 2 braided nonabsorbable suture. The tendon-to-tendon component of the repairs is performed with no. 1 braided nonabsorbable suture. Only noncutting or round needles are used for passing sutures through the rotator cuff. This decreases the potential for the needles to "cut out" as they are passed.

PATIENT POSITIONING AND PREPARATION

A vast majority of our rotator cuff repairs are performed under regional anesthesia using an interscalene block. After the induction of anesthesia, passive range of motion of the shoulder should be assessed. This includes forward elevation, external rotation with the arm at the side, and abduction in the coronal plane. If there is significant stiffness present, a gentle manipulation should be performed focusing on forward elevation and abduction. In most cases, this gentle manipulation results in full forward elevation and improvement in abduction and external and internal rotation. If range of motion cannot be easily obtained, then a capsular release should be performed during the arthroscopic evaluation. In addition, the releases performed for tendon mobilization during the rotator cuff repair also facilitates recovery of range of motion.

The patient is placed in a sitting position, using a positioning device that secures the head and neck in a stable position and allows complete access to the entire shoulder region. The sitting position should be approximately 80- to 90-degrees upright. Preparation and draping is performed in a standard fashion. It is important to have adequate exposure of the entire shoulder and upper extremity. The exposed area should allow an extension of the incision anteriorly and posteriorly if this is found to be necessary during the procedure. The procedure begins with an arthroscopic evaluation of the glenohumeral joint and subacromial space. This provides an opportunity to identify and treat intraarticular findings and perform capsular releases if necessary. The location and size of the rotator cuff tear can then be confirmed, and the tissue quality and mobility can be assessed. Based on this assessment, we decide whether an open repair is indicated or whether the repair should be performed arthroscopically or with a mini-open technique. The arthroscopic assessment is discussed in Chapters 1 and 2.

SURGICAL INCISION LANDMARKS

Different skin incisions have been described for rotator cuff surgery using a superior approach. However, we have found a strap incision based over the midportion of the acromion to be the most useful (Fig. 3-4). The incision is centered between the lateral edge of the acromion and the AC joint. It begins over the midportion of the acromion and extends anteriorly, approximately 3 to 4 cm beyond the anterior edge of the acromion. The incision should be oriented so that an anterior extension is located in the anterior axillary line and a posterior extension is in line with the posterior axillary line. The potential for an "extensile" exposure can be important if additional procedures are found to be necessary. For example, when a significant subscapularis tear occurs in association with a supraspinatus and infraspinatus tear, a re-

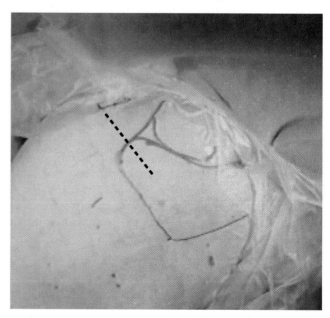

FIGURE 3-4. Superior aspect of the shoulder showing the skin incision based over the anterior one third of the acromion and extending anteriorly in the anterior axillary line.

pair is indicated. The superior incision can be extended anteriorly for a deltopectoral approach to the proximal portion of the humerus. This approach is necessary for complete subscapularis ruptures. Tears that involve the most superior portion of the subscapularis tendon can generally be repaired through a standard superior approach. Although very uncommon, the superior incision may be extended posteriorly to allow a posterior approach to the shoulder. This can be helpful when the posterior portion of the rotator cuff tear is retracted and cannot be mobilized through the superior incision.

APPROACH

The skin and subcutaneous tissues are divided and subcutaneous dissection performed to allow mobilization of the soft tissue flaps (Fig. 3-5). The bony landmarks should be palpated including the anterior and lateral portions of the acromion, the lateral clavicle, and the AC. We have found it helpful to insert a needle into the AC joint to identify this landmark throughout the exposure.

The interval between the anterior and middle portions of the deltoid is identified. This raphe can be seen originating at the anterolateral corner of the acromion. ◨ A relatively avascular interval, it is then divided from a point 3 cm distal to the anterolateral portion of the acromion and over the top of the anterior acromion to the AC joint. Care should be taken to avoid violation of the AC joint. The attachment of the anterior deltoid to the anterior acromion is elevated subperiosteally exposing the entire anterior acromion. In this manner, the coracoacromial ligament is released from the anterior/inferior acromion. The ligament should be allowed to remain contiguous with the fascia of the underside of the deltoid. Although previously, we felt that a resection of a portion of the ligament was necessary, we no longer use this approach. Instead, by allowing the coracoacromial liga-

ment to maintain its continuity with the deltoid fascia when the deltoid is reattached to the anterior acromion, there is the potential that the coracoacromial ligament will continue to function as a restraint to superior migration of the humeral head. As noted, the elevation and release of the anterior deltoid should extend to the AC joint but should not compromise the joint itself. The anterior deltoid is then retracted anteriorly to expose the subacromial space in preparation for performing the procedure.

PROCEDURE

On completing the approach, the anterior acromion is exposed and there is access to the subacromial space. The anatomy of the anterior acromion, with respect to the presence of an anterior acromial spur and the concavity of the underside of the acromion, should next be assessed. An acromioplasty is performed with the goals of (a) converting the concavity of the underside of the acromion to a flat surface and (b) recessing the anterior edge of the acromion to the same level as the anterior edge of the lateral clavicle (Figs. 3-6 and 3-7). ◨ The acromioplasty can be performed using a variety of techniques. We prefer to use a microsagittal saw and to perform the resection in one step. The saw blade should be wide enough to accomplish the resection with one pass. It should be angled posteriorly and inferiorly to exit the inferior surface at a point that converts the concavity to a flat surface. This can be determined by careful palpation of the underside of the acromion. **If the angle of the saw is too vertical, an inadequate resection will be performed. However, if the angle of the saw is too horizontal, there is a risk of an excessive resection and compromise of its structural integrity.** Therefore, the angle of the resection must be carefully determined. The resected portion of the anterior and inferior acromion is then removed. The underside of the acromion should be palpated

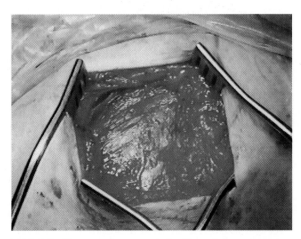

FIGURE 3-5. The use of two angled self-retaining retractors oriented perpendicularly provides excellent exposure of the deeper tissue.

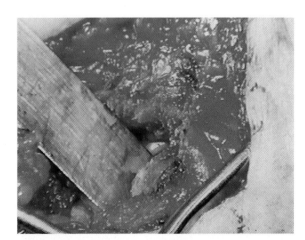

FIGURE 3-6. After exposure of the anterior acromion an elevator is placed in the subacromial space prior to acromioplasty with a micro sagittal saw.

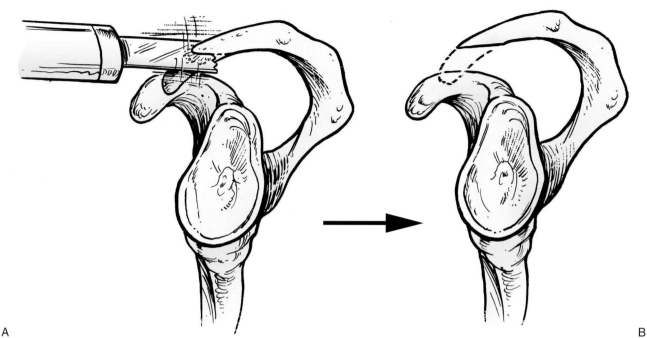

A   B

FIGURE 3-7. The acromioplasty is performed with a microsagittal saw **(A)** that recesses the anterior edge and converts the concave underside to a flat surface **(B).**

to confirm that a smooth surface is present. Often, there is some irregularity that remains, which can be corrected with a rasp (Fig. 3-8). The inferior aspect of the AC joint should also be palpated. Osteophytes in this area may be prominent and should be removed using a rongeur and/or rasp.

With completion of the acromioplasty, exposure of the subacromial space is improved (Fig. 3-9). At this point, visualization of the rotator cuff tear should be obtained and generally requires resection of a portion of the overlying

bursa. The bursal resection should be done carefully. Often, the bursa is adherent to the superior aspect of the rotator cuff and should be elevated until the edge of the rotator cuff tear can be visualized. As long as an adequate edge of the rotator cuff tendons is visualized, bursa that remains attached to the superior aspect of the rotator cuff posteriorly and medially will not be problematic.

With visualization of the tear, it is important to understand the size, shape, and location. 📹 Most tears begin at

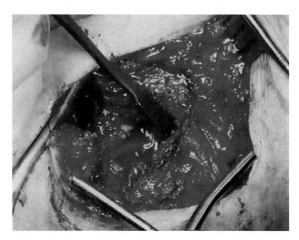

FIGURE 3-8. After the acromioplasty is completed, a small rasp is used for contouring of the undersurface of the acromion.

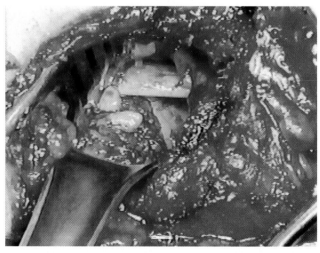

FIGURE 3-9. With the anterior deltoid retracted anteriorly and the acromioplasty completed, the subacromial space and the rotator cuff tear are well visualized.

the anterior edge of the greater tuberosity, just posterior to the bicipital groove. The biceps tendon can often be visualized within the area of the tear as it passes into the bicipital groove (Fig. 3-9). Based on tear size, the edge of the tear extends to a variable degree posteriorly along the insertion into the greater tuberosity. The anterior edge of the tear is often located in the rotator interval area. With elevation of the arm, the superior aspect of the subscapularis can be visualized. This marks the anterior edge of the rotator interval area. The mobility of the glenohumeral joint is an important factor in allowing proper visualization of the rotator cuff tear. The anterior aspect of the tear is more easily visualized with elevation and external rotation of the humerus. The posterior aspect of the tear can be visualized more easily with extension and internal rotation (Fig. 3-10). Adduction can facilitate visualization of the medial extent of the tear. However, identification of the most medial portion of the tear, particularly in large tears, is generally more difficult and requires traction on the humerus and visualization of the posteromedial aspect of the subacromial space.

As the edges of the tear are visualized, traction sutures should be placed (Fig. 3-11). We use no. 1 nonabsorbable sutures for this purpose. As the noncutting needle is passed through the edge of the tendon, tension is applied to assess the quality of the tissue by its ability to support suture material. These traction sutures are passed 3 to 4 mm from the edge of the tear or farther if necessary to achieve secure passage. Noncutting needles are used to avoid damage to the tendon. Sutures are passed through the anterior and the posterior edges of the tear. With the sutures in place, initial assessment of tendon mobility can be performed. Traction of the posterior portion of the tendon in an anterior and lateral direction will determine tissue mobility. In a similar manner, traction of the anterior portion in a posterior and lateral direction will determine its mobility. Laterally directed traction on the sutures placed in the anterior and posterior tendon allow visualization of the most medial extent of the tear or its "apex."

Based on the mobility of the tear, further mobilization techniques may or may not be necessary. This is performed in a step-by-step sequence. The first steps in mobilization are extramuscular releases. ◨ A Darrach elevator is placed over the supraspinatus tendon and advanced medially into the supraspinatus fossa. This is a relatively avascular plane.

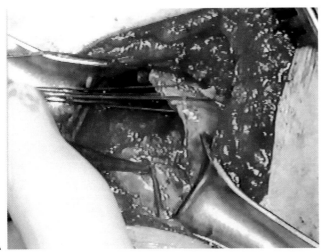

A

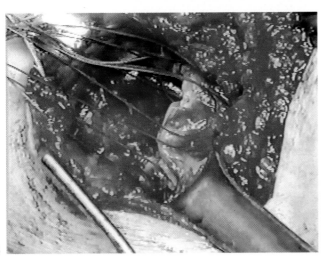

B

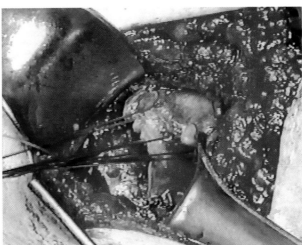

C

FIGURE 3-10. With internal rotation and extension of the humerus, the intratendinous posterior extension of the tear can be visualized **(A)**. This allows placement of sutures for the tendon-to-tendon repair **(B)**. These sutures are tied to complete this portion of the repair before performing the tendon-to-bone repair **(C)**.

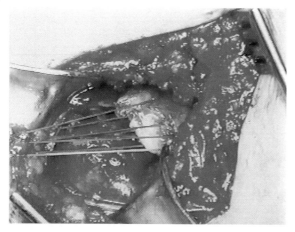

FIGURE 3-11. The retracted edge of the rotator cuff has been tagged with traction sutures. After mobilization, it can be advanced laterally to its insertion and into the greater tuberosity.

Passing the elevator releases adhesions within the coracoacromial arch. As the elevator is passed medially, lateral countertraction is placed on the tendon sutures. In a similar manner, an elevator is passed over the infraspinatus tendon into the infraspinatus fossa. When this extramuscular mobilization is completed, the mobility of the tendon is once again assessed to determine if additional mobilization is necessary. At this point, preliminary decisions can be made about the repair. Most repairs consist of a tendon-to-tendon repair combined with a tendon-to-bone repair. The shape of the tear and the mobility of the edges determine how this is performed. Because most tears are triangular, the tendon-to-tendon portion of the repair brings the anterior and posterior portions together in a medial to lateral direction. This allows the lateral edge to be brought into contact with its insertion into the greater tuberosity. If the anterior or posterior edge of the tear is relatively more mobile, an "L" or "reverse L" repair can be performed, respectively. When the anterior and posterior aspects of the tear are equally mobile, a "T" repair is performed (Fig. 3-12).

After extramuscular mobilization, if the edge of the tendons cannot be adequately mobilized to allow repair, additional mobilization techniques will be necessary. With external rotation, the adhesions at the base of the coracoid can be assessed. This area is often referred to as the "coracohumeral ligament." With external rotation of the humerus, palpation in the area of the base of the coracoid and the rotator interval may indicate the presence of dense adhesions. These can be released with scissors starting at the lateral base of the coracoid and should be done with the humerus in maximum external rotation. This release often provides additional mobility of the anterior portion of the tendon to facilitate lateral advancement of the tendon. If tendon mobilization is still not adequate to allow anatomic repair, a capsular release should be performed. This consists of release of the capsular attachment at the superior and posterior edge of the glenoid. The rotator cuff tissue is contiguous

with the capsule superiorly and posteriorly. By releasing the capsular attachments to the edge of the glenoid, the rotator cuff can be advanced laterally. With inferior traction placed on the humerus, a scalpel is used to release the capsular attachments beginning superiorly above the biceps tendon insertion and progressing posteriorly to the posterosuperior edge of the glenoid. Additional releases can be performed along the posterior superior aspect of the glenoid. **The scalpel edge should not be passed more than 5 mm beyond the edge of the glenoid margin to prevent potential injury to the neurovascular bundle.** Capsular releases further enhance the mobility of the tendon in a medial to lateral direction and facilitate the repair.

After mobilization is completed, the repair can be performed. Any bony excrescences or irregularities about the greater tuberosity should be removed and the area converted to a flat surface. A cancellous bed should be prepared. A deep trough should be avoided because it compromises bone quality for holding sutures used in the repair. In addition, a deep trough requires a greater degree of tendon advancement to achieve bony contact. The tendon reattachment should begin at the edge of the articular surface. The tendon-to-tendon portion of the repair should be planned and these sutures should be placed (Fig. 3-10). ◨ We use no. 1 or no. 2 nonabsorbable braided sutures for this purpose. These sutures are passed and usually tied to facilitate the tendon-to-bone portion of the repair. Placement of the tendon-to-tendon sutures should be performed up to the apex. When these sutures are tied, the triangular-shaped tear is essentially converted to a linear tear. We often leave the tendon-to-tendon sutures uncut so that they can be used for traction during the tendon-to-bone repair. The tendon-to-bone repair can be performed using a variety of techniques. We have used bone tunnels for placement of horizontal mattress sutures in many cases. More recently, we have used bone anchors in patients with appropriate bone quality in which anchor fixation is secure. In this chapter, we use bone tunnels for the tendon-to-bone repair.

The length of the tendon-to-bone repair determines the number of bone tunnels to be used. In our technique, which uses horizontal mattress sutures, the number of horizontal mattress sutures used in the repair is equal to the number of tunnels minus one (Fig. 3-13). For example, when four bone tunnels are used, three horizontal mattress sutures can be passed; if five bone tunnels are used, four horizontal mattress sutures can be passed. ◨ A curved awl can be used to prepare a bone tunnel through the lateral humeral cortex. This should be placed approximately 1.5 to 2 cm below the most superior aspect of the greater tuberosity. The awl is driven directly into the metaphyseal bone. In most patients, a large cutting needle can then be passed through the lateral humeral cortex and up through the greater tuberosity just lateral to the edge of the articular surface. If bone quality prevents easy passage, the awl can be used to prepare the exit portal in the cancellous bed.

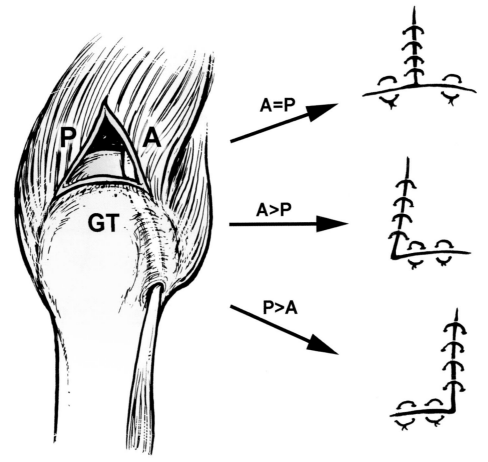

FIGURE 3-12. Triangular-shaped rotator cuff repairs consist of tendon-to-tendon and tendon-to-bone components. Based on the mobility of the tissues, the repair will resemble a "T" (when the anterior and posterior edges are equally mobile), "L" (when the anterior edge is more mobile), or "reverse L" (when the posterior edge is more mobile). A, anterior; GT, greater tuberosity; P, posterior.

A series of bone tunnels are prepared in this manner. The sutures to be used for the repair are then passed through each bone tunnel. We use no. 2 braided nonabsorbable suture. Single sutures are passed through the peripheral bone tunnels; double sutures are passed through the inferior bone tunnels (Figs. 3-13 and 3-14). The second suture through the interior bone tunnels is used as a passing suture after placement of the horizontal mattress suture through the tendon. This avoids the need for passing needles through the bone tunnels a second time when sutures are already in place. It also allows overlap of the horizontal mattress sutures with two sutures in each inferior bone tunnel being used for two adjacent horizontal mattress sutures.

After the sutures are passed through the bone tunnels a noncutting needle is used to pass the suture through the edge of the rotator cuff tendon. These sutures are passed in a horizontal mattress fashion and then passed through the bone tunnel to be tied over the lateral humeral cortex (Fig. 3-15). When all sutures have been passed, the tendon-to-

bone repair can be completed. Traction is placed on the tendon-to-tendon sutures so that the tendon can be advanced laterally. The humerus can be maintained in abduction of 20 to 30 degrees to facilitate the repair. The order of suture tying is based on the mobility of the tissue with the more mobile (less tension) areas tied first. This allows gradual advancement of the less mobile portion of the repair. As these sutures are tied, it is essential that the edge of the rotator cuff tendon be brought into direct and secure contact with the prepared bone of the greater tuberosity (Fig. 3-16).

When all sutures have been tied, the shoulder should be placed through a range of motion to assess the integrity of the repair. ▪ The movements consist of forward elevation, abduction, and internal and external rotation. The amount of external rotation obtained intraoperatively should be documented because this determines the amount of passive external rotation that can be performed during postoperative rehabilitation. The repair should be secure with the arm at the side. We do not use adduction pillows

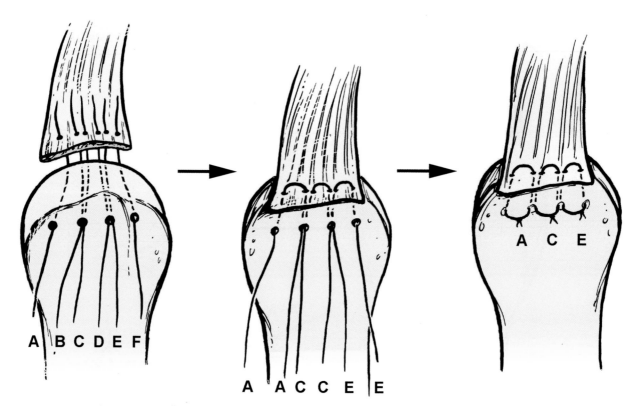

FIGURE 3-13. Following preparation of four bone tunnels, the sutures are passed. The interior bone tunnels contain double sutures, and the peripheral bone tunnels contain single sutures. This allows easier passage of the sutures and results in three horizontal mattress sutures tied over the lateral humeral cortex. With this technique, the number of horizontal mattress sutures is equal to the number of bone tunnels minus one.

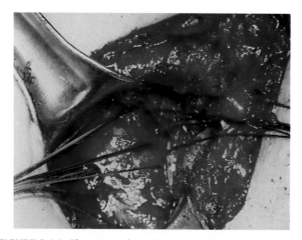

FIGURE 3-14. The sutures have been passed and three horizontal mattress sutures are in place and ready to be tied.

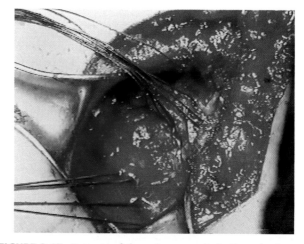

FIGURE 3-15. Passage of the sutures results in three horizontal mattress sutures. Traction on these sutures brings the tendon into contact with the previously prepared cancellous bed.

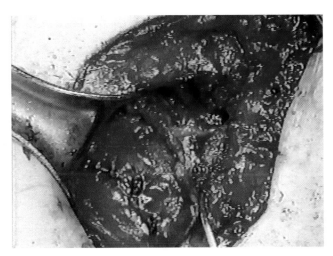

FIGURE 3-16. After the sutures are tied, the tendon-to-bone repair is completed.

or similar devices to decrease tension on the repair. These have not proven to be successful; in our experience, we have found them to result in greater postoperative stiffness.

With the repair completed, the closure is performed. <u>The most important aspect of the closure is a secure reattachment of the anterior deltoid to the anterior acromion.</u> This is done using no. 2 nonabsorbable sutures passed through bone (Fig. 3-17). A tenaculum is used to prepare bone tunnels through the anterior acromion, approximately 5 mm from the edge. Sutures are passed through the full thickness of the anterior deltoid tendon and through the bone tunnels to allow the anterior deltoid to be reattached anatomically. Additional no. 2 nonabsorbable sutures are passed through the deltoid tendon and the capsule of the AC joint, medially and through the lateral deltoid tendon, laterally. The interval between the anterior and middle portions of the deltoid

is closed with no. 1 absorbable suture. When the anterior deltoid repair is completed, it is reevaluated to confirm that it is secure. The subcutaneous tissue is then closed with nonabsorbable sutures, and the skin is closed with a running subcuticular closure using a nonabsorbable monofilament suture. Steri-Strips and a sterile dressing are applied. The upper extremity is then placed in a sling.

POSTOPERATIVE PROTOCOL

Because most rotator cuff repairs are preformed under regional anesthesia, we begin exercises immediately in the recovery room. The patient is seen by our occupational therapist who starts a program of passive range of motion of the shoulder, including forward elevation, abduction, and external rotation to a limit determined intraoperatively. This is an important component of the rehabilitation. It allows the patient to observe the range of motion that can be achieved and establishes goals as he or she begins a more formal rehabilitation program the following day. Patients are instructed in a passive range of motion exercise program and are allowed to perform active and active-assisted range of motion for the elbow, wrist, and hand. Most patients are discharged the day following open rotator cuff repair, and the remainder is able to go home the same day.

FOLLOW-UP

Patients are maintained on a passive range of motion exercise program for approximately 6 weeks following surgery. This may be extended to 7 or 8 weeks based on the size of the tear, the quality of the tissue, and the security of the repair. During this time, the patients are reevaluated approximately 10 days postoperatively for suture removal and then

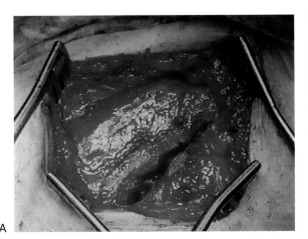

A

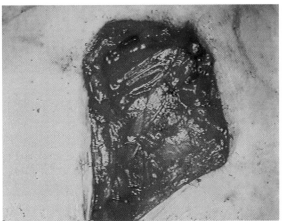

B

FIGURE 3-17. The anterior deltoid is brought back into anatomic position **(A)** and repaired to the acromion with nonabsorbable sutures passed through bone **(B)**.

again 2 to 3 weeks later. Six to 8 weeks following surgery, the sling immobilization is discontinued and the patients are progressed to an active range of motion program. Active range of motion is initially performed in a supine position. As patients improve, they are progressed to a sitting position. Active range of motion in the sitting position is true antigravity movement and can be considered the first step in a strengthening program. Isometric strengthening is begun 2 to 3 weeks after initiation of the active range of motion program. Stretching exercises are continued, even as active range of motion is initiated, until full range of motion is regained. Resistive strengthening (with weights or Thera-Band) is performed at approximately 3 months following the surgery when the patient has regained near full active range of motion. It can begin sooner if the patient has made faster progress regaining active range of motion. Patients are maintained on a maintenance program for range of motion and stretching and strengthening for 6 months following the surgery. We encourage patients to continue a strengthening program for the first year following the surgery. Our previous research has indicated that recovery of strength following rotator cuff repair, particularly after repair of large or massive tears, requires at least 1 year postoperatively.

SUGGESTED READINGS

Adamson GJ, Tibone E. Ten-year assessment of primary rotator cuff repairs. *J Shoulder Elbow Surg* 1993; 2: 57–63.

Bigliani LU, Cordasco FA, McIlveen SJ, et al. Operative repairs of massive rotator cuff tears: long-term results. *J Shoulder Elbow Surg* 1992; 1: 120–130.

Cofield RH. Rotator cuff disease of the shoulder. *J Bone Joint Surg Am* 1985; 67: 974–979

Cofield RH, Parvizi J, Hoffmeyer PJ, et al. Surgical repair of chronic rotator cuff tears: a prospective long-term study. *J Bone Joint Surg Am* 2001; 83A: 71–77.

Ellman H, Hanker G, Bayer M. Repair of the rotator cuff. End results study of factors influencing reconstruction. *J Bone Joint Surg Am* 1986; 68A: 1136–1144.

Galatz LM, Griggs S, Cameron BD, et al. Prospective longitudinal analysis of postoperative shoulder function: a ten-year follow-up study of full-thickness rotator cuff tears. *J Bone Joint Surg Am* 2001; 83A: 1052–1056.

Gupta R, Leggin BG, Iannotti JP. Results of surgical repair of full-thickness tears of the rotator cuff. *Orthop Clin North Am* 1997; 28: 241–248.

Rokito AS, Cuomo F, Gallagher MA, et al. Long-term functional outcome of repair of large and massive chronic tears of the rotator cuff. *J Bone Joint Surg Am* 1999; 81A: 991–997.

Watson EM, Sonnabend DH. Outcome of rotator cuff repair. *J Shoulder Elbow Surg* 2002; 11: 201–211.

CHAPTER 4

ANTERIOR SHOULDER REPAIR

JOSEPH D. ZUCKERMAN
ARASH ARAGHI

Recurrent anterior glenohumeral instability is an often encountered problem in orthopaedic surgery. Although it most commonly occurs in young individuals (younger than 30 years), it can be encountered in older patients, including the geriatric population. The operative management of recurrent anterior instability has evolved over the past 40 years. A significant number of well-described techniques have been used to treat this problem, ranging from bony procedures to soft tissue procedures to a combination of both approaches. More recently, it has become widely recognized that the treatment of recurrent anterior glenohumeral instability should be directed at the underlying pathoanatomy. In most patients, this involves the anterior capsule and the capsulolabral attachments. In this chapter, we discuss the operative management of recurrent anterior glenohumeral instability using this pathoanatomic approach.

ANATOMY

The literature contains many references to the "essential" lesion of recurrent anterior instability. It is now recognized that the essential lesion most likely represents a combination of findings that includes the capsule and the capsulolabral complex. Therefore, knowledge of the anatomy of the glenohumeral joint is critically important in the performance of this procedure.

The glenohumeral joint is often described as a ball and socket joint; however, it is actually a "ball on a dish." The relative flatness of the glenoid provides very little inherent constraint during glenohumeral motion. Unlike the hip joint in which the femoral head is well contained within the acetabulum, the humeral head has a much greater freedom of motion on the relatively flat glenoid. These relationships explain the wide range of motion possible at the glenohumeral joint and why the glenohumeral joint is the joint that most commonly becomes unstable.

The relatively flat glenoid is anatomically deepened by the fibrocartilaginous labrum forming a peripheral rim for the glenoid that increases both the surface area and its concavity (Fig. 4-1). The glenohumeral joint capsule attaches to the edge of the glenoid anteriorly, inferiorly, and posteriorly. Superiorly, it is contiguous with the underside of the rotator cuff and inserts just medial to the biceps labral complex.

The anterior glenohumeral capsule contains the gleno-

humeral ligaments. These are thickenings of the capsule that form the superior, middle, and inferior glenohumeral ligaments. The inferior glenohumeral ligament is the most important anterior stabilizer, particularly in the abducted and externally rotated position. The middle glenohumeral ligament is also an important anterior stabilizer. The superior glenohumeral ligament is less consistent and provides more of a restraint for inferior translation.

The continuity between the anterior capsule, the labrum, and the anteroinferior glenoid provides the important soft tissue restraint that maintains the humeral head in a reduced position on the glenoid in the abducted and externally rotated position. Disruption or compromise of these soft tissue stabilizers allows abnormal anterior translation resulting in instability. When this occurs because of a traumatic event, it most commonly results in disruption of the capsulolabral attachment to the anterior glenoid. This is often referred to as a Bankart lesion. When this disruption occurs, it may also involve a small avulsion fracture of bone that can be visualized radiographically. Avulsions occur less commonly than pure soft tissue disruption. When the capsulolabral attachment is disrupted, recurrent episodes of instability are more likely to occur. With each episode of instability, there is some additional damage to the anterior capsule. This can result in stretching or plastic deformation of the capsule (glenohumeral ligaments), further compromising the anterior stabilizers. Therefore, because the primary etiology of recurrent anterior instability is disruption of the anterior capsulolabral stabilizing mechanism, operative management should be directed at restoring the integrity of this essential support. Although recurrent anterior dislocations may also produce impression fractures of the posterolateral portion of the humeral head or anterior glenoid wear, in most cases anterior capsulolabral reconstruction will be successful in correcting the problem. In addition, there are specific situations in which the bony changes must be addressed. These instances are discussed later in the chapter.

CLASSIFICATION

Glenohumeral instability can be classified by direction, degree, frequency, etiology, and duration. The direction of dislocation can be anterior, posterior, inferior, or multidirectional. The degree of instability can represent subluxa-

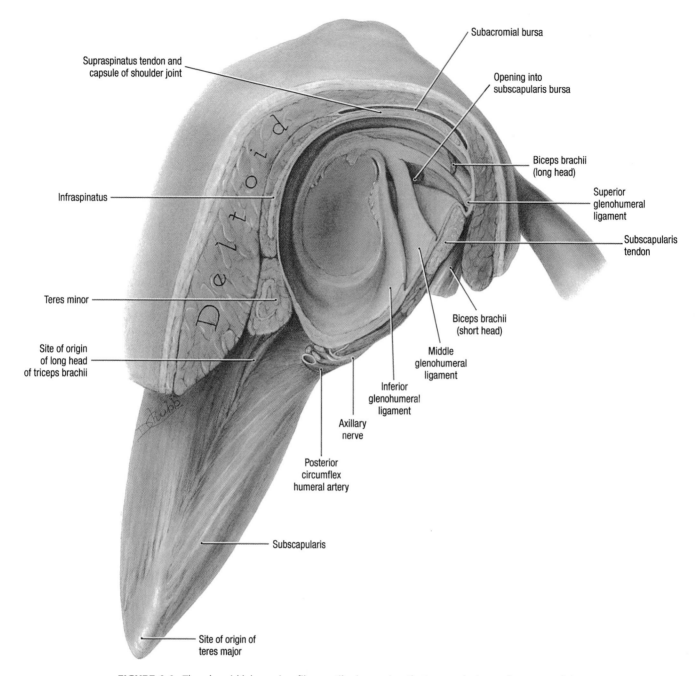

FIGURE 4-1. The glenoid labrum is a fibrocartilaginous ring that expands the surface area of the glenoid and provides a deepening affect. The glenohumeral joint capsule is characterized by thickenings anteriorly and posteriorly that correspond to the glenohumeral ligaments. The important ligaments anteriorly are the superior, middle, and inferior glenohumeral ligaments. Lateral view.

tion or dislocation. Frequency can be a single episode or recurrent episodes. The etiology can be traumatic or atraumatic. Traumatic episodes generally result from a specific significant injury. An atraumatic etiology generally indicates that instability develops in the absence of a specific injury. The atraumatic group can be further classified as vol-

untary or involuntary. Voluntary atraumatic instability occurs when an individual consciously attempts to cause the subluxation or dislocation. Involuntary episodes occur without specific voluntary actions by the individual. The duration of instability can be acute or chronic. Acute dislocations are generally considered to be those that are recognized within 24 hours of the occurrence. A dislocation that has been present for more than 24 hours is considered chronic. This aspect of classification has not been universally agreed on. Some consider any dislocation less than 3 weeks in duration as acute, and all beyond 3 weeks as chronic. Other classifications have considered acute to be less than 24 hours, subacute between 1 day and 3 weeks and chronic beyond 3 weeks. In this specific chapter, we specifically focus on the treatment of recurrent anterior glenohumeral instability in which the initial episode occurred as a result of a traumatic event and recurrent episodes occurred involuntarily.

INDICATIONS

Operative management of recurrent anterior glenohumeral instability is indicated in patients with episodes of instability that significantly interfere with their ability to perform their daily activities. The degree of disability associated with this condition varies from patient to patient. Some patients have episodes that only occur as a result of specific athletic activities, whereas others have episodes that occur with everyday activities that involve using the extremity overhead. Some patients describe episodes of instability during sleep. Each patient will describe the degree of disability associated with this condition. Some patients accept a more significant limitation of their activities in an effort to avoid surgery. The decision to proceed with surgery should be based on an in-depth discussion between the patient and the surgeon, which addresses the nature of the problem, the natural history of glenohumeral instability, the patient's lifestyle and activity needs, and operative management particularly with respect to anticipated outcomes and potential benefits and risks. With this information, the patient is able to make an informed decision.

An important consideration in deciding which patients are candidates for operative management is the frequency and ease with which episodes occur. Patients who have had three episodes of instability occurring only with athletic activity (each of which was separated by 2 or 3 years) are clearly less disabled by the condition than someone who has had six episodes of instability over the past 6 months, all of which occurred with everyday activities that include dressing and sleeping. The role of nonoperative management is generally limited. In patients with recurrent anterior instability of traumatic origin an exercise program is unlikely to resolve the problem or significantly reduce the frequency of episodes of instability. Some patients may prefer to limit their activities to avoid surgery. This may be possible with patients in whom the episodes occur during specific athletic activities, but it is certainly not feasible for those experiencing episodes with activities of daily living. This distribution further indicates the importance of a careful evaluation of

each individual patient to determine the appropriate candidates for operative management.

Operative management is contraindicated in patients who exhibit a voluntary component to the instability because these patients often have underlying psychologic problems that would preclude a successful outcome. In addition, patients who will not be compliant with postoperative management, specifically the duration of immobilization or a gradual return to activities and participation in the rehabilitation program, should also not be considered as candidates for operative management. In these subgroups of patients, the likelihood of an unsuccessful outcome is significant; thus, operative management should be avoided.

PREOPERATIVE PLANNING

The most important aspect of preoperative planning is confirmation of the diagnosis. This is accomplished with a careful history and physical examination. Standard radiographs should be obtained to identify findings that suggest recurrent anterior instability, including Hill Sachs impression fractures, anterior glenoid wear, and calcification about the anterior glenoid. If a patient has had radiographs obtained in the emergency room before closed reduction, these should be obtained and reviewed to confirm the direction of instability. In patients for whom these x-rays are not available, we prefer to obtain a magnetic resonance imaging (MRI) to document changes in the anterior capsulolabral complex. An MRI also identifies bony changes consistent with anterior instability. If standard radiographs and/or an MRI suggest significant anterior glenoid wear, a computed tomography (CT) scan should be obtained to further delineate these changes. Although it is uncommon to require anterior glenoid bone grafting, this possibility should be identified preoperatively.

EQUIPMENT

The equipment necessary to perform this procedure is not extensive. There are specific instruments that allow the preparation of the bone tunnels to be performed more easily. Currently, there are a variety of suture anchors available to reattach the anterior capsule to the glenoid if this technique is preferred. However, the technique we describe uses sutures placed through bone tunnels in the anterior glenoid to reattach the capsule.

A self-retaining retractor is very useful for retraction of the superficial and deep layers of tissue (Fig. 4-2). A modular retractor with blades of variable depth is preferable to allow for the varying amounts of soft tissue that may be encountered. Exposure of the glenoid is facilitated with use of a short-spike levering type retractor. This facilitates retraction of the anterior capsule during preparation of the bone

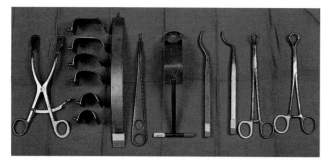

FIGURE 4-2. Equipment used during anterior shoulder repair include (from *left* to *right*): self-retaining retractor with blades of variable depth, a single spike retractor for the anterior glenoid, a small spike levering retractor, a humeral head retractor, offset awls of different sizes, and reaming tenacula of different sizes.

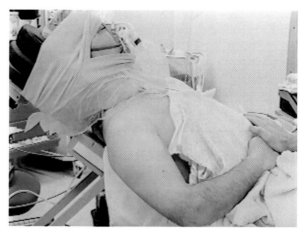

FIGURE 4-3. A patient is positioned in 30 to 40 degrees of elevation. The operative extremity is positioned to allow free mobility.

tunnels. Use of a small Hohmann retractor may also be helpful; similarly, a Fukuda humeral head retractor enhances exposure of the glenoid articular surface. Preparation of the bone tunnels is accomplished more easily with use of an offset awl and a sharp tenaculum. These are designed for this procedure and are available from different instrument manufacturers. Passage of the sutures through the bone tunnels is facilitated by using needles of varying sizes to accommodate the curvature of the bone tunnel. Although cutting needles are recommended for this portion of the procedure, we generally prefer noncutting needles for passage of the sutures through the soft tissues.

PATIENT POSITIONING AND PREPARATION

Open anterior shoulder repair can be performed under regional or general anesthesia. The vast majority of these procedures in our institution are performed under regional anesthesia. This approach is well-received by patients and has the benefit of providing early postoperative pain relief. However, the use of general anesthesia does allow for the examination of both shoulders intraoperatively. This may be the preferred approach when examination of the contralateral shoulder is important to confirm the diagnosis. However, the goal should always be to enter the operating room with a confirmed diagnosis and an established operative plan based on careful preoperative evaluation. After induction of anesthesia, the first step is the physical examination. The involved shoulder should be carefully and systematically assessed for range of motion and humeral head translation. Passive range of motion should be documented, including forward elevation: external rotation with the elbow both at the side and in 90 degrees abduction and internal rotation with the elbow at the side and in 90 degrees of abduction. Translation of the humeral head on the glenoid in anterior, posterior, and inferior directions should be assessed. The testing position should include those that

predispose to anterior, posterior, and inferior instability. Range of motion and translation should always be compared with the uninvolved shoulder.

When the examination under anesthesia is complete, the patient is positioned for the surgical procedure. The use of a specific positioning device that allows varying amounts of elevation of the head and trunk is helpful. When arthroscopy is performed before the anterior shoulder repair, we use the sitting position. Pillows should be placed under the knees to prevent sliding. Following completion of the arthroscopic component, the position should be changed to 30 to 40 degrees of elevation for the anterior shoulder repair (Fig. 4-3). The shoulder is shaved just before preparation of the skin. The area of shaving should include the anterior aspect of the shoulder and the axilla. The preparation includes the shoulder and the entire upper extremity, beginning at the base of the neck and including the shoulder girdle. Draping is performed to provide a secure sterile field that incorporates the anterior and superior aspects of the shoulder.

SURGICAL INCISION AND LANDMARKS

After preparation and draping, the bony landmarks about the anterior aspect of the shoulder are identified. A surgical marking pen is used to mark the coracoid process, the lateral clavicle, the acromioclavicular joint, and the anterior and lateral portions of the acromion. An anterior inferior incision is used in line with the axillary skin fold (Fig. 4-4). The incision is marked by placing the arm in an adducted position next to the chest wall. This allows identification of skin lines for improved cosmesis. The incision extends from the anterior aspect of the axilla superiorly toward the coracoid process. An incision of varying length can be used based on the size of the patient. Smaller incisions can be used in thin, less muscular patients, whereas a longer incision is necessary in larger more heavily muscled patients. Although some

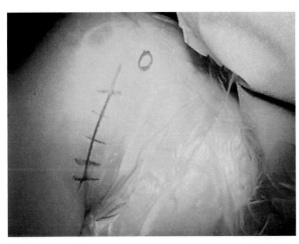

FIGURE 4-4. The anterior axillary incision extends from the axillary skin fold to the area just lateral to the coracoid process. Length of the incision vary from 5 to 7 cm depending on the patient's size.

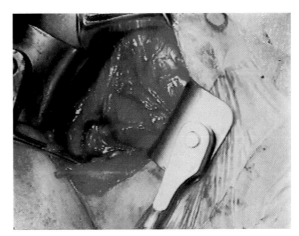

FIGURE 4-6. The vessels that mark the inferior aspect of the subscapularis tendon are cauterized to reduce bleeding.

have advocated use of an anterior/inferior axillary incision for cosmetic reasons, we prefer a more anterior incision to facilitate exposure. Although the appearance of the incision is related, in part, to its length and location, the method of skin closure and the variable tendency for the incision to spread are more important factors.

APPROACH

After incision of the skin and subcutaneous tissues, subcutaneous flaps are developed medially, laterally, superiorly (up to the coracoid process), and inferiorly. This allows identification of the deltopectoral interval. The deltopectoral interval is identified by the fat stripe covering the cephalic vein (Fig. 4-5). If difficulty is encountered identifying the interval, attention should be turned to the proximal portion of

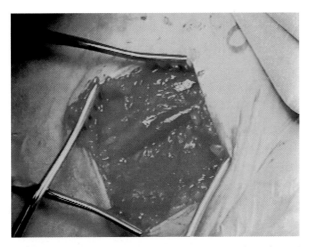

FIGURE 4-5. The deltopectoral interval is marked by a fat stripe that separates the two muscles. The cephalic vein lies within the interval.

the exposure in the area of the coracoid process. The interval is formed just distal to the coracoid process and is often easier to identify in this area. The deltopectoral interval should be carefully developed proximally and distally. The cephalic vein is more commonly retracted laterally with the deltoid because there are a number of branches that enter the vein from the deltoid. Occasionally, medial retraction of the cephalic vein with the pectoralis major is used based on anatomy of the interval. The interval is developed proximally up to the coracoid and distally to the pectoralis major insertion. The subdeltoid space is mobilized and a self-retaining retractor is used to retract the deltoid and the pectoralis major for exposure of the deeper tissues. The next layer is the clavipectoral fascia, which is divided longitudinally just lateral to the conjoined tendon muscles. This allows the conjoined tendon muscles to be mobilized and retracted medially. The release of the superior 1 cm of the pectoralis major tendon insertion can facilitate exposure in large, muscular patients. This must be done carefully and should be repaired at the completion of the procedure.

The bony and soft tissue landmarks about the proximal humerus are then identified. These include the bicipital groove, the lesser tuberosity with the insertion of the subscapularis tendon, and the rotator interval. The veins that are located at the inferior aspect of the subscapularis tendon are also identified and cauterized to prevent bleeding as the dissection progresses (Fig. 4-6).

PROCEDURE

At this point, separation of the subscapularis tendon and muscle from the underlying capsule is performed. ◖ A no. 15 blade on a long handle is preferred for this dissection. An incision is made into the subscapularis tendon, approximately 1 cm medial to its insertion into the lesser tuberosity. The incision is made in line with the humeral shaft, beginning superiorly at the rotator interval and progressing distally to the inferior aspect of the subscapularis. The most inferior aspect of the incision should curve slightly medially. The scalpel blade is beveled medially to carefully divide the tendon fibers and facilitate entrance into the interval between the tendon and the capsule. Note that the tendon fibers are striated, whereas the capsular tissue is not. This distinction is an important component of the dissection. When striated fibers are no longer visible, the capsular layer has been exposed. **If the dissection enters the deeper tissues too quickly, the capsule may be perforated.** As the tendon is elevated off the capsule, the dissection progresses medially to the musculotendinous junction. With elevation of the tendon, the muscle can be more easily separated from the capsule with a periosteal elevator. It is important to continue the dissection to the rotator interval superiorly and to the inferior portion of the subscapularis to expose the entire anterior and inferior capsule. At the inferior portion, there is less tendon and more muscle tissue. Bleeding may, therefore, occur and should be controlled by cauterization. The medial edge of the subscapularis tendon is tagged with no. 1 Mersilene sutures (Fig. 4-7). The subscapularis tendon and muscle is dissected off the underlying capsule medially until the anterior glenoid neck is palpable. The subscapularis tendon is then placed behind the self-retaining retractor. The capsular layer is now exposed. Two specific aspects of the capsule should be evaluated.

The rotator interval should be inspected to determine the size and location of the capsular fenestration (Fig. 4-8). This fenestration varies from a small lateral opening to a large opening that extends to the anterosuperior corner of the glenoid. The fenestration should be repaired using no. 1 Mersilene in simple interrupted sutures. ▧ This portion of the repair imbricates the area of the superior gleno-

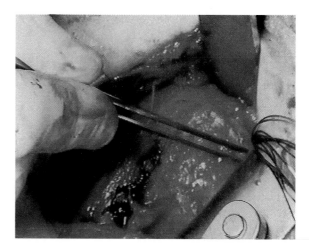

FIGURE 4-8. The rotator interval fenestration is identified superiorly. It can be variable in size, although currently it is small as shown here.

humeral ligament to the most anterior portion of the rotator cuff (Fig. 4-9). The repair can be expected to provide some degree of resistance to inferior translation in patients with a significant component of inferior laxity. The degree of capsular laxity should also be assessed. With the arm in neutral rotation, the capsule can often appear very redundant anteriorly and inferiorly. This is particularly true in patients with excessive degrees of external rotation. This finding provides a preliminary indication of the degree of capsular shift that may be necessary to achieve stability.

At this point, a capsulotomy is performed 1 cm medial and parallel to the subscapularis tenotomy (Fig. 4-10). The capsulotomy extends superiorly from the rotator interval to the anteroinferior aspect of the humeral neck. The medial edge of the capsule is tagged with two no. 1 Mersilene sutures that are placed near its midportion. A Fukuda humeral

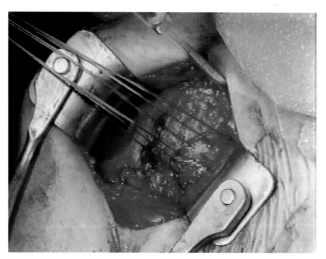

FIGURE 4-7. The medial edge of the subscapularis tendon is tagged with sutures and retracted medially to expose the underlying capsule.

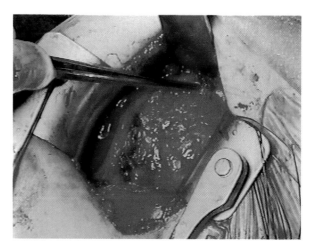

FIGURE 4-9. Closure of the rotator interval defect is performed with nonabsorbable interrupted sutures.

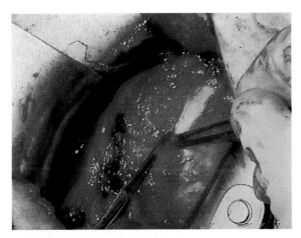

FIGURE 4-10. The vertical capsulotomy is performed 1 cm medial to the location of the subscapularis tenotomy.

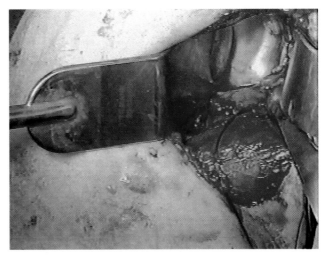

FIGURE 4-12. With the humeral head retractor and the glenoid retractor in position, the capsulolabral detachment is evident with clear visualization of the anterior glenoid.

head retractor is then inserted. This allows assessment of the anterior glenoid and the integrity of the capsulolabral insertion. The midportion of the glenoid is identified and a horizontal capsulotomy is performed (Fig. 4-11). The glenoid articular surface and the anterior glenoid can now be well visualized. With the attached sutures, the superior and inferior leaves of the capsule can be retracted superiorly and inferiorly, respectively. The capsulolabral insertion is then evaluated. Different findings are often encountered. In some patients, the capsulolabral complex is intact. This is usually encountered in patients in whom the underlying pathoanatomy is significant laxity and redundancy. These patients require only the inferior capsular shift portion of the procedure. In some patients, the capsulolabral complex is completely stripped off from its insertion into the anterior glenoid (Fig. 4-12). The anterior labrum may be absent or torn and detached from the capsule. These patients require reattachment of the anterior capsule to the anterior edge of the glenoid, with an inferior capsular shift that varies based on the amount of inferior capsular redundancy. Some patients appear to have an intact capsular insertion located medial to the anterior glenoid margin. In these cases, the anterior labrum is usually absent and the capsular attachment is generally tenuous. An elevator should be used to elevate the capsular attachment so that it can be advanced to the anterior glenoid margin and reattached in a more anatomic position.

When the anterior capsulolabral complex is detached, reattachment is an essential portion of the procedure. An anterior glenoid neck retractor is used to expose the area of reattachment. Depending on the size of the glenoid, it may be helpful to place a small Hohmann type retractor inferiorly and superiorly for additional exposure. The capsulolabral attachment is usually intact inferiorly at about the 6-o'clock position. When a left shoulder is being treated, the capsular detachment extends up to the 11-o'clock position. When a right shoulder is being treated, the capsular detachment extends to the 1-o'clock position. The goal of this portion of the procedure is to reattach the capsule to its anatomic position at the anterior margin of the glenoid to restore the soft tissue buttress to prevent anterior translation.

The anterior glenoid neck is roughened with a curette or a burr to prepare the reattachment site (Fig. 4-13). The capsular reattachment can be performed by either preparing bone tunnels for passing sutures or by using suture anchors. If suture anchors are used, it is important that they be placed directly at the junction of the anterior glenoid neck and the glenoid articular surface. This allows the capsule to be brought into its anatomic position. **It is important not to place the anchors further medially because this results in a nonanatomic capsulolabral reattachment.** This chapter focuses on the technique for preparation of bone tunnels.

There are a variety of instruments that can be used to prepare bone tunnels. ▣ We have found that the most straightforward approach is to use an offset awl combined

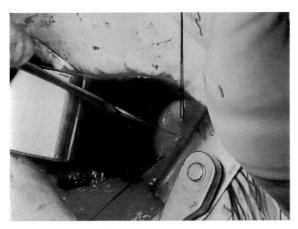

FIGURE 4-11. The horizontal capsulotomy is directed to the midpoint of the glenoid.

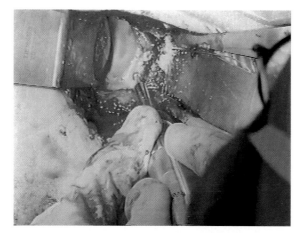

FIGURE 4-13. A motorized burr is used to decorticate the glenoid neck in the area for the capsular reattachment.

with a sharp tenaculum. These instruments can be found in the Bankart repair instrument sets that are available from different instrument manufacturers. The bone tunnel should be placed through the anterior glenoid articular surface and through the glenoid neck. Three bone tunnels are usually necessary to reattach the detached area of capsule. These are placed at the 5-o'clock, 3-o'clock, and 2-o'clock positions for a right shoulder and the 7-o'clock, 9-o'clock, and 10-o'clock positions for the left shoulder. Because restoration of the anterior/inferior capsular reattachment is critically important for success of the repair, placement of bone tunnels in this area is particularly important. The offset awl initiates the bone tunnel at the glenoid articular surface, approximately 3 to 4 mm from the edge of the bone. It is directed perpendicular to the glenoid and advanced through the subchondral bone. The awl is then placed on the anterior glenoid neck directly opposite the location on the glenoid articular surface. The awl is inserted perpendicular to the bone surface and directed toward the deepest insertion point of the previously prepared hole. **It is essential to maintain a sufficient bony bridge to prevent inadvertent fracture.** At this point, the tenaculum is used. One end of the tenaculum is placed through the entry point in the glenoid articular surface and the other is placed through the glenoid neck entry point. The tenaculum is then tightened and carefully rotated in a medial and lateral direction to form one continuous tunnel. There will be some initial resistance as the tenaculum is rotated, which will gradually decrease as the tunnel is completed and enlarged. **Excessive resistance may be an indication that the tenaculum is not in the proper position or that the prepared holes are too far apart to allow easy conversion to a tunnel.** If this occurs, proper placement of the tenaculum should first be confirmed. If this is not the problem, the awl should be reinserted to deepen and enlarge the holes. When the bone tunnels are complete, a no. 2 Mersilene suture, on a no. 5 cutting needle, is passed through the bone tunnel. In some

patients, needles can be more easily passed through the articular surface, whereas in other patients they may be more easily passed through the entry point on the glenoid neck. When the tip of the needle is visualized exiting the bone, it should be carefully advanced by following the curvature of the needle. This avoids excessive force on the bone tunnel and decreases the risk of fracture. The sutures are passed through the remaining bone tunnels in a similar fashion (Fig. 4-14).

With the three sutures in place, the capsular reattachment can be performed. ◨ The anterior glenoid neck retractor is repositioned into an extracapsular position. **The sutures previously placed in the superior and inferior leaves of the capsule should be used to advance the capsule laterally thereby avoiding passing the sutures in an undesirable lateral position; doing so could result in excessive tightening.** The Fukuda humeral head retractor remains in place while a Darrach elevator is placed below the inferior capsule to protect the axillary nerve as the needle is passed. The most inferior suture is then placed in a horizontal mattress fashion through the anterior/inferior capsule. As the sutures are passed, the capsule is advanced laterally and superiorly. The sutures are placed at the glenoid margin so that the reattachment provides the desired soft tissue buttress. The middle and superior sutures are passed in a similar fashion, with care taken to advance the capsule laterally and superiorly (Fig. 4-15). The most inferior suture is tied first. Care must be taken to ensure that the suture is tight enough to bring the capsule into direct and secure contact with the glenoid rim. The middle and superior sutures are then tied. At this point, the capsular reattachment should be assessed. A small elevator should be used to confirm that the capsulolabral detachment has been repaired and is securely in position. The Fukuda humeral head retractor is then removed and the self-retaining retractor is reinserted—

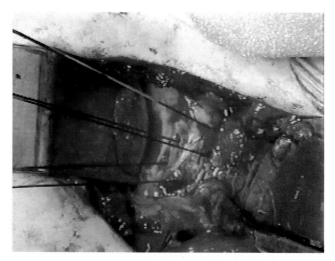

FIGURE 4-14. Three sutures have been placed through the bone tunnels that were prepared with the offset awl and reaming tenaculum.

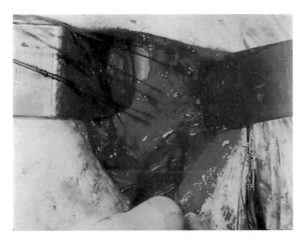

FIGURE 4-15. The sutures have been passed through the capsule as three horizontal mattress sutures.

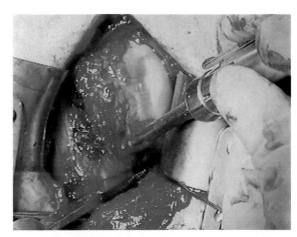

FIGURE 4-16. The motorized burr is used to decorticate the anterior-inferior humeral neck to facilitate capsular reattachment.

retracting the deltoid laterally and the subscapularis, conjoined tendon muscles, and pectoralis major medially.

At this point, the inferior capsular redundancy is assessed by palpating the size of the inferior capsular pouch. In general, all patients with recurrent anterior instability undergo some degree of inferior capsular shift. The amount of shift depends on (a) the size of the inferior capsular pouch, (b) the presence or absence of a capsulolabral detachment, (c) the degree of external rotation present preoperatively, and (d) the presence of underlying ligamentous laxity.

The inferior capsular shift should provide additional capsular support anteriorly and inferiorly but should not result in excessive capsular tightening that would restrict range of motion. To accomplish the inferior capsular shift, the anterior/inferior capsule is detached from its humeral neck insertion in an anterior to posterior direction, usually to the 6-o'-clock position. If additional capsular advancement is needed, the capsule can be detached more posteriorly. A burr is then used to decorticate the anterior/inferior glenoid neck to enhance healing of the capsule after the advancement (Fig. 4-16). The inferior capsular flap can be repaired to the remaining lateral capsule. However, inferiorly, it comes into contact with the glenoid neck, and the decortication facilitates healing. The inferior capsular flap is advanced in a superior and lateral direction (Fig. 4-17). It can usually be advanced to the most superior aspect of the original capsulotomy near or at the rotator interval. It is reattached to the lateral capsule with no. 2 Mersilene in simple interrupted sutures.

After the sutures are placed and tied, range of motion is assessed. This includes external rotation with the elbow at the side. Although the range of motion is less than preoperative, the decrease should only be 10 to 15 degrees when a capsulolabral reattachment has been performed. When the underlying pathoanatomy is capsular laxity and redundancy, a more significant decrease in external rotation is desired. However, there should always be at least 30 degrees of

external rotation present. Abduction in the coronal plane is then assessed, making certain it is at least 90 degrees and the repair is secure throughout this range.

In the position of 90 degrees of abduction, external rotation should also be evaluated. There should be at least 80 degrees of external rotation in this position without excessive stress on the repair. In patients with significant capsular laxity, we accept 10 to 15 degrees less because of the amount of soft tissue stretching that is anticipated to occur postoperatively. However, in patients who are involved in overhead throwing, 90 degrees of external rotation in the position of 90 degrees of abduction is desirable.

With completion of the repair of the inferior capsular flap, attention is turned to the superior flap. The superior flap is advanced inferiorly and laterally (Fig. 4-18). Inferior advancement is more important than lateral advancement.

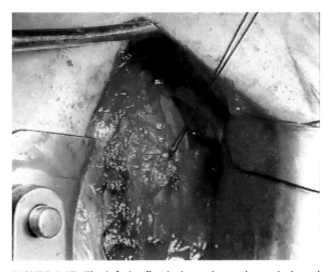

FIGURE 4-17. The inferior flap is then advanced superiorly and secured to the lateral capsule.

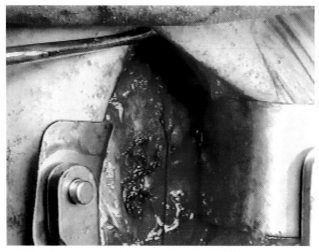

FIGURE 4-18. The superior capsular flap is advanced inferiorly and secured to the lateral capsule.

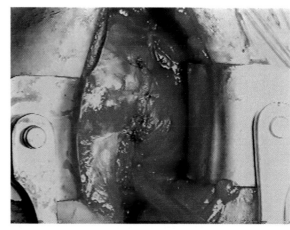

FIGURE 4-19. The subscapularis tendon is repaired directly to its remaining lateral portion. Shortening of the subscapularis should be avoided.

Excessive lateral advancement restricts external rotation, which is not desirable. The superior flap is secured to the lateral capsular tissue with no. 2 Mersilene using simple interrupted sutures. The area of overlap of the superior and inferior flaps should be imbricated with one or two horizontal mattress sutures passed first through the inferior flap and then through the overlying superior flap. Placement of these sutures reinforces the repair and provides additional anterior stability. When the repair of the superior flap is completed, range of motion should once again be assessed in the same testing sequence described previously. Range of motion should not be significantly changed from the testing performed after repair of the inferior flap.

The subscapularis tendon is next advanced to its lateral portion. An anatomic repair is performed to avoid any additional limitation of external rotation. Although older repair techniques have focused on advancement of the subscapularis as an important method of presenting recurrent instability, the repair we describe focuses on correction of the pathoanatomy. Therefore, the subscapularis, which is not an etiologic factor, should be repaired anatomically using no. 1 Mersilene in simple interrupted sutures (Fig. 4-19). It is very important that a secure subscapularis repair be performed to avoid the risk of disruption postoperatively. When the subscapularis repair is completed, external rotation should, once again, be assessed with the elbow at the side to confirm that there is no additional limitation.

The closure is completed with repair of the deltopectoral interval using absorbable sutures, subcutaneous tissue closure, and skin closure. We prefer to close the skin with a running subcuticular nonabsorbable suture (no. 3-0 Prolene) that can be removed postoperatively, because it provides improved cosmesis. Steri-Strips are applied with a sterile dressing. The operative extremity is then placed in a standard sling.

POSTOPERATIVE PROTOCOL AND FOLLOW-UP CARE

Patients are maintained in sling immobilization for 2 to 4 weeks postoperatively. The duration of sling immobilization is based on consideration of different factors that include the age of the patient, the degree of underlying ligamentous laxity, whether a capsulolabral reattachment was performed, and the security of the repair. In general, a somewhat longer period of immobilization is preferred for younger patients, those with significant underlying ligamentous laxity, and those in whom a capsulolabral detachment was not performed; conversely, a shorter period of immobilization is used for older patients, those without underlying ligamentous laxity, and those in whom a capsulolabral reattachment was performed.

Exercises are started on the day following surgery. Although shoulder range of motion is not performed, the patient is instructed in active range of motion of the elbow, wrist, and hand. In addition, isometric deltoid and external rotation exercises are performed. Isometric internal rotation exercises are not performed because of the subscapularis detachment and repair. These exercises are continued during the period of immobilization. When the sling is discontinued, an active range of motion program is initiated, focusing on forward elevation, external rotation, and internal rotation behind the back. Passive stretching exercises are not performed initially; instead, we rely on the patient's active exercise to regain range of motion. If recovery of range of motion is slower than desired, gentle stretching may be performed 6 to 8 weeks postoperatively. When active range of motion is started, isometric internal rotation exercises are added. Resistive strengthening exercises are begun when the patient has progressed in regaining active range of motion.

This generally occurs 6 to 8 weeks postoperatively. Patients are monitored for recovery of active range of motion that includes forward elevation and external rotation with the arm at the side and at 90 degrees of abduction and internal rotation behind the back. Strength recovery is also monitored as the patients are gradually progressed through isometric, isotonic, and then isokinetic-type exercises. Strengthening is performed below the shoulder level for the first 4 to 6 months postoperatively. Strengthening overhead can then be safely added.

Patients are allowed to gradually return to activities and encouraged to return to their everyday activities as soon as possible. They are allowed to jog 6 to 8 weeks postoperatively. Aerobic exercise is permitted before that time but is limited to an exercise bicycle as long as the operative extremity is not used to grasp the handle bars. Six months following the surgery, patients can return to overhead noncontact athletic activity. This specifically includes swimming, tennis, and other overhead racket sports. Basketball and baseball activities can be resumed 6 to 9 months following the surgery. Full activity basketball, which involves a significant amount of contact, should be resumed closer to 9 months following surgery. Patients can return to full unrestricted activity 9 to 12 months following the surgery. This includes football, snow skiing, and water skiing. Some modifications can be made for sports based on the position played and whether the dominant or nondominant extremity is involved.

SUGGESTED READINGS

Berg EE, Ellison AE. The inside-out Bankart procedure. *Am J Sports Med* 1990; 18: 129–133.

Bigliani L, Kurzweil P, Schwartzbach C, et al. Inferior capsular shift procedure for anterior-inferior shoulder instability in athletes. *Am J Sports Med* 1994; 22: 578–584.

Jobe FW, Giangarra CE, Kvitne RS, et al. Anterior capsulolabral reconstruction of the shoulder in athletes in overhand sports. *Am J Sports Med* 1991; 19: 428–434.

Loomer R, Fraser J. A modified Bankart procedure for recurrent anterior-inferior shoulder instability. *Am J Sports Med* 1989; 17: 374–379.

Romeo AA, Cohen BS, Carreira DS. Traumatic anterior shoulder instability. *Orthop Clin North Am* 2001; 32: 399–409.

Rowe CR, Patel D, Southmayd WW. The Bankart procedure; a long-term end-result study. *J Bone Joint Surg Am* 1978; 60A: 1–16.

Thomas SC, Matsen FA III. An approach to the repair of avulsion of the glenohumeral ligaments in the management of traumatic anterior glenohumeral instability. *J Bone Joint Surg Am* 1989; 71A: 506–513.

Wirth MA, Blatter G, Rockwood CA Jr. The capsular imbrication procedure for recurrent anterior instability of the shoulder. *J Bone Joint Surg Am* 1996; 78A: 246–259.

CHAPTER 5

ORIF: THREE-PART FRACTURE OF THE PROXIMAL HUMERUS

KENNETH J. KOVAL

Eighty-five percent of proximal humerus fractures are minimally displaced and can be treated with protected immobilization and early range of motion dependent on fracture stability. However, controversy exists regarding the optimal treatment of displaced proximal humerus fractures. Many internal fixation techniques have been advocated for the treatment of these difficult fractures including percutaneous pins, intramedullary rods placed antegrade or retrograde, figure-of-8 tension band wire or suture, and plate and screws. This chapter illustrates open reduction and internal fixation of a displaced proximal humerus fracture using Ender nails and a tension band construct.

ANATOMY

The proximal humerus can be considered to consist of the humeral head, the tuberosities, and the humeral shaft (Fig. 5-1). The anatomic neck is the junction between the

humeral head and the tuberosities. The surgical neck lies between the tuberosities and the shaft. The rotator cuff (see Figs. 3-2 and 4-1) is composed of four muscular divisions: (a) the subscapularis, which inserts on the lesser tuberosity and acts as an internal rotator of the glenohumeral joint; (b) the supraspinatus tendon, which inserts on the greater tuberosity and acts to depress the humeral head into the glenoid during elevation of the arm; (c) the teres minor and infraspinatus muscles, which are the external rotators of the shoulder and also insert on the greater tuberosity; and (d) the biceps tendon, which lies in the anteriorly directed bicipital groove and provides a useful anatomic landmark for judging rotational deformity of the humeral head during operative management. The terminal branches of the ascending division of the anterior humeral circumflex artery enter the humeral head through the bicipital groove. Fractures that split the tuberosities from the head disrupt this small arterial complex and can result in osteonecrosis of the humeral head (Fig. 5-2).

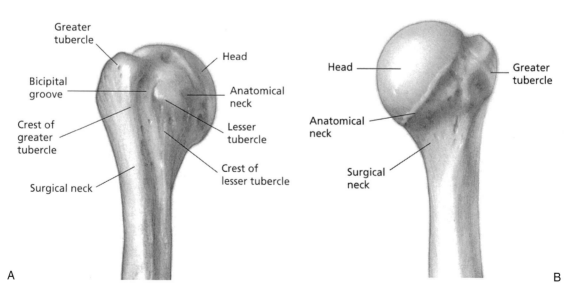

A   B

FIGURE 5-1. A: Right proximal humerus, anterior aspect. **B:** Right proximal humerus, posterior aspect.

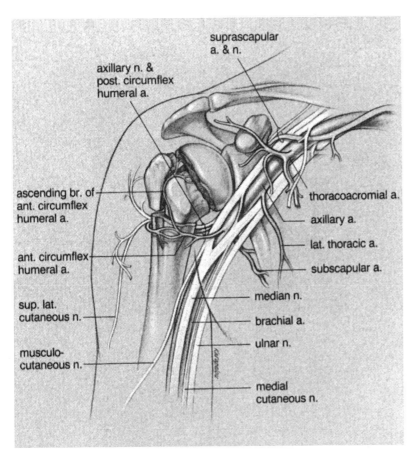

FIGURE 5-2. Right proximal humerus, arteries, nerves, and brachial plexus.

CLASSIFICATION

The Neer classification is the most widely used system in clinical practice (Fig. 5-3). This system is based on the anatomic relationship of the four major anatomic segments: articular segment, greater tuberosity, lesser tuberosity, and the proximal shaft beginning at the level of the surgical neck. Fracture types are based on the presence of displacement of one or more of the four segments. For a segment to be considered displaced, it must be either greater than 1 cm displaced or angulated more than 45 degrees from its anatomic position. The number of fracture lines is not important in this classification system. For example, one-part fractures, or minimally displaced fractures, are the most common type of proximal humeral fractures and account for up to 85% of all proximal humerus fracture. Although these fractures may have multiple fracture lines, they are characterized by the fact that none of the four segments fulfill the criteria for displacement. Hence, they are considered one part or minimally displaced.

Displaced fractures include two-part, three-part, and four-part fractures. A two-part fracture is characterized by displacement of one of the four segments, with the remaining three segments either not fractured or not fulfilling the criteria for displacement. Four types of two-part fractures can be encountered (greater tuberosity, lesser tuberosity, anatomic neck, and surgical neck). A three-part fracture is characterized by displacement of two of the segments from the remaining two nondisplaced segments. Two types of three-part fracture patterns are encountered. The more common pattern is characterized by displacement of the greater tuberosity and the shaft from the lesser tuberosity, which remains with the articular segment. The much less commonly encountered pattern is characterized by displacement of the lesser tuberosity and shaft from the greater tuberosity, which remains with the articular segment. A four-part fracture is characterized by displacement of all four segments.

Neer also categorized fracture-dislocations, which are displaced proximal humeral fractures—two-part, three-part, or four-part—associated with either anterior or posterior dislocation of the articular segment. Neer also described articular surface fractures that were of two types: impression fractures or head-splitting fractures. Impression fractures of the articular surface most often occur in association with chronic dislocations. As such, they can be either anterior or posterior and involve variable amounts of the articular surface. Head-splitting fractures are usually associated with other displaced fractures of the proximal humerus in which the disruption or "splitting" of the articular surface is the most significant component.

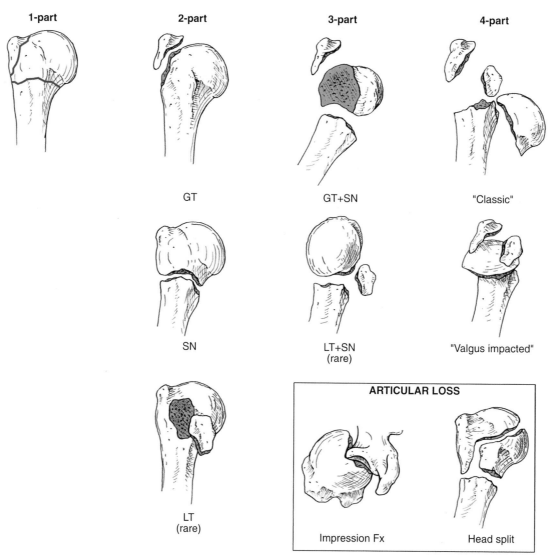

| 1-part | 2-part | 3-part | 4-part |

GT   GT+SN   "Classic"

SN   LT+SN
(rare)   "Valgus impacted"

ARTICULAR LOSS

LT
(rare)   Impression Fx   Head split

FIGURE 5-3. The Neer classification of proximal humerus fractures. This system is based on the anatomic relationship of the four major anatomic segments: the humeral head, greater tuberosity, lesser tuberosity, and the proximal humeral shaft beginning at the level of the surgical neck. Fracture types are based on the presence of displacement of one or more of the four segments. For a segment to be considered displaced, it must be either greater than 1 cm displaced or angulated more than 45 degrees from its anatomic position. (After Neer CS. Displaced proximal humeral fractures: part I. Classification and evaluation. *J Bone Joint Surg Am* 1970;52A:1077–1089, with permission.)

INDICATIONS

Functional outcome following fracture is correlated to residual deformity after healing. Healed fractures with angular deformity greater than 45 degrees or displacement greater than 1 cm have poorer results than those with more anatomic reduction. Most current reports in the literature suggest that the traditional closed methods of treating displaced proximal humerus fractures have been disappointing. Therefore, I feel that displaced proximal humerus fractures are best treated operatively.

Open reduction and internal fixation is the treatment of choice for most displaced two-part fractures. Currently, open reduction and internal fixation is the treatment of choice for displaced three-part fractures of the proximal humerus in younger individuals and prosthetic replacement in older individuals. Different techniques of internal fixation have been used for these fractures including plate and screws, percutaneous pins, tension band wires, and intramedullary devices. In general, the trend for three-part fractures has been toward avoidance of plate and screw fixation because of the difficulties in obtaining adequate fixation in osteoporotic bone. I prefer use of Ender nails augmented with a tension band suture for stabilization of three-part proximal humerus fractures. Four-part fractures are usually treated with prosthetic replacement.

PREOPERATIVE PLANNING

A shoulder trauma series consists of anteroposterior (AP) and lateral views of the shoulder obtained in the plane of the scapula and an axillary view (Fig. 5-4). The scapular AP view offers a general overview of the fracture and is usually evaluated first. The scapular lateral assists in delineating the position of the humeral head relative to the glenoid and is particularly useful in showing dislocations or posteriorly displaced fragments. The axillary view also permits assessment of the glenohumeral relationship. Computed tomography (CT) scans of proximal humeral fractures and fracture dislocations may be indicated when the trauma series radiographs are indeterminate. CT scans have also been recommended to evaluate the rotation of fragments and the degree of tuberosity displacement, as well as articular impression fractures, head-splitting fractures, and chronic fracture-dislocations.

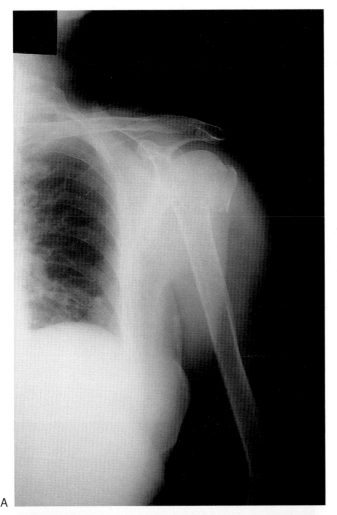

A

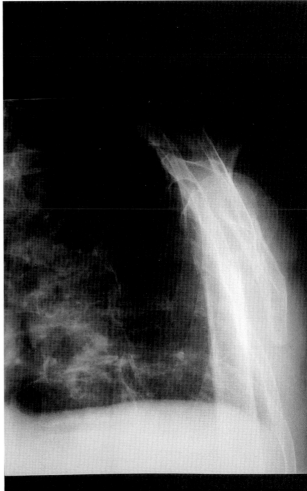

B

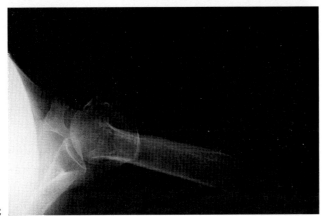

C

FIGURE 5-4. Anteroposterior **(A)**, Y view **(B)**, and axillary **(C)** revealing a displaced three-part fracture of the proximal humerus.

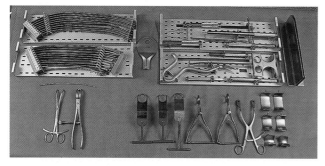

FIGURE 5-5. The equipment needed for open reduction and internal fixation of a three-part proximal humerus fracture: Ender nail instrumentation and nail set *(top row)*, large reduction forceps (2) *(bottom left)*, shoulder retractors *(bottom right)*.

EQUIPMENT

The following equipment is needed (Fig. 5-5):

- Ender nail instrumentation and nail set
- Small fragment set
- Air drill
- Heavy suture
- Large reduction forceps
- Shoulder retractors

PATIENT POSITIONING

The patient is placed on the operating table in a supine position. The head of the operating table is elevated approximately 30 degrees in a modified beach chair position (Fig. 5-6). A small bolster is placed behind the involved shoulder.

The patient is moved off to the side of the table so that the upper extremity can be placed into maximum extension without obstruction by the operating table. The patient is secured to the operating table to minimize any changes in position intraoperatively. The entire upper extremity is prepped and draped to allow full mobility during the procedure.

APPROACH

I have found that open reduction and internal fixation of most displaced proximal humerus fractures is most easily performed through a deltopectoral approach. A straight incision is used; it begins just lateral to the tip of the coracoid process and extends distally and laterally to the insertion of the deltoid (Fig. 5-7). The subcutaneous tissues are divided, and medial and lateral flaps elevated to expose the deeper muscular layers. The deltopectoral interval is identified by localization of the cephalic vein. ◼ The cephalic vein is usually retracted laterally with the deltoid muscle (Fig. 5-8). In some instances, the cephalic vein is more easily retracted medially with the pectoralis major. In either case, care should be taken to preserve the cephalic vein throughout the procedure. The subdeltoid space is mobilized as is the pectoralis major. The conjoined tendon muscles are identified, and the clavipectoral fascia divided at the medial edge of the conjoined tendon muscles. The conjoined tendon muscles and the pectoralis major are retracted medially, and the deltoid is retracted laterally. This can be most easily accomplished with the use of a self-retraining type retractor (Fig. 5-9). ◼ By evacuating the fracture hematoma, the deeper structures can be visualized.

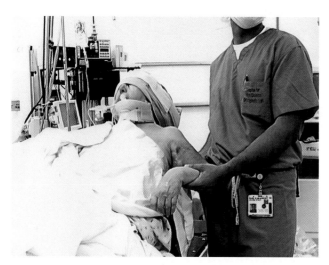

FIGURE 5-6. The patient is placed on the operating table in a supine position. The head of the operating table is elevated approximately 30 degrees in a modified beach chair position. The patient is moved off to the side of the table so that the upper extremity can be placed into maximum extension without obstruction by the operating table.

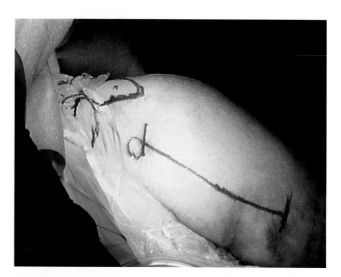

FIGURE 5-7. The deltopectoral incision begins just lateral to the tip of the coracoid process and extends distally and laterally to the insertion of the deltoid.

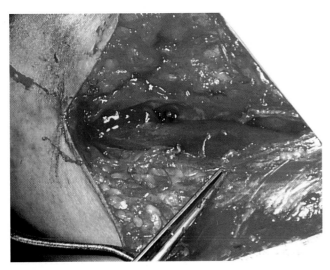

FIGURE 5-8. Identification of the cephalic vein, as indicated by the forceps.

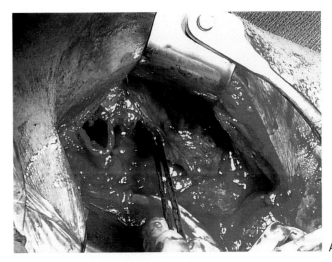

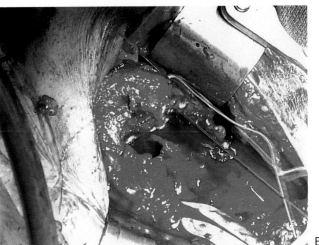

FIGURE 5-10. Mobilization of the displaced greater tuberosity **(A)** and placement of the nonabsorbable sutures at the tendon insertion site **(B)**.

PROCEDURE

The biceps tendon is identified and tagged with a suture or Penrose drain. ◼ <u>The biceps tendon provides an orientation to the greater and lesser tuberosities. The lesser tuberosity is located medial to the biceps tendon and the greater tuberosity is located superiorly and laterally.</u> ◼ Once located, the biceps tendon is followed up to the bicipital groove and rotator interval, which is incised to the glenoid rim if the fracture displacement has not already accomplished this. Dividing the rotator interval enhances exposure and fragment mobilization.

The displaced tuberosity is then mobilized with heavy nonabsorbable suture at the tendon insertion site (Fig. 5-10). ◼ <u>This incorporates the stronger rotator cuff tendon rather than placing the suture through what is usually the</u>

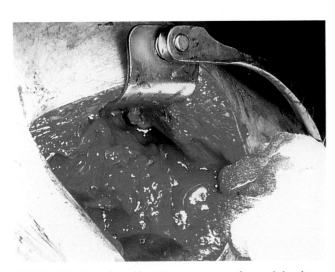

FIGURE 5-9. Use of a self-retainer to retract the conjoined tendon and the pectoralis major medially and the deltoid laterally.

<u>osteoporotic bone of the tuberosity where it may easily cut out.</u> The greater tuberosity fragment is usually displaced superiorly into the subacromial space if the supraspinatus is involved or posteriorly if the infraspinatus or teres minor is the primary deforming force. The head and attached tuberosity are mobilized with skin hooks and sutures at the bone tendon interface. The fracture site is curetted and irrigated. The three fragments are reduced to two by securing the displaced tuberosity to the head and intact tuberosity via heavy nonabsorbable suture (Fig. 5-11).

The displaced surgical neck fracture is exposed, the humeral shaft and head is mobilized, and the fracture site is curetted. A heavy suture is placed into the posterior aspect of the rotator cuff for manipulation of the humeral head fragment. Drill holes are placed in the humeral shaft fragment, 1 to 2 cm distal to the surgical neck fracture on either side of the bicipital groove (Fig. 5-12). Heavy sutures are

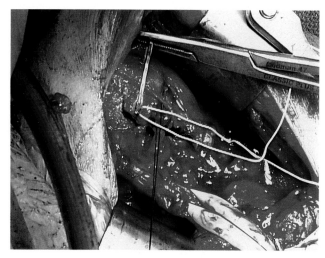

FIGURE 5-11. Stabilization of the greater tuberosity to the humeral head and intact tuberosity using heavy nonabsorbable suture.

passed through these drill holes; they will be used to provide a tension band after flexible nail insertion. Eighteen-gauge wire may be substituted for heavy nonabsorbable suture; however, although it provides greater immediate stability, it is more difficult to handle and carries the risk of breakage and migration, which can irritate the subacromial space.

The humeral head is reduced to the humeral shaft. Fracture reduction is obtained by forward elevation of the humeral shaft while gently pulling on the sutures controlling the proximal fragment. The fracture is then impacted and the arm is extended while maintaining tension on the sutures to prevent loss of reduction. Placement of tension on the sutures placed through the posterior rotator cuff extends the proximal fragment while the arm is extended and prevents apex anterior angulation.

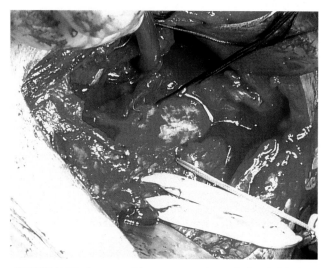

FIGURE 5-12. Passage of heavy suture through the drill holes.

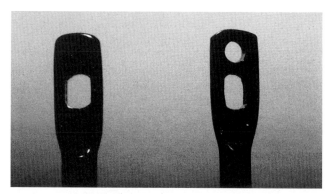

FIGURE 5-13. Modification of the Ender nail with placement of an additional hole above the slot.

Once adequate reduction is achieved, fixation is accomplished using a combination of tension band suture and flexible intramedullary nails. Ender nails (3.5 mm) are superior to straight rods or pins such as Rush rods because they afford three-point fixation, which enhances rotational stability. Furthermore, with use of Ender nails, one can place a figure-of-eight suture or wire through the eyelet to prevent proximal migration and impingement that often occurs with nonfenestrated straight rods. However, the slot of the Ender nail is long and a significant amount of metal may still protrude proximally. Therefore, the nail can be modified with placement of an additional hole above the slot (Fig. 5-13). This allows for deeper insertion of the nail into the humeral head placing the tip well below the rotator cuff tendon. The addition of the tension band configuration with intramedullary nails has been found to add even greater longitudinal and rotational stability over that of either tension banding or intramedullary nailing alone.

While maintaining reduction, small longitudinal incisions are made at the insertion of the rotator cuff fibers into the greater and lesser tuberosities. The two Ender nails are inserted through the anterior and posterior aspect of the greater tuberosity in two-part surgical neck fracture; one Ender nail is inserted through the greater tuberosity and one through the lesser tuberosity and humeral head in three-part fractures. An awl or drill bit is used to penetrate the bone. The posterior nail is best placed initially because levering on this partially inserted nail will aid in holding the reduction and preventing the humeral head from falling posteriorly (Fig. 5-14). ◼ The second nail is then inserted 1.0 to 1.5 cm anterior to the first Ender nail (Fig. 5-15). It is best to use nails of different lengths to prevent the possibility of a distal stress riser. Nails between 22 and 27 cm in length are generally adequate. Before completely burying the nails, the previously placed suture is placed through the eyelets of the nails, passing deep to the rotator cuff between the two nails (Fig. 5-16). The nails are impacted below the rotator cuff, and the suture tied in a figure-of-eight manner (Fig. 5-17); this helps to prevent proximal nail migration. Before tying the suture, the fracture reduction is evaluated.

Once the figure-of-eight is secured, range of shoulder motion and fixation stability are assessed to carefully guide

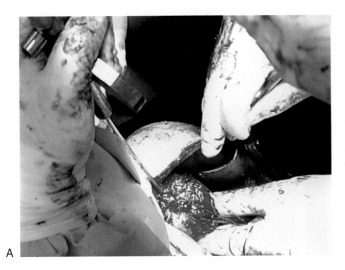

A

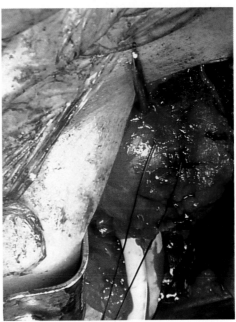

B

FIGURE 5-14. Insertion of the first Ender nail. The arm is extended with the fracture held reduced while the Ender nail is placed posterior in the proximal fragment (**A** and **B**).

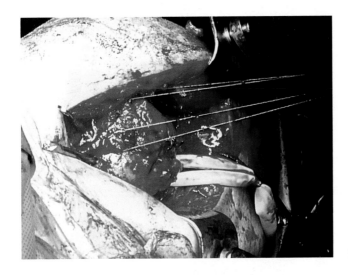

FIGURE 5-15. Placement of the second Ender nail.

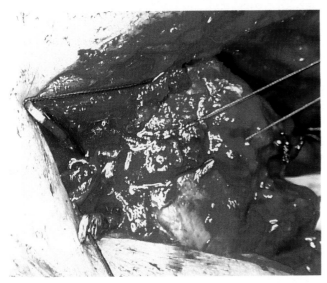

FIGURE 5-16. Before completely burying the nails, the previously placed suture is placed through the eyelets of the nails, passing deep to the rotator cuff between the two nails.

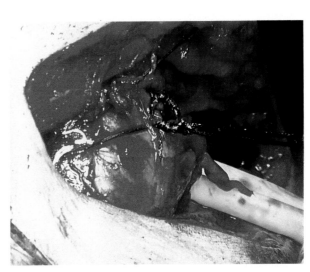

FIGURE 5-17. The nails are impacted below the rotator cuff, and the suture tied in a figure-of-eight manner.

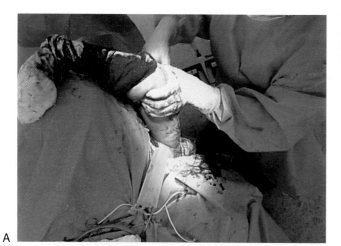

A

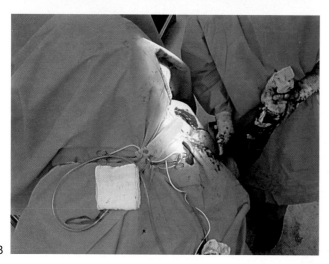

B

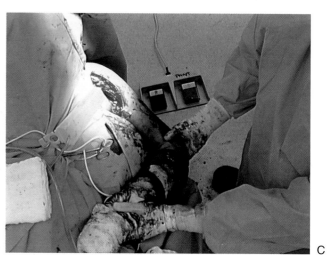

C

FIGURE 5-18. Once the figure-of-eight is secured, range of shoulder motion and fixation stability are assessed to carefully guide the postoperative rehabilitation without stressing the repair (**A** to **C**).

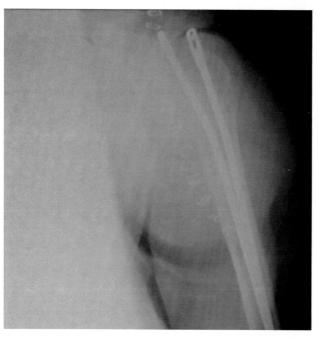

A

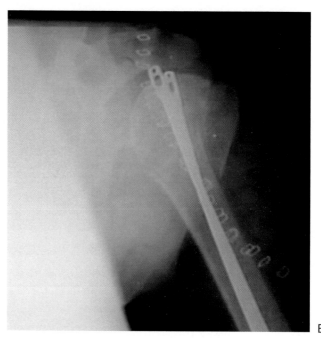

B

FIGURE 5-19. Intraoperative anteroposterior view of the shoulder with the humerus in internal rotation **(A)**, external rotation **(B)**, and axillary **(C)**. *(continued)*

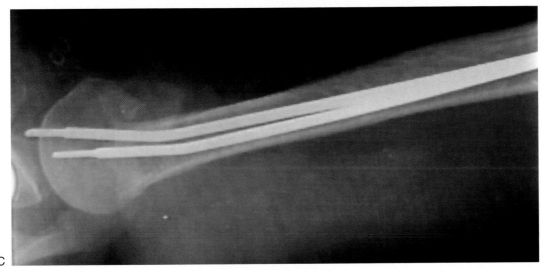

C

FIGURE 5-19. *(continued).*

the postoperative rehabilitation without stressing the repair (Fig. 5-18). ▣ The rotator cuff incisions and deltopectoral interval are closed, usually over suction drainage. A sterile dressing is applied and the upper extremity is placed in a sling.

It is very important to obtain a complete set of radiographs in the operating room (Fig. 5-19). This includes an AP view of the shoulder with the humerus in internal rotation (on the chest) and maximum external rotation as defined by the intraoperative assessment. An axillary view is also obtained.

POSTOPERATIVE PROTOCOL

On the first postoperative day, the patient is started on a rehabilitation program that consists of active range of motion of the elbow, wrist, and hand and passive range of motion of the shoulder. External rotation is limited based on the intraoperative evaluation. This is important to avoid any excess stress on the fracture repair that may compromise healing. Internal rotation is allowed to the chest. These exercises are continued for the first 6 to 8 weeks. Radiographs are obtained approximately 2 weeks following surgery to confirm the fracture position. Additional radiographs are obtained at 6 to 8 weeks following surgery. If fracture healing is sufficient, the sling is discontinued and an active range-of-motion program is begun. The patient is encouraged to use the involved upper extremity for activities of daily living. Passive range of motion is continued with gentle stretching to increase the overall range. At 8 weeks following surgery, isometric deltoid and internal and external rotator strengthening exercises are begun. Vigorous strengthening exercises are not begun until active forward elevation of at least 90 degrees is obtained. Our experience has shown that patients can expect continued recovery during the first year following surgery, although most recovery occurs during the first 6 months.

SUGGESTED READINGS

Bigliani LU. Fractures of the humerus. In: Rockwood CA, Matsen FA III, eds. *The shoulder.* Philadelphia: WB Saunders, 1990: 278–334.

Cuomo F, Flatow EL, Maday MG, et al. Open reduction and internal fixation of two- and three-part displaced surgical neck fractures of the proximal humerus. *J Shoulder Elbow Surg* 1992; 1: 287–295.

Hawkins RJ, Angelo RL. Displaced proximal humeral fractures: selecting treatment, avoiding pitfalls. *Orthop Clin North Am* 1987; 18: 421–431.

Hawkins RJ, Bell RH, Gurr K. The three-part fracture of the proximal part of the humerus: operative treatment. *J Bone Joint Surg Am* 1986; 68A: 1410–1414.

Hawkins RJ, Kiefer GN. Internal fixation techniques for proximal humeral fractures. *Clin Orthop* 1987; 223: 77–85.

Kristiansen B, Christensen SW. Plate fixation of proximal humeral fractures. *Acta Orthop Scand* 1986; 57: 320–323.

Lentz W, Meuser P. The treatment of fractures of the proximal humerus. *Arch Orthop Trauma Surg* 1980; 96: 283–285.

Moda SK, Chadha NS, Sangwan SS, et al. Open reduction and fixation of proximal humeral fractures and fracture-dislocation. *J Bone Joint Surg Br* 1990; 72B: 1050–1052.

Mouradian WH. Displaced proximal humeral fractures: seven years' experience with a modified Zickel supracondylar device. *Clin Orthop* 1986; 212: 209–218.

Neer CS II. Displaced proximal humeral fractures: part I. Classification and evaluation. *J Bone Joint Surg Am* 1970; 52A: 1077–1089.

Neer CS II. Displaced proximal humeral fractures: part II. Treatment of three-part and four-part displacement. *J Bone Joint Surg Am* 1970; 52A: 1090–1103.

Norris TR. Fractures of the proximal humerus and dislocations of the shoulder. In: Browner, BD, Jupiter JB, Levine AM, et al., eds. *Skeletal trauma.* Philadelphia: WB Saunders, 1992: 1201–1290.

Paavolainen P, Bjorkenheim JM, Slatis P, et al. Operative treatment of severe humeral fractures. *Acta Orthop Scand* 54: 374–379.

Pankovich AM. Update 1987—flexible intramedullary nailing of long bone fractures: a review. *J Orthop Trauma* 1987; 1(1): 78–95.

Sturzenegger M, Fornaro E, Jakob RP. Results of surgical treatment of multifragmented fractures of the humeral head. *Arch Orthop Trauma Surg* 1982; 100: 249–259.

Weseley MS, Barenfeld PA, Eisenstein AL. Rush pin intramedullary fixation for fractures of the proximal humerus. *J Trauma* 1977; 17(1): 29–37.

CHAPTER 6

HEMIARTHROPLASTY OF THE PROXIMAL HUMERUS

KENNETH J. KOVAL
JOSEPH D. ZUCKERMAN

The treatment of complex proximal humeral fractures presents a challenge to orthopaedic surgeons. First, these fractures are "osteoporotic" fractures that by definition represent metaphyseal fractures that occur primarily in women older than the age of 50. This results in compromised bone quality, which limits the potential to achieve secure internal fixation. Second, the muscular attachments of the proximal humerus and the associated deforming forces make it difficult to obtain and maintain an acceptable closed reduction. Third, the radiographic evaluation of the fractures can also be challenging because of the displacement patterns and the overlapping bony structures. Fourth, fractures that result in displacement of the articular segment and the tuberosities are at significant risk for the development of osteonecrosis. Therefore, hemiarthroplasty has become an important treatment option for complex proximal humerus fractures in the elderly. This chapter illustrates hemiarthroplasty of the proximal humerus.

ANATOMY

The proximal humerus consists of the humeral head, the tuberosities, and the humeral shaft (see Fig. 5-1). The anatomic neck is the junction between the humeral head and the tuberosities. The surgical neck lies between the tuberosities and the shaft. The rotator cuff is composed of four muscular divisions: (a) the subscapularis, which inserts on the lesser tuberosity and acts as an internal rotator of the glenohumeral joint; (b) the supraspinatus tendon, which inserts on the greater tuberosity and acts to depress the humeral head into the glenoid during elevation of the arm; (c) the teres minor, and (d) infraspinatus muscles, which are the external rotators of the shoulder and also insert on the greater tuberosity (Fig. 6-1). The biceps tendon, which lies in the anteriorly directed bicipital groove, provides a useful anatomic landmark for judging rotational deformity of the humeral head during operative management (see Fig. 3-2).

CLASSIFICATION

The Neer classification is the most widely used system in clinical practice (see Fig. 5-3). This system is based on the anatomic relationship of the four major anatomic segments:

the humeral head, greater tuberosity, lesser tuberosity, and the proximal humeral shaft beginning at the level of the surgical neck. Fracture types are based on the presence of displacement of one or more of the four segments. For a segment to be considered displaced, it must be either greater than 1 cm displaced or angulated more than 45 degrees from its anatomic position.

Displaced fractures include two-part, three-part, and four-part fractures. A two-part fracture is characterized by displacement of one of the four segments, with the remaining three segments either not fractured or not fulfilling the criteria for displacement. Four types of two-part fractures can be encountered (greater tuberosity, lesser tuberosity, anatomic neck, and surgical neck). A three-part fracture is characterized by displacement of two of the segments from the remaining two nondisplaced segments. Two types of three-part fracture patterns are encountered. The more common pattern is characterized by displacement of the greater tuberosity and the shaft from the lesser tuberosity, which remains with the articular segment. The much less commonly encountered pattern is characterized by displacement of the lesser tuberosity and shaft from the greater tuberosity, which remains with the articular segment. A four-part fracture is characterized by displacement of all four segments.

Neer also categorized fracture-dislocations, which are displaced proximal humeral fractures associated with either anterior or posterior dislocation of the humeral head. Six types of fracture-dislocation patterns can occur. In addition, Neer described articular surface fractures: impression fractures and head-splitting fractures. Impression fractures of the articular surface most often occur in association with chronic dislocations. Head-splitting fractures are usually associated with other displaced fractures of the proximal humerus in which the disruption or "splitting" of the articular surface is the most significant component.

INDICATIONS

Indications for prosthetic replacement following acute proximal humeral fractures include (a) four-part fractures and fracture-dislocations, (b) three-part fractures and fracture-dislocations in elderly patients with osteopenic bone, (c) head-splitting fractures, (d) anatomic neck fractures that

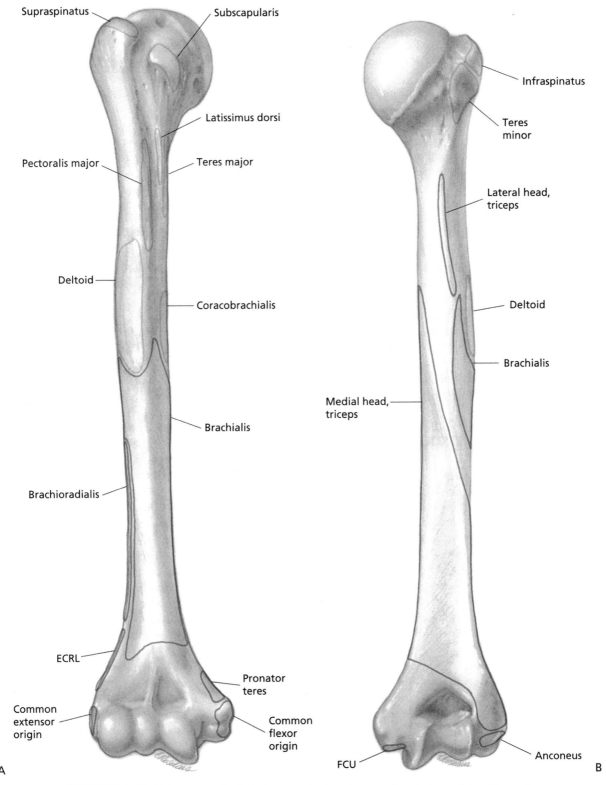

FIGURE 6-1. Right humerus. **A:** Anterior aspect, showing muscle origins and insertions. **B:** Posterior aspect, showing muscle origins *(red)* and insertions *(blue)*. (From Botte MJ. Muscle anatomy. In: Doyle JR, Botte MJ, eds. *Surgical anatomy of the hand and upper extremity.* Philadelphia: Lippincott Williams & Wilkins, 2003:92–184, with permission.)

cannot be adequately reduced and internally fixed, and (e) chronic anterior or posterior humeral head dislocations with impression fractures that involve more than 40% of the articular surface.

PREOPERATIVE PLANNING

A shoulder trauma series consists of anteroposterior (AP) and lateral views of the shoulder obtained in the plane of the scapula and an axillary view (Fig. 6-2). The scapular AP view offers a general overview of the fracture and is usually eval-

uated first. The scapular lateral assists in delineating the position of the humeral head relative to the glenoid and is particularly useful in showing dislocations or posteriorly displaced fragments. The axillary view also permits assessment of the glenohumeral relationship.

Before proceeding to hemiarthroplasty, it is important to perform preoperative templating to determine the approximate humeral and head size. Using templates, magnified to account for radiographic magnification, a stem of appropriate size is chosen. For cemented insertion, adequate space must be maintained around the stem to accommodate the cement mantle (usually 2 mm).

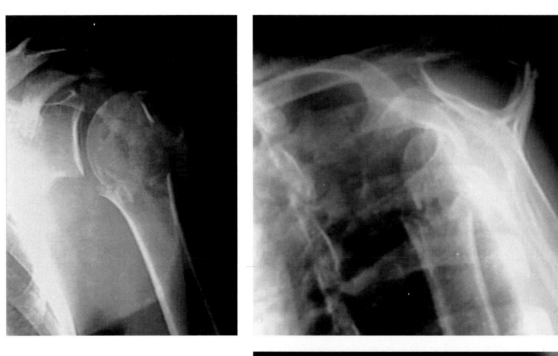

A

B

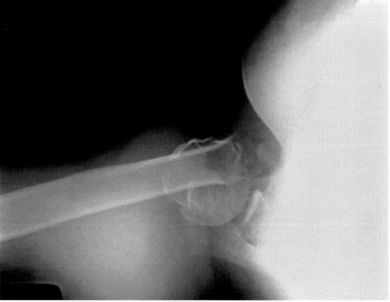

FIGURE 6-2. Anteroposterior **(A)**, Y view **(B)**, and axillary **(C)** revealing a displaced proximal humerus fracture.

C

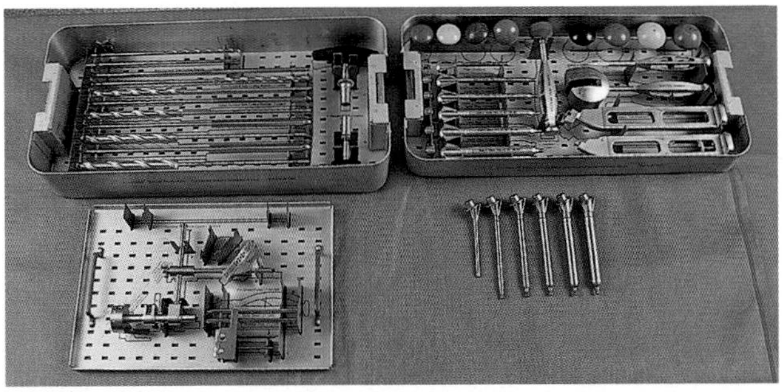

FIGURE 6-3. The equipment needed for hemiarthroplasty of the shoulder. Hemiarthroplasty set for humerus: reamer set *(top left tray)*, accessory instruments *(bottom left tray)*, trials *(top right tray)*, trials *(bottom right)*.

EQUIPMENT

Equipment is shown in Figure 6-3.

PATIENT POSITIONING

The patient is placed on the operating table in a supine position. The head of the operating table is elevated approximately 30 degrees in a modified beach chair position (Fig. 6-4). A small bolster is placed behind the involved shoulder. The patient is moved off to the side of the table so that the upper extremity can be placed into maximum extension without obstruction by the operating table. The patient is secured to the operating table to minimize any changes in position intraoperatively. The entire upper extremity is prepped and draped to allow full mobility during the procedure.

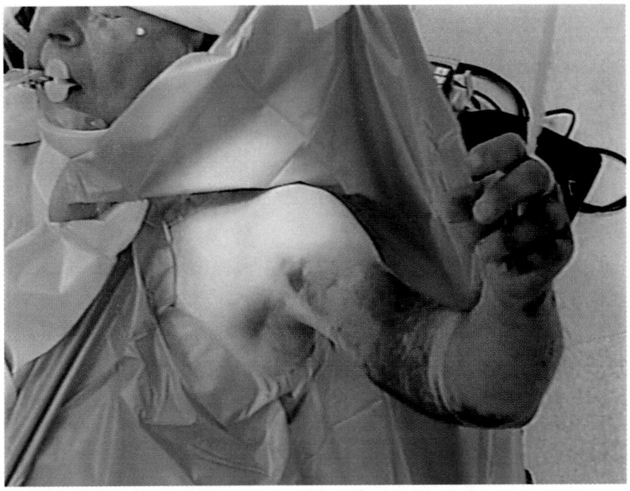

FIGURE 6-4. The patient is placed on the operating table in a supine position. The head of the operating table is elevated approximately 30 degrees in a modified beach chair position.

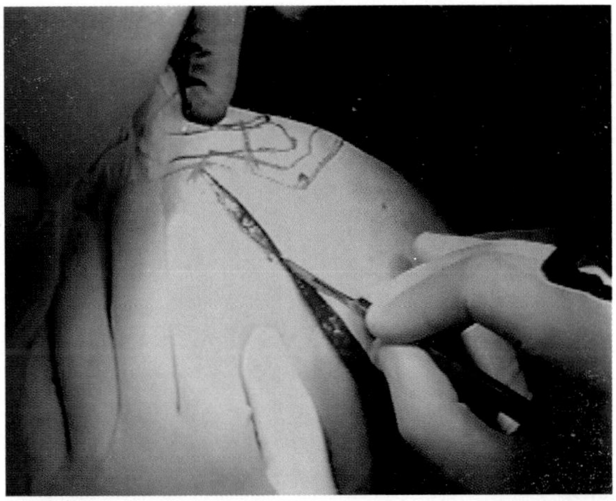

FIGURE 6-5. A straight deltopectoral incision is used that begins just lateral to the tip of the coracoid process and extends distally and laterally to the insertion of the deltoid.

APPROACH

A straight deltopectoral incision is used that begins just lateral to the tip of the coracoid process and extends distally and laterally to the insertion of the deltoid (Fig. 6-5). The subcutaneous tissues are divided and medial and lateral flaps elevated to expose the deeper muscular layers. The deltopectoral interval is identified by localization of the cephalic vein (Fig. 6-6). The cephalic vein is usually retracted laterally with the deltoid muscle. In some instances, the cephalic vein is more easily retracted medially with the pectoralis major. In either case, care should be taken to preserve the cephalic vein throughout the procedure.

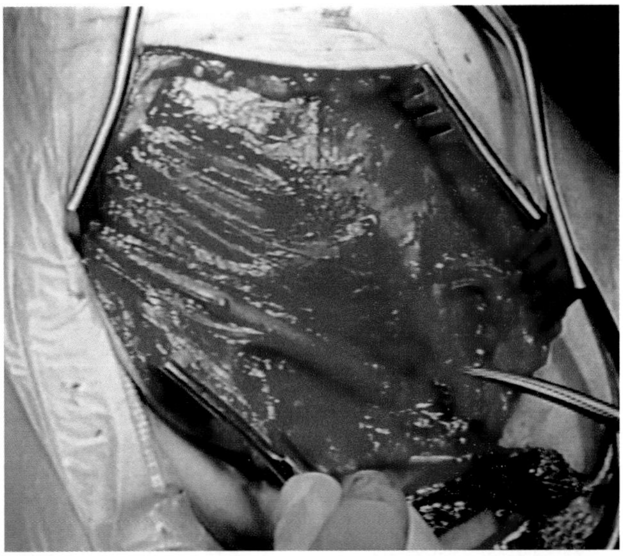

FIGURE 6-6. The deltopectoral interval is identified by localization of the cephalic vein.

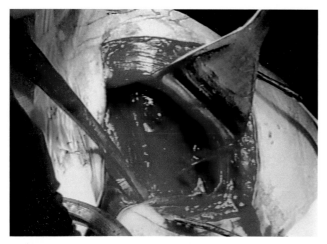

FIGURE 6-7. Retraction of the conjoined tendon and the pectoralis major medially and the deltoid laterally.

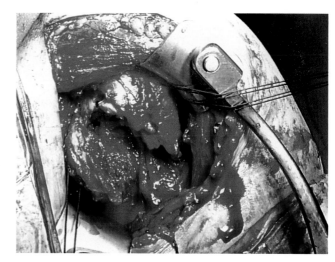

FIGURE 6-9. Each tuberosity is tagged with a heavy suture for easier mobilization.

The subdeltoid space is mobilized as is the pectoralis major. The conjoined tendon muscles are identified and the clavipectoral fascia is divided at the medial edge of the conjoined tendon muscles. The conjoined tendon muscles and the pectoralis major are retracted medially and the deltoid is retracted laterally (Fig. 6-7). This can be most easily accomplished with the use of a self-retraining type retractor. By evacuating the fracture hematoma, the deeper structures can be visualized.

PROCEDURE

The biceps tendon is identified and tagged with a suture (Fig. 6-8). ◼ The biceps tendon provides an orientation to the greater and lesser tuberosities. The lesser tuberosity is

located medial to the biceps tendon and the greater tuberosity is located superiorly and laterally. Each tuberosity is tagged with a heavy suture for easier mobilization (Fig. 6-9). ◼ These sutures are placed at the tendon insertion site because this is generally the most secure area. **Placement of the sutures through the tuberosity itself can result in fragmentation.** The lesser tuberosity is mobilized and retracted medially while the greater tuberosity is retracted laterally and superiorly. This allows visualization of the articular segment. In four-part fractures this segment is generally devoid of soft tissue attachments and is easily removed (Fig. 6-10). ◼

With the articular segment removed and the tuberosities retracted, the glenoid articular surface is inspected (Fig. 6-11). It is visualized to confirm the absence of preexisting degenerative changes or injury to the glenoid. At this point the

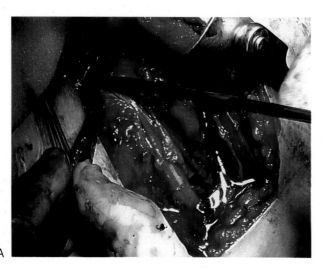

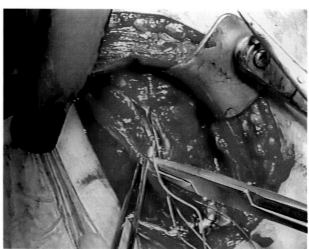

A   B

FIGURE 6-8. The biceps tendon is identified **(A)** and tagged with a suture **(B)**.

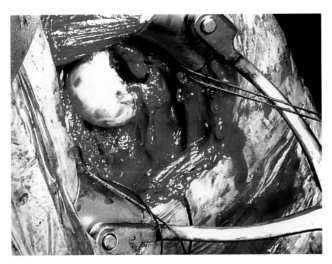

FIGURE 6-10. Visualization and removal of the articular segment.

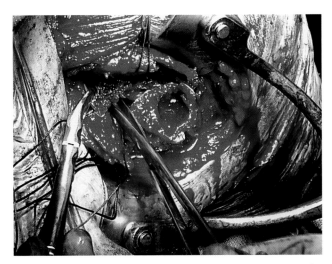

FIGURE 6-12. The humerus is placed in extension to expose the proximal portion of the humeral shaft.

humerus is placed in extension to expose the proximal portion of the humeral shaft (Fig. 6-12). A series of intramedullary reamers are used to prepare the canal (Fig. 6-13). ◼ Reaming is continued until there is cortical contact. At this point a trial component of appropriate size is inserted (Fig. 6-14). ◼ Because of proximal bone loss secondary to fracture, it is necessary to place the prosthesis in a "proud" position. However, it is usually difficult to maintain the prosthesis in this position and to control rotation during trial reductions. To overcome this problem, a surgical sponge is wrapped around the prosthesis. This fills the canal and maintains the prosthesis in proper position. The desired position of retroversion is 20 to 35 degrees. This can be modified if there is a preexisting chronic dislocation or fracture-dislocation. The position of retroversion is confirmed by comparing the position of the prosthesis with the transepicondylar axis. In addition, the position of the lateral or anterior flange of the prosthesis in relation to

the adjacent humeral cortex is marked and used to confirm proper position during cementing. The choice of head size is based upon the size of the removed humeral head regardless of whether modular or nonmodular systems are used (Fig. 6-15). With the implant in place the trial reduction is then performed.

After the humeral head is reduced onto the glenoid, the greater and lesser tuberosities are pulled into position. The biceps tendon is allowed to fall between the tuberosities. Traction on the tuberosity sutures not only maintains the tuberosities in position but also provides a more realistic assessment of stability. Assessment of posterior, inferior, and anterior stability is assessed by translating the humeral head as follows: up to 50 % of posterior translation of the humeral head on the glenoid is acceptable as is 50% of inferior translation. ◼ However, anterior translation should not exceed 25%. If these parameters are exceeded, the position of the component is reevaluated to confirm

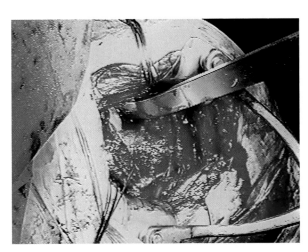

FIGURE 6-11. Inspection of the glenoid articular surface.

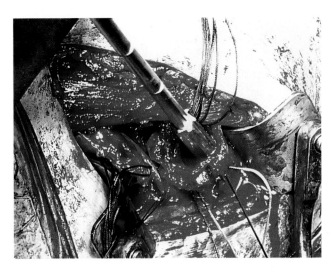

FIGURE 6-13. Reaming of the humeral canal.

FIGURE 6-14. At this point a trial component of appropriate size is inserted. Because of proximal bone loss secondary to fracture, it is necessary to place the prosthesis in a proud position **(A).** To help maintain the prosthesis in this position and to control rotation during trial reduction, a surgical sponge is wrapped around the prosthesis **(B).**

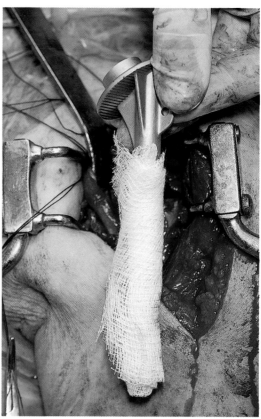

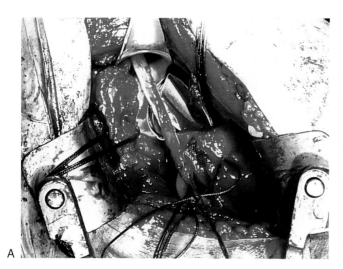

A

B

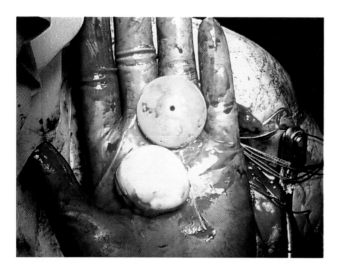

FIGURE 6-15. Comparison of the removed humeral head to the trial humeral head.

that it has not subsided or rotated in the canal. If soft tissue laxity is excessive, a larger humeral head is used. Conversely, if soft tissue tension is excessive a smaller humeral head may be necessary. In either situation, repeat assessment of stability is required to confirm that the proper components and position have been chosen. When the proper position and component size is confirmed, the trial prosthesis is removed.

At this point two drill holes are placed through the humeral cortex into the medullary canal (Fig. 6-16). These holes are placed approximately 1.5 to 2 cm distal to the level of the surgical neck component in proximity to the bicipital groove. Two heavy nonabsorbable sutures are passed through one drill hole into the medullary canal and then exit through the second drill hole (Fig. 6-17). These sutures are used for tuberosity fixation. The medullary canal is irrigated copiously and any loose cancellous bone removed. The use of the cement restrictor is based on personal preference. We generally use a cement restrictor to enhance cement distribution (Fig. 6-18). However, we avoid any formal pressurization of the cement to decrease the possibility of humeral shaft fracture. The canal is packed with a sponge to obtain adequate drying before cementing.

The cement is mixed and poured into a vented 50-cc Toomey-type syringe approximately 1 minute after mixing (Fig. 6-19). This syringe is vented by preparing a hole at the 20- to 30-cc level. This allows air to escape during insertion of the plunger so that a continuous column of cement is formed. The cement is then injected into the canal (Fig. 6-20). ◼ During insertion of the prosthesis it is essential to maintain the prosthesis in the proper proud position as well as in the desired position of retroversion. ◼ The prosthesis is held in position until the cement is completely set to avoid inadvertent subsidence or rotation into an unacceptable position (Fig. 6-21). When the cementing

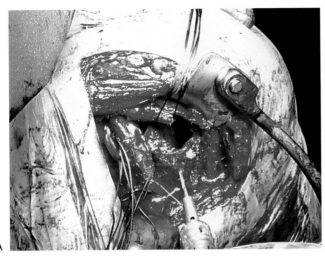
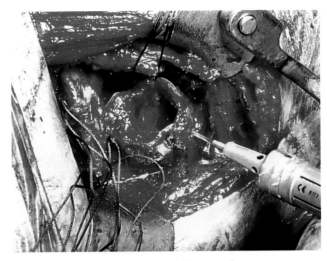

FIGURE 6-16. Two drill holes are placed through the humeral cortex into the medullary canal. These holes are placed approximately 1.5 to 2 cm distal to the level of the surgical neck component in proximity to the bicipital groove.

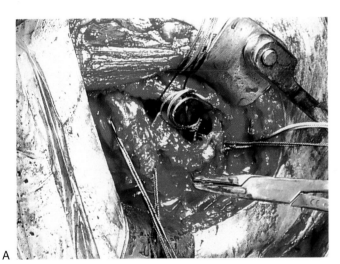
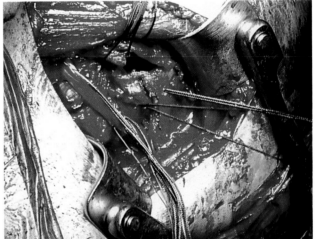

FIGURE 6-17. Two heavy nonabsorbable sutures are passed through one drill hole into the medullary canal and then exit through the second drill hole.

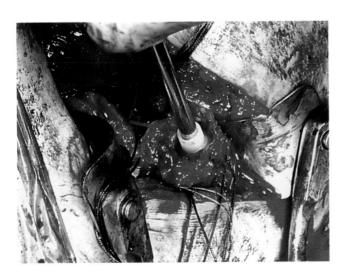

FIGURE 6-18. Placement of the cement restrictor.

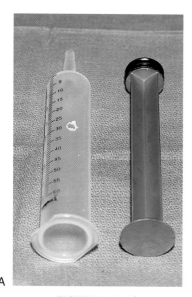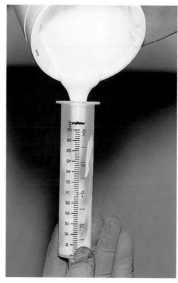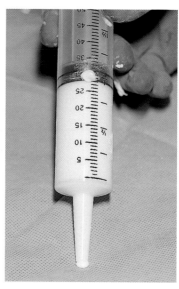

A   B,C

FIGURE 6-19. The cement is mixed and poured into a vented 50-cc Toomey-type syringe **(A)** approximately 1 minute after mixing **(B).** This syringe is vented by preparing a hole at the 20- to 30-cc level **(C).**

is complete, the position is confirmed. When a modular component is being used, the modular head is impacted into place making certain that the taper is dry and free of any debris.

Fixation of the tuberosities to the prosthesis and the shaft is a critical component of this procedure. Proper reattachment and secure fixation enhances the probability of a successful outcome in terms of range of motion and overall function. However, careful attention must be given to the technical aspects of this portion of the procedure. Heavy nonabsorbable sutures are used. These sutures are generally passed through the rotator cuff tendons just at their insertion into the tuberosities. The biceps tendon is allowed to fall between the tuberosities and is incorporated into the fixation. This results in a "functional tenodesis" but probably preserves at least a portion of its humeral head depressor function.

The principles of tuberosity fixation include (a) placement of longitudinal sutures to bring the tuberosities into a position below the prosthetic articular surface and into contact with the humeral shaft and (b) transverse suture fixation, which brings the tuberosities into contact with each other and maintains the tuberosities in the distal position obtained with the longitudinal sutures. This is analogous to the principles of fixation of the greater trochanter in hip surgery in which longitudinal wires are used to advance the trochanter distally into the proper position and transverse wires are used to secure the trochanter in this position.

At this point, the two longitudinal sutures, which have already been passed through the humeral cortex, are used

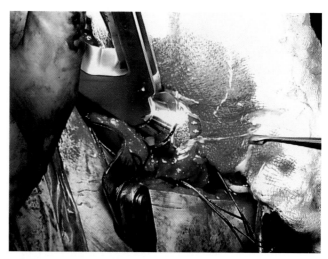

FIGURE 6-20. Injection of the cement into the humeral canal.

FIGURE 6-21. The prosthesis is held in position until the cement is completely set to avoid inadvertent subsidence or rotation into an unacceptable position.

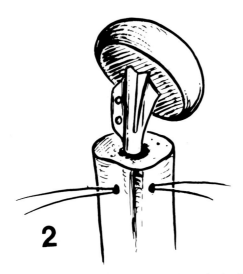

FIGURE 6-22. Placement of the sutures through the humeral shaft to reattach the tuberosities. (See text for details.)

(Fig. 6-22). The first longitudinal suture is placed in a figure-of-eight fashion through the supraspinatus tendon as it inserts into the greater tuberosity and then through the upper portion of the subscapularis tendon as it inserts into the lesser tuberosity. The second longitudinal suture is passed in similar fashion through the infraspinatus tendon as it inserts into the greater tuberosity and through the lower portion of the subscapularis tendon as it inserts into the lesser tuberosity. These sutures are passed but not tied.

The first transverse suture is then passed through the supraspinatus tendon as it inserts into the greater tuberosity, through the upper hole of the lateral keel of the prosthesis and then through the upper portion of the subscapularis tendon as it inserts into the lesser tuberosity (Fig. 6-23). The second transverse suture is passed, in similar fashion, through the infraspinatus tendon, through the lower hole in the lateral keel, and through the lower portion of the subscapularis tendon. The suture tying sequence is important.

The first longitudinal suture should be tied first. This will advance the tuberosities distally below the articular surface of the prosthesis and into contact with the humeral cortex, which is essential to obtain bone-to-bone healing. The second longitudinal suture is then tied for enhanced fixation. When the tuberosities are confirmed to be in proper position the superior transverse suture is tied followed by the inferior transverse suture. Transverse fixation brings the tuberosities into contact with each other and maintains the position obtained by the longitudinal sutures. Tuberosity reattachment is performed with the arm in approximately 20 degrees of abduction, neutral flexion, and 10- to 20-degrees external rotation. When the tuberosity fixation is completed, the stability of the fixation is carefully assessed. Range of motion in forward elevation, external rotation, internal rotation, and abduction is performed to determine the specific limits of motion that will be allowed in the postoperative rehabilitation program. In addition, we have found that bone grafting the tuberosities can enhance the healing potential. Cancellous bone from the humeral head is placed in the area of contact between the shaft and the tuberosities and between the tuberosities.

Closure includes repair of the rotator interval with nonabsorbable sutures. This is performed with the humerus in external rotation to decrease the possibility that rotator interval closure will restrict rotation. A closed suction drain is usually placed deep to the deltopectoral interval and brought out through the skin distally and laterally. The deltopectoral interval is repaired with absorbable suture as is the subcutaneous tissue. This skin closure is performed with either sutures or staples. A sterile dressing is applied and the upper extremity is placed in a sling.

It is very important to obtain a complete set of radiographs in the operating room (Fig. 6-24). This includes an AP view of the shoulder with the humerus in internal rotation (on the chest) and maximum external rotation as defined by the intraoperative assessment. An axillary view is also obtained. These radiographs provide excellent visualization of the position of the prosthesis and the position of the tuberosities.

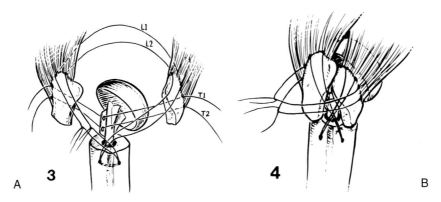

FIGURE 6-23. Schematic showing method of reattachment of tuberosities (**A** and **B**). (See text for details.)

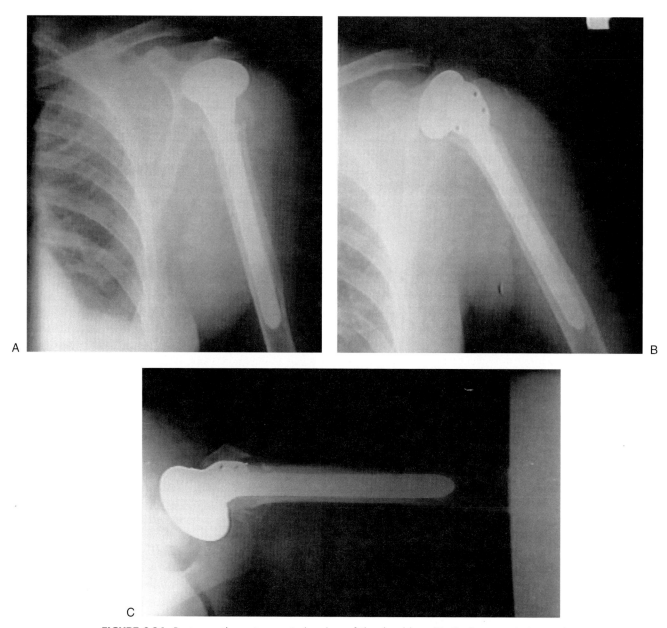

FIGURE 6-24. Postoperative anteroposterior view of the shoulder with the humerus in internal rotation **(A)**, external rotation **(B)**, and an axillary view **(C)**.

POSTOPERATIVE PROTOCOL

On the first postoperative day, the patient is started on a rehabilitation program that consists of active range of motion of the elbow, wrist, and hand and passive range of motion of the shoulder. External rotation is limited based on the intraoperative evaluation. This is important to avoid any excess stress on the tuberosity repair that could compromise healing. Internal rotation is allowed to the chest. These exercises are continued for the first 6 to 8 weeks. Radiographs are obtained approximately 2 weeks following surgery to confirm the position of the tuberosities. Additional radiographs are obtained at 6 to 8 weeks following surgery to assess the degree of tuberosity healing. If tuberosity healing is sufficient, the sling is discontinued and an active range-of-motion program is begun. The patient is encouraged to use the involved upper extremity for activities of daily living. Passive range of motion is continued with gentle stretching to increase the overall range. At 8 weeks following surgery, isometric deltoid and internal and external rotator strengthening exercises are begun. Vigorous strengthening exercises are not begun until active forward elevation of at least 90 degrees is obtained. Our experience has shown that patients can expect continued recovery during the first year following surgery, although most recovery will occur during the first 6 months.

SUGGESTED READINGS

Bigliani LU. Fractures of the shoulder. Part I: fractures of the proximal humerus. In: Rockwood CA, Green DP, Bucholz RW, eds. *Fracture in adults,* 3rd ed. Philadelphia: JB Lippincott, 1991: 871–882.

Cofield RH. Comminuted fractures of the proximal humerus. *Clin Orthop* 1988; 230: 49–57.

Fischer RA, Nicholson GP, McIlveen SJ, et al. Primary humeral head replacement for severely displaced proximal humerus fractures. *Orthop Trans* 1992; 16: 799.

Hawkins RJ, Angelo RL. Displaced proximal humeral fractures: selecting treatment, avoiding pitfalls. *Orthop Clin North Am* 1987; 18: 421–431.

Kay SP, Amstutz HC. Shoulder hemiarthroplasty at UCLA. *Clin Orthop* 1988; 228: 42–48.

Moeckel BH, Dines DM, Warren RF, et al. Modular hemiarthroplasty for fractures of the proximal part of the humerus. *J Bone Joint Surg Am* 1992; 74A: 884–889.

Neer CS II. Displaced proximal humeral fractures: part I. Classification and evaluation. *J Bone Joint Surg Am* 1970; 52A: 1077–1089.

Neer CS II. Displaced proximal humeral fractures: part II. Treatment of three-part and four-part displacement. *J Bone Joint Surg Am* 1970; 52A: 1090–1103.

Tanner MW, Cofield RH. Prosthetic arthroplasty for fractures and fracture-dislocations of the proximal humerus. *Clin Orthop* 1983; 179: 116–128.

CHAPTER 7

ORIF: HUMERAL SHAFT FRACTURE

KENNETH J. KOVAL

Humeral shaft fractures are common injuries, accounting for approximately 3% of all fractures; most can be managed nonoperatively with anticipated good to excellent results. Appropriate nonoperative and operative treatment of humeral shaft fractures, however, requires an understanding of humeral anatomy, the fracture pattern, and the patient's activity level and expectations. This chapter illustrates open treatment of a humeral shaft fracture using plate and screws.

ANATOMY

The shaft of the humerus extends proximally from the upper border of the pectoralis major insertion to the supracondylar ridge distally (Fig. 7-1). The proximal aspect of the humeral shaft is cylindrical on cross section; distally its anterior-posterior diameter narrows. The anterior border of the humerus extends from the anterior aspect of the greater tuberosity to the coronoid fossa. Its medial border extends from the lesser tuberosity to the medial supracondylar ridge. Its lateral border extends from the posterior aspect of the greater tuberosity to the lateral supracondylar ridge. The deltoid muscle inserts onto the deltoid tuberosity, located on the anterolateral surface of the proximal humeral shaft. The radial sulcus contains the radial nerve and the profunda artery. The posterior surface is the origin for the triceps and contains the spiral groove (see Fig. 6-1).

The medial and lateral intermuscular septa divide the arm into anterior and posterior compartments. The biceps brachii, coracobrachialis, and brachialis muscles are contained in the anterior compartment. The brachial artery and vein and the median, musculocutaneous, and ulnar nerves course along the medial border of the biceps. The posterior compartment contains the triceps brachii muscle and radial nerve. The lateral intermuscular septum is perforated by the radial nerve and the deep branch of the brachial artery. The medial intermuscular septum is perforated by the ulnar nerve, the superior ulnar collateral artery, and a posterior branch of the inferior ulnar collateral artery (Fig. 7-2).

CLASSIFICATION

There is no universally accepted classification system for humeral shaft fractures. Classically, humeral shaft fractures have been classified on the basis of various factors that in-

fluence treatment such as (a) fracture location (proximal, middle, or distal third of the humeral shaft), and in addition whether the fracture is proximal to the pectoralis major insertion, distal to the pectoralis major insertion but proximal to the deltoid insertion, or distal to the deltoid insertion; (b) direction and character of fracture line (transverse, oblique, spiral, segmental, or comminuted); (c) associated soft tissue injury (open or closed fracture); (d) associated periarticular injury involving the glenohumeral or elbow joints; (e) associated nerve injury involving either the radial, median, or ulnar nerves; (f) associated vascular injury involving either the brachial artery or vein; and (g) intrinsic condition of the bone (normal or pathologic)

The AO/ASIF classification of humeral shaft fractures is based on fracture comminution (Fig. 7-3). Type A are simple (noncomminuted), type B have a butterfly fragment, and type C are comminuted. These fracture types are further divided according to fracture pattern. This alphanumeric classification is used by both the AO and Orthopaedic Trauma Associations.

INDICATIONS

The indications for operative management of humeral shaft fractures are as follows:

1. Open humerus fracture. Open fractures require emergent débridement; fracture stabilization after soft tissue and osseous débridement has been reported to reduce the incidence of infection.
2. The humeral shaft fracture with associated vascular injury is best managed with internal or external fixation, either before or after vascular repair depending on the viability of the limb. When vascular repair is needed, nonoperative management is contraindicated because motion at the fracture may jeopardize the repair.
3. Ipsilateral fracture of the humerus and radius and ulna (floating elbow). Nonoperative treatment of patients with a floating elbow has resulted in high rates of nonunion, malunion, and elbow stiffness. Improved results have been reported after internal fixation of the humerus and radius and ulna fractures followed by early range of elbow motion.
4. Segmental humerus fracture. Nonoperative treatment of a segmental humerus fracture is associated with increased risk of nonunion at one or both fracture sites.

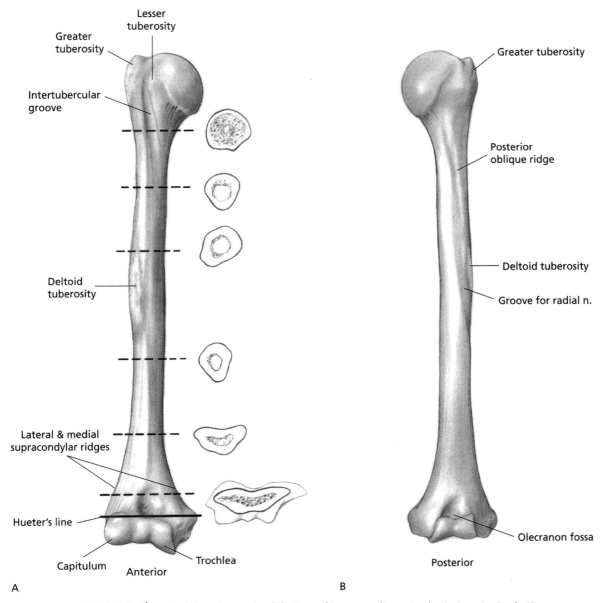

FIGURE 7-1. Anterior **(A)** and posterior **(B)** views of humerus. (From Doyle JR. Arm. In: Doyle JR, Botte MJ, eds. *Surgical anatomy of the hand and upper extremity.* Philadelphia: Lippincott Williams & Wilkins, 2003:315–364, with permission.)

5. Pathologic fractures should be internally stabilized to maximize patient comfort and to increase upper extremity function.
6. Operative stabilization of bilateral humerus fractures significantly improves patient self-care.
7. The polytrauma patient is often unable to remain in the semisitting position necessary to effect fracture reduction by nonoperative measures. Operative stabilization of the humerus is necessary to maximize the recovery and rehabilitation potential of the polytrauma patient.

8. Neurologic loss after penetrating injury is an indication for nerve exploration.
9. Fractures that cannot be maintained in acceptable alignment should be operatively stabilized. In the humeral shaft, one can accept up to 3 cm shortening, 20 degrees of anterior or posterior angulation, and 30 degrees of varus. Significant varus can, however, be cosmetically disfiguring in these individuals; and in those patients fewer degrees of varus may be accepted. Humeral shaft fractures in obese patients and women with large pendulous breasts are at increased risk of

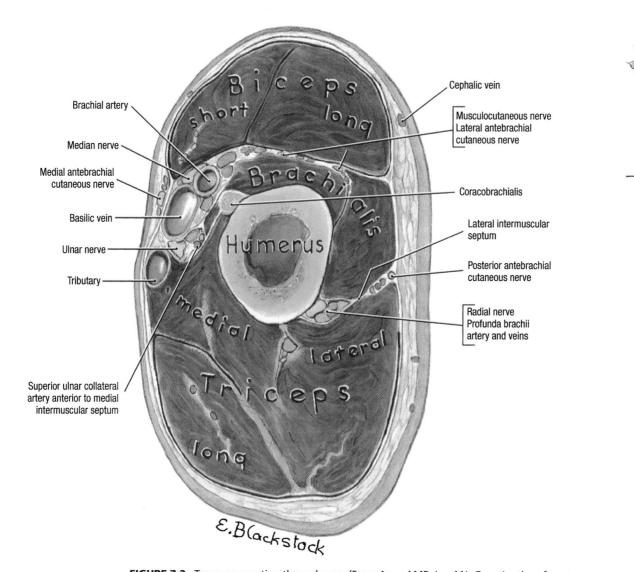

FIGURE 7-2. Transverse section through arm. (From Agur AMR, Lee MJ. *Grant's atlas of anatomy,* 10th ed. Philadelphia: Lippincott Williams & Wilkins, 1999, with permission.)

varus angulation. Malrotation is well tolerated secondary to compensatory shoulder motion.

10. Fractures of the humeral shaft associated with intraarticular fracture extension require operative treatment.

PREOPERATIVE PLANNING

A standard radiographic examination of the humerus consists of (Fig. 7-4) anteroposterior (AP) and lateral radiographs, taken at 90 degrees to one another. The shoulder and elbow joint should be included in each view.

The radiographs are obtained by moving the patient rather than simply rotating the injured extremity. In highly comminuted or displaced fractures, traction radiographs may allow better fracture definition. Comparison radiographs of the contralateral humerus are helpful for preoperative planning. Tomograms and computed tomography are rarely indicated. In pathologic fractures, additional studies (technetium bone scan, computed tomography, and magnetic resonance imaging) may be necessary to delineate the extent of disease before fracture treatment.

The exact nature of the fracture, with identification of all

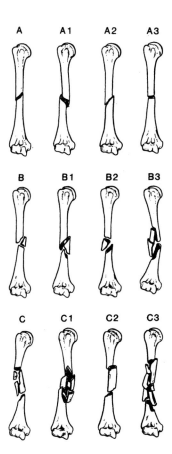

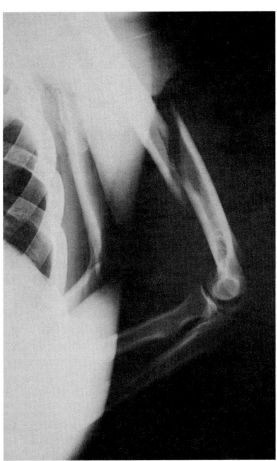

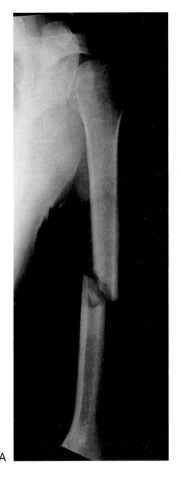

FIGURE 7-3. The AO/ASIF classification of humeral shaft fractures. (From Zuckerman JD, Koval KJ. Fractures of the shaft of the humerus. In Rockwood CA Jr, Green DP, Bucholz RW, et al., eds. *Rockwood and Green's fractures in adults,* 4th ed, vol 1. Philadelphia: Lippincott Williams & Wilkins, 1996:1025–1053, with permission.)

FIGURE 7-4. Anteroposterior **(A)** and lateral **(B)** radiographs demonstrating a displaced humeral shaft fracture.

A

B

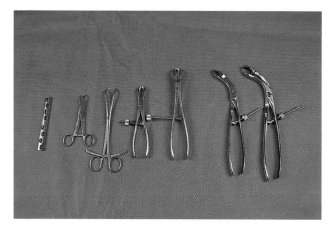

FIGURE 7-5. The instruments necessary for open reduction and internal fixation of the humeral shaft: 4.5-mm broad dynamic companion peak (DCP), small and large reduction clamps (2), Verbrugge clamps (4).

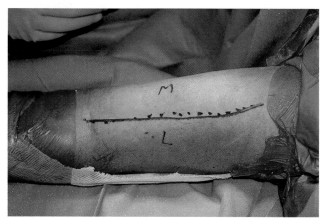

FIGURE 7-7. The incision is made along the lateral border of the biceps, ending just proximal to the elbow flexion crease.

major fracture fragments, should be determined before one attempts definitive surgical intervention. Identification of the individual fragments is often facilitated with traction radiographs. Radiographs of the opposite, uninjured extremity serve as a template for preoperative planning; the individual fracture fragments, chosen implant, and surgical tactic can be drawn on the intact humeral template. This requires the surgeon to understand the "personality of the fracture" and to mentally prepare for the operative procedure.

EQUIPMENT

The basic instruments necessary for open reduction and internal fixation of a humeral shaft fracture plate and screws include the following (Fig. 7-5):

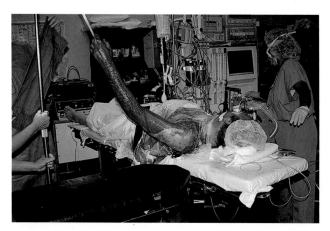

FIGURE 7-6. Supine patient positioning with use of a hand table. The upper extremity is elevated for the surgical prep.

- Small fragment plate and screws
- Large fragment plate and screws
- Large and small reduction clamps
- Verbrugge clamps

PATIENT POSITIONING AND FRACTURE REDUCTION

The patient is positioned supine with the arm placed either on a hand table or arm board (Fig. 7-6).

APPROACH

For most fractures, I prefer an anterolateral approach to the humerus. An incision is made along the lateral border of the biceps, ending just proximal to the elbow flexion crease (Fig. 7-7). The lateral border of the biceps is identified, ◙ and the muscle retracted medially (Fig. 7-8). ◙ The interval between the brachialis and brachioradialis is identified proximal to the elbow and the two muscles separated (Fig. 7-9). ◙ The brachioradialis is retracted laterally, and the brachialis and biceps muscles are retracted medially. The radial nerve lies between the brachialis and brachioradialis and must be identified (Fig. 7-10). ◙ The radial nerve is traced proximally through the lateral intermuscular septum and protected throughout the remainder of the procedure (Fig. 7-11). The periosteum is incised longitudinally at the lateral border of the brachialis muscle, and the humerus is dissected subperiosteally (Fig. 7-12). ◙ The anterolateral approach can be extended proximally into an anterior approach to the shoulder and distally to an anterior approach to the elbow.

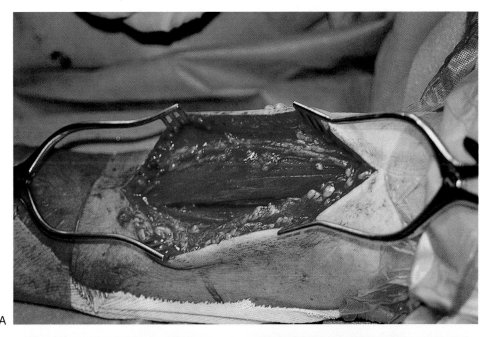

A

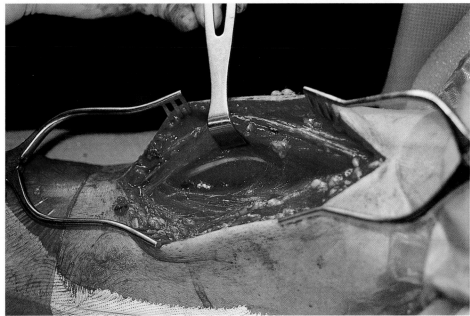

B

FIGURE 7-8. The lateral border of the biceps is identified, and the muscles are retracted medially (**A** and **B**).

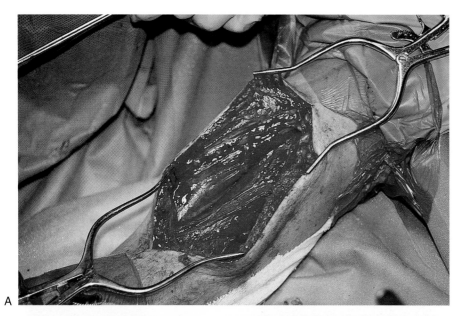

A

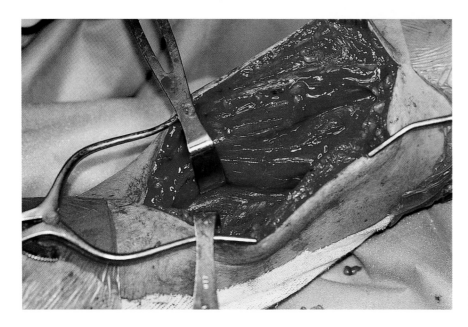

B

FIGURE 7-9. The interval between the brachialis and brachioradialis is identified proximal to the elbow and the two muscles are separated (**A** and **B**).

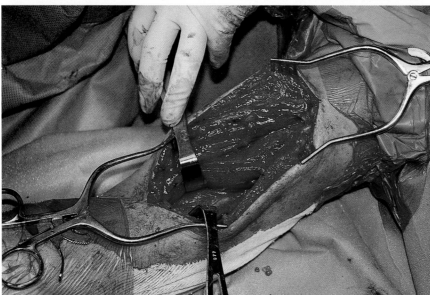

FIGURE 7-10. Identification of the radial nerve between the brachialis and brachioradialis muscles.

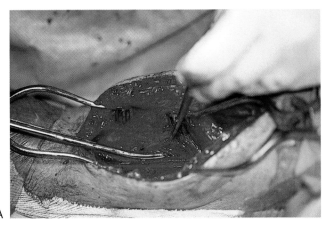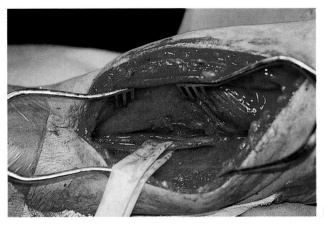

FIGURE 7-11. A: The radial nerve is traced proximally through the lateral intermuscular septum. **B:** A Penrose drain is then placed around the nerve.

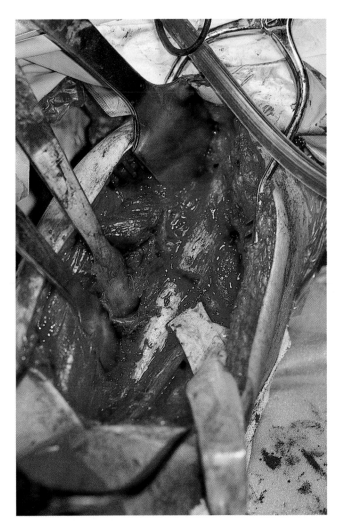

FIGURE 7-12. Exposure of the humeral shaft fracture.

PROCEDURE

The fracture is exposed, evaluated, débrided of hematoma, and anatomically reduced. Minimal soft tissue stripping should be performed; butterfly fragments must not be devitalized. Provisional stabilization is performed using reduction clamps or Kirschner wires. A 4.5-mm broad dynamic compression plate is usually selected for midshaft fractures (Fig. 7-13). ■ In smaller patients, a 4.5-mm narrow dynamic compression plate may be used. If the fracture pattern permits, the plate should be applied in compression. ■ Lag screws should be inserted through the plate whenever possible (Fig. 7-14). Eight to ten cortices fixation proximal and distal to the fracture should be obtained (Fig. 7-15). ■ Fixation stability must be assessed before closure (Fig. 7-16). ■ The need to bone graft is determined by the

amount of comminution and soft tissue stripping. In general, one should have a low threshold for cancellous bone grafting of these fractures when plates and screws are used. One should obtain final radiographs once surgery is completed (Fig. 7-17).

POSTOPERATIVE PROTOCOL

A closely monitored rehabilitation program is essential to achieve maximal functional outcome after both operative and nonoperative humeral shaft fracture management. Early and vigorous postsurgical range of motion exercises of the hand and wrist should be strongly urged. As shoulder pain diminishes, range of motion exercises for the shoulder and elbow are initiated. As union progresses, supervised exercises

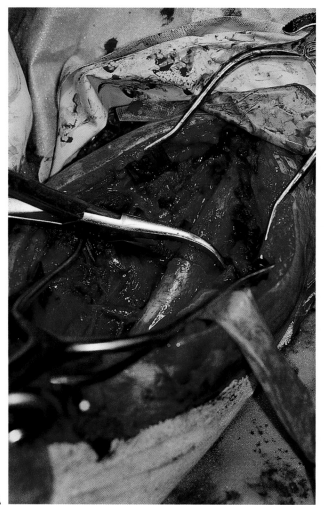
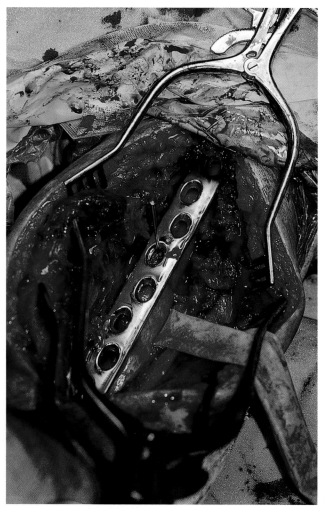

A   B

FIGURE 7-13. Provisional fracture fixation first using a reduction clamp **(A)** and then a broad compression plate **(B** and **C)**. *(continued)*

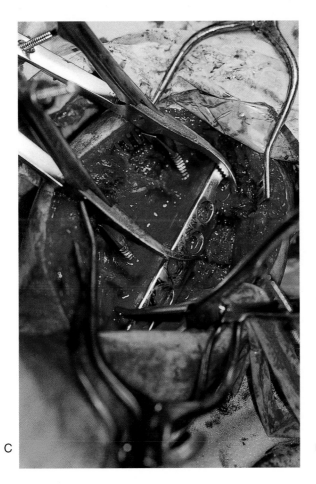

C

FIGURE 7-13. *(Continued)*

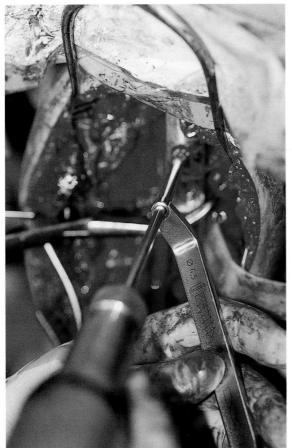

A

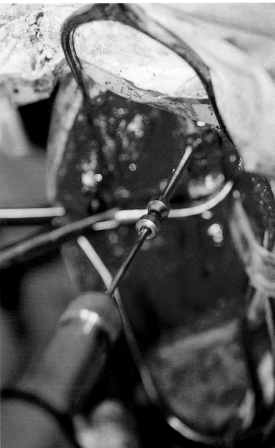

B

FIGURE 7-14. Placement of a lag screw through the plate (**A** to **C**). *(continued)*

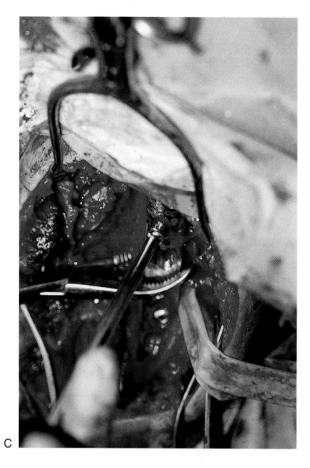

C

FIGURE 7-14. *(Continued)*

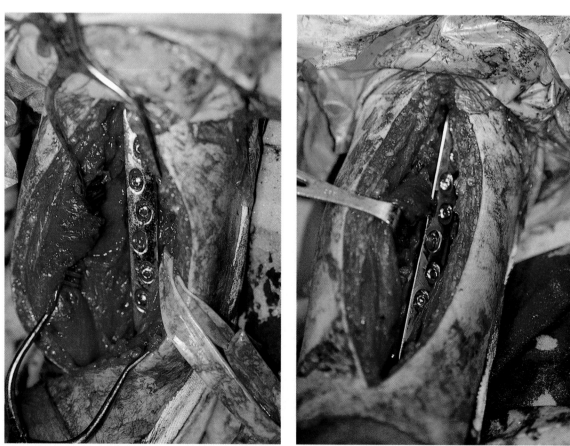

A

B

FIGURE 7-15. Final fracture fixation with insertion of the remaining screws (**A** and **B**).

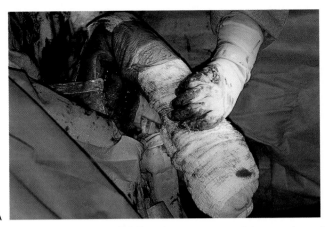
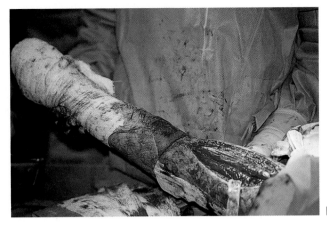

A   B

FIGURE 7-16. Placement of the arm through a range of motion to assess fracture stability.

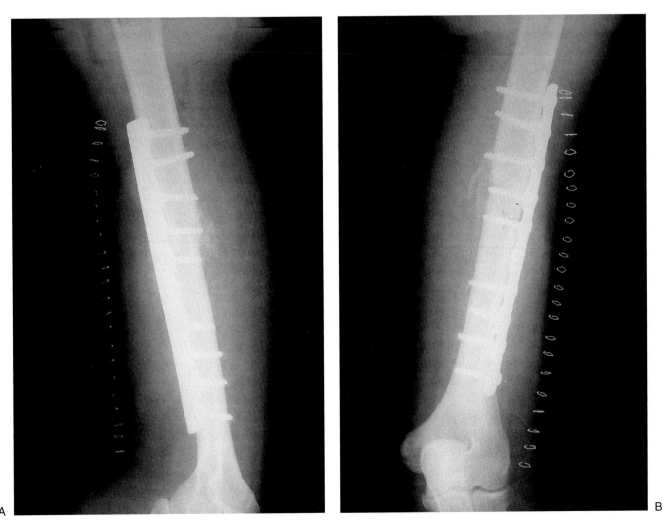

A   B

FIGURE 7-17. Final intraoperative radiographs (**A** and **B**).

to recover upper extremity strength are started. Caution is warranted relative to management of the elbow; it should not be passively stretched. Myositis ossificans, which has been reported around the elbow following humeral shaft fracture, can be prevented by exclusively using active range of motion exercises.

SUGGESTED READINGS

Bell MJ, Beauchamp CG, Kellam JK, et al. The results of plating humeral shaft fractures in patients with multiple injuries: the Sunnybrook experience. *J Bone Joint Surg Br* 1985; 67B: 293–296.

Dabezies EJ, Banta CJ II, Murphy CP et al. Plate fixation of the humeral shaft for acute fractures, with and without radial nerve injuries. *J Orthop Trauma* 1992; 6: 10–13.

Foster RJ, Dixon GL, Bach AW, et al. Internal fixation of fractures and non-unions of the humeral shaft: indications and results in a multi-center study. *J Bone Joint Surg Am* 1985; 67A: 857–864.

Heim D, Herkert F, Hess P, et al. Surgical treatment of humeral shaft fractures—the Basel experience. *J Trauma* 1993; 35: 226–232.

Klenerman L. Fractures of the shaft of the humerus. *J Bone Joint Surg Br* 1966; 48B: 105–111.

Mast JW, Spiegel PG, Harvey JP. Fractures of the humeral shaft. A retrospective study of 240 adult fractures. *Clin Orthop* 1975; 112: 254–262.

Ruedi T, Schweiberer L. Scapula, clavicle and humerus. In: Muller ME, Allgower M, Schneider R, et al., eds. *Manual of internal fixation: techniques recommended by the AO-ASIF Group.* New York: Springer-Verlag, 1991: 442–445.

Schatzker J. Fractures of the humerus. In: Schatzker J, Tile M. *The rationale of operative fracture care.* New York: Springer-Verlag, 1987: 61–70.

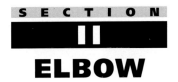

SECTION II

ELBOW

CHAPTER 8

TENNIS ELBOW RELEASE

BRIAN S. DELAY
ANDREW S. ROKITO

Tennis elbow is an eponym given to the painful condition isolated to the lateral aspect of the elbow. The condition arises from tendon degeneration at the origin of the wrist extensor tendons, most commonly the extensor carpi radialis brevis (ECRB), from the lateral humeral epicondyle. The tendon degeneration is due to repetitive wrist extension against resistance and is commonly seen in recreational tennis and racquetball players. The microscopic pathology noted in the degenerated tendon is termed angiofibroblastic hyperplasia, which demonstrates chronic tendinosis rather than acute inflammation.

Tennis elbow presents with tenderness located over the lateral humeral epicondyle, and pain is exacerbated by resisted wrist extension. Nonoperative treatment consisting of cryotherapy, activity modification, nonsteroidal antiinflammatory medication, rehabilitation, and cortisone injections generally relieves the symptoms in 85% to 90% of patients. A supervised physical therapy program focusing on flexibility, strengthening, and endurance of the wrist extensor mechanism is continued for at least 6 months before surgical consideration. Severe, persistent pain that fails to respond to conservative treatment is the main indication for surgery.

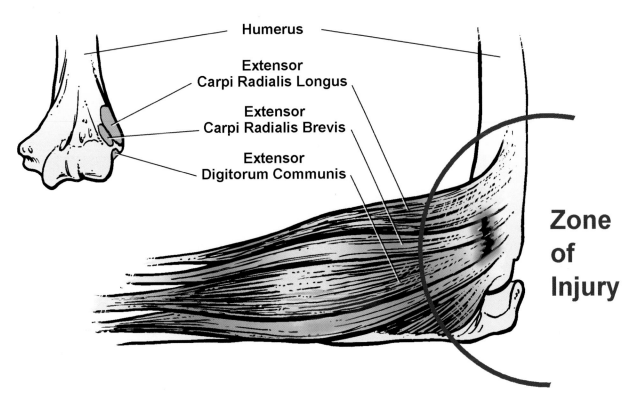

FIGURE 8-1. The forearm extensor muscles originate as a conjoined tendon from the lateral epicondyle of the elbow. Note critical zone of injury.

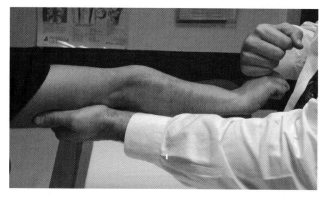

FIGURE 8-2. Physical examination reveals pain with the provocative maneuver of resisted wrist extension with the elbow in full extension.

ANATOMY

The forearm extensor musculature is comprised of the extensor carpi radialis longus, ECRB, extensor digitorum communis, extensor digiti minimi, and extensor carpi ulnaris. The extensor muscles originate as a conjoined tendon from the lateral epicondyle of the elbow. Lateral epicondylitis is most commonly localized to the ECRB tendon, and the involved area is located approximately 2 cm distal and anterior to the center of the lateral epicondyle (Fig. 8-1). It is less commonly seen in the anteromedial edge of the extensor communis or the undersurface of the extensor carpi radialis longus and is rarely present in the extensor carpi ulnaris.

CLASSIFICATION, DIAGNOSIS, AND INDICATIONS

Lateral epicondylitis is characterized by pain and tenderness over the origin of the conjoined tendon from the lateral epi-

condyle of the elbow. This condition characteristically occurs in the dominant extremity of the middle-aged athlete (e.g., tennis player) and is caused by the repetitive, eccentric contractile activity of the extensor muscles of the forearm. This overuse activity leads to ECRB degeneration and angiofibroblastic hyperplasia as described by Nirschl. Angiofibroblastic hyperplasia refers to the microscopic invasion of fibroblasts and vascular granulation-like tissue that occurs in the degenerative tendon. Three pathologic categories of lateral epicondylitis have been described by Nirschl: category I, acute, reversible inflammation without angiofibroblastic invasion; category II, partial angiofibroblastic invasion; category III, extensive angiofibroblastic invasion with or without partial or complete rupture of the tendon. The degree of angiofibroblastic hyperplasia correlates with the severity of symptoms.

Patients with lateral epicondylitis present with localized pain, which may radiate into the forearm. Physical examination reveals tenderness just distal and anterior to the lateral epicondyle, corresponding to the location of the ECRB. The provocative maneuver of resisted wrist extension with the elbow in full extension reproduces the pain (Fig. 8-2). Passive range of motion is typically preserved, and the involved extremity's neurovascular status is unaffected.

Radiographs of the elbow may demonstrate soft tissue calcifications or a lateral epicondyle exostosis in up to 25% of patients. Magnetic resonance imaging may show increased signal in the musculotendinous structures at the lateral elbow but is seldom needed to make the diagnosis.

The differential diagnosis includes posterior interosseus nerve (PIN) or radial tunnel syndrome and radiocapitellar articular disease. PIN syndrome is caused by entrapment of the posterior interosseous branch of the radial nerve at the arcade of Frohse. This condition is characterized by diffuse anterolateral elbow pain. Typically, pain is exacerbated by resisted forearm supination, and maximal tenderness to pal-

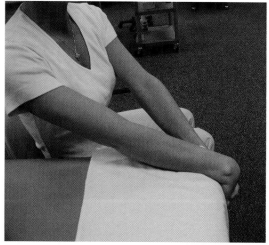
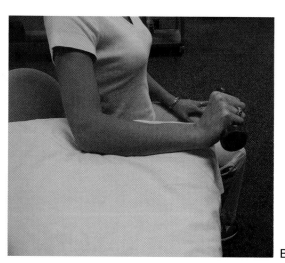

FIGURE 8-3. Rehabilitative program consists of wrist extensor stretching **(A)** and progressive strengthening **(B)** exercises.

pation is approximately 5 cm distal to the lateral epicondyle over the proximal radial forearm musculature. Patients with radiocapitellar articular disease often present with clicking and pain with elbow motion. Radiographs reveal degenerative changes at the radiocapitellar articulation. <u>A thorough history and physical examination is the key to diagnosing lateral epicondylitis.</u>

In general, nonsurgical treatment is the mainstay of treatment for lateral epicondylitis. Nonsurgical treatment consists of three phases: (a) pain relief, (b) rehabilitation, and (c) return to sports and work. The initial phase of pain relief consists of activity modification, and the use of ice, other local modalities, and antiinflammatory medication. Corticosteroid injections deep to the ECRB may be helpful during this phase by reducing pain and inflammation. **Incorrectly placed injections into the superficial tissues (resulting in subcutaneous atrophy) or into the tendon (resulting in irreversible structural changes) must be avoided.** After the initial discomfort of lateral epicondylitis has been relieved, a rehabilitation program consisting of wrist extensor stretching and progressive strengthening exercises may be started (Fig. 8-3). Concentric and eccentric resistive exercises are added as flexibility and strength improve. When exercises can be performed to fatigue without pain, the patient begins progressive exposure to sport or work-specific activities. A structured conditioning program for the elbow focusing on flexibility, strength, and endurance training eventually allows the patient's return to full activity in most cases.

Nonsurgical treatment is successful in 85% to 90% of patients. Up to 25% of patients may have a recurrence of symptoms that may respond to a similar nonsurgical therapeutic regimen. The primary indication for surgical treatment is persistent, severe pain at the epicondylar region that has failed a 3- to 6-month nonsurgical program.

SPECIAL EQUIPMENT/INSTRUMENTS

The basic instruments necessary for the surgical treatment of lateral epicondylitis include the following:

- No. 10 and no. 15 scalpel blades
- Self-retaining retractor
- Rongeur
- $^7/_{64}$-inch drill bit and power drill
- No. 1 absorbable suture

PATIENT POSITIONING

The patient should be placed supine with an arm board under the involved elbow. After administration of regional or general anesthesia, a tourniquet should be applied before standard prepping and draping. The elbow should be flexed

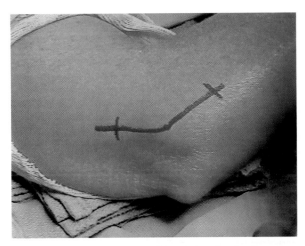

FIGURE 8-4. The curvilinear incision is longitudinally centered over the lateral epicondyle of the elbow.

to approximately 90 degrees with a rolled towel under the distal humerus.

INCISION

The surgical landmarks consist of the prominent lateral epicondyle and the lateral supracondylar ridge of the distal humerus. Palpating the forearm extensor mechanism attachment aids the identification the lateral epicondyle. A curvilinear incision centered over the lateral epicondyle is made (Fig. 8-4). The proximal limb of the incision should be centered over the supracondylar ridge of the distal humerus. Anterior and posterior subcutaneous flaps are raised to identify the origin of the conjoined tendon at the lateral epicondyle (Fig. 8-5). ◖◼◗

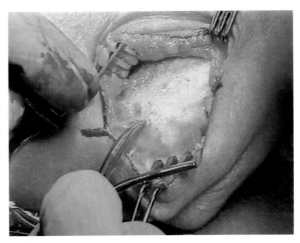

FIGURE 8-5. Thick subcutaneous flaps are developed anteriorly and posteriorly to allow identification of the origin of the conjoined tendon at the lateral epicondyle.

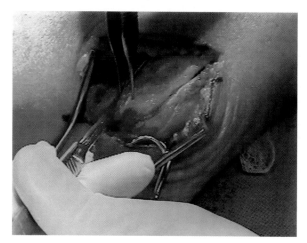

FIGURE 8-6. The anterior and posterior edges of the conjoined tendon are released from the lateral epicondyle.

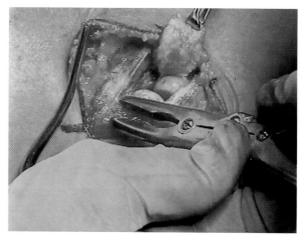

FIGURE 8-8. A rongeur is used to débride and decorticate the lateral epicondyle.

SURGICAL APPROACH AND PROCEDURE

After the origin of the conjoined tendon has been completely exposed, deep dissection begins by releasing the anterior and posterior edges of the conjoined tendon (Fig. 8-6). The extensor origin is then sharply elevated off the lateral epicondyle with the beveled edge of the no. 10 scalpel blade. Approximately a 2-cm wide area of tendon is elevated with the underlying capsule and taken distally (Fig. 8-7). Careful attention should be paid not to extend the release to the posterior aspect of the lateral epicondyle so as to avoid injury to the lateral ulnar collateral ligament. The joint is inspected for articular damage or loose bodies and irrigated. The entire lateral epicondyle can be visualized at this point. The rongeur is used to débride and gently decorticate the lateral epicondyle removing any prominent ridges of bone (Fig. 8-8). A scalpel blade is used to sharply débride the undersur-

face of the tendon aponeurosis (Fig. 8-9). The pathologic tissue is degenerative grayish-colored scar tissue (Fig. 8-10). If corticosteroid injections were given before surgery, the white granular residue may be noted during the débridement of the undersurface of the tendon. Both edges of elevated tendon should be débrided back to fresh healthy-appearing tissue. ▣

The reattachment site of the extensor origin is then prepared next. Two transosseous tunnels are made using the $^7/_{64}$-inch drill bit. Care is taken to preserve a 1-cm bone bridge between the tunnels. An additional central hole is made to enhance healing of the tendon to the epicondyle (Fig. 8-11). A heavy no. 1 absorbable suture is passed distally through the anterior tunnel and then through the tendon in a horizontal mattress fashion (Fig. 8-12). The suture is then passed proximally through the posterior tunnel and tied over the 1-cm bone bridge on the posterior aspect of the distal humerus (Fig. 8-13). The tendon edges are then reap-

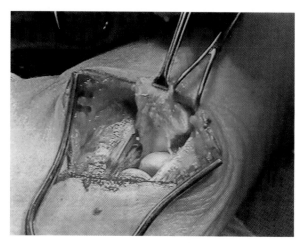

FIGURE 8-7. The conjoined tendon is elevated and taken distally with the elbow capsule. Note the degenerative scar tissue in the center of the undersurface of the tendon.

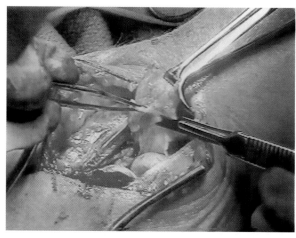

FIGURE 8-9. The degenerative scar tissue is sharply débrided off the undersurface of the extensor carpi radialis brevis tendon.

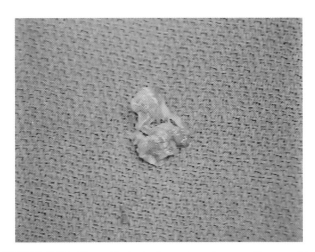

FIGURE 8-10. The pathologic tissue is a degenerative grayish-colored scar tissue.

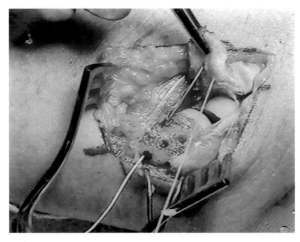

FIGURE 8-12. A suture is placed through the anterior bone tunnel and attached to the tendon in a horizontal mattress fashion.

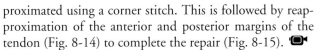

proximated using a corner stitch. This is followed by reapproximation of the anterior and posterior margins of the tendon (Fig. 8-14) to complete the repair (Fig. 8-15). ◼️

The wound is then irrigated and closed in layers. A long arm splint is placed with the elbow in 90 degrees of flexion, the forearm in neutral rotation, and the wrist free.

POSTOPERATIVE PROTOCOL

The splint and sutures are removed 1 to 2 weeks after surgery and passive range of motion exercises of the elbow, wrist, and hand are begun. Isometric exercises are begun at 3 to 4 weeks postoperatively (Fig. 8-16), and resistive wrist exercises are initiated at 6 weeks (Fig. 8-17). A progressive strengthening program ensues with return to full activity usually by 3 to 4 months (Fig. 8-3).

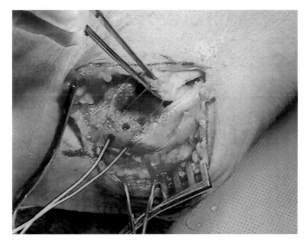

FIGURE 8-13. The extensor tendon is reattached to the decorticated lateral epicondyle by a heavy absorbable suture that is weaved through two transosseous tunnels and secured posteriorly over a 1-cm bone bridge.

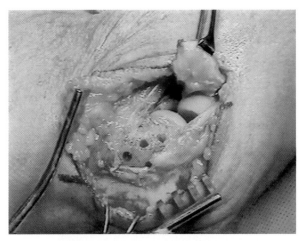

FIGURE 8-11. The lateral epicondyle is prepared by drilling two transosseus tunnels with a 1-cm bone bridge between them posteriorly. A central hole is drilled to aid tendon healing to the decorticated bone.

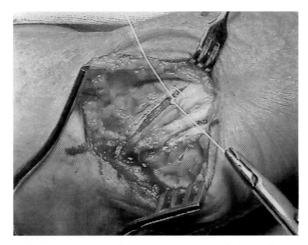

FIGURE 8-14. Closure of the anterior margin of the tendon is accomplished using a simple suture and burying the knots deep to the tendon.

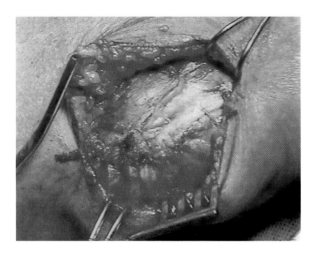

FIGURE 8-15. Final appearance of the lateral epicondyle region after the tendon repair has been completed.

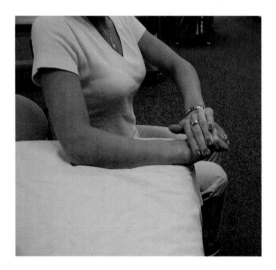

FIGURE 8-16. Postoperative rehabilitation begins with isometric exercises at 3 to 4 weeks.

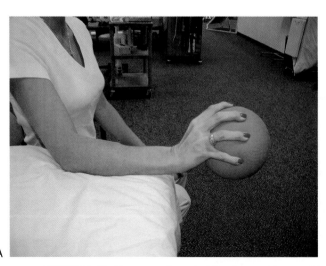

A

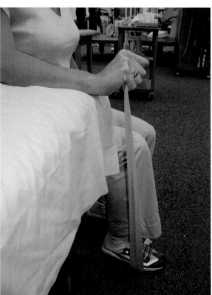

B

FIGURE 8-17. Postoperative rehabilitation continues with progressive resistive strengthening (**A** and **B**) starting at 6 weeks.

SUGGESTED READINGS

Binder AI, Hazleman BL. Lateral humeral epicondylitis: a study of natural history and the effect of conservative therapy. *Br J Rheumatology* 1983; 22: 73–76.

Ciccotti MG, Lombardo SJ. Lateral and medial epicondylitis of the elbow. In: Jobe FW, Pink MM, Glousman RE, et al., eds. *Operative techniques in upper extremity sports injuries.* St. Louis: Mosby-Year Book, 1996: 431–446.

Nirschl RP, Pettrone FA. Tennis elbow: the surgical treatment of lateral epicondylitis. *J Bone Joint Surg Am* 1979; 61A: 832–839.

Nirschl RP. Elbow tendinosis/tennis elbow. *Clin Sportsmed* 1992; 2: 851.

Price R, Sinclair H, Heinrich I, et al. Local injection treatment of tennis elbow: hydrocortisone, triamcinolone, and lignocaine compared. *Br J Rheumatol* 1991; 30: 39–44.

CHAPTER 9

ULNAR NERVE TRANSPOSITION

STEVEN M. GREEN

Compressive neuropathy of the ulnar nerve at the elbow is a very common disorder. It usually occurs as a consequence of fibrosis in the region of the medial epicondyle, which inhibits gliding of the nerve, and because the cubital tunnel narrows when the elbow is flexed. The typical symptoms include pain, paresthesia or numbness of the little and ring fingers, and weakness of pinch and grip. Relief can usually be obtained by restricting elbow flexion and avoiding pressure on the medial aspect of the elbow. If the symptoms cannot be controlled in this manner or if there is marked loss of sensibility or weakness, surgery is recommended. Many operative procedures have been described, which include neurolysis, epicondylectomy, and anterior transposition. This chapter describes the various potential sites of compression of the ulnar nerve at the elbow and the technique of submuscular anterior transposition.

ANATOMY

The eighth cervical and the first thoracic roots form the medial cord of the brachial plexus, which then divides into the ulnar nerve and the medial cutaneous nerves of the arm and forearm. In the midportion of the arm the ulnar nerve lies anterior to the medial head of the triceps and posterior to the medial intermuscular septum (Fig. 9-1). In 70% of extremities a medial musculofascial arcade, as described by Struthers, covers the nerve. This arcade is located approximately 8 cm proximal to the medial epicondyle and is composed of the deep fascia of the arm, superficial fibers of the triceps, and the internal brachial ligament arising from the coracobrachialis tendon. The nerve then passes into a fibroosseous groove that is bordered anteriorly by the medial epicondyle, posterior and laterally by the olecranon and ulnar humeral ligament, and medially by a fibroaponeurotic band. In this region numerous branches of the superior and inferior collateral and posterior ulnar recurrent arteries, as well as several veins, accompany the nerve. Also at this level, a small articular branch leaves the ulnar nerve to innervate the joint capsule. Occasionally, an anomalous muscle called the anconeus epitrochlearis is encountered covering the ulnar nerve. This muscle arises from the medial border of the olecranon and inserts onto the medial epicondyle.

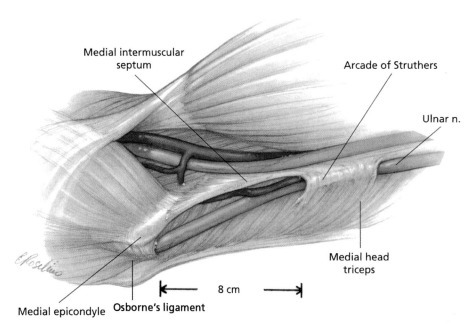

FIGURE 9-1. Anatomy of ulnar nerve and potential sites of compression. (From Doyle JR. Arm. In: Doyle JR, Botte MJ, eds. *Surgical anatomy of the hand and upper extremity*. Philadelphia: Lippincott Williams & Wilkins, 2003:389, with permission.)

After exiting the fibroosseous groove, the ulnar nerve travels between the humeral and ulnar heads of the flexor carpi ulnaris. Osborne described a fibrous band that begins at the fibroaponeurosis of the epicondylar groove and continues to the flexor carpi ulnaris. It is often very thick and is a common cause of ulnar nerve compression. (Synonyms for the ligament described by Osborne are the triangular ligament, the arcuate ligament, and humeral ulnar arch.) In this region the medial collateral ligament of the elbow lies posterior to the ulnar nerve. While lying within the muscle of the flexor carpi ulnaris, the ulnar nerve gives off motor branches to this wrist flexor. Traveling distally, the nerve pierces the flexor pronator fascia and then lies between the flexor digitorum superficialis (FDS) and the flexor digitorum profundus (FDP).

CLASSIFICATION

A popular method of recording the severity of ulnar nerve neuropathy was described by McGowan:

Grade 1—sensory changes only
Grade 2—weakness of the intrinsic muscles
Grade 3—complete intrinsic palsy

I find McGowan's classification inadequate, because there are more than three patterns of ulnar neuropathy. Therefore, I use the schema outlined in Table 9-1.

INDICATIONS

The characteristics of ulnar nerve compression at the elbow include local tenderness; alteration in the sensibility of the hypothenar eminence, the entire small finger, and the dorsal and ulnar palmar aspects of the ring finger; and weakness of the FDP of the ring and small fingers, the abductor digiti quinti, the interossei, and the adductor pollicis.

Nonoperative treatment is usually effective and involves reduction in activity, avoidance of external compression and elbow flexion, nonsteroidal antiinflammatory medications, and elbow pads and splints that inhibit elbow flexion.

In those cases in which symptoms persist or in which there is evidence of chronic sensory and/or major dysfunction, surgery is recommended. Because cervical radiculopathy, thoracic outlet syndrome, compression within Guyon's canal, and polyneuropathy can mimic ulnar nerve compression at the elbow, electrodiagnostic studies are often performed before surgery.

SPECIAL EQUIPMENT/INSTRUMENTS

- Hand table
- Calibrated tourniquet
- Bipolar coagulator
- Vessel loops or small Penrose drains
- Army/Navy retractors
- Power drill with 2-mm bit or 0.045-inch Kirschner wire

POSITIONING

The patient is placed supine on the operating table with the arm abducted 90 degrees and resting on a padded hand table (Fig. 9-2).

INCISION

Using a skin marker, an incision is planned on the medial aspect of the elbow region. The incision extends approximately 10 cm proximal to the medial epicondyle, passing 2 cm anterior to the epicondyle, and continuing 8 cm distally (Fig. 9-3).

TABLE 9-1. ALTERNATE[a] CLASSIFICATION OF ULNAR NERVE NEUROPATHY

Sensory	Motor
S-1: Episodic paresthesias	M-0: Normal motor power
S-2: Constant paresthesias	M-1-E: Weakness of FDP
S-3: Numbness as identified by abnormal 2-point discrimination or Semmes-Weinstein testing	M-1-I: Weakness of intrinsics
	M-2-E: Complete palsy of FDP
	M-2-I: Complete palsy of intrinsics

E, extrinsic muscle; FDP, flexor digitorum profundus; I, intrinsic muscle.
[a]Alternate to McGowan's.

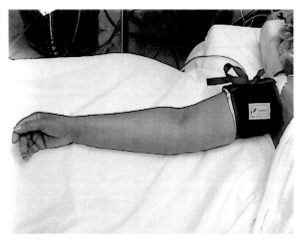

FIGURE 9-2. The patient's arm is abducted 90 degrees and rests on a padded hand table.

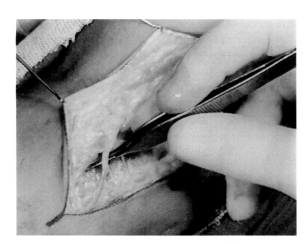

FIGURE 9-4. Medial cutaneous nerve of forearm.

SURGICAL PROCEDURE 📷

A well-padded pneumatic tourniquet is positioned as close to the axilla as possible. The upper extremity is then prepared and draped. The tourniquet is applied after exsanguination and the skin incision outlined with a marking pencil (Fig. 9-3). Subsequent to the skin incision, the dissection is continued through the adipose tissue with scissors. Numerous veins require coagulation or ligation. At this time, the medial cutaneous nerves should be identified and mobilized (Figs. 9-4 and 9-5). Colored vessel loops are placed around these nerves to both remind the surgeon of their presence and to aid in their gentle retraction (Fig. 9-6). Next, the ulnar nerve is located posterior to the medial intermuscular septum (Fig. 9-7), and the fascia is incised from the upper arm to the epicondyle (Figs. 9-8 and 9-9). Using Army/Navy retractors, the proximal subcutaneous tissue is retracted, and with blunt scissors the arcade of Struthers is released (Fig. 9-10). **If the arcade is not fully released, it may cause an iatrogenic compression of the ulnar nerve**

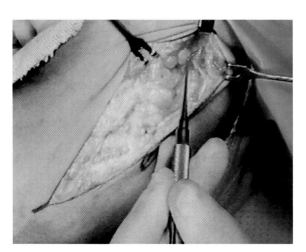

FIGURE 9-5. Medial cutaneous nerve of arm.

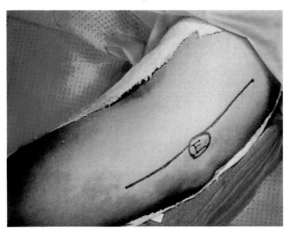

FIGURE 9-3. Incision marked. *E,* medial epicondyle.

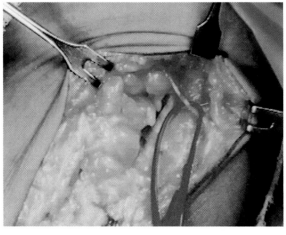

FIGURE 9-6. Vessel loop around medial cutaneous nerve of arm.

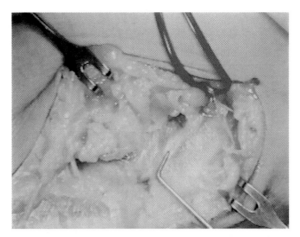

FIGURE 9-7. Probe at medial intermuscular septum.

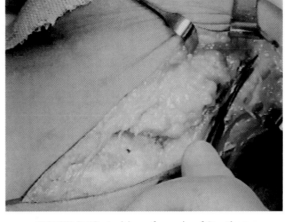

FIGURE 9-10. Incision of arcade of Struthers.

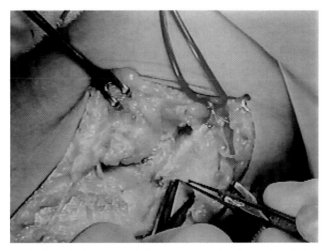

FIGURE 9-8. Exposure of ulnar nerve proximal to epicondyle.

subsequent to the anterior transposition. Next, the retro-condylar fascia is divided (Fig. 9-11), and exposure of the nerve is continued in a proximal-to-distal direction by dividing Osborne's ligament (Fig. 9-12) and separating the two heads of the flexor carpi ulnaris muscle (Fig. 9-13).

While protecting the ulnar nerve (Fig. 9-14), the intermuscular septum is fully exposed and then excised (Fig. 9-15). Many vessels are located near the attachment of the intermuscular septum to the medial epicondyle and these require coagulation. The nerve should be carefully dissected away from its bed with as much preservation as possible of any blood vessels that accompany the nerve; however, vessels can be coagulated to permit anterior transposition. During the neurolysis, the nerve is retracted gently with either vessel loops or small Penrose drains. **The small articular branches require division, but injury to the flexor carpi ulnaris motor branches should be avoided (Fig. 9-16); these are located distal to the epicondyle.** Subsequent to the neurolysis and with the elbow flexed, the nerve often subluxes anteriorly (Fig. 9-17). **The elbow should be placed**

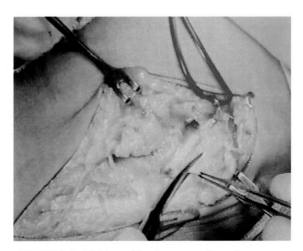

FIGURE 9-9. Division of fascia surrounding ulnar nerve.

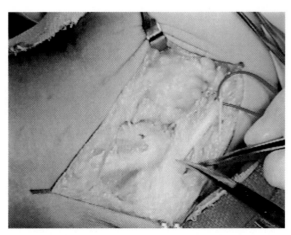

FIGURE 9-11. Division of retrocondylar fascia.

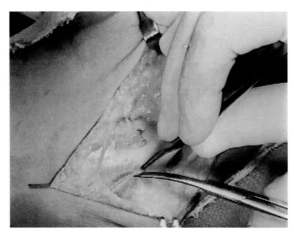

FIGURE 9-12. Release of Osborne's ligament.

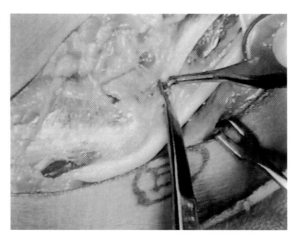

FIGURE 9-15. Excision of intermuscular septum.

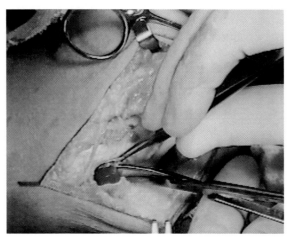

FIGURE 9-13. Separation of the two heads of the flexor carpi ulnaris.

in full flexion to ensure that the tendon of the medial head of triceps does not translate over the epicondyle. If this tendon does translate, it must be incised; otherwise, the patient will complain of persistent painful snapping despite surgery.

After a complete mobilization, the nerve is inspected for any severe fibrosis, and, if the epineurium is fibrotic, a limited epineurotomy is performed until a good fascicular pattern can be observed. Next, the origin of the flexor-pronator is sharply incised from the medial epicondyle, and the muscle group reflected off the anterior medial aspect of the elbow (Fig. 9-18). During this mobilization, the median nerve and brachial artery may be encountered, because they lie medial to the flexor-pronator muscle group. **During the dissection of the humeral head of the flexor carpi ulnaris muscle, one should be careful not to injure the medial collateral ligament** (Fig. 9-19). Once the muscle mobilization

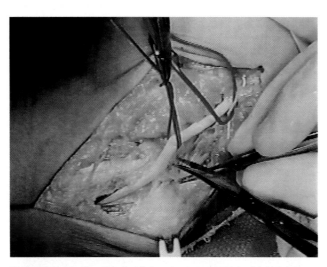

FIGURE 9-14. Neurolysis of the ulnar nerve. Vessel loops retract nerve.

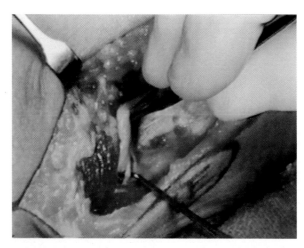

FIGURE 9-16. Probe at motor branch of the flexor carpal ulnaris muscle.

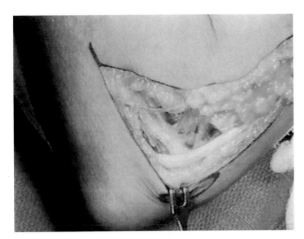

FIGURE 9-17. On flexion of the elbow, the ulnar nerve undergoes anterior subluxation.

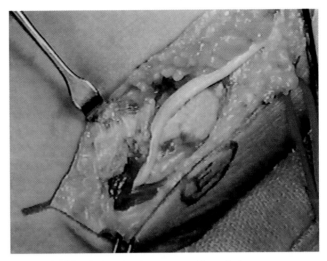

FIGURE 9-20. Anterior transposition of ulnar nerve.

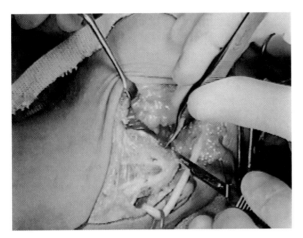

FIGURE 9-18. Dissection of the flexor pronator muscle group from its epicondylar origin.

has been completed, the ulnar nerve is transposed anteriorly and the surgeon must make sure that it lies in a straight path without kinking or impingement (Fig. 9-20). Three holes are drilled into the tip of the medial epicondyle (Fig. 9-21), and, with the elbow in full extension, the flexor pronator tendon is reattached with 2-0 sutures (Fig. 9-22). Once the submuscular anterior transposition has been completed, the nerve is reevaluated to ensure that it glides easily beneath its new muscular cover (Fig. 9-23). Although many surgeons prefer to release the tourniquet before skin closure, this has not been found necessary provided that careful hemostasis has been obtained throughout the procedure.

The adipose tissue is closed with 2-0 or 3-0 absorbable sutures, which is followed by a subcuticular closure also using an absorbable suture (Fig. 9-24). The elbow is then splinted in 90 degrees of flexion for 10 days. Active range of motion is begun at that time with intermittent protection

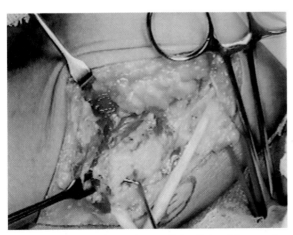

FIGURE 9-19. Probe at the medial collateral ligament.

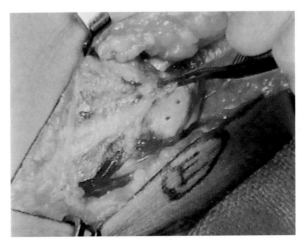

FIGURE 9-21. Holes have been drilled into epicondyle for reattachment of flexor pronator tendon, which is being held by forceps.

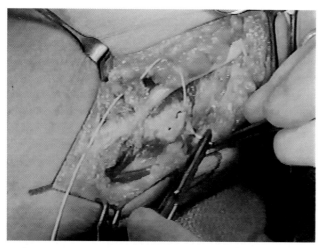

FIGURE 9-22. Suture placed through flexor pronator tendon and hole drilled into epicondyle.

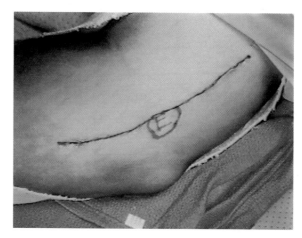

FIGURE 9-24. Subarticular closure of incision.

provided by a sling or removable splint for an additional 2 weeks.

FOLLOW-UP

Three weeks after surgery, passive range of motion exercises can be started if adequate mobility has not been obtained. Progressive strengthening can also be instituted at this time.

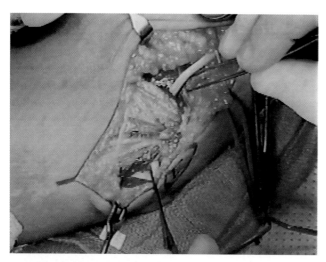

FIGURE 9-23. The gliding of the ulna nerve is tested subsequent to anterior transposition and reattachment of the flexor pronator muscle.

Several months of scar massage with a thick cream such as cocoa butter and the application of silastic skin cover are effective means of minimizing the surgical scar.

SUGGESTED READINGS

Adelaar RS, Foster WC, McDowell C. The treatment of the cubital tunnel syndrome. *J Hand Surg Am* 1984; 9: 90–95.

Broudy AS, Leffert RD, Smith RJ. Technical problems with ulnar nerve transposition at the elbow: findings and results of reoperation. *J Hand Surg Am* 1978; 3: 85–89.

Dellon AL. Operative technique for submuscular transposition of the ulnar nerve. *Contemp Orthop* 1988; 16: 17–24.

Learmonth JR. A technique for transplanting the ulnar nerve. *Surg Gynecol Obstet* 1942; 75: 792–793.

Leffert RD. Anterior submuscular transposition of the ulnar nerves by the Learmonth technique. *J Hand Surg Am* 1982; 7: 147–155.

McGowan AJ. The results of transposition of the ulnar nerve for traumatic ulnar neuritis. *J Bone Joint Surg Br* 1950; 32: 293–301.

Pasque CB, Rayan GM. Anterior submuscular transposition of the ulnar nerve for cubital tunnel syndrome. *J Hand Surg Br* 1995; 20: 447–453.

Posner MA. Compressive ulnar neuropathies at the elbow: II. treatment. *J Am Acad Orthop Surg* 1998; 6: 289–297.

Szabo RM. Entrapment and compressive neuropathies. In: Green DP, Hotchkiss RN, Pederson WC, eds. *Green's operative hand surgery*, 4th ed, vol 2. New York: Churchill Livingstone, 1999: 1422–1429.

Zemel NP, Jobe FW, Yocum LA. Submuscular transposition/ulnar nerve decompression in athletes. In: Geleberman RH, ed. *Operative nerve repair and reconstruction*. Philadelphia: JB Lippincott, 1991: 1097–1105.

CHAPTER 10

ORIF: DISTAL HUMERUS FRACTURE

KENNETH J. KOVAL

Normal function of the hand depends, in part, on a mobile and stable elbow joint. The elbow allows the hand to be positioned in space, it provides power for lifting, and it helps to stabilize the upper extremity. Distal humerus fractures comprise a small portion of upper extremity fractures but are often difficult to treat. The treatment of choice for displaced distal humerus fractures in adults is open reduction and internal fixation using plates and screws. This chapter illustrates open reduction and internal fixation of distal humerus fractures.

ANATOMY

The distal aspect of the humerus can be considered as having medial and lateral columns (Fig. 10-1). Each of these columns is roughly triangular and is bound on its outer border by a supracondylar ridge. The distal aspect of each column is defined as a condyle, each containing an articulating portion (trochlea or capitellum) and a nonarticulating portion (medial or lateral epicondyle). The forearm extensor muscles originate from the lateral epicondyle, and the flexor muscles originate from the medial epicondyle. The capitellum is hemispherical and projects anteriorly; it articulates with the radial head. The trochlea is cylindrical in shape and articulates with the proximal ulna. The articular cartilage surface of the capitellum and trochlea projects downward and forward from the end of the humerus at an angle of approximately 30 degrees. The carrying angle for the elbow (trochlea-olecranon relationship) is approximately 4 to 8 degrees of valgus.

The coronoid and radial fossae are located proximal to the articular surface on the anterior surface of the humerus; these fossae receive the coronoid process and radial head, respectively. Posteriorly, the olecranon fossa receives the tip of the olecranon, making it possible for the elbow to go into full extension.

CLASSIFICATION

Riseborough and Radin classified intraarticular distal humerus fractures based on the amount of fracture displacement and comminution (Fig.10-2):

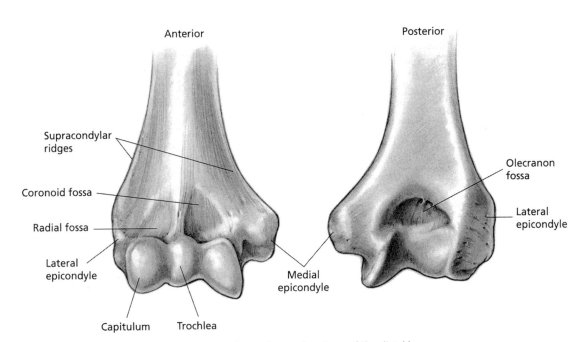

FIGURE 10-1. Anterior and posterior views of the distal humerus.

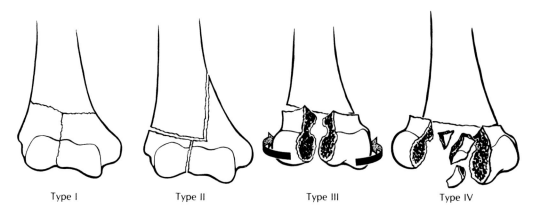

Type I   Type II   Type III   Type IV

FIGURE 10-2. The Riseborough and Radin classification of intraarticular distal humerus fractures. (From DeLee JC, Green DP, Wilkins KE. Fractures and dislocations of the elbow. In: Rockwood CA, Green DP, eds. *Fractures in adults,* 2nd ed. Philadelphia: Lippincott, 1984:559–652. Copyright 1980, Rochester, MN. By permission of Mayo Foundation for Medical Education and Research. All rights reserved.)

Type I: nondisplaced fracture between the capitellum and trochlea

Type II: slight displacement between the capitellum and trochlea without rotational malalignment

Type III: intraarticular fracture displacement with rotational malalignment

Type IV: severe comminution of the articular surface with fracture displacement

The OTA classification is comprehensive (Fig. 10-3); distal humerus fractures are divided into three main categories. Type A fractures are extraarticular, Type B fractures are partial articular, and Type C fractures are complete articular fractures. These categories are then subdivided into subtypes:

- Type A: extraarticular fracture

  A1: apophyseal avulsion
  A2: metaphyseal simple
  A3: metaphyseal multifragmentary

- Type B: partial articular

  B1: lateral sagittal
  B2: medial sagittal
  B3: frontal

- Type C: complete articular

  C1: articular simple, metaphyseal simple
  C2: articular simple, metaphyseal multifragmentary
  C3: articular, metaphyseal multifragmentary

INDICATIONS

Most intraarticular fractures of the distal humerus are best treated by open reduction and internal fixation. The favorable results of operative treatment compared with those associated with skeletal traction or cast immobilization have been well documented. Operative reduction affords the op-

portunity to accurately reduce the articular surface and restore its congruous relation to the olecranon, thereby ensuring the intrinsic stability of the humeroulnar relation. However, when determining the optimal management for fractures of the distal humerus, several factors must be taken into account. These include the amount of displacement and comminution, the presence of osteoporosis, the functional demands and expectations of the patients, the presence or absence of associated injury, the patient's overall medical condition, and finally the surgeon's experience.

PREOPERATIVE PLANNING

Initial radiographs should include an anteroposterior (AP) and lateral of the elbow (Fig. 10-4). Oblique radiographs may also be obtained for further fracture definition. Traction radiographs may better delineate the fracture pattern and may be useful for preoperative planning. Because intercondylar fractures are much more common than supracondylar fractures in adults, the radiographs should be scrutinized for evidence of intraarticular fracture extension. Comparison radiographs of the contralateral extremity are useful for preoperative planning.

The exact nature of the fracture should be understood before one attempts any form of surgical intervention. Although useful for simpler fractures, preoperative planning is critical for more complex injuries. This forces the surgeon to understand the "personality of the fracture" and mentally prepare an operative plan. All aspects of the reduction and fixation should be drawn out to help avoid technical pitfalls and ensure that all the needed equipment is available.

EQUIPMENT

The basic instruments necessary for open reduction and internal fixation of a distal humerus fracture include the following (Fig. 10-5):

Groups:

Humerus, distal segment, extra-articular (13-A)

1. Apophyseal avulsion (13-A1)

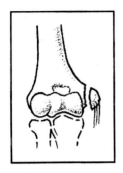

2. Metaphyseal simple (13-A2)

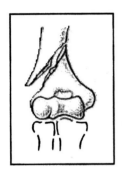

3. Metaphyseal multifragmentary (13-A3)

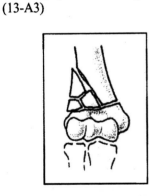

Humerus, distal segment, partial articular (13-B)

1. Lateral sagittal (13-B1)

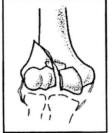

2. Medial sagittal (13-B2)

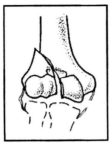

3. Frontal (13-B3)

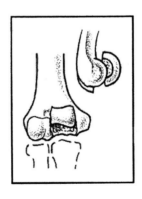

Humerus, distal segment, complete articular (13-C)

1. Articular simple, metaphyseal simple (13-C1)

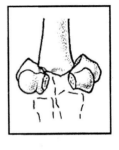

2. Articular simple, metaphyseal multifragmentary (13-C2)

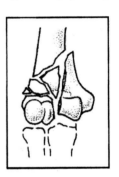

3. Articular, metaphyseal multifragmentary (13-C3)

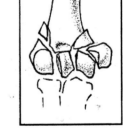

FIGURE 10-3. The OTA classification of distal humerus fractures. (From Orthopaedic Trauma/Committe for Coding and Classification. *Journal of Orthopaedic Trauma* 1996; 10 (Suppl 1).

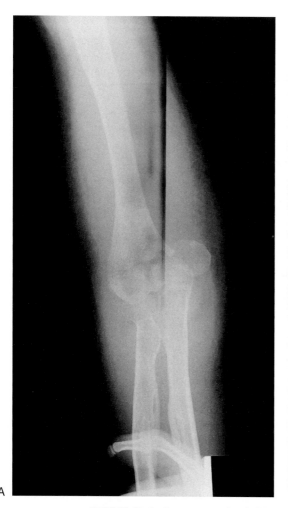

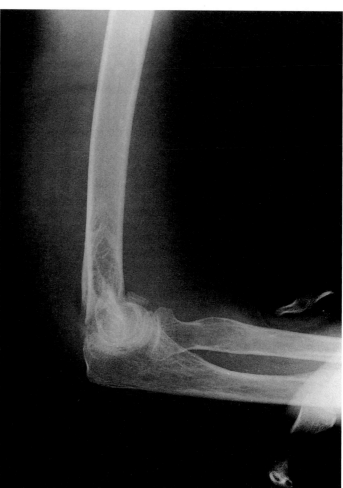

A   B

FIGURE 10-4. Anteroposterior **(A)** and lateral **(B)** radiographs demonstrating a displaced intraarticular distal humerus fracture.

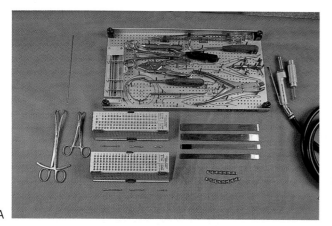

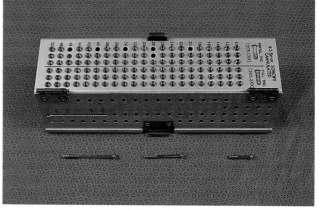

A   B

FIGURE 10-5. Instruments for ORIF of distal humerus fracture: Kirschner wire *(top left)*; cerclage wire set *(top tray)*; *(bottom row, left to right)* large- and small-pointed reduction clamps (2), small-diameter cannulated screws, osteotomes, 3.5-mm pelvic recon plates (from set), oscillating saw **(A).** Small diameter cannulated screw set (close-up) **(B).** *(continued)*

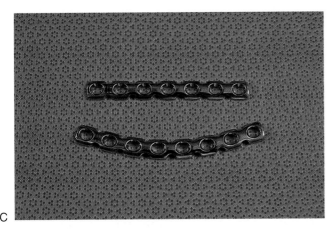

C

FIGURE 10-5. *(Continued)* Recon plates (close-up) **(C).**

- Small fragment plate and screws
- Large fragment plate and screws
- Pelvic instrument and implant sets
- Kirschner wires
- Small-diameter cannulated screws
- Large- and small-pointed reduction clamps
- Cerclage wire set
- Osteotomes
- Oscillating saw
- Herbert or Acutrac screw set (for small articular fragments)
- Mini fragment set (for small articular fragments)

PATIENT POSITIONING AND FRACTURE REDUCTION

The operative procedures can be performed under regional or general anesthesia (Fig. 10-6). I prefer to place the patient in a lateral decubitus position. The arm is held outright and

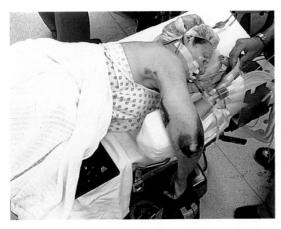

FIGURE 10-6. Placement of the patient in a lateral decubitus position with the elbow supported on pad attached to the table.

the elbow supported on blankets or on a well-padded attachment to the operating table. The iliac crest is prepped and draped if bone grafting is anticipated. Surgery is performed under tourniquet control; a sterile tourniquet is used to provide a wider sterile field and the ability to reapply the tourniquet as needed.

APPROACH

A midline skin incision is made on the posterior aspect of the distal arm, curving medially around the tip of the olecranon and extending to the subcutaneous border of the proximal ulna (Fig. 10-7). The incision is carried to the triceps retinaculum, and deep medial and lateral soft tissue flaps raised (Fig. 10-8). ◼ The ulnar nerve is identified proximally and tagged with a Penrose drain or vessel loop (Fig. 10-9). ◼ The ulnar nerve is mobilized proximally to the medial intramuscular septum and distally through the fascia of the flexor carpi ulnaris. **One must be careful to maintain the motor branches that arise at the level of the**

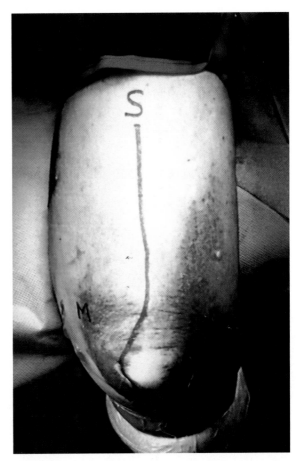

FIGURE 10-7. A midline skin incision is made on the posterior aspect of the distal arm, curving medially around the tip of the olecranon and extending to the subcutaneous border of the proximal ulna.

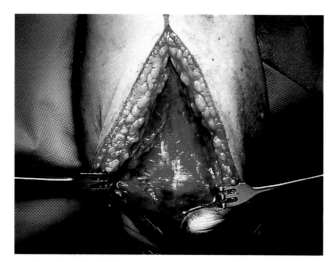

FIGURE 10-8. Exposure of the triceps retinaculum.

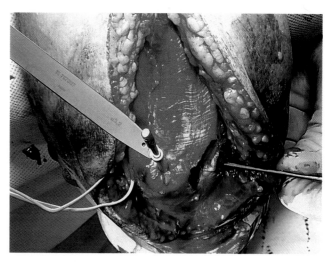

FIGURE 10-10. Before making the olecranon osteotomy, a pilot hole is made down the medullary canal from the tip of the olecranon, using a 3.2-mm drill.

distal humerus and enter into the flexor carpi ulnaris. By mobilizing the nerve proximally and distally, traction on the nerve during the postoperative rehabilitation is prevented and the nerve is kept in the soft tissues out of the way of the internal fixation. I prefer to find the nerve proximally after it pierces the intermuscular septum; it is easier to palpate and mobilize. The Penrose drain is held together with a suture, not a clamp, to avoid placing extra tension on the nerve by the weight of the clamp.

Although a number of deep surgical exposures have been described, my preference has been to use a transolecranon approach using a chevron osteotomy for intraarticular distal humerus fractures. After isolating and mobilizing the ulnar nerve, the medial and lateral border of the triceps tendon and olecranon are identified. Laterally, the anconeus muscle is elevated off the olecranon to directly visualize the articular surface. The periosteum over the proximal ulna is elevated for 1 to 2 cm distal to the planned osteotomy for later reattachment.

Before making the chevron osteotomy, the proximal ulna is drilled and tapped to facilitate later reattachment. A pilot hole is made from the tip of the olecranon down the medullary canal, using a 3.2-mm drill (Fig. 10-10); one should take care to remain within the medullary canal. The length of this drill tract is then measured and tapped (Fig. 10-11). The osteotomy is made in the center of the sigmoid notch of the olecranon sulcus; this central area can be determined by placing a clamp from lateral to media (Fig. 10-12). ◘ The chevron osteotomy is made with the V facing upright to maximize the size of the proximal fragment. **If the apex is pointed proximally toward the tip of the olecranon process, there is a risk of splitting of the olecranon.**

The osteotomy is created using a fine-bladed oscillating saw to reach the articular cartilage (Fig. 10-13) and completed with a thin osteotome (Fig. 10-14). Completion of the osteotomy with the osteotome results in irregularity of

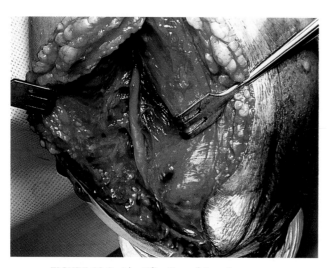

FIGURE 10-9. Identification of the ulnar nerve.

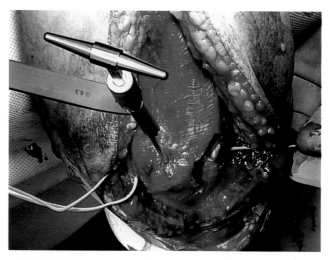

FIGURE 10-11. Tapping of the pilot hole using a 6.5-mm tap.

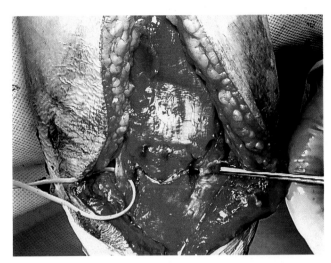

FIGURE 10-12. Use of a clamp to determine the center of the olecranon sulcus. The planned olecranon osteotomy is demonstrated.

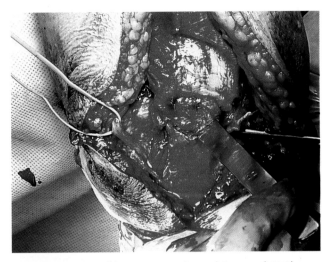

FIGURE 10-14. A thin osteotome is used to complete the osteotomy.

the articular surface, which is a guide to later reduction of the osteotomy. ◼ The tip of the olecranon and triceps tendon and muscle are then elevated proximally and protected within a moist sponge (Fig. 10-15). ◼ **It is usually not necessary to identify and mobilize the radial nerve; however, if the fracture has humeral shaft extension that would require excessive triceps mobilization, one should isolate the radial nerve to minimize the risk of traction injury.**

PROCEDURE

The exact nature of the intraarticular fracture pattern is determined (Fig. 10-16). ◼ The fracture hematoma is removed using a dental pick and irrigation. One should take care to avoid loss of small articular fragments devoid of soft

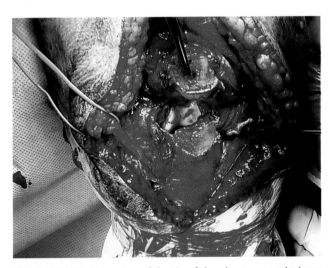

FIGURE 10-15. Retraction of the tip of the olecranon and triceps tendon proximally.

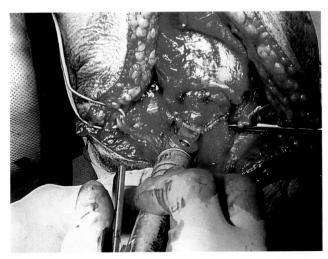

FIGURE 10-13. Use of an oscillating saw to create the osteotomy.

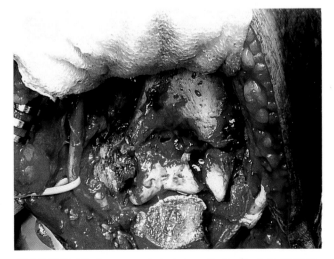

FIGURE 10-16. Exposure of the intraarticular fracture pattern.

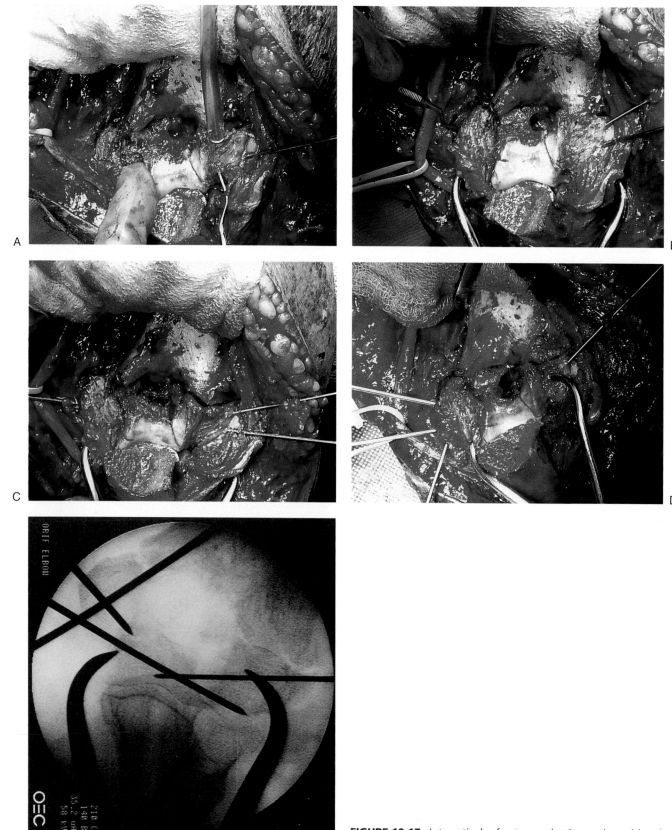

FIGURE 10-17. Intraarticular fracture reduction and provisional Kirschner wire fixation (**A** to **E**).

tissue attachments. Once the fracture anatomy is confirmed, attention is turned toward reducing and provisionally stabilizing the intraarticular fracture component (Fig. 10-17). Kirschner wires can be placed into the medial and lateral condyles; they are used as "joysticks" to help fracture reduction. Once reduced, Kirschner wires are placed across the fracture for provisional fixation.

Definitive fixation for the intraarticular fracture component involves use of lag screws. One or two 3.5-mm cortical or 4.0-mm cancellous screws are placed across the fracture surface (Fig. 10-18). I usually place the screws from medial to lateral to direct the drill bit away from the ulnar nerve. If there is intraarticular fracture comminution, these screws should be inserted as holding screws not lag screws to prevent narrowing the articular surface. If there are coronal fracture lines, it may be necessary to use minifragment screws, threaded Kirschner wires, or headless screws (Herbert, Acutrac screws) placed from posterior to anterior, to provide fracture fixation. Occasionally, one may find that

the articular reconstruction may be facilitated by securing one of the articular components directly to one of the bony columns of the distal humerus. This would be followed by restoration of the remaining articular element to this stable skeletal and articular unit.

Once the articular surface has been reconstructed and stabilized, the distal articular block is reduced to the humeral shaft. Provisional fracture fixation can be provided by Kischner wires inserted up the medial and lateral columns. **One should verify that the distal articular-humeral shaft relationship has been restored: (a) the valgus carrying angle and (b) the capitellum and trochlea project downward and forward from the end of the humerus at an angle of approximately 30 degrees.**

Definitive fixation of the articular segment to the humeral shaft involves use of two plates, one along each column. Although the most stable mechanical construct has the two plates 90 degrees to each other, it is technically easier to place both plates posteriorly. The lateral plate (3.5 dy-

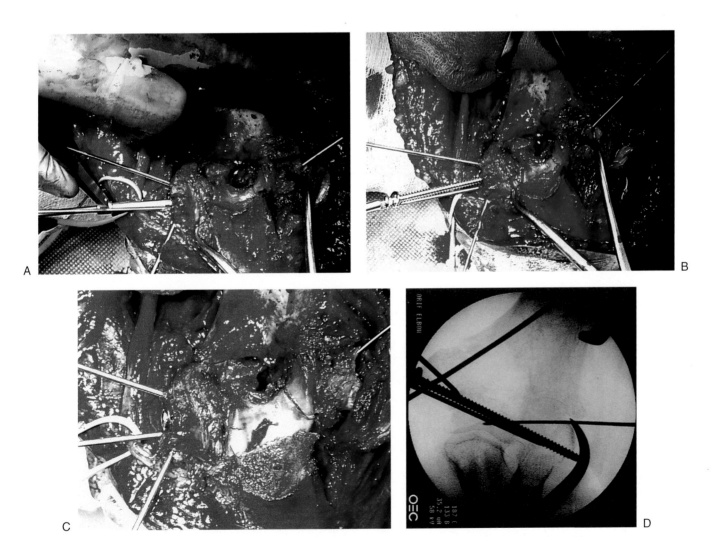

FIGURE 10-18. Placement of a lag screw across the intraarticular fracture component (**A** to **D**).

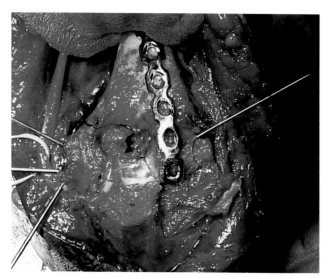

FIGURE 10-19. The lateral plate is placed posteriorly along the lateral column.

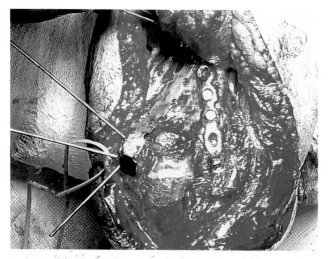

FIGURE 10-20. Placement of the medial plate posteromedially with contouring around the tip of the medial epicondyle.

namic compression plate [DCP] or reconstruction plate) is placed posteriorly along the column and needs minimal contouring (Fig. 10-19). ◼ The distal aspect of the plate can extend to the articular surface of the capitellum. The medial plate (3.5 reconstruction or ¹/₃ tubular plate) is placed medial or posteromedial and usually must be contoured around the tip of the medial epicondyle (Fig. 10-20). ◼ Wrapping the plates around the posterior aspect of the capitellum and the medial epicondyle allows placement of "homerun" screws through the plate and up the columns. These long screws, which traverse the columns and exit the cortex proximally, are useful when the fracture line is distal (transcondylar) because they provide bicortical fixation. One must verify that the plates do not impinge on the olecranon fossa to prevent loss of elbow extension secondary to mechanical block.

Once satisfied with the plate positioning, holding screws are inserted into the proximal and distal fracture fragments (Fig. 10-21). I generally attach the lateral plate before the medial plate, because it is technically easier to apply. If the fracture pattern permits, screws should inserted as lag screws. The medial plate is then applied. Bone graft is applied if there is comminution in the supracondylar or humeral shaft region.

The elbow is placed through a range of motion to assess fracture stability and verify full range of elbow motion without hardware encroachment in the olecranon fossa. The proximal ulna is then prepared for reattachment of the olecranon osteotomy. A 2-mm hole is drilled perpendicular to the long axis of the ulna approximately 3 to 4 cm distal to the osteotomy. This drill hole is approximately halfway between the volar and dorsal surfaces of the ulna. I generally make the distance from the osteotomy to this drill hole similar to that from the osteotomy to the olecranon tip. Placement of this drill hole in an excessively dorsal location increases the risk for drill hole fracture when the ten-

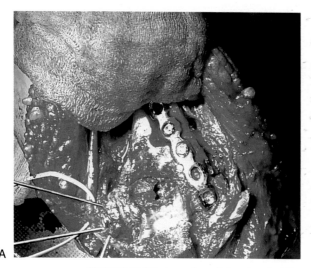

A

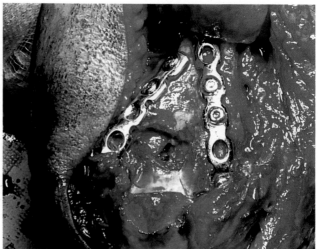

B

FIGURE 10-21. Insertion of the plate holding screws into the medial and lateral plates (**A** and **B**).

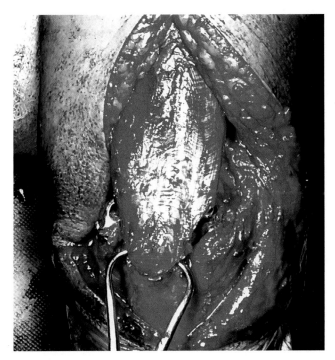

FIGURE 10-22. Reduction of the olecranon osteotomy.

sion band wire is tightened. An 18- or 20-gauge wire is then passed through this drill hole.

The olecranon osteotomy is reduced and provisionally stabilized using a tenaculum clamp (Fig. 10-22). ◼ A 6.5-mm cancellous lag screw with washer is inserted from the tip of the olecranon into the ulnar shaft through the previously drilled hole. ◼ One should verify fracture reduction dur-

ing lag screw insertion because there is a tendency for the osteotomy to translate and rotate as the screw is advanced into the distal fragment.

Before final seating of the lag screw, a 14-gauge angiocatheter is passed deep to the triceps tendon and washer, anterior to the 6.5-mm screw (Fig. 10-23). The tension band wire is crossed over the posterior surface of the olecranon, threaded through the tip of the angiocatheter, and pulled out through the opposite side of the triceps tendon. Two loops are made in this wire, one knot on each side of the ulna.

The wire knots are then tightened sequentially with the elbow in extension. This provides more uniform tension to the bone-implant construct. The knots are cut to a length of 3 to 4 mm, bent down, and buried in the soft tissue (Fig. 10-24). A slit is made in the triceps tendon, in line with its fibers, and the 6.5-mm lag screw and washer are seated under the triceps tendon.

The tourniquet is released. The need for ulnar nerve transposition is assessed. I do not routinely transpose the ulnar nerve unless there is impingement of the ulnar nerve within the cubital tunnel. If I feel transposition is necessary, I perform a subcutaneous transposition with the ulnar nerve protected by a facial sling.

Final radiographs are obtained (Fig. 10-25). One should confirm that the tension band wire passes anterior to the lag screw and deep to the washer. The fracture is examined through a full range of elbow motion to verify fracture stability and ascertain that there is no tension on the ulnar nerve with elbow flexion and extension. The wound is irrigated and closed in layers. The arm is placed into a posterior plaster splint with the elbow in extension. The elbow is splinted in extension because I have found that the most common deformity after distal humerus fracture is residual flexion contracture.

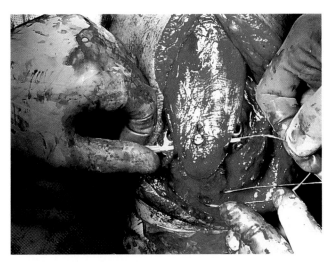

FIGURE 10-23. Passage of a 14-gauge angiocatheter deep to the triceps tendon and washer, anterior to the 6.5-mm screw. The tension band wire is crossed over the posterior surface of the olecranon, threaded through the tip of the angiocatheter, and pulled out through the opposite side of the triceps tendon.

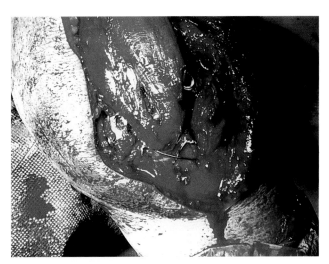

FIGURE 10-24. Clinical photograph after the wire knots have been tightened and the lag screw seated.

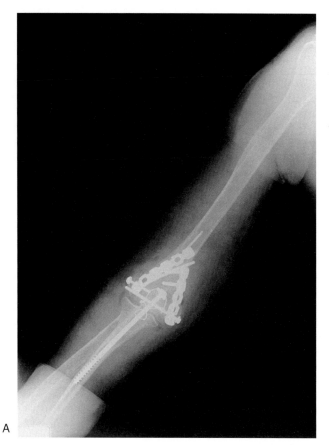
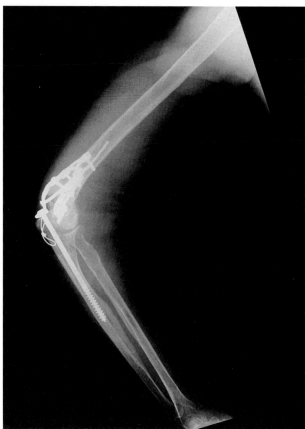

A

B

FIGURE 10-25. Final anteroposterior **(A)** and lateral **(B)** radiographs.

POSTOPERATIVE PROTOCOL

Active motion is initiated on the first postoperative day. The patient is instructed to lie supine and forward flex the involved shoulder to bring the elbow overhead. With the uninjured arm supporting the involved forearm, gravity is used to assist elbow flexion. A similar approach is used for elbow-extension exercises, but, in this case, the patient sits upright and gently assists the forearm into extension. Two splints are fabricated by the occupational therapy department—one in full extension and the other in 90 degrees of flexion. Use of these splints is alternated by the patient, particularly at night, to help minimize the risk of flexion and extension contractures.

Active and patient-assisted flexion-extension exercises are continued throughout the first 3 to 4 weeks. At 6 weeks postoperatively, if radiographic union is progressing satisfactorily, the patient is allowed light resisted exercises.

SUGGESTED READINGS

Gabel GT, Hanson G, Bennett JB et al. Intraarticular fractures of the distal humerus in the adult. *Clin Orthop* 1987; 216: 99–107.

Holdsworth BJ, Mossad MM. Fractures of the adult distal humerus. Elbow function after internal fixation. *J Bone Joint Surg Br* 1990; 72: 362–365.

Johansson H, Olerud S. Operative treatment of intercondylar fractures of the humerus. *J Trauma* 1971; 11: 836–843.

Jupiter JB. Trauma to the adult elbow. In: Browner BD, Jupiter JB, Levine AM, eds. *Skeletal trauma.* Philadelphia: WB Saunders, 1992: 1125–1145.

Jupiter JB, Neff U, Holzach P, et al. Intercondylar fractures of the humerus. An operative approach. *J Bone Joint Surg Am* 1985; 67A: 226–239.

Letsch R, Schmidt-Neuerburg KP, Stürmer, KM et al. Intraarticular fractures of the distal humerus. Surgical treatment and results. *Clin Orthop* 1989; 241: 238–244.

Müller ME, Allgöwer M, Schneider R, et al. *Manual of internal fixation. Techniques recommended by the AO-ASIF group,* 3rd ed. Berlin: Springer-Verlag, 1991: 451.

Perry CR, Gibson CT, Kowalski MF. Transcondylar fractures of the distal humerus. *J Orthop Trauma* 1989; 3: 98–106.

Riseborough EJ, Radin EL. Intercondylar T fractures of the humerus in the adult. A comparison of operative and non-operative treatment in twenty-nine cases. *J Bone Joint Surg Am* 1969; 51A: 130–141.

Schatzker J. Fractures of the distal end of the humerus. In: Schatzker J, Tile M, eds. *The rationale of operative fracture care.* Berlin: Springer-Verlag, 1987: 71–87.

Zagorski JB, Jennings JJ, Burkhalter WE, et al. Comminuted intraarticular fractures of the distal humeral condyles. *Clin Orthop Rel Res* 1986; 202: 197–204.

CHAPTER 11

OLECRANON FRACTURES: TENSION BAND WIRING

KENNETH J. KOVAL

Fractures of the olecranon are relatively common in adults. The prominence of the olecranon, its subcutaneous position, and the attachment of the triceps make it particularly vulnerable to injury. The articular surface of the olecranon articulates with the trochlea, with motion allowed only in the anteroposterior plane. These articulating surfaces provide a major component of elbow stability. Therefore, intraarticular olecranon fractures have the potential to disrupt the stability of the elbow joint. This chapter illustrates open reduction and internal fixation of a displaced olecranon fracture.

ANATOMY

The olecranon, the proximal aspect of the proximal ulna, is a subcutaneous structure and is, therefore, vulnerable to direct trauma. Together with the coronoid process, the olecranon forms the greater sigmoid (semilunar) notch of the ulna, a deep depression that serves as the articulation with the trochlea (Fig. 11-1). This articulation allows rotational motion only about the flexion-extension axis, pro-

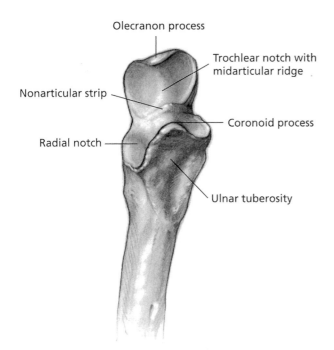

Olecranon process

Trochlear notch with midarticular ridge

Nonarticular strip

Coronoid process

Radial notch

Ulnar tuberosity

FIGURE 11-1. The proximal ulna.

viding intrinsic stability to the elbow joint. The articular cartilage surface of the olecranon is interrupted by a transverse ridge known as the "bare area." Posteriorly, the triceps tendon envelops the articular capsule before it inserts onto the olecranon; the fascia overlying the triceps muscle spreads out medially and inserts into the deep fascia of the forearm and into the periosteum of the olecranon and proximal ulna. A fracture of the olecranon with displacement represents a functional disruption of the triceps mechanism, resulting in loss of active extension of the elbow. The ulnar nerve is located on the medial aspect of the elbow, posterior to the medial epicondyle and medial collateral ligament.

CLASSIFICATION

There is no universally accepted classification system for olecranon fractures. Colton classified olecranon fractures into two major groups: nondisplaced (type I) and displaced (type II). A type I fracture has less than 2 mm of separation and no increase in displacement with flexion to 90 degrees, with the patient able to extend the elbow against gravity. Colton further subdivided the displaced fractures into type IIA, avulsion; IIB, oblique and transverse; IIC, comminuted; and IID, fracture-dislocation.

Schatzker classified olecranon fractures as either nondisplaced or displaced (Fig. 11-2). Displaced fractures can be either extraarticular or intraarticular. Intraarticular fractures are further divided into transverse, oblique, comminuted, or fracture-dislocation. Transverse fractures can be simple or complex (associated with joint depression). Oblique fractures can be proximal (tip to the midpoint of the semilunar notch) or distal (midpoint of the semilunar notch to the coronoid process). Comminuted fractures have multiple fracture lines and may be associated with a radial head fracture or dislocation.

INDICATIONS

The indications for operative treatment include olecranon fractures with greater than 2-mm articular displacement or step-off, injuries with elbow-extensor mechanism disruption,

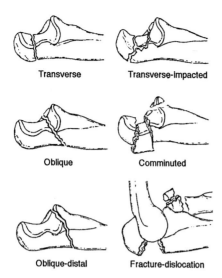

FIGURE 11-2. The Schatzker classification of olecranon fractures. (From McKee MD, Jupiter JB. Trauma to the adult elbow and fractures of the distal humerus. In: Browner BD, Jupiter JB, Levine AM, eds. *Skeletal trauma.* Philadelphia: WB Saunders, 1998:1470, with permission.)

and open fractures. The inability to extend the elbow against gravity suggests loss of elbow-extensor mechanism integrity.

The choice of implant to stabilize an olecranon fracture is based on the fracture pattern and location. A tension band wire construct can be used for simple and complex transverse fracture patterns proximal to the coronoid. The tension band wire converts the extensor force of the triceps to a dynamic compressive force across the fracture. Beyond the level of the coronoid, however, a tension band wire construct cannot provide sufficient rotational control. A plate and screw fixation is used for proximal oblique fractures and fractures distal to the coronoid.

PREOPERATIVE PLANNING

Radiographic evaluation for an olecranon fracture includes an anteroposterior (AP) and lateral view (Fig. 11-3). When the olecranon fracture is part of an elbow fracture-dislocation, traction radiographs may be used to evaluate the injury as well. The lateral radiographs reveal the extent of the frac-

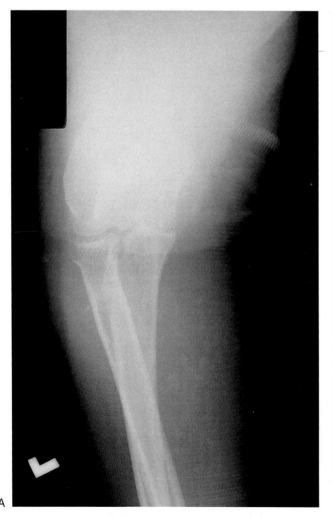

A

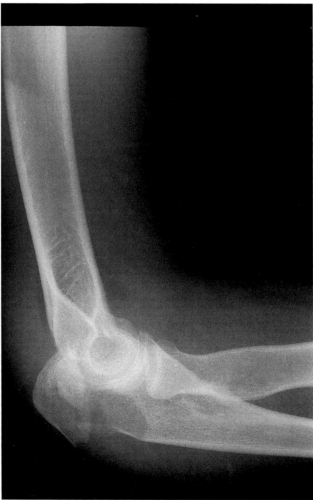

B

FIGURE 11-3. Anteroposterior **(A)** and lateral **(B)** view of the elbow showing a displaced olecranon fracture.

ture and the presence of comminution or joint depression. The integrity of the radial head-capitellar articulation is examined, and subluxation or dislocation of the semilunar notch from the trochlea is noted. The anteroposterior radiograph is examined for sagittal fracture lines that are not well displayed on the lateral view. The integrity of the radial head-capitellar and semilunar notch-trochlea articulation are also determined on this view. Comparison radiographs are helpful in complex fracture patterns.

EQUIPMENT

The equipment necessary for tension band wiring of the olecranon include the following (Fig. 11-4):

- 0.062-inch Kirschner wires
- Wire driver
- Cerclage wire set
- 14-gauge angiocatheter
- Large- and small-pointed reduction clamps
- Small fragment set

PATIENT POSITIONING AND FRACTURE REDUCTION

The patient can be positioned supine or lateral. I prefer a supine position with the arm placed across the patient's chest (Fig. 11-5). The procedure is usually performed under tourniquet control.

INCISION

The incision begins distally on the subcutaneous border of the ulna. It is continued proximally in line with the sub-

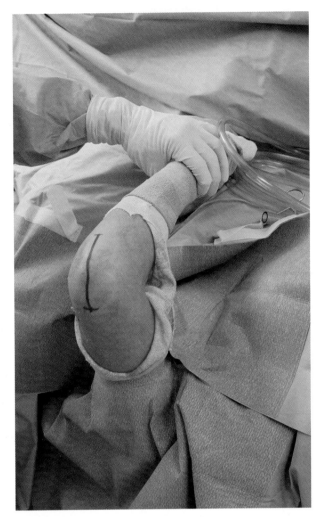

FIGURE 11-5. Supine patient positioning with the arm placed across the chest.

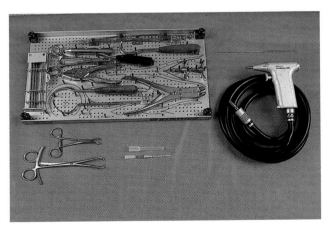

FIGURE 11-4. Equipment for tension band wiring of the olecranon: cerclage wire set *(top left tray)*, 0.062-inch Kirschner wire *(top right)*, large- and small-pointed reduction clamps (2) *(bottom left)*, 14-gauge angiocatheter *(bottom middle)*, and wire driver *(bottom right)*.

cutaneous border to the ulna of the olecranon area, where it is curved radially around the tip of the olecranon and then extended proximally in the midline 3 to 5 cm (Fig. 11-6).

APPROACH

The incision is developed down to the fascia. A subcutaneous flap is elevated over the tip of the olecranon (Fig. 11-7). The location of the ulnar nerve can be determined by palpation; it is not usually necessary to isolate and transpose the ulnar nerve. Distally, muscle origins are reflected extraperiosteally as needed. ◉ The posterior aspect of the fracture line is now usually visible. The fracture lines are cleaned of clot and debris. ◉ Two millimeters of periosteum is reflected from either side of the fracture lines to help visualization and fracture reduction. ◉ The joint is visualized by retracting the proximal fragment (Fig. 11-8).

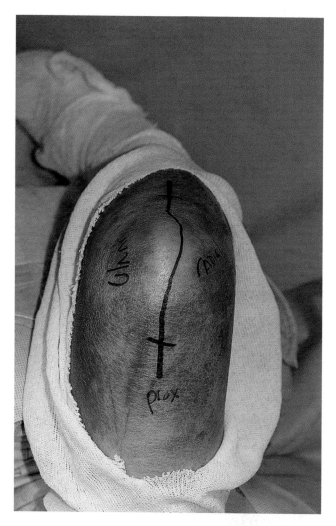

FIGURE 11-6. The skin incision for open reduction of the ole-cranon.

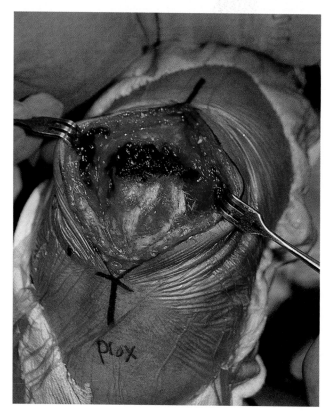

FIGURE 11-7. The incision is developed down to the fascia. A subcutaneous flap is elevated over the tip of the olecranon.

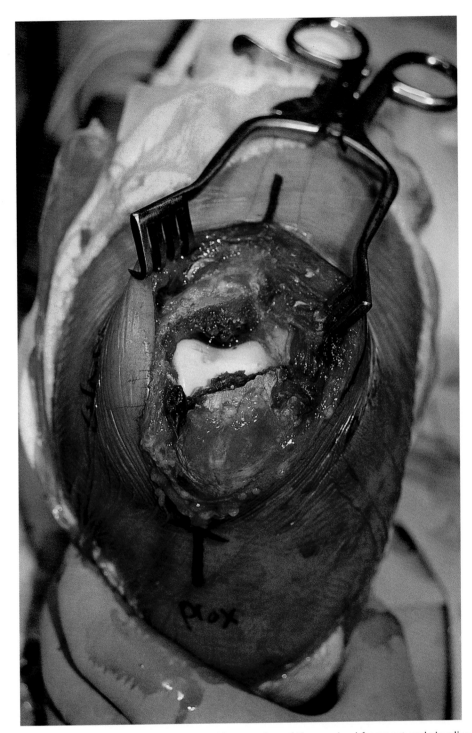

FIGURE 11-8. The exposed fracture site with retraction of the proximal fragment and visualization of the elbow joint.

PROCEDURE

Fracture reduction begins with elevation of any depressed articular component, if present. Bone graft is used if necessary to support the depressed fragments. These reduced articular fragments can be stabilized using Kirschner wires or small-diameter screws. The main fracture fragments are then reduced and temporarily held in place with pointed reduction clamps (Fig. 11-9). Fracture reduction can be facilitated with (a) use of a tenaculum clamp on the proximal fragment for manipulation, (b) the elbow extended, and (c) placement of a drill hole in the proximal ulnar shaft to anchor the distal prong of the pointed reduction clamp.

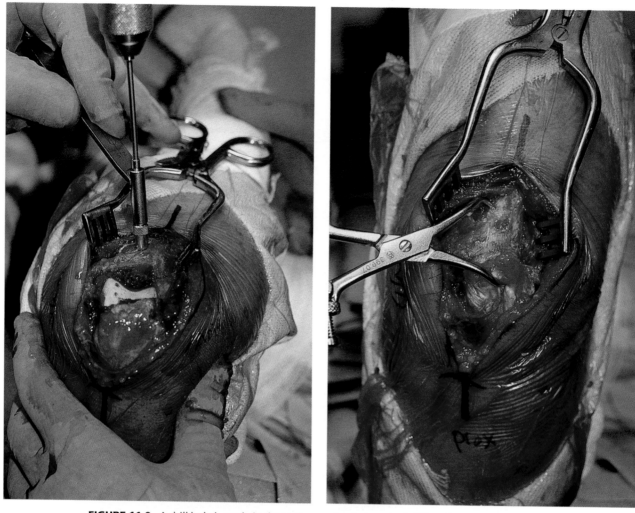

A

B

FIGURE 11-9. A drill hole is made in the in the proximal ulnar shaft **(A)** and a pointed tenaculum clamp used to provisionally stabilize the fracture reduction **(B).**

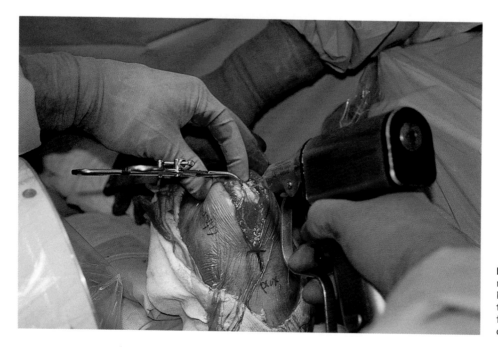

FIGURE 11-10. Following fracture reduction, two parallel 0.062-inch Kirschner wires are inserted from the tip of the olecranon, across the fracture, and out the anterior cortex of the distal fragment.

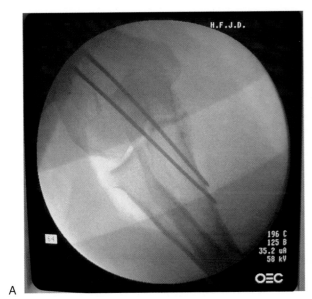 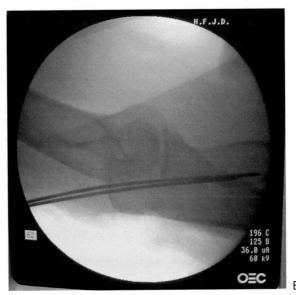

A   B

FIGURE 11-11. Anteroposterior **(A)** and lateral **(B)** radiographs verifying implant position.

The fracture reduction is then verified by visual inspection and fluoroscopic evaluation. Once satisfied with the fracture reduction, two parallel 0.062-inch Kirschner wires are inserted from the tip of the olecranon, across the fracture and driven out the anterior cortex of the distal fragment (Fig. 11-10). ▣ <u>Engaging the anterior cortex may diminish pin migration.</u> The wire position is checked fluoroscopically (Fig. 11-11), and the wires are then backed out to anterior cortex to prevent excessive anterior soft tissue penetration when the wires are fully seated.

A 2-mm hole is drilled perpendicular to the long axis of the ulna and approximately 3 to 4 cm distal to the fracture (Fig. 11-12). ▣ I generally make the distance from the fracture to this drill hole similar to that from the fracture to the olecranon tip. This drill hole is approximately halfway between the volar and dorsal surfaces of the ulna. **Placement of this drill hole in an excessively dorsal location increases the risk for drill hole fracture when the tension band wire is tightened.**

An 18- or 20-gauge wire is passed through this drill hole (Fig. 11-13). A 14-gauge angiocatheter is then passed deep to the triceps tendon and the tip of the olecranon, anterior to the Kirschner wires (Fig. 11-14). ▣ The tension band wire is crossed over the posterior surface of the olecranon, threaded through the tip of the angiocatheter, and pulled out through the opposite side of the triceps tendon (Fig. 11-15). Two loops are made in this wire, one knot on each side of the ulna (Fig. 11-16).

The wire knots are then tightened sequentially with the elbow in extension (Fig. 11-17). ▣ This provides more uniform tension to the bone-implant construct. The knots are cut to a length of 3 to 4 mm, bent down, and buried in the soft tissue. The Kirschner wires are bent dorsally just past 90 degrees with a metal suction tip and cut, leaving 3 to 4 mm of wire remaining past the bend. By using a wire pliers, the K-wires are bent over to 180 degrees (Fig. 11-18) and rotated until the short portion of the bent wire is anterior. The fibers

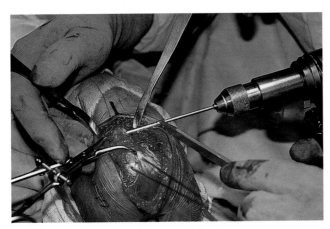

FIGURE 11-12. A 2-mm hole is drilled perpendicular to the long axis of the ulna approximately 3 to 4 cm distal to the fracture.

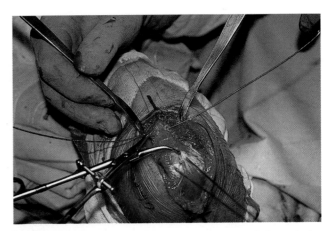

FIGURE 11-13. An 18- or 20-gauge wire is passed through the drill hole in the proximal ulna.

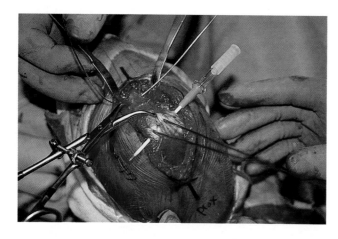

FIGURE 11-14. A 14-gauge angiocatheter is passed deep to the triceps tendon and the tip of the olecranon, anterior to the Kirschner wires.

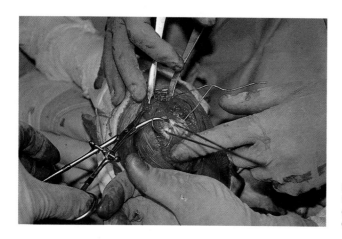

FIGURE 11-15. The tension band wire is crossed over the posterior surface of the olecranon, threaded through the tip of the angiocatheter, and pulled out through the opposite side of the triceps tendon.

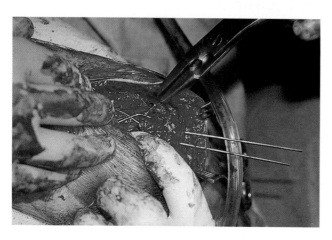

FIGURE 11-16. Two loops are made in the tension band wire, one knot on each side of the ulna.

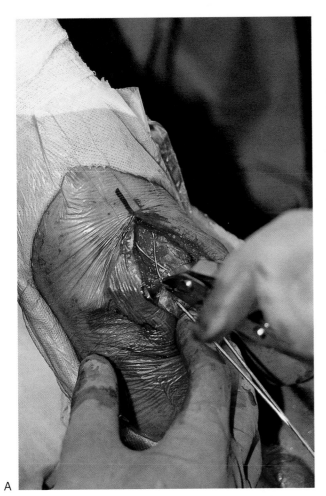
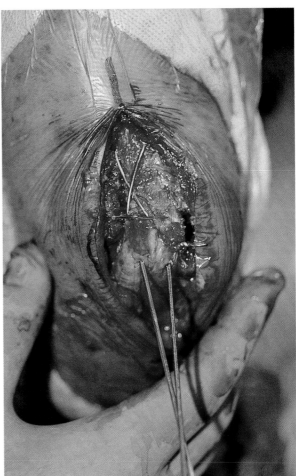

FIGURE 11-17. Tightening the wire knots with the elbow in extension **(A)**. Appearance of the tension band wire after tightening **(B)**.

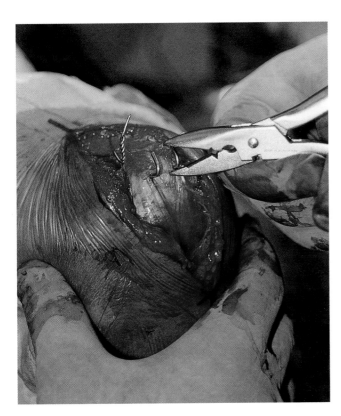

FIGURE 11-18. Use of a pliers to bend the Kirschner wires 180 degrees.

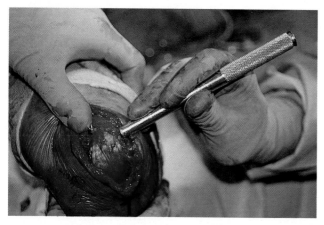

FIGURE 11-19. Final seating of the tension band wire knots and Kirschner wires.

of the triceps tendon are split sharply with a scalpel at the entry point of the bent K-wires, and the wires are then seated using a mallet and bone tamp (Fig. 11-19). It is important to verify that the bent proximal aspect of the wire is buried under the triceps to minimize the risk of wire backout (Fig. 11-20).

The tourniquet is released. Final radiographs are obtained (Fig. 11-21). One should confirm that the tension band wire passes anterior to both K-wires. The fracture is examined through a full range of elbow motion to verify stability and ascertain that the far end of the K-wires that engage the far cortex do not restrict forearm rotation (Fig. 11-22). ◼️ The wound is irrigated and closed in layers. A drain is not used if adequate hemostasis is obtained after tourniquet release. The arm is placed into a posterior plaster splint.

POSTOPERATIVE PROTOCOL

Initially, the limb is splinted at 90 degrees for 3 to 5 days to promote soft tissue healing. Fractures fixed with the tension band principle begin early active motion once the incision is clean and dry. Active and active-assisted motion exercises continue until there is radiographic evidence of progression to union, clinical evidence of union (no pain with physiologic stress), and an active range of motion of at least 75%

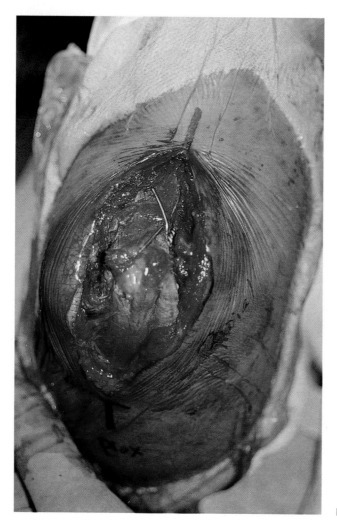

FIGURE 11-20. Final clinical appearance.

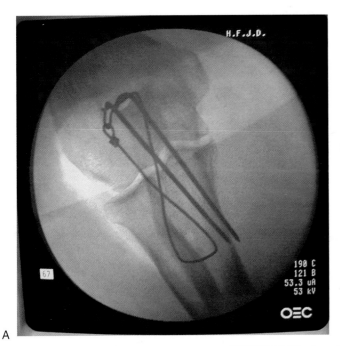
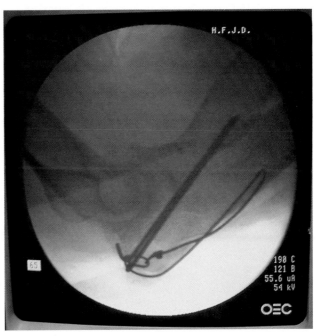

A

B

FIGURE 11-21. A and B. Final radiographs.

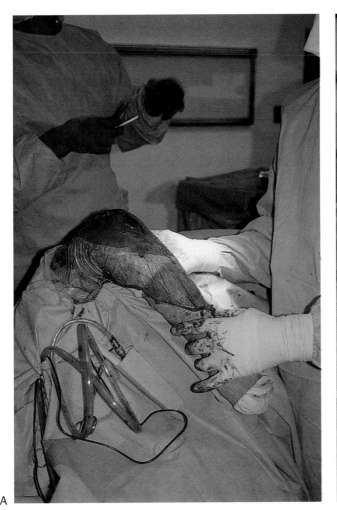
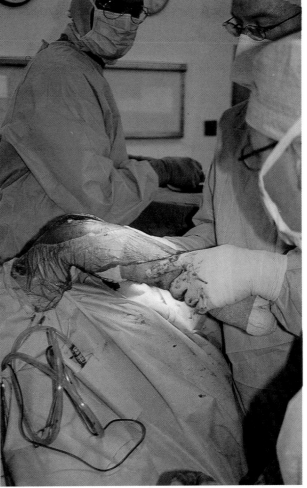

A

B

FIGURE 11-22. Placement of the extremity through a range of motion to verify stability and ascertain that the far end of the K-wires that engage the far cortex do not restrict forearm rotation.

of the contralateral elbow (75% of normal with bilateral injuries). The patient begins a progressive-resistance program designed to strengthen the entire upper extremity. Functional-capacity evaluations are used for return to work for manual laborers.

SUGGESTED READINGS

Cabanela M. Olecranon fractures. In: Morrey BF, ed. *The elbow and its disorders.* Philadelphia: WB Saunders, 1987.

Colton CL. Fractures of the olecranon in adults: classification and management. *Injury* 1973–1974; 5: 121–129.

Gartsman GM, Sculco TP, Otis JC. Operative treatment of olecranon fractures—excision or open reduction with internal fixation? *J Bone Joint Surg Am* 1981; 63A: 718–721.

Hume MC, Wiss DA. Olecranon fractures: a clinical and radiographic comparison of tension band wiring and plate fixation. *Clin Orthop* 1992; 285: 229–235.

Macko D, Szabo RM. Complications of tension-band wiring of olecranon fractures. *J Bone Joint Surg Am* 1985; 67A: 1396–1401.

Morrey BF. Current concepts in the treatment of fractures of the radial head, the olecranon, and the coronoid. *Instr Course Lect* 1995; 44:175–185.

Murphy DF, Greene WB, Dameron TB. Displaced olecranon fractures in adults. *Clin Orthop* 1987; 224: 215–223.

Rowland SA, Burkhart SS. Tension band wiring of olecranon fractures: a modification of the AO technique. *Clin Orthop* 1993; 277: 238–242.

Schatzker J. Olecranon fractures. In: Schatzker J, Tile M, eds. *The rational basis of operative fracture care.* New York: Springer-Verlag, 1987.

Wolfgang G, Burke F, Bush D, et al. Surgical treatment of displaced olecranon fractures by tension band wiring technique. *Clin Orthop* 1987; 224: 192–204.

SUPRACONDYLAR HUMERUS FRACTURES: OPERATIVE MANAGEMENT

DAVID S. FELDMAN

Supracondylar fractures are the most common pediatric fractures about the elbow and have a peak incidence in the first decade of life. These fractures often instill fear in the treating physician because of the young age of the child, the often gross displacement, and the risk of neurovascular compromise from the injury and treatment. Taking a careful systematic approach to the operative care and postoperative management of these fractures helps alleviate these concerns. This enables the surgeon to have confidence in the operating room and enables the child to have the best possible outcome.

ANATOMY

Isolated supracondylar fractures are extraarticular, lying beyond the proximal extensions of the joint capsule. Appreciation of the anatomic relationships between the structures that make up the elbow complex while in extension is paramount to understanding the mechanisms of injury responsible for these fractures.

The anterior capsule is appreciable thickened and its fibers become most taut with hyperextension of the humeroulnar joint. Remodeling of the metaphysis peaks during the second half of the first decade of life creates a radiographic picture dominated by poorly defined trabeculae, thinned cortices, and metaphyseal flaring. Specifically, there is structural insufficiency about the coronoid and olecranon fossae because of deficiency in the thickness of the anterior and posterior cortices of the medial and lateral supracondylar columns. Furthermore, normal ligamentous laxity of childhood contributes to the mechanisms of injury implicated in supracondylar fractures. In hyperextension, the linear force vector transmitted along the olecranon is converted into a bending force that becomes concentrated in the supracondylar region and propagates through the supracondylar columns as the olecranon, acting as a fulcrum, is driven into the olecranon fossa (Fig. 12-1). Supracondylar fractures are typically transverse and are located at the level of the olecranon fossa.

With complete displacement (see the section on classification), the risk of neurovascular complication is significant. The regional anatomy includes the brachial artery and median nerve located anteriorly in the antecubital fossa, the ulnar nerve coursing posterior to the medial epicondyle, and the radial nerve anterolaterally. Injuries to these neurovascular structures have all been reported.

CLASSIFICATION

Gartland's three-stage classification of extension supracondylar humeral fractures is based on degree of displacement:

Type I: nondisplaced or minimally displaced; the anterior humeral line still passes through the middle third of the ossification center of the capitellum.

Type II: displaced in extension with posterior cortex intact and rotation of the distal fragment (Fig. 12-2).

Type III: completely displaced with both cortices fractured; type III supracondylar fractures can be subclassified (Wilkins' subclassification) based on the position of the distal fragment in the coronal plane, that is, posteromedial and posterolateral (Fig. 12-3).

INDICATIONS

Although stable supracondylar fractures can be managed with closed reduction and casting above the elbow, unstable types II and III fractures require closed reduction with percutaneous pinning to maintain the reduction.

DIAGNOSIS AND PREOPERATIVE PLANNING

A standard radiographic evaluation of the pediatric elbow includes the following:

Anteroposterior (AP) view of the elbow complex with the elbow extended.

■ Evaluation of Baumann's angle, the humeroulnar angle, and the metaphyseal-diaphyseal angle. Baumann's angle is the angle created between the physeal line of the lateral condyle and the long axis of the humerus. An increased

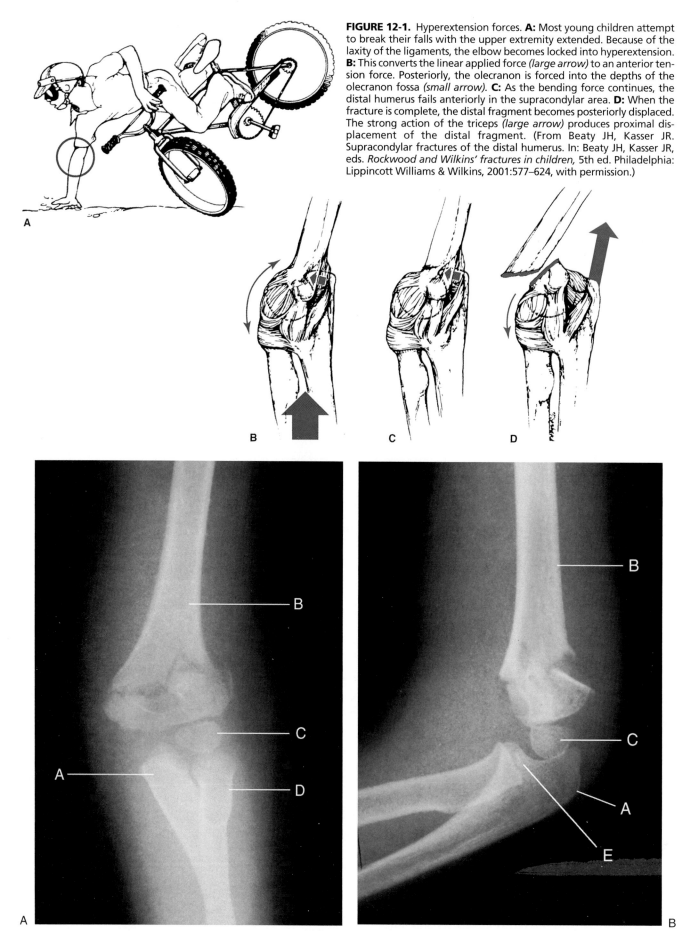

FIGURE 12-1. Hyperextension forces. **A:** Most young children attempt to break their falls with the upper extremity extended. Because of the laxity of the ligaments, the elbow becomes locked into hyperextension. **B:** This converts the linear applied force *(large arrow)* to an anterior tension force. Posteriorly, the olecranon is forced into the depths of the olecranon fossa *(small arrow)*. **C:** As the bending force continues, the distal humerus fails anteriorly in the supracondylar area. **D:** When the fracture is complete, the distal fragment becomes posteriorly displaced. The strong action of the triceps *(large arrow)* produces proximal displacement of the distal fragment. (From Beaty JH, Kasser JR. Supracondylar fractures of the distal humerus. In: Beaty JH, Kasser JR, eds. *Rockwood and Wilkins' fractures in children,* 5th ed. Philadelphia: Lippincott Williams & Wilkins, 2001:577–624, with permission.)

FIGURE 12-2. Type II extension supracondylar humerus fracture (left elbow). **A:** Anterior-posterior. **B:** Lateral. A, ulna; B, humerus; C, capitellar epiphysis; D, radius; E, radial head.

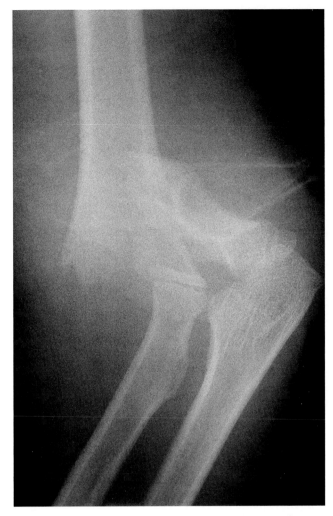

FIGURE 12-3. Type III extension supracondylar humerus fracture (right elbow).

angle compared with the opposite side signifies a varus deformity (Fig. 12-4).

■ Translation as well as comminution of the medial and lateral columns should be assessed on the AP film. The presence of translation of the fracture fragment represents an unstable fracture, because translation requires disruption of both anterior and posterior cortices (Fig. 12-5).

■ Full elbow extension is a prerequisite for obtaining a true AP of the elbow. Often the child's elbow is swollen, painful, and difficult to range. In these circumstances, an AP of the distal humerus can be obtained despite incomplete elbow extension. The distal humerus can be placed on the cassette without forcing the patient to extend the elbow. In addition, an AP of the proximal radius can also be obtained by placing the forearm on the cassette.

Lateral view with the elbow flexed and the forearm in

neutral is best achieved with the shoulder in external rotation.

■ The distal end of the teardrop is formed by the ossific center of the capitellum. An obscured teardrop may represent a displaced fracture.

■ The shaft-condylar angle decrease with extension-type supracondylar fractures as the distal fragment is displaced posteriorly; this angle increases in the less common flexion-type fractures as the distal fracture fragment with the capitellum is driven anteriorly.

■ With extension-type supracondylar fractures, the anterior humeral line passes anterior to the to the middle of the capitellum. Similarly, the coronoid line passes anterior to the lateral condyle with these fractures. Conversely, the anterior humeral and coronoid lines line pass posteriorly with respect to their described landmarks with flexion-type supracondylar fractures (Fig. 12-4).

Oblique View

An oblique view may be necessary to demonstrate a nondisplaced or minimally displaced supracondylar fracture. A high index of suspicion in the setting of negative AP and lateral ra-

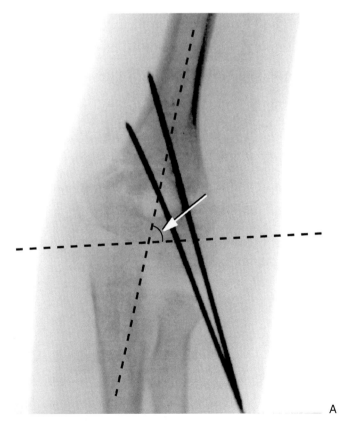

A

FIGURE 12-4. A: Two lateral pins used to obtain fixation for supracondylar humerus fracture. Note divergence of pins and Baumann's angle *(arrow)*. **(continued)**

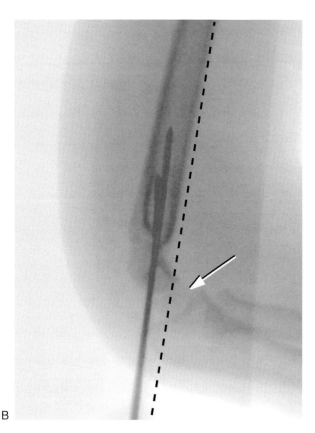

B

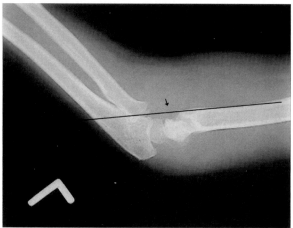

C

FIGURE 12-4. *(Continued)* **B:** Note lateral reduction of fracture on lateral film. Note anterohumeral line and relationship with capitellum *(arrow)*. **C:** Anterior humeral line falling in front of capitellum (left elbow).

diographs warrants this view. This view is also used during the pinning of a fracture to see the reduction of the columns.

MEDIAL-LATERAL CROSSED-PIN FIXATION VERSUS LATERAL PARALLEL PIN CONSTRUCT

The optimal configuration of pin fixation continues to be debated in the literature. Contemporary textbooks of pediatric orthopaedics describe the crossed-pin configuration as the preferred treatment, except when the medial epicondyle

or the ulnar nerve cannot be palpated. Several studies report that lateral pin fixation performed correctly is effective in maintaining reduction (Fig. 12-5).

EQUIPMENT

The following equipment is needed (Fig. 12-6):

- Power wire driver
- 0.062-inch Kirschner wires (K-wires) for percutaneous pin fixation
- C-arm fluoroscopic image intensifier

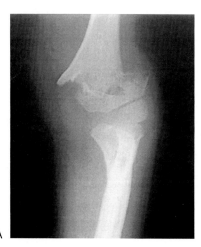

A

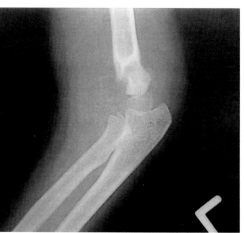

B

FIGURE 12-5. Supracondylar humerus fracture demonstrating lateral translation of the distal fragment: **A:** Anteroposterior. **B:** Lateral (left elbow).

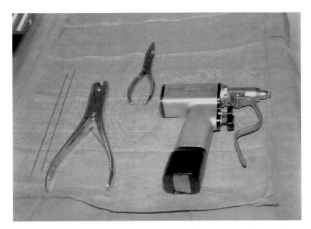

FIGURE 12-6. Instruments *(left to right):* 0.062 K-wires, wire cutter, needle-nose pliers, and power wire driver.

- 3-inch plaster slabs
- Webril/Ace bandages

OPERATIVE TECHNIQUE

Patient Positioning

The patient is positioned supine so that the shoulder is at the edge of the table. No tourniquet is applied; however, a

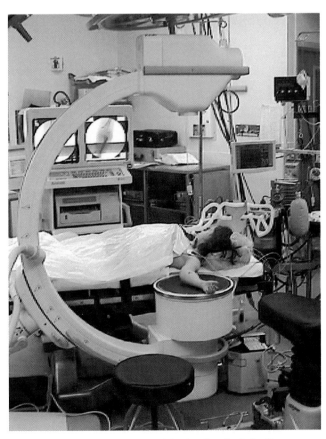

FIGURE 12-7. Patient positioning for the left elbow.

sterile one should be available. The affected upper extremity is prepped and draped in a sterile fashion. The C-arm image intensifier is positioned adjacent, parallel to the table and covered with a sterile drape. The patient's elbow is placed on the image intensification machine. The image intensifier is used as the operating table so further radiographs can be obtained to reevaluate the fracture pattern, assess the closed reduction, and confirm K-wire placements. The monitor is placed on the opposite side of the table in the surgeon's direct line of vision. The surgeon and assistant are seated for the procedure. The surgeon sits on the lateral side of the elbow (Fig. 12-7).

Closed Reduction

Closed reduction of extension-type supracondylar fractures uses the following technique:

- Correction of medial/lateral displacement. Medial or lateral translation is corrected by applying a translational force with or without a valgus or varus moment in the coronal plane to the distal fragment. Confirmation of fragment placement is achieved with image intensification with the elbow in extension. Minimal traction is used to achieve this reduction (Fig. 12-8).
- Correction of rotation. Posteromedial displacement usually may require pronation of the forearm and posterolateral displacement may require supination of the forearm. The correction of medial/lateral translation and rotation must be corrected before the elbow is flexed.
- Correction of posterior displacement/angulation. Minimal traction is maintained. Posterior displacement is corrected as the distal fragment is lifted anteriorly as the surgeon places a thumb on the olecranon, slowly pushing it distally and anteriorly. The elbow is flexed during this maneuver to tighten the posterior periosteal hinge and reduce the fracture. Pronation may be needed in full flexion in order to lock the fracture fragments (Fig. 12-9).
- Confirmatory radiographs—four views. AP and lateral films should be obtained to document acceptable reduction. The AP view is often unobtainable for fractures with the elbow in full flexion; therefore, oblique medial and lateral column views should be used instead. Any residual medial/lateral angulation in the coronal plane must be corrected to prevent cubitus varus and valgus. Residual malrotation of the distal fragment, suggested when the two segments at the fracture appear to have different diameters, should also be corrected, although the patient often compensates clinically because of the multiple degrees of freedom available at the glenohumeral joint. The lateral view should be used to check flexion-extension alignment and confirm restoration of the shaft-condylar angle. The presence of the crescent sign, created with overlap of the ossification center of the lateral condyle and olecranon, suggests residual angulation in the distal fragment.

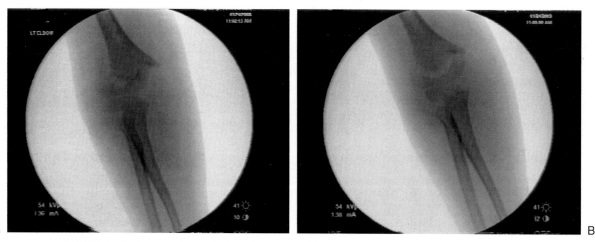

FIGURE 12-8. A: Lateral translation of supracondylar humerus fracture. **B:** Post reduction in extension (right elbow).

Percutaneous Pinning

Percutaneous fixation is indicated for reduced types II and III fractures. After closed reduction is achieved, 0.062-inch K-wires are introduced under image intensification control to secure the reduction.

Pin Fixation

The K-wires must engage the distal fragment and should pass through the medial and lateral columns, cross proximal to the fracture site, and penetrate the opposite cortices (Fig. 12-10). In the coronal plane, the pins should be oriented 30 to 40 degrees to the long axis of the humerus so that they are fixed in the center of the supracondylar columns. Less stable fixation is achieved when the pins cross at the fracture site.

■ ▣ The lateral K-wire is introduced first while the surgeon holds the elbow in acute flexion while palpating the lateral condyle. Under image intensification, a lateral column view can be used to ensure that the K-wire enters the cortex distal to the fracture. Confirmation of the position of the pin is performed on the lateral view. The

medial cortex must be penetrated to achieve adequate stability. A second lateral pin should be inserted more medial and this pin may go through the olecranon fossa and then through the medial cortex. The pins should be slightly convergent proximal to distal (Fig. 12-4). This

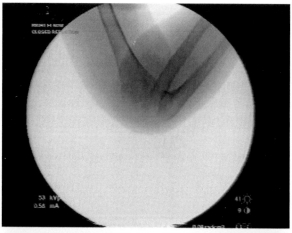

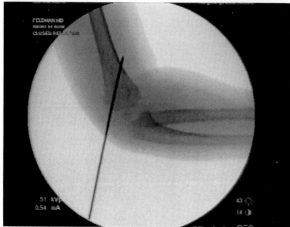

A,B

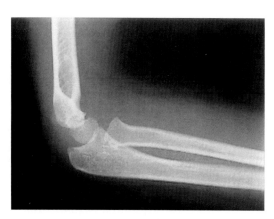

FIGURE 12-9. Post reduction lateral.

FIGURE 12-10. A: Demonstration of lateral column closed reduction. **B:** Pin fixation of lateral column.

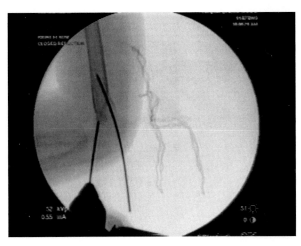

FIGURE 12-11. Medial pin being inserted. Note anterior to posterior direction on lateral film.

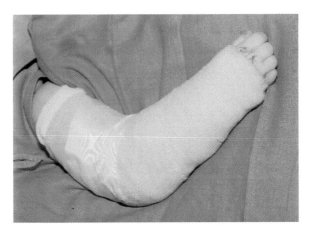

FIGURE 12-13. Post surgical splint in 60 degrees of elbow flexion.

may be the only fixation that is required, or one can insert a medial pin for added fixation if the fracture is noted to be unstable on fluoroscopy.

For the preferred cross-wire fixation, insertion of the lateral pin first allows the surgeon to introduce the medial pin with the elbow maintained in less than full flexion, thus reducing potential injury to the ulnar nerve. ◨ The thumb of the left hand of the (right-handed) surgeon palpates the inferior edge of the medial epicondyle and drops into the ulnar groove to palpate the ulnar nerve before the medial K-wire is introduced. The medial pin begins at the center of, or anterior to, the medial epicondyle and is directed from anteromedial to posterolateral. As reported in clinical studies, the ulnar nerve is at risk during placement of the medial pin (Fig. 12-11).

Following pin fixation, the elbow is reexamined in all four views (AP, lateral, internal oblique, and external oblique) to confirm reduction. ◨ Motion at the fracture site should be evaluated under image intensification (Fig.

12-12). Following acceptable reduction, the pins are cut and bent over to facilitate easy removal on follow-up.

Immobilization

The arm is immobilized in a safe amount of flexion. This is determined by the degree of swelling. No pressure on the antecubital fossa skin or soft tissue is allowed. If the arm is very swollen one may immobilize the arm in as little as 20 to 30 degrees of flexion. The forearm is in neutral position. Remember that the pins not the splint are maintaining reduction. The arm is wrapped with generous padding that may then be split, and the plaster splint is appropriately secured with a loose Ace bandage. Care must given to secure the splint to allow for postoperative swelling (Fig. 12-13).

POSTOPERATIVE PROTOCOL

Postoperatively, neurovascular examinations are made and the patient is checked for any signs of compartment syndrome.

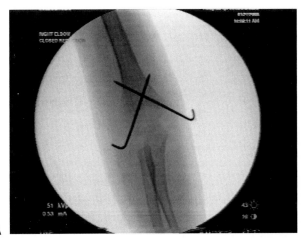

A

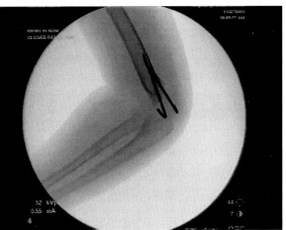

B

FIGURE 12-12. **A:** Post reduction anteroposterior with pins crossing above the fracture. **B:** Post reduction lateral.

The patient often goes home the next day if he or she is comfortable. At 1 week, AP and lateral radiographs are obtained to ensure that the reduction has been maintained. If the patient was placed in a splint with little flexion, the splint can be changed at this time. The patient is then seen again 2 weeks later (3 weeks postoperatively), and radiographs are obtained with the splint off. If there is evidence of healing, which is almost uniformly the case, the pins are removed in the office. The parents are asked to encourage the child to flex and extend the elbow but not to do it for the child, that is, no assisted or passive range of motion. A sling or removable splint may be used to protect the child when he or she is playing or in danger of injury. For the most part immobilization is not used.

The child is then seen again 3 weeks later to assess range of motion. Most often, radiographs are not needed at that time, and physical and occupational therapy are rarely needed. Further follow-up depends on the outcome and specific case.

SUGGESTED READINGS

Herring JA. Upper extremity injuries. In: Herring JA, Mihran O, eds. *Tachdjian's pediatric orthopedics,* 3rd ed. Philadelphia: WB Saunders, 2002: 2139–2168.

Wilkins KE. Fractures and dislocations of the elbow region. In: *Fractures in children,* vol 3. Philadelphia: Lippincott-Raven, 1996: 655–744.

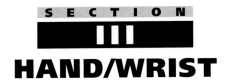
CHAPTER 13

OPEN CARPAL TUNNEL RELEASE

MARTIN A. POSNER

Carpal tunnel syndrome is the most commonly encountered compressive neuropathy in the upper extremity. It is not a single disease entity but rather a constellation of symptoms. Although some of these symptoms were reported in 1854 by Sir James Paget in a patient who had sustained a fracture of his distal radius, it was not until the 1930s that numbness following distal radius fractures was associated with median nerve compression. The term *carpal tunnel syndrome* was coined by Moersch in 1938, but it was not until Phalen published a series of articles beginning in 1950 that the condition was popularized. It is estimated that approximately 1 million adults in the United States are diagnosed each year with carpal tunnel syndrome.

ANATOMY

The carpal tunnel is a well-defined anatomic channel that topographically extends from the wrist flexion crease to the midpalm, a distance of about 4 cm. It is a semirigid channel whose floor and sides are formed by a concave arch of carpal bones and whose roof or palmar surface is the transverse carpal ligament (Fig. 13-1). The ligament, whose proximal margin blends into the antebrachial fascia of the forearm, measures 3 to 4 cm in width and 2.5 to 3.5 cm in thickness. It attaches radially to the scaphoid tubercle and trapezial ridge and ulnarly to the hook of the hamate and pisiform. The carpal tunnel is the conduit for the median nerve and digital flexor tendons from the forearm into the hand. Nine flexor tendons pass through the tunnel, the flexor superficialis and profundus to each finger and the flexor pollicis longus to the thumb. The median nerve lies immediately beneath the transverse carpal ligament and at this site is comprised of 30 to 35 fascicles. The sensory fascicles to the middle finger are usually the most superficial (volar), and the motor fascicles to the thenar intrinsic muscles are situated volar and radial.

The anatomic course of the motor branch of the median nerve is variable and is classified according to its relationship to the transverse carpal ligament. In most cases (47%) the nerve branches just distal to the ligament and takes a *recurrent* or *extraligamentous* course to the muscles. Less often (31%), it branches within the tunnel and takes a *subligamentous* course to the muscles, and in 23% of cases it actually penetrates the ligament and takes a *transligamentous* course. The median artery travels on the volar surface of the median nerve. It is usually a thin vestigial structure but occasionally it is sizable and makes a significant contribution to the superficial palmar arterial arch.

CLASSIFICATION AND INDICATIONS

Compression of the median nerve in the carpal tunnel is the most commonly encountered compressive neuropathy in the upper extremity. It generally worsens with time and can,

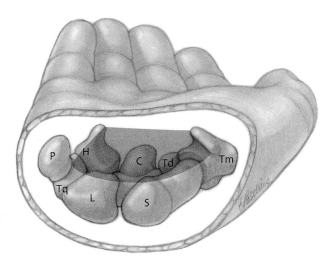

FIGURE 13-1. The carpal tunnel is a fibroosseous canal. Associated bones which contribute to its boundaries include the hook process of the hamate (*H*), capitate (*C*), trapezoid (*Td*), pisiform (*P*), triquetrum (*Tq*), lunate (*L*), scaphoid (*S*), and trapezium (*Tm*). The roof is formed by the flexor retinaculum. (From Berger RA, Doyle JR, Botte MJ. Wrist. In: Doyle JR, Botte MJ, eds. *Surgical anatomy of the hand and upper extremity.* Philadelphia: Lippincott Williams & Wilkins, 2003:486–531, with permission.)

therefore, be classified into early, intermediate, and advanced stages based on symptoms, physical findings, and electrodiagnostic studies. The early stage of the disease is when symptoms have been present for less than one year. There is rarely any intrinsic muscle weakness during this stage. Electrodiagnostic studies usually show some delay in sensor conduction, although the studies are often negative. Treatment for the early stage is generally nonoperative. If the patient has nighttime paresthesias, the use of a wrist splint while sleeping is usually effective. In the absence of thenar muscle weakness, the indication for surgery depends solely on the magnitude of discomfort that only the patient can determine. If that discomfort interferes with the patient's work and/or leisure time activities, surgery is recommended.

Surgery is almost always indicated for the intermediate stage because there is usually thenar muscle weakness. A decrease in strength of these muscles, as demonstrated on physical examination, is the key indication for surgery even when the patient's sensory complaints are not disabling or even when nighttime paresthesias are eliminated with the use of a wrist splint. A wrist splint provides only symptomatic improvement; it is not therapeutic and does not reduce or reverse the deleterious effects of compression on the motor fascicles.

The advanced stage is usually characterized not only by thenar muscle weakness but also by atrophy of these muscles. In some cases, the atrophy is so severe that there is complete wasting of the thenar eminence and there is no longer any muscle mass covering the radial side of the thumb metacarpal. Although surgery is unlikely to improve this situation, especially in elderly patients, it usually relieves some of the sensory complaints, particularly nighttime paresthesias. Numbness, however, often persists. Paresthesias and numbness are separate and distinct symptoms, and patients often have difficulty distinguishing between them, particularly preoperatively. It is not uncommon for patients to report that following surgery their paresthesias were relieved but that their fingers remained "numb." Consequently, they believe that the operation was unsuccessful or, worse, that the surgeon was negligent and failed to decompress the carpal tunnel. Actually, the persistence of numbness is related to the severity and chronicity of median nerve compression that has resulted in permanent damage to the sensory fascicles. Before surgery it is important to explain to patients the limited objectives of the operation. They should be informed that the primary objective is to prevent further nerve damage and that, although paresthesias will probably diminish, any improvement in sensibility and/or thenar muscle strength depends on the ability of the nerve to recover. In all likelihood, that improvement will be incomplete and in advanced cases there may not be any improvement. Surgery should, therefore, be performed before irreversible nerve changes develop. It is for that reason that patients whose carpal tunnel

is in the intermediate stage are advised to undergo surgery without any undue delay. Although delaying surgery for weeks is not detrimental, deferring it for months is ill-advised.

PREOPERATIVE PLANNING

As with any medical condition, a comprehensive history and physical examination are important. A history of an endocrine disorder such as diabetes mellitus or thyroid dysfunction may be indicative of a demyelinating polyneuropathy rather than a localized compressive neuropathy. Electrodiagnostic studies are useful to differentiate between the two types of neuropathies. Even in the absence of a polyneuropathy, endocrine disorders can "sensitize" nerves to the effects of even mild compression. Carpal tunnel syndrome, therefore, tends to be more common in diabetic than nondiabetic patients. Patients with carpal tunnel syndrome are also prone to develop compressive neuropathies at other sites (e.g., ulnar nerve at the elbow). They are also likely to develop trigger fingers. The frequency of these associations gives added importance to obtaining a complete history and conducting a comprehensive physical examination each time that the patient is seen. Even in the absence of any concomitant problem, the patient should be informed that other compressive neuropathies and/or trigger fingers could develop at some future time. It is important to emphasize that these problems are not a complication of surgery and that they are as likely to develop in patients who opt not to have surgery.

EQUIPMENT/INSTRUMENTS

A hand operating table is preferable to operating on an armboard. The greater width of a hand table facilitates better instrument control by the surgeon and surgical assistant because they are able to rest their forearms on the table. Surgical instruments are standard hand instruments.

POSITIONING AND PLANNING

The patient is placed in a supine position on the operating room table with his or her arm outstretched on the operating hand table. The hand table is positioned so that the patient's arm is abducted about 70 degrees at the shoulder. **Abduction greater than 90 degrees should be avoided because it can result in postoperative shoulder discomfort and possibly a traction injury to the brachial plexus.** The operation is usually performed under regional block anesthesia, either an axillary block or infraclavicular block, and tourniquet control (Figs. 13-2 and 13-3).

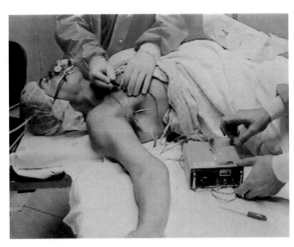

FIGURE 13-2. With the patient in the supine position and the arm on the operating hand table, the anesthesiologist administers an infraclavicular anesthetic block. A nerve stimulator facilitates localization of the brachial plexus.

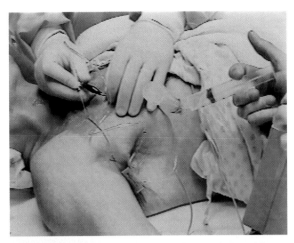

FIGURE 13-3. With the needle in the correct position, the anesthetic is injected.

SURGICAL APPROACH AND PROCEDURE

An incision is made in the thenar crease in the palm or in the crease that often lies just ulnar to the thenar crease. The incision is made directly in the crease and not adjacent to it, and it is carried proximally to stop at the wrist flexion crease (Fig. 13-4). ◼ In most cases, this surgical approach provides excellent visualization of the entire carpal tunnel. However, in the patient whose carpal tunnel syndrome is secondary to a proliferative tenosynovitis of the flexor tendons, as seen in rheumatoid arthritis for which a tenosynovectomy is required, the incision is carried more proxi-

mally into the distal forearm. When the incision is extended proximally, it should not cross the wrist flexion crease at a right angle because it will likely result in a hypertrophic, unsightly scar. Instead, the incision is continued ulnarly within the wrist flexion crease for a distance of 1 to 2 cm and it is then curved proximally. A similar surgical approach is sometimes necessary to achieve satisfactory exposure in nonrheumatoid patients who have thick, beefy hands.

After the skin incision is completed, the subcutaneous tissues are incised and care is taken to avoid injury to the palmar cutaneous nerve that branches from the main body of the median nerve proximal to the wrist flexion crease (Fig. 13-4). ◼ Usually, the palmar cutaneous nerve is not seen because it is radial to the incision. However, it sometimes crosses the incision site and should be protected. The palmar fascia is then incised, and in the proximal portion of the operative field the palmaris longus tendon is retracted radially. Cutting the palmaris longus tendon should be avoided because it can retract proximal to the wrist flexion crease and leave a ball of tissue that the patient may complain is unsightly. Following incision of the palmar fascia, the proximal portion of the transverse carpal ligament is usually obscured by fat tissue extending from the hypothenar area. Rather than cutting through this fat tissue, it is mobilized by sectioning one or two vertical septa of the palmar fascia. The fat tissue can then easily be retracted ulnarly, which permits excellent visualization of the entire length of the transverse carpal ligament. ◼ The transverse carpal ligament is then incised (Fig. 13-5); this should be done slowly to avoid injury to the median nerve and its motor branch. A motor branch that takes a transligamentous course to the thenar muscles is especially vulnerable to injury. A clue to the presence of a motor branch that takes this route is a small clump of fat tissue at the site where the branch penetrates the ligament. It is important to ensure

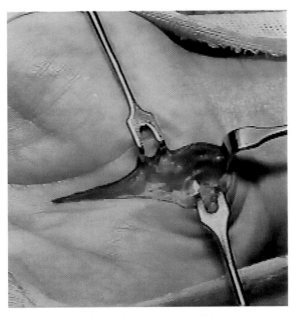

FIGURE 13-4. The skin incision is made within a skin crease adjacent to the thenar crease and is carried proximally to stop at the wrist flexion crease.

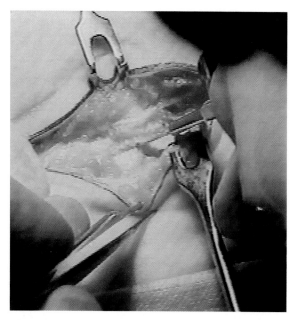

FIGURE 13-5. The transverse carpal ligament is divided and care is taken to avoid injury to a motor branch that has a transligamentous approach to the thenar muscles.

that the entire length of the transverse carpal ligament has been divided. It is also advisable to release the distal portion of the antebrachial fascia (Fig. 13-6). ◖▶

The median nerve usually lies immediately beneath the divided ligament. However, in some cases it is adherent to the radial side of the ligament and is not immediately visualized. **The median nerve must be mobilized from this position; in doing so the surgeon rather than the surgical assistant should position the retractor to avoid injuring the nerve by inadvertently placing the retractor, particularly a rake retractor, directly into or around the nerve (Figs. 13-7 and 13-8).** ◖▶ The motor branch is then visualized; this is facilitated by blunt dissection along the radial border of the median nerve. The first branch is usually the motor branch.

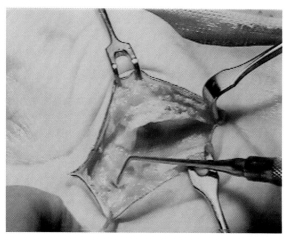

FIGURE 13-6. With the transverse carpal ligament divided, the superficial arterial palmar arch is visualized.

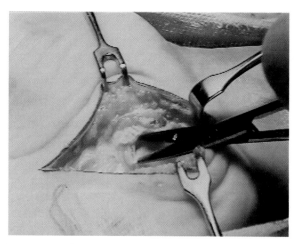

FIGURE 13-7. Thickened fibrotic tenosynovium tissue is excised to visualize the compressed median nerve.

When dissecting along the ulnar border of the median nerve, a thin nerve branch is sometimes encountered. This is a sensory branch that connects with the common digital nerve from the ulnar nerve and should be protected. As with a transligamentous motor branch of the median nerve, a clue to the presence of this thin sensory branch is some fat tissue along the ulnar border of the median nerve.

In some cases, nerve compression is secondary to hypertrophic tenosynovitis and a tenosynovectomy is performed (Figs. 13-9 and 13-10). ◖▶ The indication for an epineurolysis (epineurotomy or epineurectomy) at the site of nerve compression is controversial. Although some believe it is unnecessary, it is probably beneficial when there is a severe

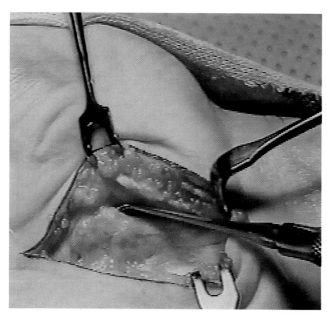

FIGURE 13-8. The motor branch is identified. It is situated just distal to the transverse carpal ligament, which is the most common location (recurrent or extraligamentous) for a motor branch.

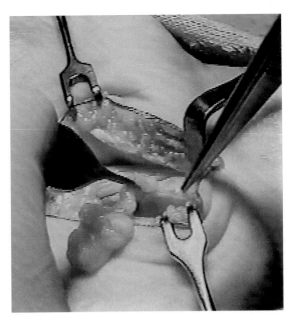

FIGURE 13-9. Thickened fibrotic tenosynovium is excised.

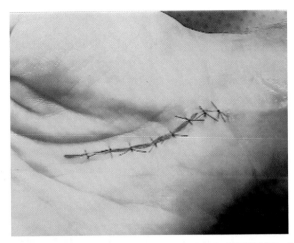

FIGURE 13-11. The skin is closed with interrupted 4-0 nylon sutures.

compression and the epineurium is thickened. The entire carpal tunnel, including the floor of the tunnel deep to the tendons, should be inspected. Occasionally, a mass such as a ganglion arising from the floor of the tunnel is the cause for nerve compression. At the conclusion of surgery, the tourniquet is released and any bleeding points cauterized. It is unnecessary to lengthen the transverse carpal ligament by any Z-plasty procedure, and only the skin incision must be sutured (Fig. 13-11). A gauze dressing is applied to the hand and wrist. A bulky dressing that interferes with digital flexion or extension should be avoided (Fig. 13-12). The use of a wrist splint depends on the personal preference of the surgeon. It is rarely necessary, but if one is applied it should be discontinued after a week or two.

POSTOPERATIVE PROTOCOL

Elevation of the limb is recommended to minimize postoperative swelling. To be effective, elevation must be constant; to emphasize this point, patients are told that keeping their hand in a dependent position for 1 minute negates keeping it elevated for hours. Digital exercises are encouraged as soon as the effects of the anesthetic block have worn off. Patients are instructed to actively flex and extend their fingers and thumb on a regular basis. They are encouraged to perform these exercises 10 times each hour. The frequency of exercising is much more important than the duration of

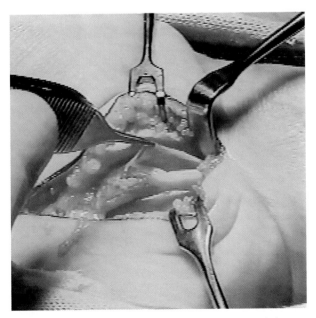

FIGURE 13-10. In this patient the epineurium around the compressed portion of the nerve was abnormally thick and it was also excised.

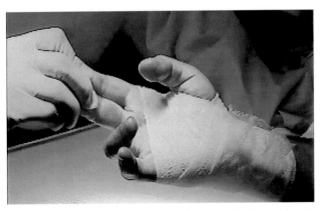

FIGURE 13-12. The postoperative bandage is thin and only around the palm and wrist to avoid interfering with digital motions.

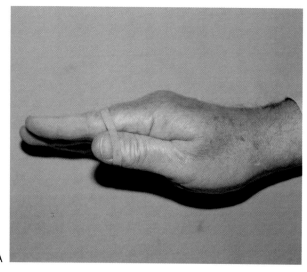

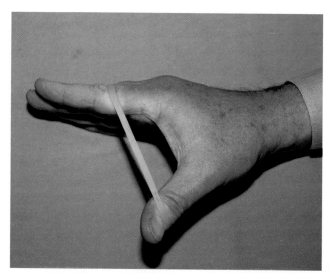

FIGURE 13-13. A and **B:** Resistive exercises are used to improve thenar strength.

each session. Patients who exercise effectively usually regain complete digital mobility within the first week. Active range of motion exercises are also encouraged for the shoulder, elbow, and wrist.

FOLLOW-UP

The sutures are generally removed the second week, and active resistive exercises are then instituted. Resistive exercises for the thenar muscles involve abducting the thumb against resistance. This is best achieved by wrapping a rubber band around the palm and thumb, at the level of the interphalangeal joint, and abducting the thumb against the resistance of the rubber band (Fig. 13-13). Similar to digital exercises, 10 repetitions are encouraged each hour. As thenar muscle strength improves, the exercises are performed against greater resistance using thicker rubber bands or multiple rubber bands. Swelling and induration at the operative site are common but gradually diminish over the ensuing weeks. Application of a thin silicone pad to the area hastens the normal maturation process of the scar. Patients can usually resume light work activities 2 to 3 weeks after surgery and strenuous activities, including sports activities, within 6

to 8 weeks. Serious amateur and professional athletes often return to their sport as early as 1 week after surgery.

SUGGESTED READINGS

Bleecker ML, Bohlman M, Moreland R, et al. Carpal tunnel syndrome: the role of carpal canal size. *Neurology* 1985; 35: 1599–1604.

Clayburgh RH, Beckenbaugh RD, Dobyns JH. Carpal tunnel release in patients with diffuse peripheral neuropathy. *J Hand Surg Am* 1987; 12A: 380–382.

Cobb TK, Dalley BK, Posteraro RH, et al. Anatomy of the flexor retinaculum. *J Hand Surg Am* 1993; 18A: 91–99.

Cobb TK, Cooney WP, An KN. Pressure dynamics of the carpal tunnel and flexor compartment of the forearm. *J Hand Surg [Am]* 1995; 20A: 193–198.

Dellon AL, Kallman CM. Evaluation of functional sensation in the hand. *J Hand Surg [Am]* 1983; 8: 865–870.

Ditmars DM. Patterns of carpal tunnel syndrome. *Hand Clin* 2993; 9: 241–252.

Kerwin G, Williams CS, Seiler JG. The pathophysiology of carpal tunnel syndrome. *Hand Clin* 1996; 12: 243–251.

Lanz U. Anatomic variation of the median nerve in the carpal tunnel. *J Hand Surg [Am]* 1977; 2A: 44–53.

Stevens JC, Beard M, O'Fallon WM, et al. Conditions associated with carpal tunnel syndrome. *Mayo Clin Proc* 1992; 67: 541–548.

CHAPTER 14

DE QUERVAIN'S RELEASE

MICHAEL E. RETTIG

Tenosynovitis of the first dorsal compartment was initially described by de Quervain in 1895. The abductor pollicis longus (APL) and the extensor pollicis brevis (EPB) are inflamed as they pass under the extensor retinaculum of the first dorsal compartment. Localized tenderness and swelling in this region with a positive Finkelstein test confirm the diagnosis of de Quervain's tenosynovitis. Initial nonoperative treatment consists of splinting and local cortisone injection. If conservative modalities fail to relieve the symptoms, surgical decompression of the first compartment is indicated.

ANATOMY

The extensor tendons on the dorsum of the hand and wrist are contained in six compartments (Fig. 14-1). The first extensor compartment, which is the most radial compartment, contains the tendons of the APL and the EPB. The extensor retinaculum covers the tendons in the first compartment and holds them adjacent to the radial styloid. Proximal to the wrist, these tendons cross superficial to the radial wrist extensors in the second dorsal compartment, and they then form the palmar border of the anatomic snuff box. The APL originates from the posterior surface of the radius and ulna and inserts onto the base of the thumb metacarpal. The APL is an abductor and extensor of the thumb and is innervated by the posterior interosseous nerve. The EPB originates from the posterior surface of the radius and interosseous membrane and inserts onto the dorsal base of the thumb proximal phalanx. The EPB extends the thumb proximal phalanx and is also innervated by the posterior interosseous nerve.

Within the anatomic snuffbox, the radial artery passes deep from the volar forearm into the interosseous space between the thumb and index finger metacarpals. The radial sensory nerve branches superficial to the first compartment tendons, as it innervates the skin over the dorsum of the thumb and fingers.

Many variations within the first dorsal compartment have been described, and these must be known before surgical treatment is performed to ensure complete release of both the APL and EPB. These include multiple slips of the APL, variable insertions of the APL, and separate compartments for the APL and EPB tendons. Failure to recognize these variations and subsequent incomplete release of the APL or EPB will result in persistence of symptoms after surgical decompression of the first dorsal compartment.

INDICATIONS

Initial management of de Quervain's tenosynovitis consists of splinting with a thumb spica splint to immobilize the involved tendons. Corticosteroid is also injected into the first compartment. Oral nonsteroidal antiinflammatory medication can be helpful in mild cases in conjunction with splinting. If the patient fails to respond adequately to these modalities, surgical release of the first dorsal compartment is indicated.

SPECIAL EQUIPMENT AND PATIENT POSITIONING

The patient is positioned supine on the operating room table, with the upper extremity on an arm board or hand table. A pneumatic tourniquet is placed on the proximal aspect of the upper extremity, over a layer of padding, and is preset to 250 mm Hg (Fig. 14-2). The surgeon sits within the corner made by the arm board and the operating room table. The skin and subcutaneous tissue just proximal to the radial styloid is infiltrated with 2% lidocaine without epinephrine, and the extremity is then prepped and draped in the usual sterile fashion.

INCISION

Before incising the skin, the radial styloid is palpated, and the skin incision is marked with a sterile marking pen or methylene blue. A variety of skin incisions have been described for exposure and release of the first compartment. The skin incision must provide adequate exposure to identify and protect the radial sensory nerve branches that lie superficial to the extensor retinaculum covering the first dorsal compartment.

Typically, a 2-cm transverse incision is marked 1 cm proximal to the radial styloid, at the radial aspect of the wrist (Fig. 14-3). This incision allows for exposure and safe retraction of the radial sensory nerve branches before incision of the retinaculum. Other potential incisions include a short oblique incision, zigzag incision, and a chevron incision, with the apex volarly to allow for retraction of a dorsal flap of skin and subcutaneous tissue. A transverse incision proximal to the radial styloid in a natural skin crease provides adequate exposure and heals well. A longitudinal skin incision is more likely to result in an unsightly painful hypertrophic scar.

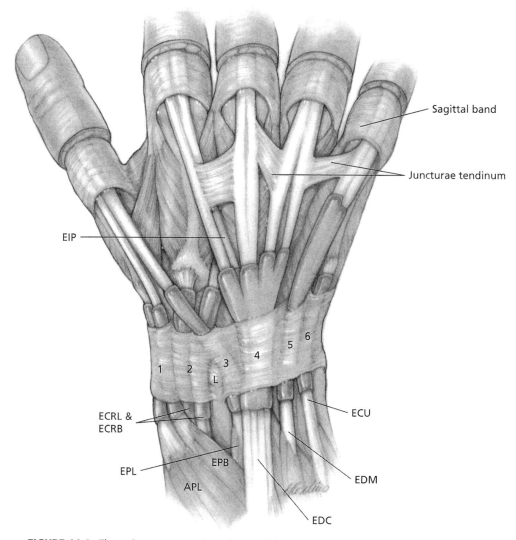

FIGURE 14-1. The wrist extensor retinaculum and the most common arrangement of the extensor tendons and juncturae. The wrist, thumb, and finger extensors gain entrance to the hand beneath the extensor retinaculum through a series of six tunnels, and at this level are covered with a synovial sheath. (From Doyle JR. Hand. In: Doyle JR, Botte MB, eds. *Surgical anatomy of the hand and upper extremity.* Philadelphia: Lippincott Williams & Wilkins, 2003:532–666, with permission.)

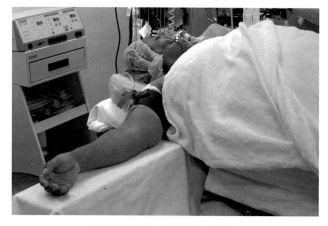

FIGURE 14-2. Patient position.

SURGICAL APPROACH AND PROCEDURE 📷

After satisfactory local anesthesia, the upper extremity is exsanguinated, and the tourniquet is inflated to 250 mm Hg. The skin is sharply incised with a no. 15 scalpel along the marked incision line. After sharply incising the skin (Fig. 14-4), the subcutaneous dissection is performed with a blunt-tipped scissors to the level of the extensor retinaculum over the first dorsal compartment. The branches of the radial sensory nerve are identified and carefully retracted dorsally and volarly to expose the extensor retinaculum (Fig. 14-5).

Injury to the radial sensory nerve can result in a greater problem for the patient than was the first-compartment

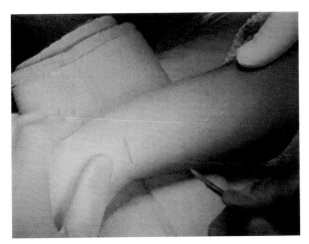

FIGURE 14-3. Transverse skin incision marked 1 cm proximal to radial styloid.

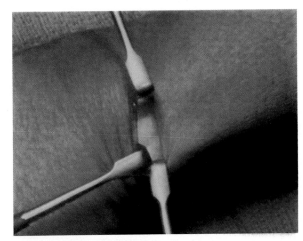

FIGURE 14-6. Proximal extent of the extensor retinaculum.

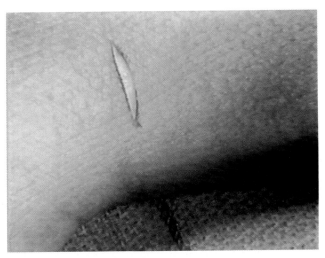

FIGURE 14-4. Skin incision completed, before subcutaneous dissection and identification of radial sensory nerve.

tenosynovitis. The radial sensory nerve and its branches are superficial and are prone to injury with a deep skin incision. After sharply incising the skin, the subcutaneous tissue should be bluntly dissected off the retinaculum and retracted, before the retinaculum is divided. It is not necessary to identify and dissect all of the branches of the radial sensory nerve; this will result in symptomatic neuropraxia and possibly loss of sensation over the dorsal aspect of the thumb and index finger.

The most distal and proximal edge of the extensor retinaculum can be identified by careful distal and then proximal retraction of the skin (Figs. 14-6 and 14-7). Again, the branches of the radial sensory nerve are carefully retracted. With a scalpel, the extensor retinaculum is then incised longitudinally along the length of the first compartment, in the dorsal aspect of the retinaculum (Fig. 14-8). By incising the extensor retinaculum in this fashion, a palmar-based flap of

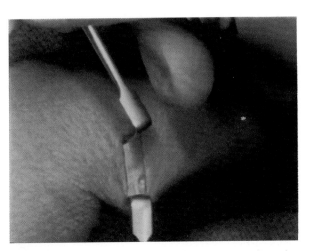

FIGURE 14-5. Identification of radial sensory nerve branches.

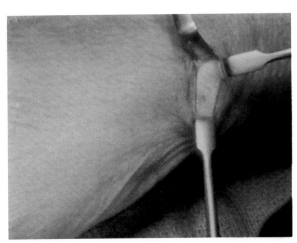

FIGURE 14-7. Distal extent of the extensor retinaculum.

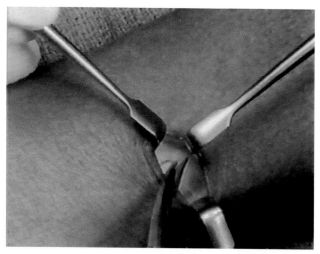

FIGURE 14-8. Incision in the dorsal aspect of the extensor retinaculum.

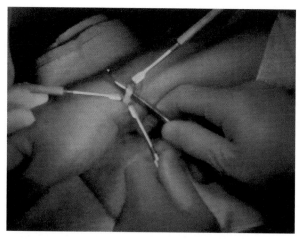

FIGURE 14-11. Traction on the decompressed extensor pollicis brevis tendon.

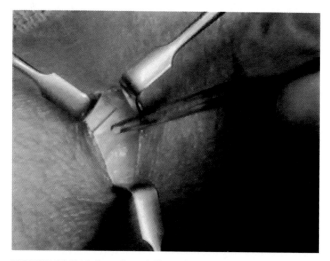

FIGURE 14-9. Palmar-based flap of extensor retinaculum prevents volar subluxation.

retinaculum remains to prevent volar subluxation of the tendons of the first compartment.

Division of the retinaculum in the dorsal aspect with preservation of a palmar-based flap minimizes potential volar subluxation of the extensors that can occur with wrist flexion (Fig. 14-9). Postoperative splinting with the wrist in extension may also limit this complication.

The tendons of the first compartment, the EPB and the APL, are then inspected (Fig. 14-10). The EPB lies dorsal in the first compartment and typically has a more distal muscle belly. The APL is more volar in the first compartment and typically has multiple slips. The tendons may be housed in two separate compartments within the first compartment, and if there is a septum dividing the first compartment, both tendons must be relieved of constriction.

There are many variations of the anatomy of the first dorsal compartment. These include multiple slips of the APL, anomalous insertions of the tendons, and the presence of a

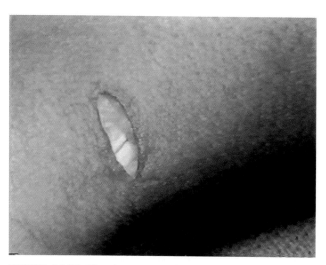

FIGURE 14-10. The decompressed tendons of the dorsal compartment.

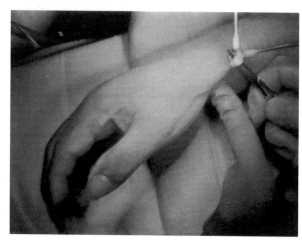

FIGURE 14-12. Traction on the released abductor pollicis longus tendon.

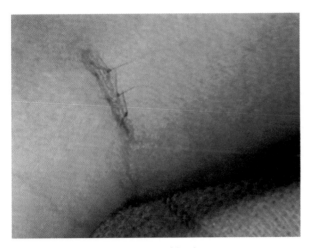

FIGURE 14-13. Skin closure.

septum within the first compartment separating the APL and EPB. Inadequate operative release of the retinaculum can be avoided by careful identification and decompression of both the APL and EPB during the surgical procedure.

Gentle traction to the two tendons is applied by a hemostat to verify their release. Traction on the EPB tendon extends the metacarpophalangeal joint (Fig. 14-11), and tension on the APL abducts and extends the thumb metacarpal shaft (Fig. 14-12). Release of both tendons must be completed before wound closure.

After release of the first compartment, the tourniquet is deflated. Hemostasis is obtained with electrocautery. The wound is irrigated and closed with 5-0 nylon suture (Fig. 14-13). A bulky hand dressing is then applied, with a thumb spica plaster splint in wrist extension. The patient is transferred to the recovery room to be discharged later in the day. The patient is given a prescription for analgesia and is instructed on strict elevation of the hand for several days.

POSTOPERATIVE PROTOCOL AND FOLLOW-UP

The patient is seen approximately 10 days after the surgical procedure. The dressing and the sutures are removed. A removable thumb spica splint is provided and used intermittently for 2 weeks, with the patient gradually weaning from the splint as the discomfort resolves.

SELECTED READINGS

Finkelstein H. Stenosing tendovaginitis at the radial styloid process. *J Bone Joint Surg* 1930;12:509–540.

Harvey FJ, Harvey PM, Horsley MW. De Quervain's disease: surgical or nonsurgical treatment. *J Hand Surg (Am)* 1990; 15A: 83–87.

Jackson WT, Viegas SF, Coon TM, et al. Anatomic variations in the first extensor compartment of the wrist: a clinical and anatomical study. *J Bone Joint Surg Am* 1986; 68A: 923–926.

Weiss APC, Akelman E, Tabatabai M. Treatment of de Quervain's disease. *J Hand Surg (Am)* 1994; 19A: 595–598.

CHAPTER 15

TRIGGER FINGER RELEASE

ANN-MARIE R. PLATE

Stenosing tendovaginitis, or trigger finger, is a common clinical condition characterized by a painful "locking" or "clicking" of the digit. It can occur in any digit, but most commonly occurs in the thumb (30% to 60%), followed by the index and ring fingers and, occasionally, in the little finger. Many conditions have been associated with "triggering" including rheumatoid arthritis, diabetes, Dupuytren's disease, and partial tendon lacerations. In addition, an infant or toddler may have a congenital trigger digit.

Trigger finger was first described by Notta in 1850. He coined the term *Notta's nodule* as the palpable thickening in the flexor tendon overlying the metacarpophalangeal joint. The exact pathobiology is unknown.

ANATOMY

The flexor tendon sheath is composed of two parts: (a) an inner membranous synovial portion and (b) an outer retinacular pulley portion. The synovial portion has a visceral layer and a parietal layer. The visceral layer is intimate with the tendon, known as the epitenon layer, and the parietal layer is the outer layer that constitutes the synovial pouch.

The retinacular portion of the tendon sheath is composed of a series of pulleys or fibrous bands overlying the

synovial portion. The pulleys are named by their shape (transverse, annular, and cruciate) within a proximal to distal numbering system. Specifically, there are annular (A) 1 through 5 and cruciate (C) 1 through 3. The arrangement of the pulleys in a proximal to distal orientation are as follows: A-1 over the metacarpophalangeal joint, A-2 over the proximal portion of the proximal phalanx, C-1 at the level of the distal aspect of the proximal phalanx, A-3 over the proximal interphalangeal joint, C-2 at the proximal portion of the middle phalanx, A-4 over the middle portion of the middle phalanx, C-3 at the distal aspect of the middle phalanx, and A-5 over the distal interphalangeal joint (Fig. 15-1). The most proximal pulley is a transverse pulley formed by the palmar aponeurosis. The transverse fascicular fibers of the palmar aponeurosis that overlie the proximal flexor tendon sheath are anchored on either side of the tendon to the deep palmar interosseous fascia by thick, vertical fibrous bands. Consequently, a proximal pulley is formed around the flexor tendon, approximately 1 cm in length.

The pulley arrangement in the thumb is slightly different. The thumb has an A-1 pulley overlying the metacarpophalangeal joint, followed by the oblique pulley (an extension of the adductor aponeurosis) over the proximal phalanx and an A-2 pulley. There are no cruciate pulleys (Fig. 15-2).

The portion of the tendon sheath involved in a trigger

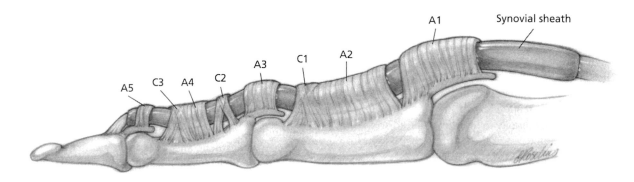

FIGURE 15-1. Digital flexor sheath. The digital flexor tendon sheath is composed of synovial (membranous) and retinacular (pulley) tissue components. The membranous portion is a synovial tube sealed at both ends. The retinacular (pulley) portion is a series of transverse (the palmar aponeurosis pulley), annular, and cruciform fibrous tissue condensations, which begin in the distal palm and end at the distal interphalangeal (DIP) joint. The floor or dorsal aspect of this tunnel is composed of the palmar plates of the metacarpophalangeal, proximal interphalangeal, and DIP joints and the palmar surfaces of the proximal and middle phalanges. (From Doyle JR. Hand. In: Doyle JR, Botte MJ, eds. *Surgical anatomy of the hand and upper extremity.* Philadelphia: Lippincott Williams & Wilkins, 2003:522–666, with permission.)

digit is the A-1 pulley and the palmar aponeurosis. In the thumb, it consists only of the A-1 pulley. Histologic changes have been shown to occur in these portions of the retinacular sheath and in the tendon itself. A normal A-1 pulley has a convex, well-vascularized outer layer and a concave, avas-cular inner gliding surface. The inner layer is fibrocartilaginous, composed of type I collagen, fibroblasts, and chondrocytes. The number and type of chondrocytes in the A-1 pulley of a trigger digit is abnormal. The normal A-1 pulley is predominately composed of type I collagen, whereas trig-

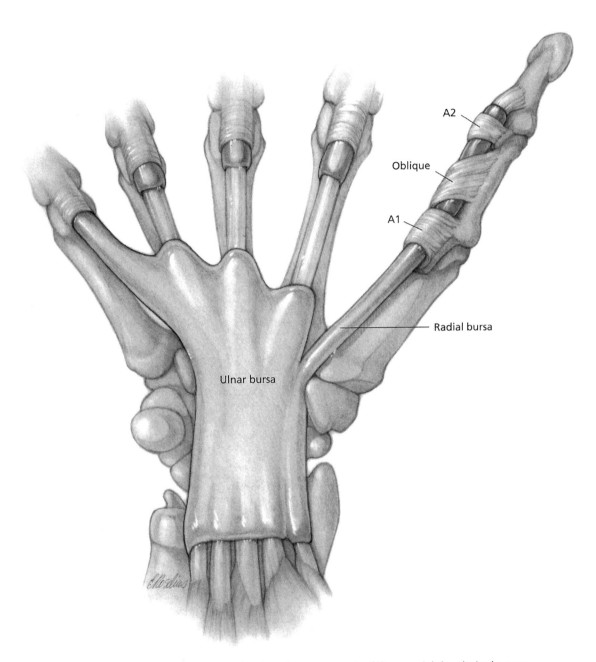

FIGURE 15-2. The membranous and retinacular components of the synovial sheaths in the proximal fingers, thumb, palm, and wrist. Note that the retinacular portion of the thumb flexor sheath is comprised of only two annular and one oblique pulley. The radial bursa is a continuation of the flexor pollicis longus synovial sheath, which extends from the region of the interphalangeal joint of the thumb to 2.5 cm proximal to the wrist flexion crease. In the index, long, and ring fingers, the membranous portion of the sheath begins at the neck of the metacarpals and continues distally to end at the distal interphalangeal joint. In most instances, the membranous portion of the small finger synovial sheath continues proximally to the wrist. (From Doyle JR. Hand. In: Doyle JR, Botte MJ, eds., *Surgical anatomy of the hand and upper extremity.* Philadelphia: Lippincott Williams & Wilkins, 2003:522–666, with permission.)

ger digit pulleys are composed mainly of type III collagen. Also, the number of chondrocytes is greatly increased from normal. Hence, the pathology is a proliferation of chondrocytes not synovial cells.

The initiating factor in chondrocyte proliferation is unclear. Studies have shown that increased compressive forces on connective tissue can produce fibrocartilaginous metaplasia. With full finger flexion, the pressure on the A-1 pulley is 500 to 700 mm Hg, whereas in the neutral position the pressures are only 0 to 50 mm Hg. The repetitive compressive loads caused by frequent finger flexion may be the mechanical factor leading to increased chondrocyte proliferation. A similar metaplasia occurs in the corresponding adjacent portion of the flexor tendon superficialis with the formation of Notta's nodule.

CLASSIFICATION/DIAGNOSIS

Trigger digits are commonly divided into acquired and congenital. The acquired trigger digit most commonly occurs in the fifth or successive decades. There is a predilection for females, with a 6:1 female to male incidence. Adults (acquired triggers) most often present with snapping or intermittent locking, especially in the morning. The patient often complains of pain over the metacarpophalangeal joint, aggravated with applied pressure on the A-1 while the patient actively flexes and extends the digit. The digit may "lock" prohibiting active extension of the proximal interphalangeal joint. In the case of a locked trigger digit, the joints are passively extended one at a time, beginning with the distal interphalangeal joint and then the proximal interphalangeal joint. Alternatively, the digit may become locked in extension not allowing active flexion. This is not as common, but when it does occur, it is usually in the thumb.

Congenital trigger digits are usually not noted until the first pediatric visit or later as the child begins to use his or her thumbs. Therefore, it is speculated that they are not true congenital triggers but rather acquired in the first weeks to months. The frequency of congenital trigger digits ranges from 1 in 2,000 (0.05%) to as high as 1 in 50 (2%). In contrast to adults, children have an equal distribution by sex and present with a locked digit. The thumb is the most common in either group, but much more so in children, especially bilateral trigger thumbs that occur about 25% of the time.

PREOPERATIVE PLANNING

Standard radiographs are recommended to evaluate the metacarpophalangeal and interphalangeal joints. Antero-

posterior (AP), lateral, and oblique views of the hand and individual digit are obtained.

EQUIPMENT

- Lead hand (optional)
- Small right-angle retractors (at least three)
- Blunt-tipped dissecting scissors
- Surgical arm board
- Tourniquet

POSITIONING AND PREPARATION

The surgery is usually performed under a local anesthetic with sedation as needed for the patient's emotional and physical comfort. The patient is supine on the operating table with his or her arm comfortably positioned on the hand table, fully supinated (Fig. 15-3). The digital block is given after the patient is sedated by the anesthesiologist. The block is performed at the level of the distal palmar crease in line with the affected digit. The injection site is prepped with an alcohol swab and the lidocaine is injected into the tendon sheath and, with a small adjustment of the needle tip, into the subcutaneous tissue overlying the tendon sheath. A tourniquet is applied to the forearm, not the upper arm, because it is less painful for the awake patient to have compression across the smaller muscle mass of the forearm as opposed to the larger muscle mass of the upper arm. The tourniquet is usually applied 100 mm Hg above the patient's systolic blood pressure (about 250 mm Hg). The hand is then prepped as to the surgeon's preference. Perioperative antibiotics are usually not required in surgery of the hand that involves only the soft tissues unless the patient is immunocompromised (i.e., diabetic, immune deficiency disease, steroid use), but this is governed by the surgeon's preference as well. Depending on the patient's degree of sedation, the hand may be positioned in the lead hand for control of the other digits and elimination of sudden movements.

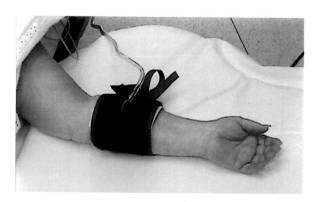

FIGURE 15-3. Patient position.

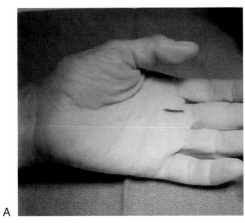
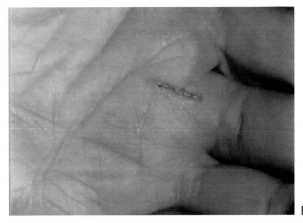

A

B

FIGURE 15-4. A: Guide for palmar incision. **B:** Longitudinal skin incision for middle-digit trigger release.

SURGICAL INCISION AND LANDMARKS

The classic operative approach is through a transverse skin incision at the level of the A-1 pulley parallel to the distal palmar crease. The A-1 pulley is then divided longitudinally. However, the principle of an extensile approach is not easily performed using this type of incision. A more pliable incision is a longitudinal skin incision over the A-1 pulley located between the distal palmar crease and the proximal digital crease (Fig. 15-4). **Care must be taken not to extend the incision into either the distal palmar crease or the proximal digital crease, because this would violate the rule of never crossing a crease at a right angle and may lead to contractures.** The palmar skin has multiple longitudinal skin creases that can be used as a guide for the incision, and, thus, cosmetic scarring is reduced.

A single incision through the skin is followed by dissection straight down to the tendon sheath with a pair of blunt-tipped scissors. The neurovascular bundles lie parallel and on either side of the tendon sheath. To protect the neurovascular bundles, the dissection is performed with the scissor tips positioned perpendicular and directly over the tendon, with spreading performed in a longitudinal fashion only (i.e., in line with the course of the tendon) (Fig. 15-5). Also, blunt retractors are placed to hold the subcutaneous fat aside, along with the neurovascular bundles. <u>As long as the dissection is maintained over the tendon, the bundles are protected.</u> This technique allows easy and full visualization of the A-1 pulley for a complete release (Fig. 15-6). The pulley is incised longitudinally up to the level of the A-2 distally. 📹 The proximal subcutaneous tissue is dissected by spreading above and below the palmar aponeurosis. The palmar aponeurosis is seen as white fibrous bands fanning out above the tendon. This transverse pulley is incised bluntly with the scissors. 📹

Some surgeons prefer to excise, as opposed to incise, the A-1 pulley. This decision is governed solely by surgeon's preference unless a retinacular cyst exists. If this is the case, the cyst with the pulley should be excised and sent to the pathology department. Also, occasionally there is an abundance of tenosynovium present on the tendons, which may be excised and sent to the pathology department as well.

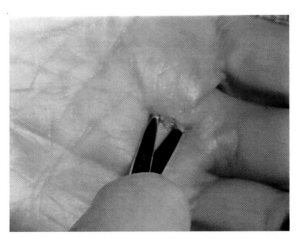

FIGURE 15-5. Longitudinal dissection performed perpendicular to and directly over the tendon.

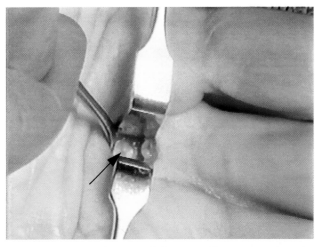

FIGURE 15-6. Visualization of the A-1 pulley. Note retinacular cyst *(arrow)* on A-1 pulley of flexor tendon sheath.

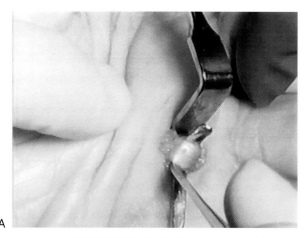
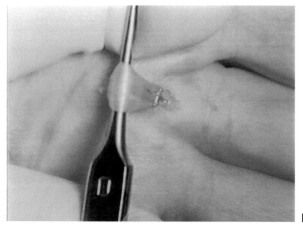

A   B

FIGURE 15-7. A: A retractor is passed beneath the flexor digitorum superficialis tendon. **B:** The retractor is used to gently elevate the tendon to lyse adhesions.

After the pulley is released, the flexor digitorum superficialis (FDS) tendon is clearly seen with the flexor digitorum profundus (FDP) tendon lying beneath. ◼ Occasionally, adhesions between these tendons occur and must be lysed. A right-angle retractor is passed beneath the FDS tendon (Fig. 15-7A), and the tendon is gently pulled up and out of the incision to separate it from the FDP tendon (Fig. 15-7B). **One must check that both slips of the FDS tendon are retracted, because the FDS divides into Campers' chiasm at this level. Extreme care must be taken that the neurovascular bundles are not accidentally retracted out of wound during this step.** The finger is passively extended at the proximal interphalangeal joint while maintaining traction on the FDS tendon. ◼ Often, the lysis of the adhesions is audible. Finally, because this procedure is often performed with local anesthesia, the patient is asked to actively flex the affected finger to confirm full resolution of the tendon locking.

The trigger thumb requires a little more delicacy regarding the neurovascular bundles and the initial skin incision. The common digital nerve of the thumb arises from the radial division of the median nerve and lies on the superficial surface of the flexor pollicis brevis before it divides into the

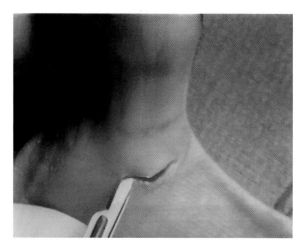

FIGURE 15-9. Incision on left trigger thumb.

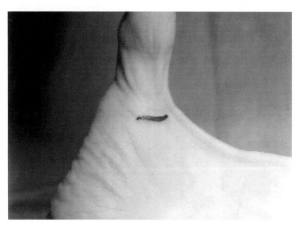

FIGURE 15-8. Guide for thumb incision.

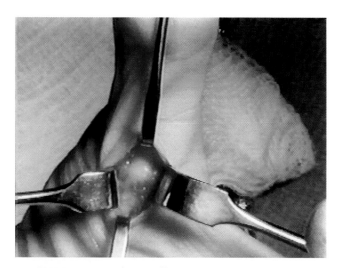

FIGURE 15-10. Flexor pollicis longus tendon in sheath.

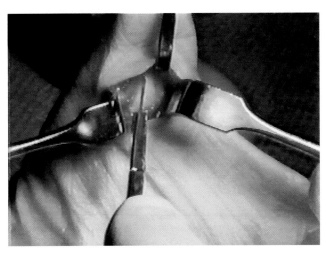

FIGURE 15-11. Incising A-1 pulley.

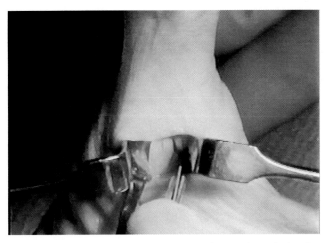

FIGURE 15-12. Flexor pollicis longus tendon as viewed after incision of the A-1 pulley.

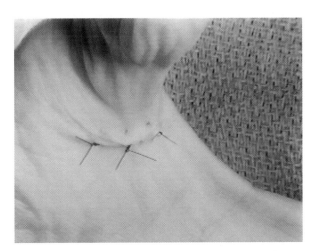

FIGURE 15-13. Skin closure of thumb after trigger release.

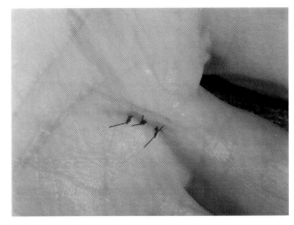

FIGURE 15-14. Skin closure of middle digit after trigger release.

ulnar and radial digital nerves. The ulnar branch continues along its distally directed course up the ulnar border of the thumb, whereas the radial digital nerve must cross superficial to the flexor pollicis longus (FPL) tendon to reach the subcutaneous tissue on the radial side of the thumb. **This crossing occurs just beneath the deep dermis at the level of the metacarpophalangeal crease, leaving the radial digital nerve prone to injury.** <u>A transverse incision is recommended at the thumb digital crease to limit the vulnerability of the radial digital nerve</u> (Figs. 15-8 and 15-9). Similar to a trigger finger, dissection is performed longitudinally over the FPL tendon with the neurovascular bundles retracted on either side (Fig. 15-10). The A-1 pulley is then released in a longitudinal fashion (Fig. 15-11). There is no need to manually retract the FPL tendon because there is only one tendon present in the sheath, unlike a trigger finger and, therefore, no intertendinous adhesions to lyse (Fig. 15-12).

The incision is irrigated and the skin is closed with nylon sutures (Figs. 15-13 and 15-14). A postoperative dressing consisting of a gauze and a 2-inch kling is applied (Fig. 15-15). All the other digits and the proximal interpha-

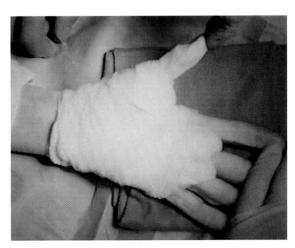

FIGURE 15-15. Final postoperative dressing after release of thumb and middle-digit triggers.

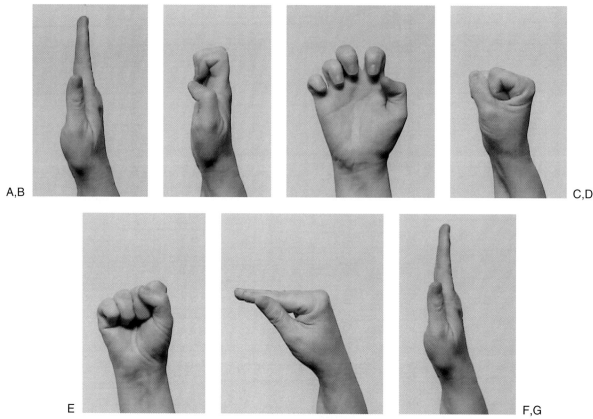

FIGURE 15-16. Stretching exercise called "tendon gliding" (see video for correct motion sequence). Points to remember for different positions: **(A)** start with fingers pointing straight-up; **(B)** "curl" fingers until the tips touch the palm (lateral view); **(C)** palmar view; **(D)** roll knuckles all the way down into a tight fist; **(E)** palmar view; **(F)** maintain straight fingers; and **(G)** extend fingers fully. Repeat exercise 10 times, at least six times per day, until full motion returns.

langeal joint of the involved digit should remain free with unobstructed motion.

POSTOPERATIVE PROTOCOL AND FOLLOW-UP

The patient is encouraged to use the fingers immediately following surgery and as much as possible postoperatively but to keep the dressing clean and dry. The patient returns to the office 1 week later for dressing and suture removal. All patients require postoperative therapy but may not require a therapist. The patient is taught to massage the incisional scar and to perform range of motion and stretching exercises (Fig. 15-16) ■◀ and gradual strengthening exercises.

Depending on the patient, a therapist may be required to assist in these therapeutic exercises.

SELECTED READINGS

Benson LS, Ptaszek AJ. Injection versus surgery in the treatment of trigger finger. *J Hand Surg [Am]* 1997;22:138–144.

Cardon LJ, Ezaki M, Carter PR. Trigger finger in children. *J Hand Surg [Am]* 1999; 24: 1156–1161.

Griggs SM, Weiss AP, Lane LB, et al. Treatment of trigger finger in patients with diabetes mellitus. *J Hand Surg [Am]* 1995; 20: 787–789.

Saldana MJ. Trigger digits: diagnosis and treatment. *J Am Acad Orthop Surg* 2001; 9: 246–252.

Steenwerckx A, De Smet L, Fabry G. Congenital trigger digit. *J Hand Surg [Am]* 1996; 21: 909–911.

CHAPTER 16

DISTAL RADIUS FRACTURES: EXTERNAL FIXATION AND SUPPLEMENTAL K-WIRES

KEITH B. RASKIN

Fractures of the distal radius are one of the most commonly encountered injuries presenting to the emergency room setting. Understanding the normal distal radius anatomy is essential for the treating physician. The outcome of management of the unstable distal radius fracture is directly related to successfully identifying, reducing, and stabilizing the various fragments. Restoring articular congruity and the relation between the distal radius and the surrounding skeletal structures, while avoiding the complications of treatment, are key considerations.

ANATOMY

The radial length is defined as the distance between the medial articular surface of the radius and the corresponding articular head of the ulna. There is a considerable normal variation in length, defined as positive ulnar variance (ulna length is greater than the radius) and negative ulnar variance (ulna length is less than the radius). Radial inclination is the angle of the surface, as identified from the radial styloid to the medial articular surface. Normal is 22 degrees with a range of 13 to 30 degrees. The volar tilt is the angle of the surface from the dorsal to the volar surface as seen on the lateral radiograph. The average is 11 degrees with a range of 0 to 28 degrees. The scaphoid and lunate fossas are the articular surfaces that correspond with their adjacent carpal bones, and the sigmoid notch is the articulating surface with the ulna head (Fig. 16-1).

CLASSIFICATION

Many classifications exist for fractures of the distal radius. Most of these classifications attempt to subdivide this injury into predictable fracture patterns that may be useful in de-

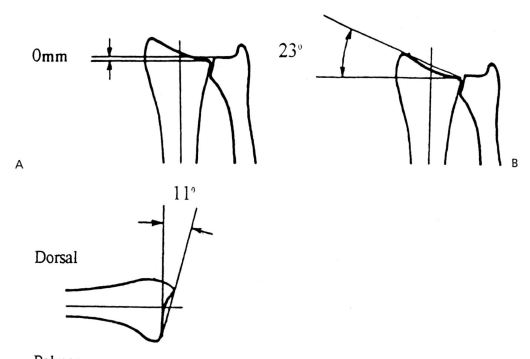

FIGURE 16-1. Radiographic parameters of radial length (also referred to as ulnar variance) **(A)**, radial inclination **(B)**, and volar tilt **(C)** used for purposes of description and treatment.

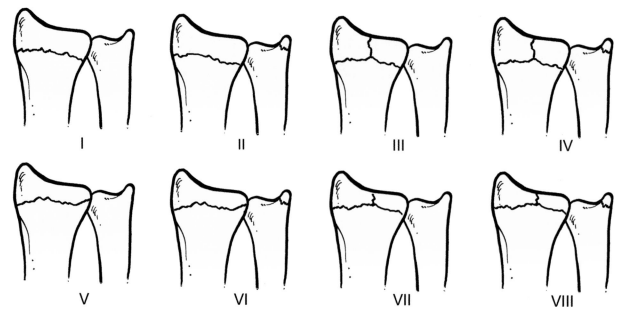

FIGURE 16-2. Frykman classification. The distal ulna is not fractured in types I, III, V, and VII. Intraarticular fractures are represented by types III, IV, V, VI, VII, and VIII.

termining treatment options. The earliest and most common classification is the Frykman classification in which the radius fracture is assessed with respect to articular involvement and whether there is an associated ulnar styloid fracture (Fig. 16-2). Despite the popularity of this classification, there is little gained toward insight into treatment planning or prediction of outcome. Eight types of fractures were described.

The AO classification similarly describes various intraarticular and extraarticular fractures with nine patterns of increasing complexity. Other classifications are the Rayhack, Mayo, and Fernandez systems.

All of the classifications require memorization of various numbers or combinations of numbers. The basic concept of most distal radius classifications is to establish three factors, which is also the basis of my classification: articular involvement, direction of displacement, and stability. These can be easily remembered and apply to most frac-

tures of the distal radius, allowing an effective treatment plan.

Raskin Classification

E/I: extraarticular versus intraarticular
D/V: dorsal versus volar displacement
S/U: stable versus unstable

After an initial attempted reduction, instability is defined as residual shortening of greater than 5 mm, dorsal angulation greater than 10 degrees, comminution of greater than 50% of the metaphyseal region, or bicortical fragmentation. Based on this three letter classification, the treatment plans outlined in Table 16-1 have been developed and are recommended.

With the increasing popularity of high-speed activities, such as in-line skating, snow boarding, and mountain bik-

TABLE 16-1. RECOMMENDED TREATMENT PLANS

Description		Treatment
EDS	Extraarticular dorsal angulated stable fracture	Cast
EDU	Extraarticular dorsal angulated unstable fracture	Intrafocal pins or plate
EVS	Extraarticular volar angulated stable fracture	Cast
EVU	Extraarticular volar angulated unstable fracture	Buttress plate ORIF
IDS	Intraarticular dorsal angulated stable fracture	Cast and close observation
IDU	Intraarticular dorsal angulated unstable fracture	External fixation
IVS	Intraarticular volar angulated stable fracture	Cast
IVU	Intraarticular volar angulated unstable fracture	Buttress plate ORIF

ing, there has been a higher associated incidence of more comminuted unstable distal radius fractures in younger active patients. The majority of these fractures are of the intraarticular dorsal displaced unstable (IDU) type, requiring closed reduction and external fixation.

PREOPERATIVE PLANNING

Clinical assessment of the wrist deformity in conjunction with radiographic correlation is essential initial management. Standard radiographs are obtained in the posteroanterior (PA), lateral, and oblique views (Fig. 16-3). Comparative views of the unaffected contralateral side are also recommended. This enables the surgeon to determine the normal radial length, inclination, and volar tilt for each individual patient, because an acceptable degree of variability exists within the population. If an associated intercarpal ligament injury is suspected, then a magnetic resonance imaging (MRI) or intraoperative arthroscopy may be warranted (Fig. 16-4). It is essential to encourage the patient to begin active range of motion exercises for the digits, elbow, and shoulder before surgi-

cal intervention. This diminishes the likelihood of progressive stiffness and functional limitations.

EQUIPMENT

Equipment needed is as follows (Fig. 16-5):

- External fixator
- Blunt-tipped external fixation half-pins
- Appropriately sized drill bit and power drill
- 0.062-inch smooth K-wires
- Bone graft substitute as needed
- Intraoperative fluoroscopy
- Surgical arm board

Intraoperative radiographic assessment of the radius fracture with respect to restoration of radial length, inclination, volar tilt, and articular alignment mandates the use of fluoroscopic equipment. Application of the external fixation device requires the appropriate drills, blunt skeletal half-pins, and ex-

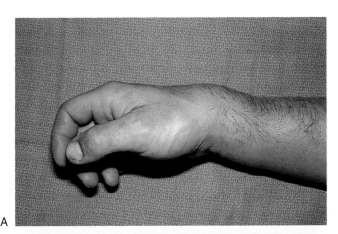
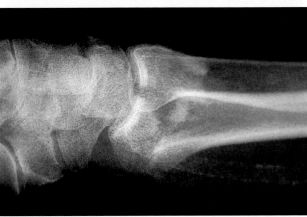
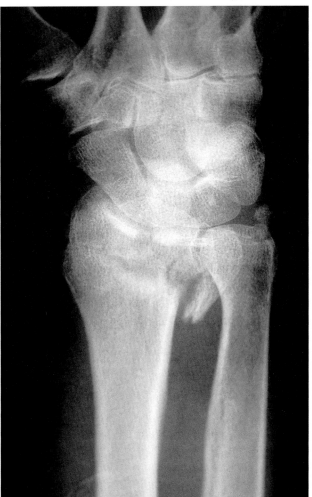

FIGURE 16-3. A: Clinical appearance of acute displaced distal radius fracture. Anteroposterior view **(B)** and lateral view **(C)** of underlying unstable distal radius fracture.

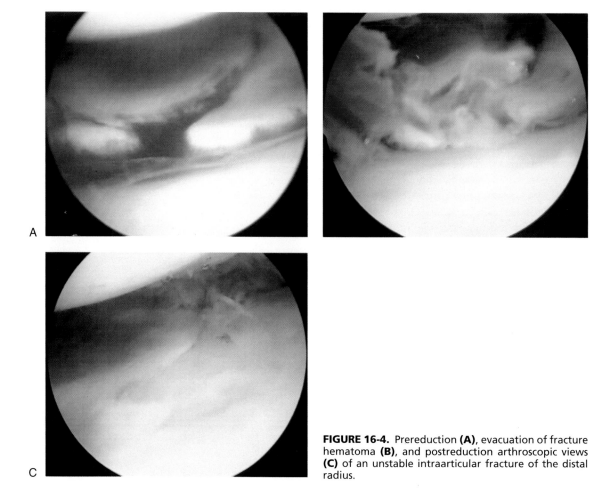

FIGURE 16-4. Prereduction **(A)**, evacuation of fracture hematoma **(B)**, and postreduction arthroscopic views **(C)** of an unstable intraarticular fracture of the distal radius.

ternal fixation frame of the surgeon's choice. Supplemental Kirschner wire fixation has proven to add to fracture stability and is straightforwardly inserted with a power wire driver. If bone graft or bone graft substitute is needed, one should confirm that the proper surgical tools or products are available.

POSITIONING AND PREPARATION

The surgery is most commonly performed under a regional anesthetic with supplemental intravenous sedation. The patient is in a supine position with the arm abducted to the side of the body at 90 degrees. The surgeon can comfortably sit within the inner side of the arm table extension, with the assistant opposite (Fig. 16-6). The surgeon must avoid placing the forearm in a position of hyperpronation in an attempt to improve visualization during pin insertion, because this can lead to poor pin placement or malreduction at the fracture site.

SURGICAL INCISION LANDMARKS

Although external fixation frames have previously been inserted using a percutaneous technique, the unacceptably

high incidence of associated complications related to malpositioning of the pins and related soft tissue injury have led to the more commonly used limited incision technique of half-pin insertion. The pins are inserted into the index metacarpal proximal shaft and the radial shaft, approximately 3 to 4 cm proximal to the fracture.

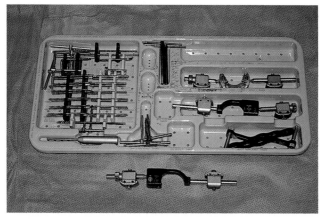

FIGURE 16-5. Equipment for distal radius fracture: tray consists of drills, screws, trocar, clamps, wrist templates, and T-wrenches. The external fixator is shown below.

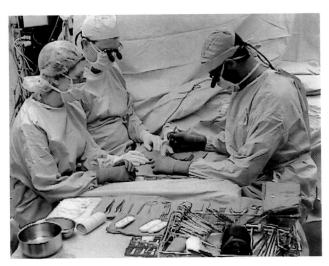

FIGURE 16-6. Customary operative setup and patient arm position for surgical management of distal radius fracture.

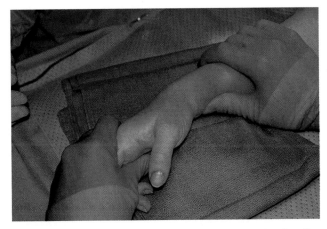

FIGURE 16-8. Initial closed manipulation of the distal radius fracture for gross reduction before application of external fixation frame.

The length of the external fixator should be clearly identified before making the skin incisions, because this will determine the amount of distraction that the fixator is able to achieve. If the proximal incision site along the radial shaft is too proximal in location, the fixator length may prohibit obtaining sufficient ligamentotaxis (Fig. 16-7). ◙

SURGICAL APPROACH AND PROCEDURE

After an adequate anesthetic level has been achieved, the entire arm is prepped and draped in a standard manner. More severely deformed wrists are initially aligned through primary, gentle closed manipulation (Fig. 16-8). The arm is exsanguinated with a compressive elastic bandage, and a well-padded tourniquet is then inflated over the proximal arm to an appropriate level. The planning of pin placement for the fixator is aided through the proper positioning of the fixation device along the radial side of the forearm before in-

cisions (Fig. 16-9). ◙ The index metacarpal is approached through a 2-cm longitudinal incision over the dorsal radial base (Fig. 16-10). ◙ The terminal branches of the radial sensory nerve are well protected, because the first dorsal interosseous muscle and periosteum are minimally reflected. ◙

The drill guide is carefully aligned with the surface of the metacarpal to ensure bicortical pin insertion. ◙ This decreases the likelihood of unicortical drilling with the related complications of potential pin loosening, infection, or iatrogenic metacarpal fracture. After predrilling the pin sites, ◙ the pins are manually inserted while maintaining the correct pin alignment. ◙

The radial shaft pins are then placed using a similar technique of insertion. Again, a 2-cm longitudinal incision is created along the radial shaft proximal to the fracture site, with the lateral antibrachial cutaneous nerve branches protected. ◙ The deeper dissection reveals the radial sensory nerve as it pierces the fascial layer between the brachioradialis and the extensor carpi radialis longus (Fig. 16-11). ◙ The pins are inserted between the extensor carpi radialis

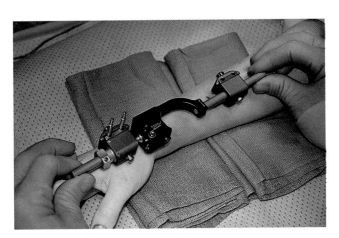

FIGURE 16-7. Use of external fixation device to ensure proper proximal pin placement.

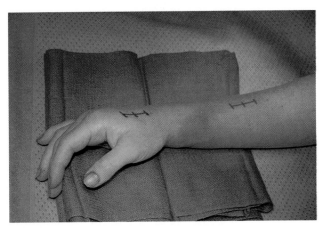

FIGURE 16-9. Marked incision sites for external fixation pin placement.

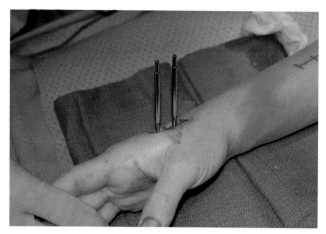

FIGURE 16-10. Distal half-pin placement along the dorsoradial border of index metacarpal.

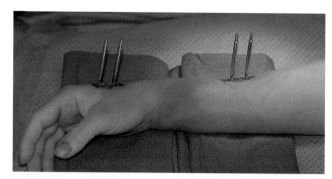

FIGURE 16-12. Completion of half-pin placement for the external fixation frame.

longus and brevis, thereby avoiding the radial sensory nerve. ◼️ Accurate bicortical pin insertion is equally important at this location (Fig. 16-12).

Once the pins have been inserted ◼️ and placement confirmed with the intraoperative fluoroscopy unit (Fig. 16-13), the wounds are irrigated and closed before application of the external fixation frame. This allows for better wound repair without interfering with the closure (Fig. 16-14).

The external fixation frame is secured to both sets of half pins while the wrist is maintained in a relatively aligned posture. ◼️ Most frames have a sliding clamp component that allows for distraction (ligamentotaxis) across the wrist joint (Fig. 16-15). I have found it useful assisting in the reduction with gentle longitudinal traction applied to the fingers, while countertraction is maintained at the 90-degree flexed elbow. Finger trap apparatus along with a weight and pulley system has also been previously described with similar success.

After the compressive force of the carpus has been neutralized from the surface of the radius through ligamentotaxis,

closed manipulation of the fracture can be performed. Often, the residual dorsal angular deformity prevails, despite restoration of radial length and inclination. The fixator is temporarily adjusted in a flexed position, allowing for a greater correction of a volar tilt. By manual reduction of the distal fragments, with possible intrafocal pinning, the correction of volar tilt can be obtained. Several of the newer external fixators have a mechanical ability to assist in restoring volar tilt and radial inclination and rotational alignment (Fig. 16-16).

Smooth Kirschner wires are percutaneously inserted from the radial styloid fragment and into the intact radial shaft, acting as a buttress support for the fracture. If intrafocal pins are to be added, care is taken to avoid penetrating the extensor tendons. This may require a small stab incision and blunt surgical spreading through the soft tissue before pin placement.

I prefer to insert two to three wires in a diverging pattern from the styloid or from the dorsal radial border of the distal fragment into the radial shaft to add to the stability of the configuration and thereby lessen the demands of the external fixator (Fig. 16-17). ◼️ Although a transverse wire can be safely placed from the radial styloid to the medial fracture fragment, oftentimes this medial fragment is comminuted with little or no cortical bone purchase.

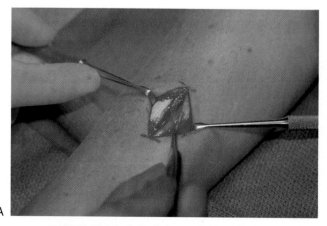

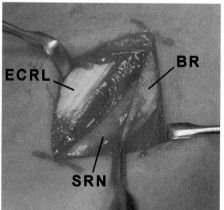

A

B

FIGURE 16-11. A: Radial nerve is identified and protected before placement of the proximal half-pins. **B:** *BR*, brachioradialis tendon; *ECRL*, extensor carpi radialis longus tendon; *SRN*, radial sensory nerve.

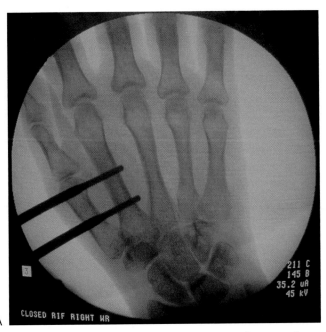

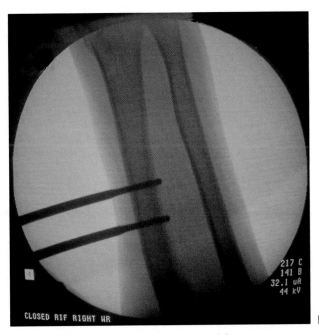

A   B

FIGURE 16-13. Intraoperative fluoroscopic assessment of distal pins **(A)** and proximal pins **(B)** with good alignment.

Once the wires are placed and intraoperative radiographs confirm placement (Fig. 16-18), the fixator can be restored to a neutral alignment, avoiding the flexed posture required for primary fracture reduction. If the radiographs reveal malreduction of the fracture despite optimal frame and wire application, a limited open reduction and additional bone graft or bone graft substitute is strongly suggested. This can be performed through a small incision over Lister's tubercle with blunt surgical spreading through the soft tissue until the fracture is encountered. The extensor pollicis longus should be decompressed from within Lister's tubercle to prevent potential attritional rupture. Often a Freer elevator can augment the elevation of the fracture fragments before insertion of the bone graft. Fluoroscopic imaging or direct inspection of the articular surface through a dorsal capsulectomy confirms final reduction.

One of the more common pitfalls of this procedure is to overdistract the carpus through excessive ligamentotaxis. This commonly leads to the complications of stiff digits with residual loss of motion, loss of wrist flexion and extension arc, and possibly reflex sympathetic dystrophy (RSD).

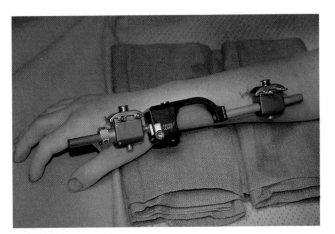

FIGURE 16-14. Pin incision sites are repaired before application of frame.

FIGURE 16-15. Initial placement of external fixation fame after distraction is achieved through the sliding couple clamp.

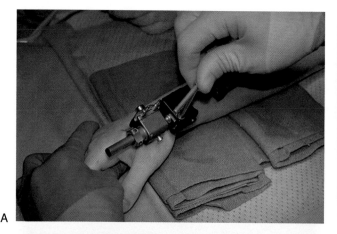

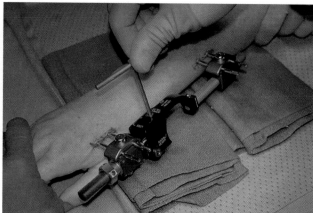

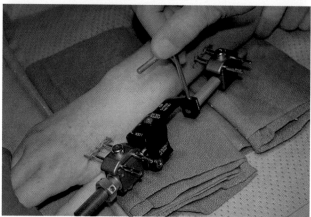

FIGURE 16-16. Frame allows for radial and ulnar deviation **(A)**, dorsal and volar alignment **(B)**, and pronation and supination **(C)** at the fracture site.

There are two basic intraoperative techniques that I have routinely performed to ensure avoidance of overdistraction and the subsequent complications.

The most reliable technique is a passive finger flexion test. Once the fixator is in place and the fracture is reduced, the surgeon passively flexes the patient's metacarpophalangeal joints along with simultaneous flexion of the interphalangeal joints. If the fingers can be passively flexed to the level of the proximal palmar crease without excessive force,

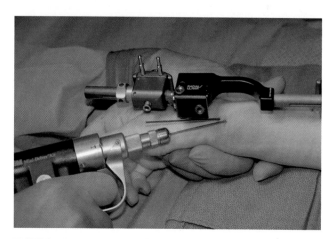

FIGURE 16-17. Insertion of 0.062-inch K-wires from styloid into intact radial shaft.

there is no excessive distraction across the wrist joint. However, if there is a great degree of difficulty in passively flexing the digits, then extrinsic extensor tendon tightness is present, which is directly related to overdistraction.

The intraoperative radiographic assessment is an additional secondary evaluation tool of ligamentotaxis after fracture reduction. Based on my experience, the distance of the radiocarpal (RC) joint space and the midcarpal (MC) joint space should be measured on standard anteroposterior (AP) fluoroscopic views. If the ratio of the RC:MC joint was 2:1 to 1:1, most patients fell within the safe zone of distractive force across the wrist (Fig. 16-19). If there was greater than a 1:1 RC:MC ratio (i.e., 1:2 RC:MC), then the volar radioscaphocapitate and radiolunotriquetral ligaments may be overdistracted and can potentially lead to the common complications of stiffness.

POSTOPERATIVE PROTOCOL

There are various methods of postoperative management of the external fixators, each of which have their proponents. I have found that a dry sterile bandage surrounding the fixator half-pins, along with dressing changes and pin care every 2 weeks, has eliminated the need for daily patient care and has allowed for successful healing with a paucity of compli-

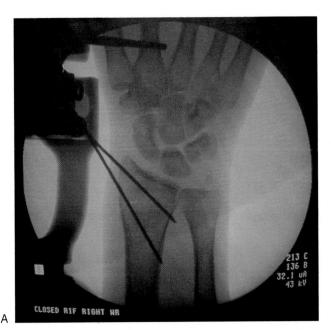

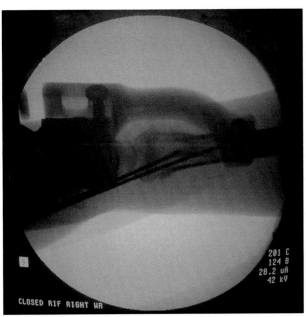

A

B

FIGURE 16-18. Postreduction intraoperative fluoroscopic assessment of posteroanterior **(A)** and lateral **(B)** views, confirming restoration of radial length, inclination, volar tilt, and articular congruity.

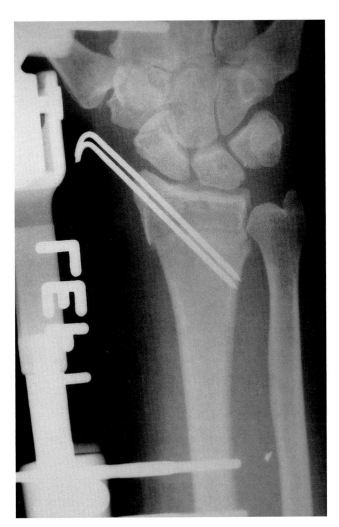

FIGURE 16-19. Anteroposterior radiograph of distal radius fracture after closed reduction and external fixation with supplemental Kirschner wire. Radiocarpal and midcarpal articulations are seen without overdistraction.

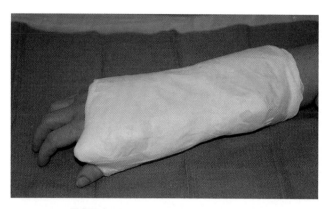

FIGURE 16-20. Postoperative dressing.

cations in most patients (Fig. 16-20). In the unlikely event that a superficial infection is encountered, local wound care is performed on a daily basis with oral antibiotics prescribed. It is rare to encounter a case of osteomyelitis and the need for premature removal of the fixator along with debridement and intravenous antibiotics.

During the early postoperative period, it is imperative that finger, elbow, and shoulder range of motion exercises be instituted (Fig. 16-21). If there appears to be slow progress in regaining an acceptable arc of motion, then a more comprehensive occupational therapy program is begun.

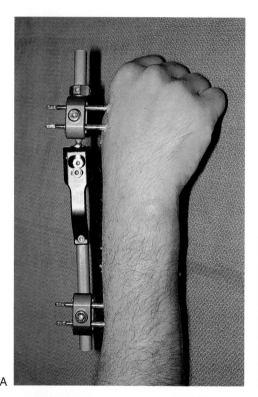

A

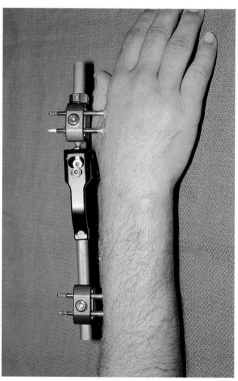

C

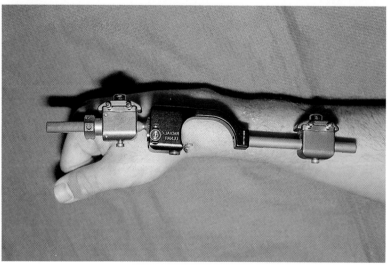

B

FIGURE 16-21. Postoperative clinical views of maintained flexion (**A** and **B**) and extension of digits (**C**) after proper application of external fixation with appropriate ligamentotaxis.

FOLLOW-UP

Distal radius fractures often heal within 6 to 8 weeks. Once adequate healing is observed clinically and radiographically, the fixator and pins can be removed under a local anesthetic. It is not uncommon for the radiographic appearance of fracture bridging to lag behind clinical assessment of healing without point tenderness at the previous fracture site. Therapy is advanced to include wrist range of motion and subsequent strengthening.

SUGGESTED READINGS

Broos PL, Fourneau IA, Stoffelen DV. Fractures of the distal radius. Current concepts for treatment. *Acta Orthop Belg* 2001; 67: 211–218.

Cooney WP. Distal radius fractures: external fixation proves best. *J Hand Surg [Am]* 1998; 23: 1119–1121.

Huch K, Hunerbein M, Meeder PJ. External fixation of intra-articular fracture of the distal radius in young and old adults. *Arch Orthop Trauma Surg* 1996; 115: 38–42.

Kaempffe FA, Walker KM. External fixation for distal radius fractures: effect of distraction on outcome. *Clin Orthop* 2000; 380: 220–225.

Kapoor H, Agarwal A, Dhaon BK. Displaced intra-articular fractures of distal radius: a comparative evaluation of results following closed reduction, external fixation and open reduction with internal fixation. *Injury* 2000; 31: 75–79.

Raskin KB. Management of fractures of the distal radius: surgeon's perspective. *J Hand Ther* 1999; 12(2): 92–98.

Raskin KB, Rettig ME. Distal radius fractures and malunions: skeletal realignment through external fixation. *Atlas Hand Clin* 2000; 5(1): 59–77.

Rettig ME, Raskin KB. Acute fractures of the distal radius. *Hand Clin* 2000; 16: 405–415.

Rikli DA, Kupfer K, Bodoky A. Long-term results of the external fixation of distal radius fractures. *J Trauma* 1998; 44: 970–976.

Seitz WH Jr. External fixation of distal radius fractures. Indications and technical principles. *Orthop Clin North Am* 1993; 24: 255–264.

Weiland AJ. External fixation, not ORIF, as the treatment of choice for fractures of the distal radius. *J Orthop Trauma* 1999; 13: 570–572.

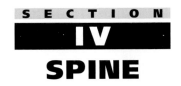
CHAPTER 17

LUMBAR MICRODISCECTOMY

THOMAS J. ERRICO

Lumbar microdiscectomy has become the gold standard of discectomy techniques for the treatment of low back pain from nerve root compression related to disc trauma or degenerative disc disease. Approximately 300,000 microdiscectomy procedures of the lumbar spine are performed annually. The incidence of males undergoing lumbar microdiscectomy can be up to twice that of females, in part because of the higher load burden on the male lumbar spine.

Patients have benefited enormously from the use of the surgical microscope to treat lumbar disc disease, first applied over 25 years ago. Benefits include further reduced trauma to spinal muscles; decreased manipulation of nerve structures; smaller closure scars; and diminished morbidity, anesthesia, and operative time.

Microdiscectomy is typically performed on an outpatient basis or with one overnight hospital stay. The procedure has proved to be an effective surgery, with 85% to 95% of patients receiving significant pain relief or abatement, depending on the series. There is a reoperation rate of approximately 5% to 10%. Because the integrity of all the muscles, ligaments, and joints is maintained, the mechanical aspect of the lower back, as well as the function, is kept intact.

ANATOMY

The normal lumbar spine is composed of the five lumbar vertebrae (L1 to L5) and the first sacral vertebra (S1); the latter vertebra is fused to the sacrum. As with all spinal vertebrae, lumbar vertebrae are separated by an intervertebral fibrocartilage disc. The name of each disc is derived from the two adjacent vertebral bodies. Therefore, the disc between L4 and L5 is the L4-5 disc. The most caudal intervertebral disc of the lumbar spine is the L5-S1 disc. The posterior bony elements of vertebrae include paired pedicles, transverse processes, inferior and superior articular processes, and laminae and a spinous process. The laminae are continuous with the articular processes, which join with the articular processes of the respective bodies, above and below, to form the bilateral facet joints. The laminae unite posteriorly to form the spinous process. At any vertebral level, the combi-

nation of the intervertebral disc and pair of facet joints is often referred to as the trijoint complex. The space between laminae is the interlaminar space; throughout the spine, these spaces are connected by the relatively elastic ligamentum flavum (yellow ligament) (Fig. 17-1). The kinematics of disc movement are defined by the relationships of the disc, of the facet joints, and of the strong ligaments, with their attachments to the posterior elements.

The stability and flexibility of the vertebral column is made possible by strong ligamentous support. The anterior longitudinal ligament (ALL), a broad ligament that extends from the occipital bone to the sacrum, unites the anterior aspects of the lumbar vertebrae. The posterior longitudinal ligament (PLL) begins at the axis and continues the entire length of the spine. It joins the posterior aspect of the vertebral bodies widening slightly at each intervertebral space to directly reinforce the respective discs.

The neural elements of the lumbar spine include the distal termination of the spinal cord, known as the conus medullaris/cauda equina complex, which travels within the spinal canal and is demarcated similar to the cord in other spinal regions: anteriorly by the posterior vertebral bodies, laterally by the pedicles, and posteriorly by the laminae and facet joints. At the inferior aspect of the body of L1, the spinal cord with its lumbar and sacral nerve roots form the cauda equina complex. A nonnervous thread, the filum terminale, continues to the base of the coccyx, essentially attaching the distal cord to the coccygeal ligament. The dural sac containing the lumbar and sacral nerve roots provides bilateral exits through bony neural foramina that are formed by superior and inferior notches on the adjacent pedicles or, more distally, within the lateral walls of the sacrum. Each nerve root derives its name from the pedicle above. Therefore, the L3 roots exit underneath the L3 pedicles.

Anatomy Particularly Relevant to Disc Herniation

A classic disc herniation occurs on one side (unilaterally) off-center of the midline and compresses one root. Typically, the lower nerve root is affected; for example, in an L4-5 disc

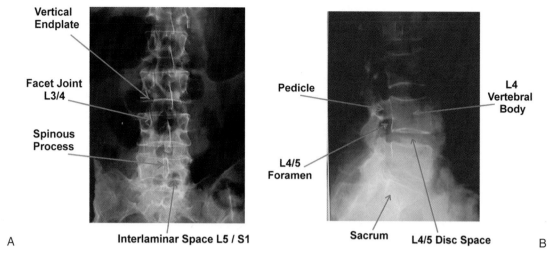

Vertical
Endplate

Facet Joint
L3/4

Spinous
Process

A

Interlaminar Space L5 / S1

Pedicle

L4/5
Foramen

Sacrum

L4/5 Disc Space

L4
Vertebral
Body

B

FIGURE 17-1. Anteroposterior **(A)** and lateral **(B)** x-ray film views of lumbar vertebrae.

herniation, the traversing L5 nerve root is compressed. The L4 root would generally be spared compression, as it exits beneath the higher L4 pedicle, just above the herniating L4-5 disc. Similarly, a typical L5-S1 herniation compresses the S1 nerve root.

Pathoanatomy of Disc Degeneration

The trijoint complex accumulates various amounts of trauma from normal use and with age-related conditions (arthritis) and progressive disorders (spondylolisthesis, scoliosis). Initial disc changes may present as peripheral tears of the annular fibers, delamination of the outer layers (annulus), or nuclear degeneration with diminished water-holding properties. Disc bulging without herniation can also occur. With progressive trauma and diminishment of the functional integrity of the trijoint complex, affected vertebrae may become unstable.

Annular tears of different types (radial, circumferential) typically occur in conjunction with nuclear degeneration, resulting in loss of disc height. Similar bony and cartilage degenerative changes in the facet joints result in joint subluxation and capsular laxity. Herniation of a disc can occur either early or late in this degenerative process. Further disc resorption with narrowing of the disc space and development of disc fibrosis and osteophyte formation ensues, along with the development of spinal stenosis.

Definition of Disc Herniation

The most problematic concept in the definition of a disc herniation is to differentiate a true herniation from a bulging disc. As discs degenerate during the normal aging process they lose water content and disc height. Naturally the lateral wall of the disc bulge outward in a symmetrical fashion much as the sides of a tire low on air bulge outward as the rim gets closer to the ground. A true herniation is not merely a symmetrical bulging but rather an *asymmetrical protrusion* of disc material outward from the normal circumference of the disc. The asymmetry of the protrusion is the key differentiation factor between bulge and herniation.

CLASSIFICATION

The most common classification for herniated discs focuses on the manner in which the disc herniates. Herniations are (a) contained (annulus or the PLL prevents the nuclear material from escaping), (b) extruded (nuclear material has escaped through the annulus or the PLL but remains in contact with the nucleus pulposus), or (c) sequestered (one or several separate pieces of nuclear material have escaped the annulus and are separated from the remainder of the nucleus pulposus, usually migrating further upward or downward within the canal).

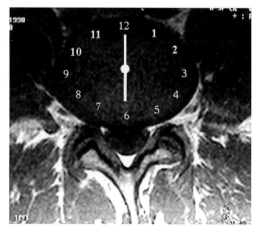

FIGURE 17-2. Magnetic resonance imaging. 6-o'clock position, central disc; 5:30 or 6:30, posterolateral disc; 5-o'clock or 7-o'clock position, intraforaminal disc; 3:30 to 4:30, extraforaminal disc; 7:30 to 8:30, far-lateral disc.

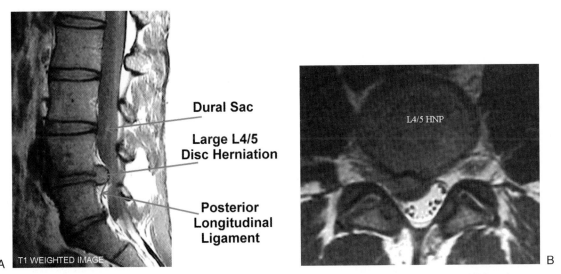

FIGURE 17-3. Magnetic resonance imaging views of a large L4-5 disc herniation, sagittal **(A)** and axial **(B)**.

An alternative classification focuses on location. Herniations are central, posterolateral, intraforaminal, or extraforaminal. Each type has a specific position on a clock face that is visually "templated" over the cross-sectional view of a disc (Fig. 17-2). The 12-o'clock position is the disc's anterior midline; similarly, the 6-o'clock position is the posterior midline. The apex of a central herniation occurs at the 6-o'clock position, and the apex of posterolateral herniations are at the 5:30 (left) or 6:30 (right) position, depend-ing on if the herniation occurs on the left or right. The apex of intraforaminal herniations are centered at the 5-o'clock or 7-o'clock position, and the apex of extraforaminal disc herniations are positioned between 3:30 and 4:30 on the left or 7:30 and 8:30 on the right. The latter type is also termed far-lateral herniations and is notable for affecting the upper root. For example, a far-lateral L4-5 herniation affects the upper L4 root after it exits from under the L4 pedicle, rather than affecting the more medial L5 root (Figs. 17-3 to 17-5).

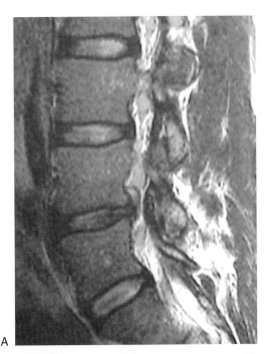

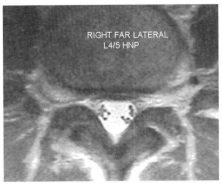

FIGURE 17-4. Magnetic resonance images of large right L4-5 extraforaminal disc herniation, sagittal **(A)** and axial **(B)**. Note that a large fragment of disc material has migrated upward from the disc space and is compressing the L4 root against the inferior aspect of the pedicle. Compared to the L5-S1 foramen below almost the entire foramen of L4-5 is occupied by disc material *(arrow)*.

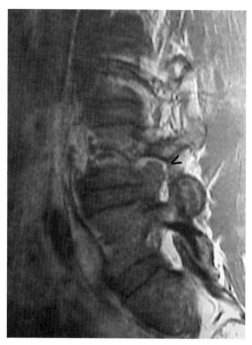

FIGURE 17-5. Magnetic resonance image of foraminal herniation.

CONSERVATIVE TREATMENT

Only a severe neurologic deficit (significant progressive leg pain or weakness and extremity numbness) or cauda equina syndrome (including bowel and bladder dysfunction) is a contraindication for a trial of conservative therapy. Most patients improve following adequate conservative care lasting 2 to 3 months. Although the definition and course of conservative therapy can differ across physicians and patients, in general, it may include an initial 24- to 72-hour period of bed rest, nonsteroidal antiinflammatory drugs (NSAIDs) and other pharmacologic agents, physical therapy, and a trial of oral steroids or a consideration of epidural steroid injections. Patients who either fail to improve or plateau at a level of symptoms that are unacceptable to them may wish to consider a surgical option.

INDICATIONS FOR SURGERY

Proper patient selection is the best predictor of surgical outcome in discectomy, as with most other surgical procedures. The ideal candidate for disc surgery presents with a predominance of leg pain over back pain. Classically, the leg pain radiates below the knee in a single dermatomal pattern. The patient typically demonstrates positive root tension signs with the straight-leg raising test or a cross straight leg raise. If a neurologic deficit is present, it should correlate with the clinical presentation and the radiographic findings. Magnetic resonance imaging (MRI) is the imaging proce-

dure of choice. Plain radiographs are helpful in ruling out concurrent diagnoses such as spondylolysis or spondylolisthesis. In some cases, flexion and extension radiographs may be ordered to rule out instability. Although the absolute indications for surgery are diagnosis of a severe neurologic deficit or cauda equina syndrome, most surgical patients are indicated for failure to improve after adequate conservative therapy.

SPECIAL EQUIPMENT

The operating room microscope provides superb magnification and illumination for performing a microdiscectomy and is my preference (Fig. 17-6). Some surgeons prefer the use of the headlamp with loupe magnification systems. Microscopes offer the additional advantage of a "built-in" option to connect the scope to a video camera to record the surgery and/or a monitor for observation and teaching purposes. Using a microscope, the first assistant and surgeon have identical views of the field, which facilitates coordination in the surgical technique (Fig. 17-7) and resident education.

Specialized instruments usually include a microretractor, a collection of small Kerrisons, pituitaries, and curettes, although surgeons often have other personal preferences for

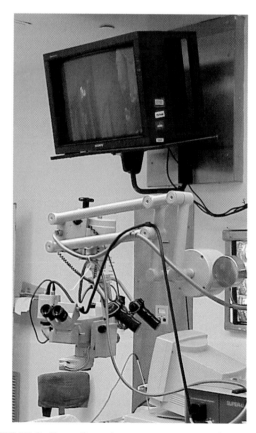

FIGURE 17-6. Operating microscope, camera, and TV monitor.

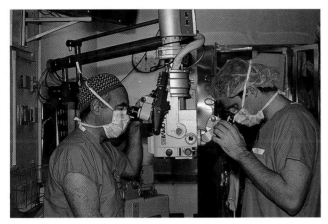

FIGURE 17-7. The operating scope permits the surgeon and first assistant to have virtually the same view of the operative field.

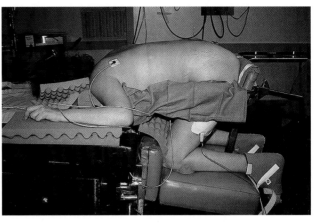

FIGURE 17-9. Patient placed in the knee-chest position, using the Andrews attachment to a standard Amsco surgical table.

instruments to use through the small incision (Fig. 17-8). Small microretractors have a tendency to tilt, lateral side up, in small wounds. To correct this tendency, one can hook a chain with a weight over the lateral blade of the retractor system and hang it off the edge of the table. A good resource for a hook, chain, and weight is a hip self-retractor system (see the section on surgical procedure for further detail).

Preference for operating tables also varies. A standard Amsco surgical table with the Andrews attachment is a frequent choice of surgeons. This particular table has a heavy base that makes it possible to position the patient eccentrically and maintain a stable operative field. Alternatively, some surgeons use large gel rolls or a Jackson table.

SURGICAL PROCEDURE

Patients are administered general anesthesia and placed prone on the surgical table in the knee-chest position.

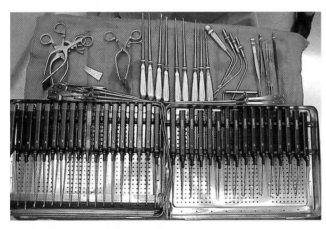

FIGURE 17-8. These sterile operating room trays hold the typical assortment of instruments required to perform microdiscectomy. Upper left are William's retractors, a wide assortment of curettes, Kerrisons (usually angled with narrow shoes), and various nerve root retractors and "feelers" for peridural work.

Placed thus, the lumbar spine flexes slightly and the interlaminar spaces widen a bit (Fig. 17-9). The knee-chest position allows the patient's abdomen to hang free, which decreases intraabdominal pressure. Placing the abdomen in a pressure-free state improves the prone patient's ventilation and also significantly lessens epidural bleeding during surgery. Less epidural bleeding improves the surgeon's vision of the surgical field and contributes to a more controlled procedure and benefits the patient in reduced blood loss.

Localizing the surgical incision is always of paramount importance in spinal surgery. When the incision is as small as 1 to 2 inches, localization takes on added critical significance. One must precisely locate the correct interlaminar space to avoid wrong level surgery. Localization begins with palpation of the interspinous spaces (Fig. 17-10). The L4-5 interspace can usually be located on a line visualized perpendicular to the spine and at the level of the top of the iliac crests. The vertebral levels and interlaminar space can then be confirmed with a lateral intraoperative radiograph taken with a sterile needle placed about 1 inch from the midline but opposite to the planned laminotomy. On pal-

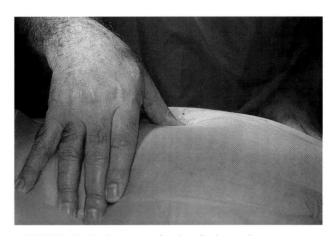

FIGURE 17-10. Surgeon palpating the interspinous spaces.

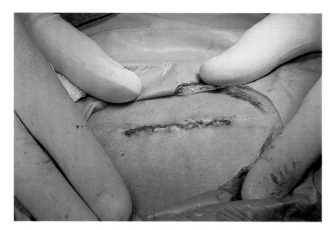

FIGURE 17-11. The incision, the length of which may vary from 1 to 2 inches, depending on the size of the patient.

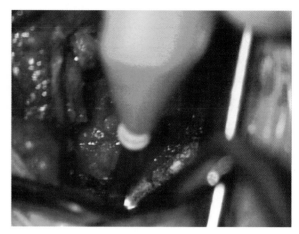

FIGURE 17-13. Electrocautery is used to clear the soft tissue from the lamina.

pation, the L5 spinous process is the first mobile process, working cranially from the fixed sacral processes. Furthermore, the L5-S1 interspace is usually larger than the L4-5 interspace.

The length of incision varies based on the size of the patient and should be carefully considered. Most often, a 1.25-inch incision is sufficient and well tolerated (Fig. 17-11). **However, if the incision is too small for a patient, excessive retraction of the skin edges in an attempt "to make the field work" can adversely impact wound healing. It also produces unnecessary frustration for the surgeon in maneuvering instruments and tissues and attempting to visualize structures.**

Following the initial incision of the skin and soft tissues, an off-midline fascial incision is performed. The fascial incision must be done off the midline to maintain the integrity of the spinous ligament. A completely intact ligament is mandatory, because all spine retractor systems employ the interspinous ligament complex for countertraction while retracting the paravertebral muscles (Fig. 17-12). **If the medial blade of the retractor system slips between the spinous processes and disrupts the interspinous ligament, adequate**

countertraction is not available, and the exposure is reduced. The surgeon must enlarge the incision or use another type of retractor, such as a Taylor retractor. As with small microretractors, Taylor retractors have a tendency to tilt, lateral side up, in small wounds. Some surgeons tie the Taylor retractor down to the base of the operating room table. Alternatively, one can hook a chain with a weight over the Taylor retractor.

Once the interlaminar space is exposed and the soft tissues are removed with a pituitary and electrocautery, the operating scope is brought into position (Figs. 17-13 and 17-14). Using the operative scope, a laminotomy is done next to expose the canal and the spinal nerves. An enlarged view of the laminotomy can be achieved by minor adjustments: upward, downward, medial, and lateral tilting of the scope (Fig. 17-15). Once the dural tube is exposed, remaining ligament and lamina can be safely removed using Kerrison rongeurs. The blunt posterior aspect of the Kerrisons should always be positioned in contact with the dura when performing these tasks; in that way, one again minimizes the possibility of accidentally injuring the dura with the cutting edges of the instrument.

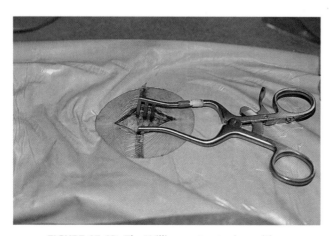

FIGURE 17-12. The Williams retractor in position.

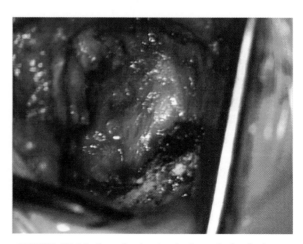

FIGURE 17-14. Superior lamina is cleared of soft tissue.

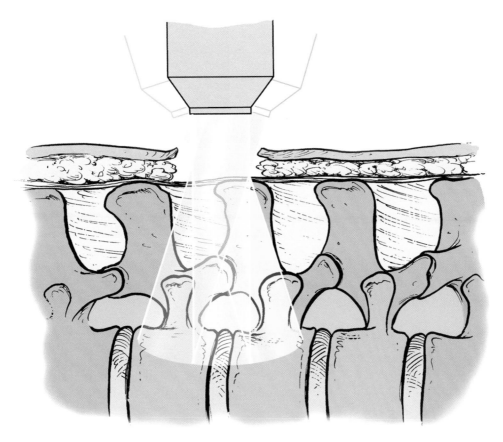

FIGURE 17-15. Graphic demonstrating operating microscope illumination. The microscope can be tilted upward, downward, medially, and laterally, offering a significantly larger view of the field than one might expect through such a small incision.

After the dural tube and near root are exposed, the surgeon must gently retract the exiting nerve root medially to find the disc space and the offending herniation. The surgeon must appreciate that the position of the disc varies relative to the position of the interlaminar space at different levels of the spine. For example, the L5-S1 disc lies directly beneath a relatively large L5-S1 interlaminar space; the surgeon may not need to remove any lamina to proceed or only a very small amount. However, with each more cephalad intervertebral disc space, the disc is incrementally higher relative to the interlaminar space, increasing the amounts of lamina that must be removed to access the disc.

The large ligamentum flavum at L5-S1 allows for easy entry into the spinal canal with a small scalpel blade and forceps. By lifting the ligamentum flavum upward, the surgeon minimizes an incidental durotomy. Once the dura is exposed, further removal of ligamentum flavum and lamina can be performed with Kerrison rongeurs.

At the L4-5 level and higher, the interlaminar space is not sufficiently large to allow for the opening of the ligamentum with a scalpel. Because the ligamentum inserts underneath the superior lamina, removal of the inferior edge of the superior lamina enlarges the interspace (Fig. 17-16). This can be performed with a Kerrison or a burr (Fig. 17-17). 📷

Bleeding from the cancellous bone of lamina can be controlled with the application of bone wax (Fig. 17-18). 📷 Entry into the spinal canal is accomplished by enlarging the laminotomy above the insertion of the ligamentum flavum with a Kerrison 📷 on the undersurface of the lamina (Figs. 17-19 to 17-21), or alternatively once again employ-

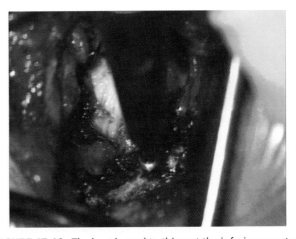

FIGURE 17-16. The burr is used to thin out the inferior aspect of the superior lamina.

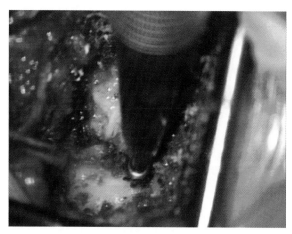

FIGURE 17-17. The lamina is thinned with the burr, down toward the underlying ligamentum flavum.

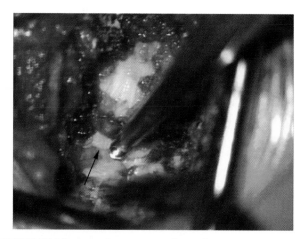

FIGURE 17-20. A Kerrison rongeur *(arrow)* removes the remaining thinned out lamina.

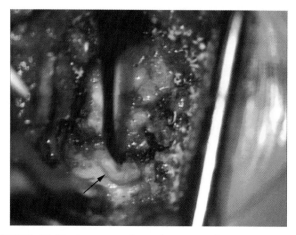

FIGURE 17-18. Bone wax *(arrow)* on a small elevator can be used to control bleeding from cancellous bone.

ing a scalpel (Fig. 17-22). ◖▪ The lateral edge of the laminotomy may safely remove up to 50% of the medial aspect of the facet joint, exposing the underlying nerve root (Fig. 17-23). ◖▪ Removal of greater than 50% of the medial facet may lead to postoperative facet fracture with resultant pain and/or instability.

In this situation, microdissectors or nerve hooks are used to retract the nerve root medially, positioning it medial to the herniation where it can be protected using a right-angle nerve retractor (Fig. 17-24). Traction must be relaxed on the protected "medialized" nerve root by the first assistant at every opportunity, such as when the surgeon has briefly removed instruments from the field. Placing the nerve root under tension may cause a temporary intraneural ischemia, with a potential of injury. Intermittent relaxation of the root likely lessens any potential damage occurring from the ischemia by shortening the ischemic state and allowing recovery in between periods of stretch and tension.

With the root retracted, the surgeon can incise the disc vertically to allow for entry of a pituitary into the disc space

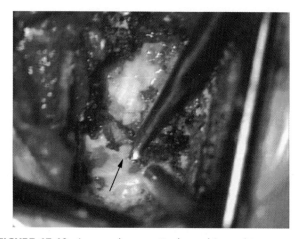

FIGURE 17-19. An upgoing curette *(arrow)* is used to separate the underlying ligamentum flavum from the undersurface of the lamina.

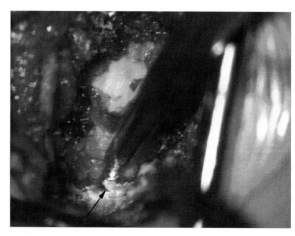

FIGURE 17-21. The Kerrison *(arrow)* removes the lamina above the insertion of the ligamentum flavum exposing the epidural fat in the spinal canal.

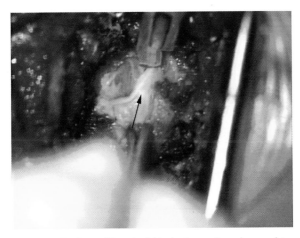

FIGURE 17-22. A no. 15 scalpel blade *(arrow)* can be used to cut the ligamentum flavum aiding removal.

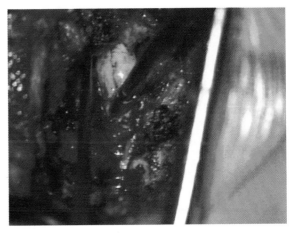

FIGURE 17-25. A pituitary rongeur is used to remove disc material from the disc space.

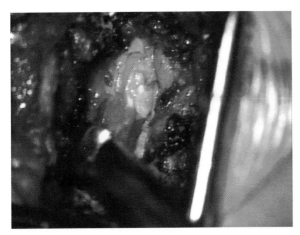

FIGURE 17-23. The Kerrison sequentially removes approximately the lateral half of the ligamentum flavum.

and removal of the herniated portion of the disc material (Fig. 17-25). A single vertical incision is preferable to a rectangular annulotomy. A thin, healed annular scar is probably a stronger barrier to recurrent disc herniation than a broad fibrous scar over a large annulotomy. The pituitaries and curettes allow for local, aggressive removal of disc material from directly under the nerve root. Aggressive "radical" discectomy of the entire disc space with scraping of the endplates is not indicated. There is no evidence that this prevents recurrence or promotes a spontaneous interbody fusion over the course of time.

When an adequate amount of disc material has been removed from the actual disc space, the surgeon must examine the spinal canal for additional extruded fragments that may have migrated. A thorough review of preoperative MRI scans at this time is essential. Removal of all extruded disc fragments is highly dependent on (a) interpretation of the preoperative MRI scans, (b) sufficient lamina removal, and (c) correlation of intraoperative findings with preoperative images (Fig. 17-26). ◼️ It is this correlation that helps min-

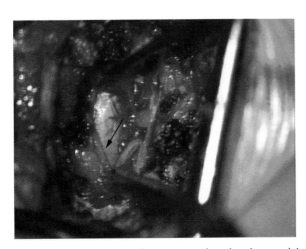

FIGURE 17-24. The dural tube is exposed under the overlying epidural fat *(arrow)*.

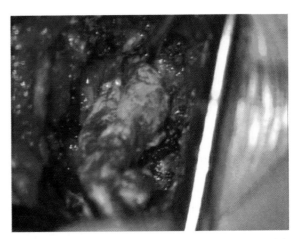

FIGURE 17-26. Large extruded fragment being removed from under the nerve root.

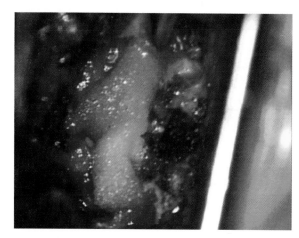

FIGURE 17-27. Gelfoam is placed over the nerve root.

imize the risk of retained fragments. Illumination and magnification of the microscope greatly minimizes the risk.

When removal of the herniated material is complete and the surgeon is satisfied with the nerve root decompression, a fat graft or Gelfoam is used to cover the laminotomy (Fig. 17-27). ◼ Currently, there is no consensus on the risks and benefits of postoperative scar barriers. Bupivacaine (Marcaine) may be used to infiltrate wound edges to reduce postoperative pain at the incision site just before closure. **The fascia is closed before injecting the skin with bupivacaine. If bupivacaine drips onto the nerve root it may cause numbness of the affected root that will be difficult to differentiate from a neural deficit.** The surgical wound is closed in a standard manner: a subcuticular stitch with Steri-Strips and a sterile dressing. The dressed incision is protected by a sterile eye patch, which is usually large enough to cover the small incision. At the time of closure, ketorolac (Toradol), a nonnarcotic injectable analgesic, may be given to the patient and continued postoperatively for comfort to ease early mobilization and prevent the side effects of narcotic medications.

COMPLICATIONS

Potential risks of microdiscectomy surgery are low and include incidental durotomy, infection, bowel and bladder dysfunction, and nerve root injury. Although incidental durotomy is best avoided during disc surgery, adequate intraoperative repair has not been shown to adversely affect long-term outcome.

POSTOPERATIVE CARE

Early mobilization of the patient and discharge (as an outpatient surgery or on the first postoperative morning) is

beneficial to the patient. Pain right after discharge is usually best managed with NSAIDs. Only if necessary, mild narcotic pain medication such as hydrocodone bitartrate and acetaminophen (Vicodin) or propoxyphene and acetaminophen (Darvocet) can be prescribed. I prefer to use a nonaddictive medication or restrict narcotic analgesics to only several weeks for mild to moderate pain relief. After that, over-the-counter medications are appropriate.

FOLLOW-UP CARE

Patients are usually seen in 7 to 10 days for a wound check. At this time, a formal physical therapy program is prescribed to enhance patient recovery. They are custom designed to include exercise to any weak lower extremity muscle groups secondary to neurologic deficits. General trunk strengthening and aerobic exercise is encouraged.

SUGGESTED READINGS

Abramovitz JAN, Neff SR. Lumbar disc surgery: results of the prospective lumbar discectomy study of the joint section on disorders of the spine and peripheral nerves of the American Association of Neurological Surgeons and the Congress of Neurological Surgeons. *Neurosurgery* 1991; 29: 301–308.

Andrews DW, Lavyne MH. Retrospective analysis of microsurgical and standard lumbar diskectomy. *Spine* 1990; 15: 329–335.

Caspar W, Campbell B, Dragos BD, et al. The Caspar microsurgical diskectomy and comparison with a conventional standard lumbar disk procedure. *Neurosurgery* 1991; 28: 78–87.

Errico TJ, Fardon DF, Lowell TD. Open discectomy as treatment for herniated nucleus pulposus of the lumbar spine. *Spine* 1995; 20: 1829–1833.

Goald HJ. Microlumbar diskectomy: follow up of 147 patients. *Spine* 1978; 3: 183–185.

Johnson MG, Errico TJ. Lumbar disc herniation. In: *Orthopaedic knowledge update, spine 2.* Rosemont, IL: American Academy of Orthopaedic Surgeons, 2002: 323–332.

Kahanovitz N, Viola K, Muculloch J. Limited surgical diskectomy and microdiskectomy. A clinical comparison. *Spine* 1989; 14: 79–81.

Lowell TD, Errico TJ, Fehlings MG, et al. Microdiskectomy for lumbar disk herniation: a review of 100 cases. *Orthopedics* 1995; 18: 985–990.

Maroon JC, Abla AA. Microlumbar diskectomy. *Clin Neurosurg* 1986; 33: 407–417.

Nyström B. Experience of microsurgical compared with conventional technique in lumbar disk operations. *Acta Neurol Scand* 1987; 76: 129–141.

Striffeler H, Gröger U, Reulen HJ. "Standard" microsurgical lumbar diskectomy vs. "conservative" microsurgical diskectomy. A preliminary study. *Acta Neurochir* 1991; 112: 62–64.

Williams RW. Microlumbar diskectomy. A 12-year statistical review. *Spine* 1986; 11: 851–852.

Wilson DH, Harbaugh R. Microsurgical and standard removal of the protruded lumbar disk: a comparative study. *Neurosurgery* 1981; 8: 422–427.

CHAPTER 18

LUMBAR SPINAL LAMINECTOMY

JOHN A. BENDO
AMIR HASHARONI

Lumbar spinal stenosis is a narrowing of the spinal canal, most often caused by degenerative changes, that produces compression of the neural elements. The narrowing may involve a single or multiple motion segments. Symptoms created by lumbar stenosis usually have an insidious onset and progress slowly. Vague complaints of low backache and stiffness are typical and are related to degenerative disc disease; in addition there are symptoms of osteoarthritis that are often poorly localized discomfort in the lumbosacral region. This pain, when associated with changes in position and with lifting or bending may be indicative of underlying spinal instability associated with degenerative scoliosis or spondylolisthesis. Back symptoms tend to worsen with activity (mechanical pain) and improve with rest. There are two categories of leg pain symptoms associated with lumbar spinal stenosis. One type of stenosis presents as unilateral leg pain along with numbness, burning, and paresthesias radiating in a dermatomal distribution. This radicular type of presentation is present in less than 20% of symptomatic stenosis patients and is more often seen with severe foraminal or lateral recess stenosis. Neurogenic claudication is defined as the onset of lower extremity pain, paresthesias, or weakness on walking. Symptoms are typically bilateral and consist of an aching, cramping, or burning sensation in the legs. The discomfort starts in the buttocks and often progresses distally to the thighs, calves, and feet. These symptoms are classically exacerbated by standing and by exercising in an erect or extended posture and are relieved by sitting and forward flexion. Patients often assume a hunched or "simian" posture when walking. This phenomenon can be explained by the fact that the size of the spinal canal varies with different postures. Physical examination most commonly reveals a normal neurologic examination. Lumbar extension may exacerbate lower extremity symptoms. Range of motion (ROM) evaluation of the hips and knees should always be performed to rule out degenerative joint disease as a cause of leg pain. Groin pain is not characteristic of lumbar spinal stenosis and should alert the examiner to the possibility of hip arthritis or dysfunction of the sacroiliac joint. An abdominal examination should be performed to rule out an aortic aneurysm. Palpation of distal pulses is necessary to evaluate the possibility of peripheral vascular disease.

ANATOMY

Two distinct anatomic areas, the central spinal canal and the intervertebral nerve root foramen, can potentially compromise the neural elements. The cauda equina is bound anteriorly by the disc, the posterior longitudinal ligament (PLL), and the vertebral body. The pedicles, together with the lateral margins of the ligamentum flavum, create the lateral margins; the laminae, facet joints, and ligamentum flavum form the posterior margins. The spinal nerve-root canal lies within the lateral recess zone, beginning with the origin of the nerve root sleeve at the disc level and ending as the nerve root passes along the inferomedial border of the pedicle at the cephalad aspect of the intermediate level. The intervertebral foramen lies within the pedicle zone. The superior portion of the foramen is located at the intermediate level, and the inferior portion is located at the disc level. The intraspinal pathway of the nerve root and the spinal nerve is formed by the lateral recess zone at the disc level, the pedicle level as it extends to the cephalad aspect of the intermediate level, and the intervertebral foramen at the intermediate level. These three areas correspond to the entrance zone, the midzone, and the exit zone (Fig. 18-1).

CLASSIFICATION

Lumbar spinal stenosis can be classified on the basis of either cause or anatomy. The original etiologic classification, distinguishes congenital or developmental from acquired or degenerative spinal stenosis. Congenital lumbar spinal stenosis is seen in patients of normal stature with congenital short pedicles or in those with a bone dysplasia, such as in achondroplastic dwarfs. Other rare disorders that may manifest congenital stenosis include hypochondroplasia, diastrophic dwarfism, Morquio's syndrome, hereditary exostosis, and cheirolumbar dysotosis. These individuals often first experience symptoms in their 30s and 40s. Acquired stenosis is most likely degenerative, usually starting in the sixth or seventh decade of life.

Anatomic classifications of lumbar spinal stenosis are used to identify specific areas of narrowing of the spinal canal and are particularly helpful as guides for operative decompression. The anatomy of the spinal canal at each vertebral segment can be understood better by dividing the canal into a series of transverse regions (three levels from cephalad to caudad) and sagittal regions (three zones from midline laterally). From cephalad to caudad, the three transverse levels are the pedicle level, the intermediate (vertebral body) level, and the disc level. The pedicle level extends from the

ZONES

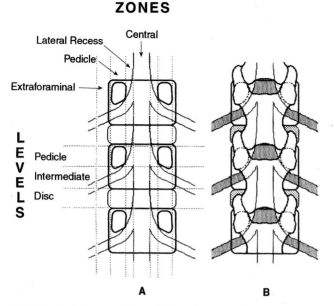

FIGURE 18-1. Coronal plane of spine demonstrating neural pathway zones. Lateral recess, entrance zone; pedicle (foraminal), midzone; extraforaminal, exit zone. Spivak JM. Degenerative lumbar spinal stenosis. *J Bone Joint Surg Am* 1998;80(7):1054, with permission.

superior to the inferior cortical margin of the pedicle. The intermediate level begins at the inferior border of the pedicle and extends caudally to the inferior end plate of the vertebrae. The disc level begins at the inferior end plate and extends caudally to the superior border of the next pedicle. From the midline laterally, the three sagittal zones are the central zone, the lateral-recess zone, and the pedicle zone. The central zone is the area between the normal lateral borders of the noncompressed dural sac. The lateral recess zone is the area between the lateral border of the dural sac medially and a longitudinal line connecting the medial edges of the pedicles laterally. The pedicle zone is the area between the medial and lateral borders of the pedicle.

Lumbar spinal stenosis may be subclassified into central and lateral stenosis (Fig. 18-2). Central spinal stenosis commonly occurs at the disc level, as a result of a bulging disc, facet joint overgrowth (mainly from the inferior articular process of the cephalad vertebrae), and thickening and redundancy of the ligamentum flavum. Lateral stenosis includes both lateral recess and foraminal stenosis. Lateral recess stenosis, which occurs as a result of the degenerative changes similar to those associated with central spinal steno-

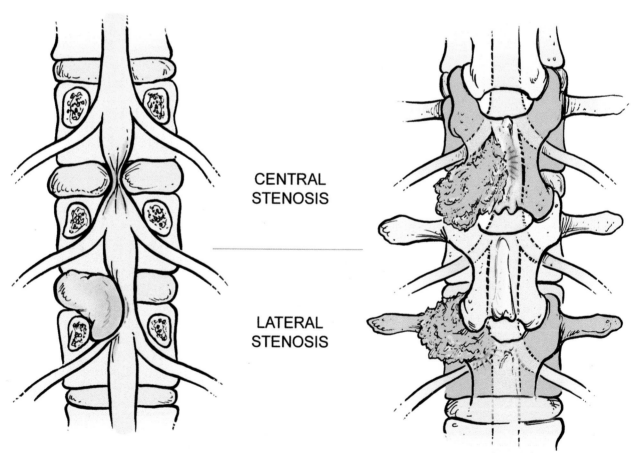

FIGURE 18-2. Central stenosis (*top, left* and *right*) usually develops at the disc level from a bulging disc with facet joint overgrowth from the inferior articular process of the cephalad vertebrae and thickening and redundancy of the ligamentum flavum. Lateral stenosis (*bottom, left* and *right*) includes both the lateral recess and foraminal stenosis resulting from overgrowth from the superior articular process of the caudad vertebra and other degenerative changes similar to those of central stenosis. Lateral recess stenosis affects the spinal nerve root at the disc level.

sis, affects the spinal nerve root canal at the disc level and the superior aspect of the pedicle level. Lateral recess stenosis is uncommon at the inferior aspect of the pedicle but may exist with hypertrophic granulation tissue from the posteriorly located pars interarticularis in patients with spondylolytic defects. Foraminal stenosis is most common at the disc level. Thus, it usually begins in the inferior portion of the intervertebral level. It is at this level that the exiting nerve root may be compressed by disc material, an osteophyte from the inferior aspect of the cephalad vertebrae, or from the superior articular process of the caudad vertebrae.

INDICATIONS

In the past, early operative treatment was recommended for the treatment of symptomatic lumbar stenosis because it was thought that this disorder was always progressive. However, more recent information has suggested a more favorable natural history. The disease has been shown to be relatively stable for 70% of patients with symptomatic spinal stenosis. Long-term follow-up has indicated a 15% incidence of worsening of symptoms and a 15% incidence of improvement of symptoms.

Because lumbar spinal stenosis is not life threatening and rapid catastrophic neurologic deterioration is very rare, the decision to perform an operation should be made after failure of nonoperative treatment, such as physical therapy, epidurals, and oral medication. The presence of a nonprogressive neurologic deficit has been shown to poorly correlate with physical function and thus is not an absolute surgical indication. Progression of a functionally disabling neurologic deficit or cauda equina syndrome, although rarely associated with lumbar spinal stenosis, are two indications for urgent operative intervention. Surgery should be reserved for those patients who have evidence of severe spinal stenosis on imaging studies and have a preponderance of lower extremity symptoms. Patient expectations should be thoroughly discussed before surgery. The goals of surgery are to decrease pain and improve function.

PREOPERATIVE EVALUATION

Before surgery, the following medical workup is required for general anesthesia: electrocardiogram (ECG), complete blood count (CBC), erythrocyte sedimentation rate (ESR), liver and renal function studies, and urinalysis. Any preexisting medical condition should be followed and worked up. The preoperative imaging studies carry great importance in determining the anatomic site of compression and the proper extent of the decompression.

Radiographic examination of a patient in whom lumbar spinal stenosis is suspected often demonstrates multilevel spondylosis. This may or may not be associated with steno-

sis of the spinal canal. Degenerative spondylolisthesis and degenerative lumbar scoliosis are radiographic findings suggestive of lumbar spinal stenosis. Anteroposterior and lateral radiographs should be taken in the standing position; dynamic flexion and extension radiographs taken in the recumbent position are useful for determining whether there is abnormal motion, or instability, at the affected level. For those patients who have associated degenerative scoliosis, weight-bearing anteroposterior and lateral radiographs taken on a long plate are particularly helpful for assessing curve magnitude as well as the overall balance of the entire spine in the coronal and sagittal planes (Fig. 18-3).

Computed tomography (CT) scan is the most cost-effective single test for establishing the diagnosis of lumbar spinal stenosis. It provides excellent osseous detail, especially in the region of the lateral recess. Limitations include ionizing radiation, inferior soft tissue visualization, and inability to visualize the conus medullaris (Fig. 18-4). Magnetic resonance imaging (MRI) provides superior visualization of the soft tissue elements of the spinal canal and is especially useful for the evaluation of abnormalities of the intervertebral disc. Its diagnostic accuracy is superior to those of myelography and plain CT, and it is as accurate and sensitive as myelography followed by CT. The combination of axial and sagittal images allows for complete evaluation of the central spinal canal and the neural foramen. Regions of very low signal intensity on T2-weighted images caused by sclerotic osteophytes can lead to overestimation of the amount of true osseous stenosis. MRI of the scoliotic lumbar spine often is suboptimal because axial images are often not made in the proper plane parallel to the involved disc spaces. The combination of high-quality MRI and plain CT can provide complete evaluation of the spinal canal and often obviates the need for preoperative myelography (Fig. 18-5).

Lumbar myelography followed by CT is also an effective way to obtain a complete anatomic evaluation of compression of the neural elements within the lumbar spine. Lateral myelograms made with the spine in flexion and extension often demonstrate a dynamic component of the stenosis that may be due to segmental instability (in flexion) or encroachment on the spinal canal by bulging discs and ligamentum flavum (in extension). Its main disadvantage includes its invasive nature and insensitivity to foraminal disease. Recent studies have suggested that MRI and CT myelography provide complementary information. However, postmyelographic CT is superior to MRI as a single study for the preoperative planning of decompression for lumbar spinal stenosis.

Electrophysiologic studies, including electromyography (EMG), nerve conduction velocities (NCVs), and somatosensory evoked potentials (SSEPs), are not considered part of the routine assessment for establishing the diagnosis of lumbar spinal stenosis. It is not uncommon to have normal electromyograms and NCVs in a case of classic lumbar spinal stenosis. However, the more typical pattern in symp-

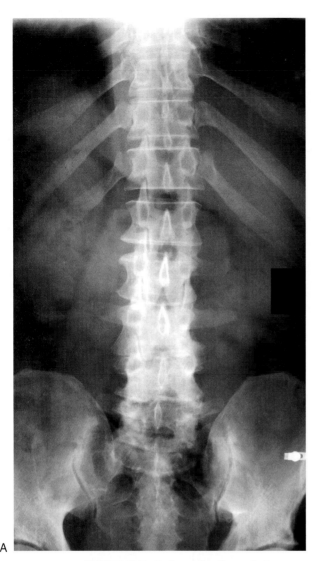
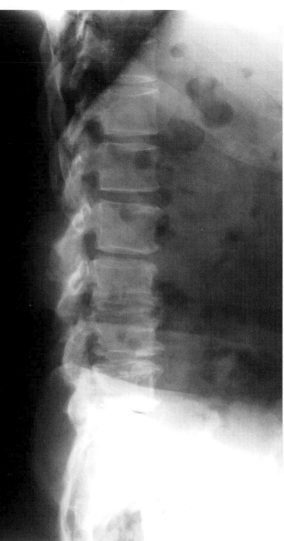

A

B

FIGURE 18-3. A: Coronal radiograph demonstrating sclerosis of the facet joints and vertebral body osteophyte formation. **B:** Lateral radiograph revealing typical findings associated with advanced lumbar spondylosis: loss of lumbar lordosis and multilevel intervertebral disc space narrowing.

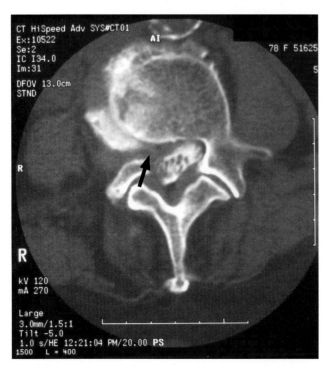

FIGURE 18-4. Axial computed tomography demonstrating high-grade right lateral recess stenosis.

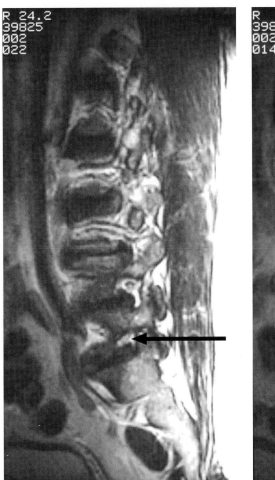

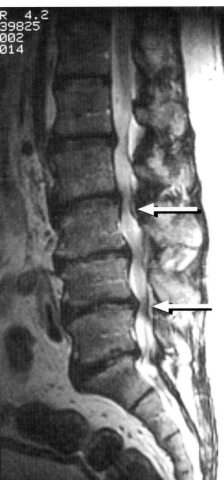

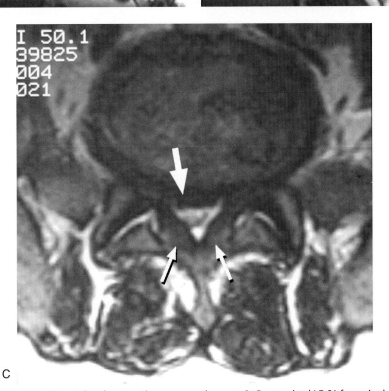

FIGURE 18-5. T2-weighted magnetic resonance images. **A:** Parasagittal L5-S1 foraminal stenosis *(arrow)* with L5 nerve root compression. **B:** Myelogram-like effect of T2-weighted sagittal image demonstrating multiple levels of severe central canal stenosis *(arrows)*. **C:** Axial image revealing redundant ligamentum flavum (small arrows), and a significant bulging of the disc *(large arrow)* posteriorly, creating a severe degree of central and lateral recess stenosis.

tomatic patients is that of a polyradiculopathy, often with bilateral involvement of multiple levels. The NCV, which measures the speed at which the nerve impulse travels, is particularly useful in differentiating peripheral neuropathy (prolonged) from radiculopathy (normal).

EQUIPMENT AND INSTRUMENTS

The following equipment is needed (Fig. 18-6):

- Frazier suction with stylet (8, 10, 12 French)
- Cobb elevators
- Cobb curettes
- Stille-Horseley bone cutter
- Leksell rongeur (narrow, 3 mm; medium, 5 mm; large, 8 mm)
- Assortment of Kerrison rongeurs
- Deep Gelpi retractor or McCullough retractors
- Pituitary rongeur
- Penfield (no. 2, no. 3, no. 4)
- Ball dissector
- Woodson elevator and spatula
- Scoville nerve root retractor
- Bone wax
- Gelfoam soaked in thrombin

PATIENT POSITIONING AND PREPARATION

After adequate anesthesia is obtained, the patient is positioned prone, either on a Jackson table or a four-poster frame, or in a knee-chest position (on the Andrews frame) with the abdomen hanging free (Fig. 18-7). We prefer the abdomen to be free of compression, thus lowering central venous and inferior vena cava pressures and diminishing intraoperative blood loss. The Jackson table allows for hip extension, thus maximizing lumbar lordosis. This is particularly effective when internal fixation is planned. All pressure points should be checked and padded well. The facial struc-

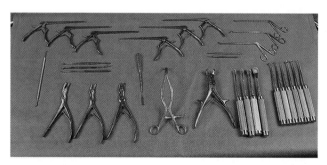

FIGURE 18-6. Equipment: Kerrison rongeurs (6), pituitary rongeurs (3) *(top row);* Woodson elevator and spatula, Penfields (no. 2, no. 3, no. 4), Scoville nerve root retractor, ball dissectors (2) *(middle row);* Leksell rongeurs (narrow, 3 mm; medium, 5 mm; large, 8 mm), deep Gelpi retractor, Stille-Horseley bone cutter, Cobb elevators, Cobb curettes *(bottom row).*

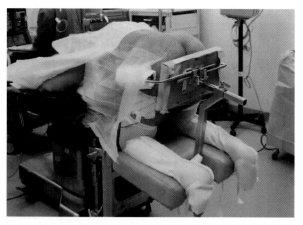

FIGURE 18-7. Patient is prone and placed in a knee-chest position with the abdomen hanging free.

tures particularly the eyes should be free of pressure. Compression stockings and intermittent pneumatic compression boots are routinely used to decrease the incidence of deep venous thrombosis (DVT). Bladder catheterization should be employed for cases lasting longer than 2 hours or when excessive blood loss is anticipated. Perioperative antibiotics should be administered in the form of one preoperative dose in the holding area and postoperative doses over 24 hours.

SURGICAL INCISION LANDMARKS, APPROACH, AND PROCEDURE

Anatomic landmarks used to design an appropriate midline skin incision are the top of the iliac crest (usually L4-5) and the lowest interspinous region palpated (usually L5-S1) (Fig. 18-8). One should consider using an operating microscope or loupe magnification with headlight illumination to

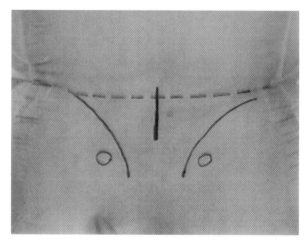

FIGURE 18-8. Preoperative bony landmarks. Circles are posterior superior iliac spines, curved lines are the iliac crests, and the center vertical line represents the incision.

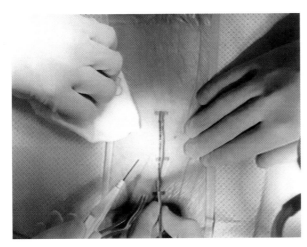

FIGURE 18-9. Incision.

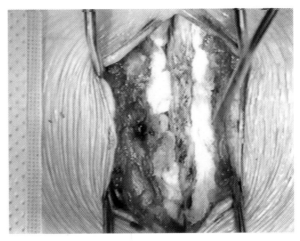

FIGURE 18-11. Exposure of spinous processes, laminae, and facet joints. Blunt dissection with Cobb elevators and packing with gauze.

facilitate the decompression. Placement of a needle followed by a lateral radiograph is helpful to localize the correct level. ◼ A standard midline incision (Fig. 18-9) is then made, and the underlying fascia is identified. The midline fascia is then split with an electrocautery, and the paraspinal musculature is stripped in a subperiosteal manner with Cobb elevators (Fig. 18-10). ◼ The paraspinal gutters are then packed with gauze sponges for hemostasis (Fig. 18-11). After the sponges are removed, self-retaining cerebellar retractors are placed (Fig. 18-12). ◼

Several techniques have been described for decompression of the degenerative stenotic lumbar spine (Figs. 18-13 and 18-14). The standard wide decompressive laminectomy includes removal of the central lamina and ligamentum flavum (Figs. 18-15 to 18-17), ◼ along with a partial facetectomy to decompress the lateral recesses and foramina, bilaterally. One should begin the decompression in the least stenotic area, progressing to the more stenotic areas (Fig.

18-18). In addition, a central trough should be created first (Fig. 18-19), ◼ followed by lateral decompression of the recesses and foramen (Fig. 18-20). ◼ Compressed nerve roots are then directly visualized and decompressed from their origin at the thecal sac and throughout their course as they exit the neural foramina (Fig. 18-21). ◼

Lateral decompression should be performed in line with the nerve roots as they move through the foramen, thereby avoiding amputation of the roots. As each level is decompressed, one should consider packing the neural structures with Gelfoam soaked in thrombin (Fig. 18-22) along with paddies to maintain adequate hemostasis (Fig. 18-23). The electrocautery should be set at a low level when working in the spinal canal. A sharp 0.25-inch osteotome is particularly effective for performing a partial facetectomy in the presence of severe stenosis. The discs should be directly inspected following a laminectomy to exclude significant anterior compression secondary to herniation. Small disc-osteophyte

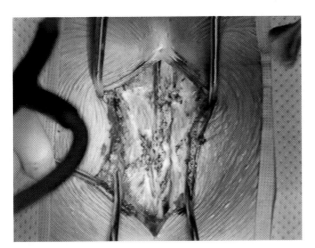

FIGURE 18-10. Opening of fascia and exposure of spinous processes.

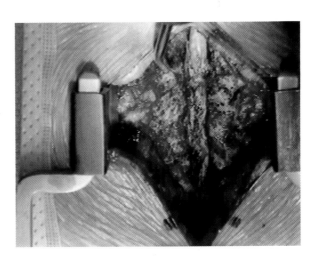

FIGURE 18-12. Spinous processes, laminae, and facet joints are exposed.

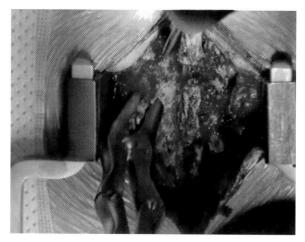

FIGURE 18-13. Spinous process resection.

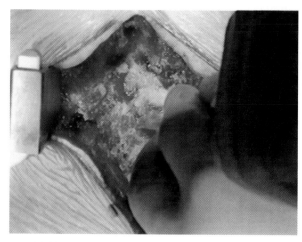

FIGURE 18-16. Curette introduced sublaminally.

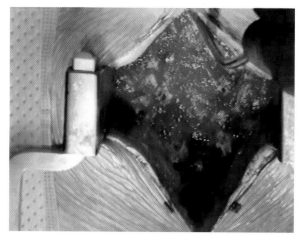

FIGURE 18-14. Spine following resection of spinous processes.

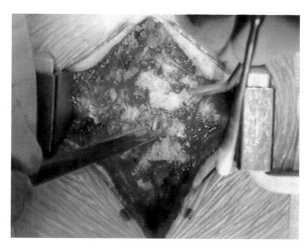

FIGURE 18-17. Beginning the laminectomy.

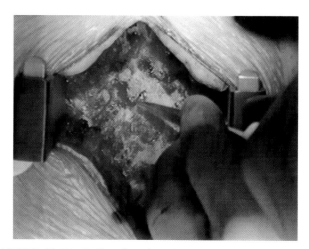

FIGURE 18-15. Finding the edge of the lamina with an "upgo-ing" curette.

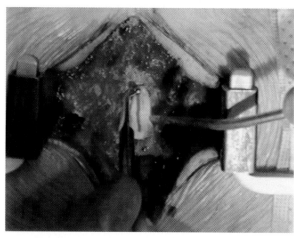

FIGURE 18-18. Introducing patty between the lamina and dural sac using a ball-point probe.

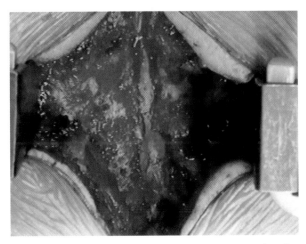

FIGURE 18-19. Central trough laminectomy completed.

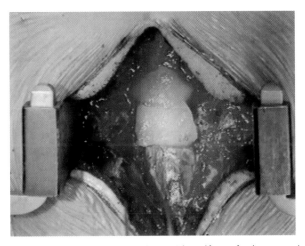

FIGURE 18-22. Covering the dura with Gelfoam for hemostasis.

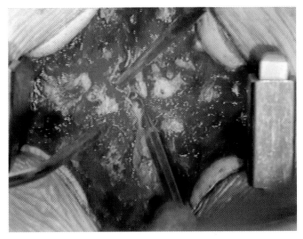

FIGURE 18-20. Lateral recess decompression initiation.

complexes should be ignored; however, larger soft herniations may require excision. Alternative techniques of decompression for the treatment of degenerative central and lateral recess stenosis have been designed in an attempt to preserve more of the osteoligamentous arch, theoretically diminishing the problem of postoperative instability. These techniques include a beveled laminectomy with angular resection of only the anterior portion of the lateral aspect of the lamina, selective single or multiple unilateral or bilateral laminotomy (fenestration procedure), multiple partial laminectomy, and lumbar laminoplasty. **The problem of regrowth of bone with clinically important recurrent stenosis may be more frequent in association with methods of decompression involving limited resection of bone.** Incidental durotomy should be primarily repaired when encountered. Nonbraided 6-0 nonabsorbable suture is our suture of choice. Placing the patient in a Trendelenburg position, while instructing the anesthesiologist to hold an inspiration to prevent movement, is helpful when repairing the defect. Fibrin glue or tissue seal

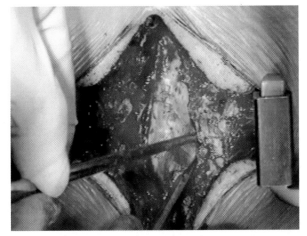

FIGURE 18-21. Widening of the laminectomy while keeping a close watch to avoid injuring the pars interarticularis. Care is taken to avoid too much resection of the medial facet.

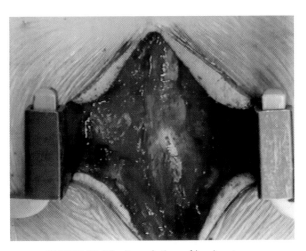

FIGURE 18-23. Completion of laminectomy.

is particularly useful for small dural defects not reparable. If persistent postoperative cerebrospinal fluid leakage is anticipated, one should consider placing a subarachnoid diverting drain for 2 to 3 days postoperatively. When closing the wound, consider a medium-size Hemovac drain to prevent postoperative compressive hematoma formation. Drains should be avoided with persistent leakage of cerebrospinal fluid to avoid an arachnoid-cutaneous fistula. Avoid overzealous decompression around the area of the pars interarticularis to prevent intraoperative or postoperative iatrogenic pars fractures.

The role of arthrodesis in the operative treatment of lumbar spinal stenosis has been the subject of many debates in the recent literature. Following routine decompression in the absence of spinal deformity or instability, concomitant spinal arthrodesis generally does not provide additional clinical benefit. Instability created by resection of the facet joints at the time of operation may be an indication for arthrodesis to prevent postoperative instability and pain. It is generally accepted that stability will be maintained if greater than 50% of each facet joint is left intact. However, biomechanical evidence has suggested that instability may occur after unilateral total facetectomy, even if the remaining facet has been left completely intact.

The role of arthrodesis in the operative treatment of lumbar spinal stenosis with associated degenerative spondylolisthesis has also been extensively studied. Most studies indicated that there is an improvement in clinical outcome in these patients when an arthrodesis is performed at the time of initial decompression. Investigators have discovered that there is a higher chance of reformation of spinal stenosis and instability following laminectomy without fusion in patients with spondylolisthesis. Preoperative radiographic and anatomic risk factors associated with the postoperative development or progression of spondylolisthesis at the level of the fourth and fifth lumbar vertebrae include a well maintained disc height, the absence of degenerative osteophytes, and a smaller, sagittally oriented facet joint.

The surgical management of spinal stenosis in association with degenerative scoliosis is not as clear cut a picture as that of degenerative spondylolisthesis. Not all patients with surgically significant spinal stenosis within a lumbar scoliosis require a simultaneous posterolateral fusion procedure. Certain factors should be assessed preoperatively. The flexibility of the curve should be evaluated by side-bending radiographs. A flexible curve that lacks osteophytes may require arthrodesis to avoid postoperative progression following laminectomy. In some instances, a single symptomatic nerve root can be isolated by means of selective diagnostic injections, allowing for a more limited decompression. A documented history of curve progression should also prompt concomitant arthrodesis. In addition, arthrodesis with curve correction is often necessitated with radiculopathy within the concavity of the curve. Also, a lateral listhesis

is an indication of instability and should be fused. Lastly, a patient with significant loss of lordosis and sagittal imbalance may prompt an arthrodesis to prevent further postoperative kyphosis and increasing back pain.

Simultaneous discectomy and laminectomy raises some concerns. When combined with a laminectomy, "radical" disc excision may lead to iatrogenic spondylolisthesis because it potentially destabilizes the anterior column. A unilateral discectomy performed in addition to a total laminectomy should not lead to postoperative instability when the spine is stable preoperatively. However, if bilateral discectomy is performed along with laminectomy, consideration should be given to concomitant arthrodesis to prevent postoperative instability.

The use of instrumentation in arthrodesis for lumbar spinal stenosis remains controversial. Earlier studies suggested superior clinical results and improved fusion rates when instrumentation was employed. Rigid constructs have been associated with a better clinical result than semirigid constructs, which allow more motion between the fixation screws and the rod or plate. More recent studies suggest that adding instrumentation may improve the fusion rate, although this seldom correlates with clinical outcome. In the face of a degenerative scoliosis, after removal of compressive bone and ligamentous tissue, additional decompression can be accomplished by realignment of the spine with use of segmental distraction via instrumentation along the concavity of the curve. This is done after setting of the convex rod first, with mild compression between screws to preserve or improve lumbar lordosis. For the rare presentation of a painful, collapsing, degenerative scoliosis with back pain only, there may be a role for corrective instrumentation and fusion alone.

POSTOPERATIVE CARE AND FOLLOW-UP

Patients are mobilized immediately following surgery. They are encouraged to remain out of bed, and ambulation training is begun on the first postoperative day. Occasionally, a lumbosacral corset is prescribed for excessive back pain, although it is not part of the routine recommendation. A patient who had a durotomy is advised to remain flat on the back for 24 to 48 hours to prevent headache and leakage of cerebrospinal fluid. Most patients are discharged home on the second postoperative day.

OUTCOME

The results of operative decompression for lumbar spinal stenosis have been generally good. However, more recent studies suggest that the long-term outcome may not be as good as originally thought. The initial favorable clinical outcome seems to deteriorate over time. Factors associated with a poorer outcome include multiple comorbidities, single-level decompressions, a predominance of low back pain, diabetes with neuropathy, osteoarthrosis of the hip, and preoperative degenerative scoliosis. There is a 5% incidence of symptomatic degeneration at levels adjacent to the decompression. Recurrent symptoms may be caused by recurrence of stenosis at a level that was previously decompressed, progression of stenosis at an adjacent level, or mechanical back pain with instability.

Although primarily done to relieve pain, decompression for lumbar spinal stenosis also can affect the function of the bladder. The results of cystomanography and electromyography do not change after decompression, but the postvoiding residual volume often improves in those patients in whom it had been elevated preoperatively.

SUGGESTED READINGS

Booth KC, Bridwell KH, Eisenberg BA, et al. Minimum 5-year results of degenerative spondylolisthesis treated with decompression and instrumented posterior fusion. *Spine* 1999; 24: 1721–1727.

Fischgrund JS, Mackay M, Herkowitz HN, et al. Degenerative lumbar spondylolisthesis with spinal stenosis: a prospective, randomized study comparing decompressive laminectomy and arthrodesis with and without spinal instrumentation. *Spine* 1997; 22: 2807–2812.

Herkowitz HN, Kurz LT. Degenerative lumbar spondylolisthesis with spinal stenosis: a prospective study comparing decompression with decompression and intertransverse process arthrodesis. *J Bone Joint Surg Am* 1991; 73A: 802–808.

Johnson KE, Rosen I, Uden A. The natural course of lumbar spinal stenosis. *Clin Orthop* 1992; 79: 82–86.

Katz JN, Lipson SJ, Chang LC, et al. Seven-to-ten year outcome of decompressive surgery for degenerative lumbar spine disorders. *Spine* 1996; 21: 92–98.

Katz JN, Stucki G, Lipson SJ, et al. Predictors of surgical outcome in degenerative lumbar spinal stenosis. *Spine* 1999; 24: 2229–2233.

Kirkaldy-Willis WH, Paine KWE, Cauchoix J, et al. Pathology and pathogenesis of lumbar spondylosis and stenosis. *Spine* 1978; 3: 319–328.

Postacchini F. Management of lumbar spinal stenosis. *J Bone Joint Surg Br* 1996; 75B: 154–164.

Riew KD, Yin Y, Gilula L, et al. The effect of nerve-root injections on the need for operative treatment of lumbar radicular pain. A prospective, controlled, double-blind study. *J Bone Joint Surg Am* 2000; 82A: 1589–1593.

Spivak JM. Current concepts review: degenerative lumbar spinal stenosis. *J Bone Joint Surg Am* 1998; 80A: 1053–1066.

CHAPTER 19

LUMBAR FUSION

JEFFREY M. SPIVAK
PETER BONO

The purpose of lumbar spinal fusion is to immobilize vertebral motion segments that have become unstable and/or painful because of a variety of conditions (degenerative disc disease; trauma; and isthmic or degenerative spondylolisthesis, among others). All fusion surgery involves bone graft to provoke a biologic response and cause the graft to fuse with the vertebral elements, thereby stopping motion between vertebrae at the affected level(s). Optimally, spinal fusion for the reduction of pain involves one or more motion segments; however, fusing more segments excessively reduces the normal spinal movement and may place too much stress on adjacent vertebral joints. In recent decades, the introduction of spinal instrumentation has enhanced the rate of successful fusion, in part because of the added stability that they provide at the fusion site during healing.

Spinal stability is defined as the ability of the spine under physiologic loads to maintain normal relationships between vertebrae, in such a way that there is neither damage nor subsequent irritation to the spinal cord or nerve roots. Many authors have attempted to define instability. Frymoyer presented a clinical definition stating "a loss of spinal motion segment stiffness, such that force application to that motion segment produces greater displacement(s) than would be seen in a normal structure, resulting in a painful condition, and placing neurologic structures at risk." This is a fairly thorough clinical description of instability. The term segmental instability, coined by McNab, has been used to describe greater than normal angulatory and translatory motion as a result of degenerative disc disease. Through cadaveric studies, White and Panjabi have attempted to quantify instability and as a result have developed radiographic criteria for instability. Using flexion and extension radiographs, translational motion of 3.5 mm or angular motion of 11 degrees of one vertebra over another is indicative of segmental instability.

Approaches to spinal fusion surgery include posterolateral intertransverse fusion, posterior lumbar interbody fusion (PLIF), anterior lumbar interbody fusion (ALIF), and anterior/posterior spinal fusion. This chapter is limited to discussion of posterior approaches, most particularly the gold standard of spinal fusion, posterolateral intertransverse process fusion (using transpedicular screw instrumentation and posterior iliac crest bone grafting).

ANATOMY

Understanding the relationships of the anatomic structures of the posterior lumbar spine is important for performing a safe and successful spinal fusion. Posterior bony elements of a lumbar vertebra include the spinous process, laminae, pars interarticularis, facets, transverse processes, and pedicles (Fig. 19-1). Posterior soft tissue structures include the supraspinous ligament, interspinous ligament, ligamentum flavum, and facet capsules. The pedicles are cylindrical bony projections off the posterosuperolateral aspect of the vertebral body that connect the vertebral body with the posterior bony arch. The pedicles are oriented in an anteromedial direction when viewed from the posterior. This angulation progressively increases from L1 through L5. Also, the cylindrical diameter of the pedicles progressively increases from the upper to the lower lumbar spine. This knowledge of pedicle anatomy is extremely vital for safe and successful insertion of screws into the pedicle. The spinous process of each vertebra extends caudally and overlaps the vertebra below by about one half of a segment. For example, the tip of the spinous process of L4 is actually over the body of L5.

At the base of the spinous process are the laminae, which project laterally both cranially and caudally, to form the superior and inferior facets, respectively (Fig. 19-2). The portion of bone found between the superior and inferior facets is the pars interarticularis and is named for its location between the articular processes. The lateral most part of the pars interarticularis is C-shaped and easily found between the facet joints (Fig. 19-2). It is important to identify the lateral border of the pars interarticularis. Excessive bone removal during laminectomy decompression can lead to destabilization of the vertebra. Once the pars interarticularis is found, the C-shaped lateral border can be followed superiorly to the inferior edge of the transverse process and the accessory process (on the posteroinferior aspect of the root of the transverse process) is found. These are important landmarks for pedicle screw insertion, which is discussed later. The superior articular process is found adjacent to the transverse process and accessory process and is directly over the pedicle (Fig. 19-2). The convergence of these three structures is important in the identification of the pedicle. The accessory process and mammillary process (rough elevation on posterior border of superior facet) may be difficult to locate and can be absent in some patients. The superior articular process is oriented in an anterolateral position relative to the inferior articular process of the cephalad vertebra. For example, when examining the L4-5 facet joint the superior facet of L5 is found anterior and lateral to the inferior facet of L4.

The posterolateral gutter is an important region to identify, as this is where bone graft is laid for a posterolateral

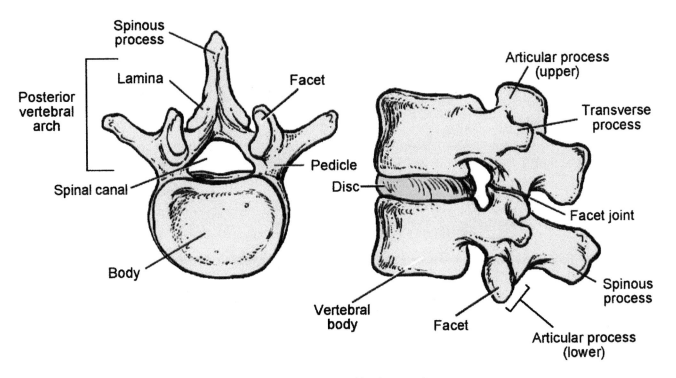

FIGURE 19-1. Anatomy of lumbar vertebrae.

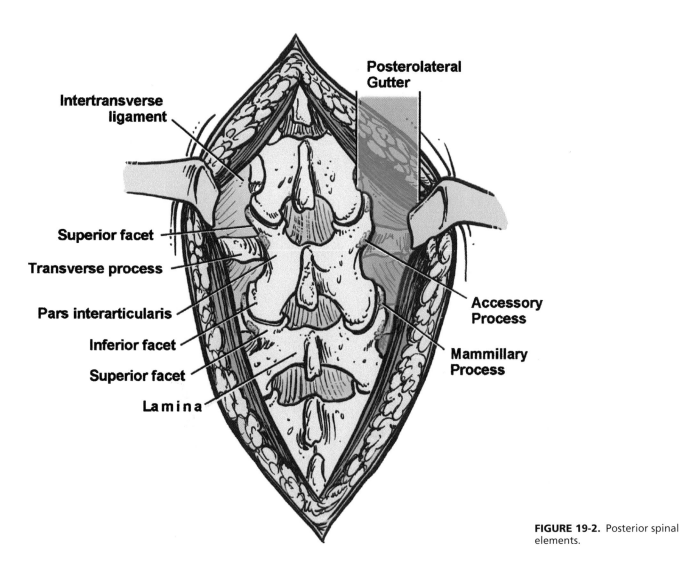

FIGURE 19-2. Posterior spinal elements.

fusion (Fig. 19-2). The gutter is generally defined as the area lateral to the facet joints, supported anteriorly by the transverse processes and the intertransverse ligament.

Posterior ligaments important for spinal stability include the supraspinous ligament, which runs along the dorsal aspect of the spinous processes, and the interspinous ligament, which segmentally attaches between spinous processes (Fig. 19-3). These two ligaments aid in resisting flexion moments. The ligamentum flavum is a strong, elastic structure that runs in a shingle pattern. It originates on the ventral surface of the cephalad lamina and inserts onto the dorsal surface of the caudal lamina.

The muscles of the lumbar spine are divided into three layers. The latissimus dorsi is the most superficial muscle and is covered centrally by the lumbodorsal fascia. The deep muscle layer is subdivided into the superficial layer and deep layer, which contain the transversocostal group and the transversospinal group, respectively. The transversocostal group consists of the iliocostalis, the longissimus, and the spinalis muscles forming the erector spinae group. The transversospinalis group consists of the short rotators: multifidus, rotatores, interspinalis, and intertransversarii.

CLASSIFICATION

Classification is not applicable in lumbar fusion.

INDICATIONS

The role of arthrodesis in the treatment of degenerative disorders of the lumbar spine is still not fully defined. Agreement concerning specific indications for spinal fusion

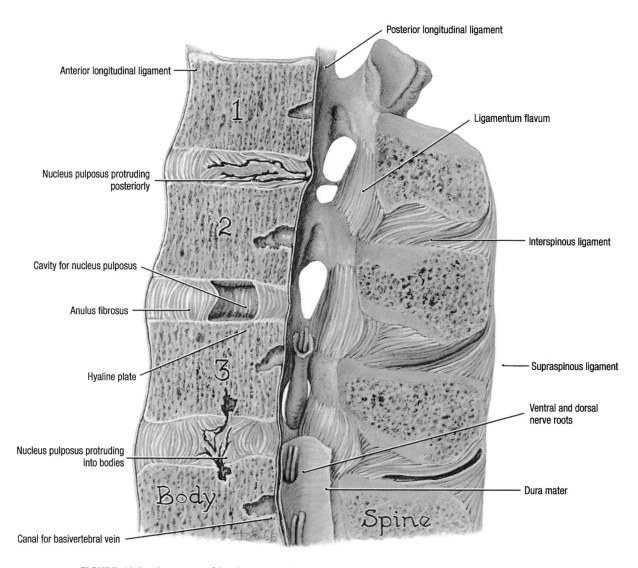

FIGURE 19-3. Ligaments of lumbar spine. (From Agur AMR, Lee MJ. *Grant's atlas of anatomy,* 10th ed. Philadelphia: Lippincott Williams & Wilkins, 1999, with permission.)

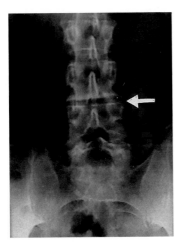

FIGURE 19-4. Preoperative anteroposterior x-ray film. L3-4 disc space collapse *(arrow)*.

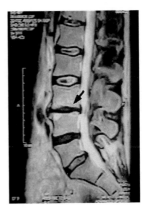

FIGURE 19-6. Preoperative T2-weighted sagittal magnetic resonance imaging. At L3-4, note decreased disc height *(arrow)*, decreased signal, and endplate changes.

has evolved slowly. Posterior spinal fusion is commonly used to stabilize lumbar motion segments in spinal stenosis, degenerative spondylolisthesis, isthmic spondylolisthesis, recurrent disc herniation, scoliosis (degenerative or idiopathic), kyphosis, and back pain.

The common denominator in all of these conditions is back pain. Spinal pain can originate from mechanical, inflammatory, or neurochemical sources. The exact mechanisms are not clearly understood, but vertebral motion plays an important role. The purpose of spinal fusion is to eliminate pathologic motion and thereby eliminate pain. In cases of deformity, the goal of spinal fusion is to maintain correction and prevent progression of deformity.

Indications for Instrumented Fusions

Spinal arthrodesis is associated with complications, particularly with the addition of instrumentation. Therefore, the

benefits to be obtained must be weighed against the risks. The primary indications for use of instrumentation in lumbar spinal fusions are segmental instability, deformity correction, unstable spinal trauma, and improvement in the healing rate of the fusion. This last indication is particularly important in repeat fusions in cases of pseudoarthrosis. Added risks associated with the use of instrumentation include increased blood loss, possible iatrogenic neural injury, and a higher postoperative wound infection rate.

PREOPERATIVE PLANNING

A fundamental objective of preoperative planning is to confirm the correct vertebral level or levels of fusion and to localize the incision. Anteroposterior (AP) and lateral radiographs (Figs. 19-4 and 19-5), as well as axial computerized tomography (CT) or magnetic resonance imaging (MRI) (Figs. 19-6 and 19-7) are used for the purpose of identifying the injured vertebra or vertebrae and to estimate the position, orientation, and width of the vertebral pedicle; the latter pedicle information is important for later instrumen-

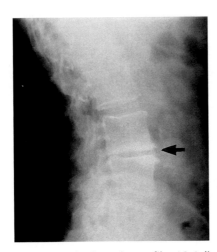

FIGURE 19-5. Preoperative lateral x-ray film. L3-4 disc space collapse *(arrow)*.

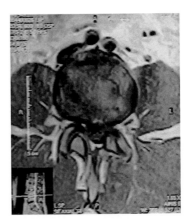

FIGURE 19-7. Preoperative T1-weighted axial magnetic resonance imaging. L3-4 central disc bulge.

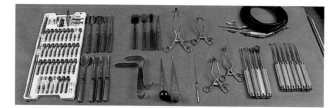

FIGURE 19-8. Equipment. (*left* to *right*): transpedicular implant system (pedicle screw system), gouges (autograft procedure); *(top row)* curved osteotomes (autograft procedure), two Gelpi retractors, high-speed burr; *(bottom row)* Taylor retractors, straight and curved blunt-tipped pedicle finders, flexible ball-tipped probe, two cerebellar retractors, Cobb elevators, and curettes.

tation of the vertebrae. There are several techniques for localization of the incision and these are discussed within the section on patient position and preparation section.

EQUIPMENT AND INSTRUMENTS

Needed equipment is as follows (Fig. 19-8):

- Frame choices:
  Andrews frame/kneeling
  Jackson table/hip extension
  Four-post Relton-Hall frame/hip extension
- Cerebellar retractors
- Cobb elevators
- Curved osteotome (autograft procedure)
- Curettes and gouges (autograft procedure)
- Gelpi retractors
- Taylor retractor
- Radiopaque marker pins
- High-speed burr or awl
- Straight or curved blunt-tipped pedicle finder
- Flexible ball-tipped probe

- Transpedicular implant system (pedicle screw system)
- Bone wax
- Gelfoam

PATIENT POSITIONING AND PREPARATION

Proper patient position in the operating room is important for several reasons. First, adequate relief of intraabdominal pressure reduces epidural venous pressure and decrease intraoperative bleeding. Second, several positioning frames exist that allow for varying amounts of lumbar lordosis. Each type of frame has advantages and disadvantages. Kneeling frames, such as the Andrews frame, flex the hips and reduce lumbar lordosis (Fig. 19-9). This has the effect of opening the interlaminar space and thus may facilitate decompression of the spinal canal. However, the reduced lumbar lordosis may be undesirable if an instrumented lumbar fusion is being performed. Frames that allow for full hip extension, such as the Jackson table or the four-post Relton-Hall frame, allow for full lumbar lordosis and subsequently narrow the interlaminar space. This may make central canal and lateral recess decompression more difficult and also presents a "worst case scenario" to ensure an adequate decompression. **Caution must always be taken when positioning a patient on any prone positioning frame because injury to the skin overlying bony prominences is more likely if not thoroughly padded. In addition, abduction of the arms should be limited to 90 degrees to the trunk axis to avoid a possible stretch injury to the brachial plexus.**

SURGICAL INCISION AND LANDMARKS

Several bony landmarks can easily be palpated to help one obtain a rough approximation of the operative level in the lumbar spine (Fig. 19-10). The top of the iliac crests gener-

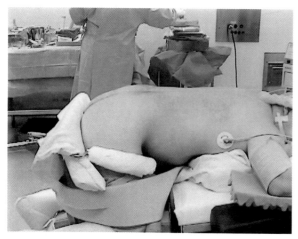

FIGURE 19-9. Knee-chest patient position using Andrews kneeling frame.

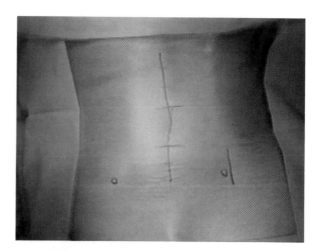

FIGURE 19-10. Surgical markings for midline posterior lumbar incision and a separate iliac crest incision. Left and right circles mark each posterior superior iliac spine.

ally are seen at the L4-5 level on lateral radiograph. With palpation of the top of the crests, the thumbs can be brought to the midline at the crest level and the L4 spinous process is generally found. Alternatively, the sacrum may be palpated over the midline in a cephalad direction. The first notable prominence is the L5 spinous process. It is reiterated that these landmarks are approximations only and it is our recommendation that an intraoperative cross-table lateral radiograph with markers be obtained to establish the correct level of the operation.

A preoperative lateral radiograph with a needle placed using sterile technique can be useful for localization of the incision. For a lumbar discectomy, an 18-gauge needle is placed along the superior aspect of the spinous process of the cephalad vertebra. This usually corresponds to the superior pole of the incision for approaching the operative disc level. For example, the needle placement for an L4-5 lumbar discectomy would be along the superior aspect of the L4 spinous process. A second lateral radiograph is obtained for level confirmation following exposure and before decompression.

For more extensive exposures, we often obtain a cross-table lateral radiograph with two 18-gauge needles positioned to mark the superior and inferior poles of the incision before sterile preparation (Fig. 19-11). This is generally along the spinous processes two levels above the cephalad vertebra and one level below the caudal vertebra to be fused. Once the exposure is completed, a second intraoperative lateral radiograph is taken with a straight clamp placed on an interlaminar area. Alternatively, an 18-gauge spinal needle can be placed into the exposed mamillary processes. This aids in identifying the insertion point and direction for pedicle screw placement if instrumentation will be used. Generally, we always try to obtain as much information as possible from intraoperative radiographs.

SURGICAL APPROACH

The posterior approach to the lumbar spine is through a posterior midline incision (Fig. 19-10). This midline skin incision can be followed by one of two different fascial exposures: a direct posterior approach and an intermuscular posterolateral approach to the lateral facets, transverse processes, and intertransverse space. The posterior approach, the workhorse of the lumbar spine, is the subject of this chapter. It provides access to all of the posterior spinal elements by means of a single longitudinal midline fascial incision. Direct exposure of the spinous process, laminae, and facets at all levels can be achieved. In addition, further lateral dissection and retraction of the paraspinal musculature can also reach the transverse processes and posterolateral gutter. If necessary, exposure of the posterior wall of the vertebral body and disc space can be achieved following laminotomy or laminectomy. This requires mobilization and medial retraction of the thecal sac or a more lateral exposure of the disc space, either via the neural foramen or more laterally (extraforaminal). The conus medullaris in the upper lumbar segments prevents safe medial retraction of the thecal sac.

Technique

Once the length of the incision is determined, the skin incision is marked (Fig. 19-10). A midline incision is made over the spinous processes of the operative levels (Fig. 19-12). Dissection proceeds through subcutaneous adipose tissue either sharply or with electrocautery to the lumbodorsal fascia. Cerebellar retractors placed in the subcutaneous tissue allow tension to be applied to the tissues and expedite dissection. Meticulous hemostasis is imperative. To facilitate closure and to ensure midline dissection, a Cobb elevator can be used to gently clear adipose tissue from the midline, thereby clearly exposing the midline fascia. The lumbodorsal fascia is then incised with electrocautery over the bulbous tip of the

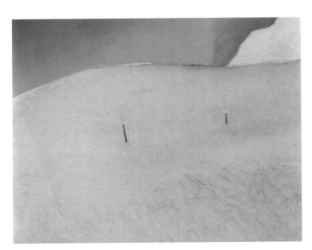

FIGURE 19-11. Localization of incision. Placement of two 18-gauge needles at superior and inferior poles of incision, followed by cross-table lateral radiograph.

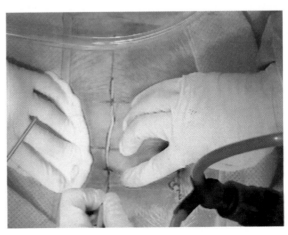

FIGURE 19-12. Midline incision through skin.

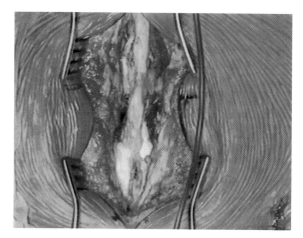

FIGURE 19-13. Lumbosacral fascial incision.

spinous process (Fig. 19-13). This is carried out through all the spinous processes to be removed. We recommend leaving intact the midline fascia and supraspinous ligament of the spinous processes that are not part of the planned decompression. This allows for stability of the posterior column of the remaining vertebrae and also provides a midline structure for reattachment of the fascia during wound closure. Once the fascia is incised, the musculature is elevated subperiosteally along the lamina with electrocautery. This is best done in a caudal to cephalad direction, because the paraspinous muscles originate obliquely on the midline interspinous ligament. Packing sponges helps facilitate the dissection and also aids in hemostasis. ▣ Sponges are removed and cerebellar retractors are placed deeper in the wound to retract the paraspinal muscles. Next, dissection proceeds laterally to identify the facet joint capsule. Care must be taken to avoid disruption of the facet capsule if spinal instrumentation is not to be used. Once the facets are identified, the pars interarticularis is exposed between the joints. Identification of this landmark is crucial during canal decompression, because overzealous widening of the central

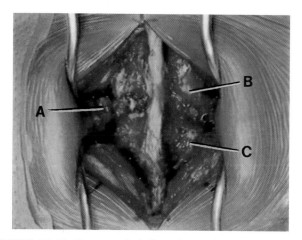

FIGURE 19-14. Deep surgical dissection. *A:* L3 transverse process. *B:* L2-3 facet joint. *C:* L3-4 facet joint.

canal can lead to violation of the pars interarticularis and subsequent iatrogenic fracture and instability. If the surgical plan is to perform a fusion limited to the posterior spinal structures, then surgical exposure to this point is generally satisfactory. If a posterolateral fusion is planned, then further lateral dissection is necessary to expose the transverse processes and intertransverse spaces (lateral gutters) (Fig. 19-14).

Further lateral exposure begins with subperiosteal removal of soft tissue overlying the pars using a Cobb elevator to sweep the muscle laterally away from the pars. **Bleeding is routinely encountered during pars dissection and should be anticipated. Caution should be used to avoid dissecting anteriorly around the lateral border of the pars because the dorsal root ganglion is beneath the pars.** Next, dissection of the paraspinal muscles off the facet capsule is facilitated by gentle retraction of the muscles with a Cobb elevator up and over the facet joint capsule. The last obstacle to overcome is exposure of the transverse processes. These can be palpated laterally at the caudal aspect of each facet joint. As mentioned earlier, the superior articular process (of the caudal vertebra) lies anterolateral relative to the inferior articular process (of the cephalad vertebra) and the transverse process (part of the caudal vertebra) is adjacent to the superior articular process. Also, the transverse process can be found by following the lateral border of the pars superiorly, where an accessory process is often found near the base of the transverse process. A Cobb elevator is used, along with electrocautery, to subperiosteally release and laterally sweep muscle attachments from the transverse processes. **Bleeding is routinely encountered during dissection along the lateral wall of the superior articular process. The facet bleeder has a predictable course over the lateral wall of the facet, and the electrocautery can be held over this position to stop the bleeding.** Once the transverse processes have been identified, gentle retraction with a Cobb elevator in a lateral sweeping motion allows for exposure of the intertransverse ligament. This ligament will serve as an anterior sling along which to span bone graft from one transverse process to another for achieving an intertransverse process fusion. **Caution must be taken to avoid anterior penetration through this ligament because the retroperitoneal space, containing nerve roots and vascular structures, is immediately anterior. Bleeding from anterior to the intertransverse ligament may be difficult to control, but attempts to control it should be made with bipolar electrocautery and hemostatic agents rather than uncontrolled unipolar electrocautery.** Once sufficient lateral exposure is obtained, self-retaining retractors are placed over the transverse processes at the cephalad and caudal ends of the exposure, and the lateral gutters are tamponaded with packing sponges.

SPINAL FUSION PROCEDURES

There are essentially two commonly used posterior lumbar fusion techniques in spinal surgery today. A *posterior spinal fusion* refers to a fusion limited to the posterior elements including spinous processes, facets, and laminae. An *intertransverse process fusion* (posterolateral fusion) refers to a fusion between the transverse processes of adjacent vertebrae within the posterolateral gutter, including the lateral borders of the pars interarticularis and superior articular facet processes. Fusion levels can also be provisionally stabilized with the use of metallic internal fixation (spinal instrumentation).

Posterior Spinal Fusion Technique

With this technique the fusion surfaces are limited to the posterior spinal structures, excluding the transverse processes and posterolateral gutters. Once the surgical approach is completed, preparation for bone grafting and fusion can be initiated. Thorough denuding of the spinous processes and laminae is performed with curettes, rongeurs, or a motorized burr. The spinous processes and laminae can also be split and shingled using a sharp osteotome, creating additional living, bleeding bone surfaces for healing. Facet joints involved in the fusion should be denuded of their capsule and articular cartilage. Once decortication is completed, local and harvested iliac crest bone graft is placed along the interlaminar spaces to bridge the laminae. Caution must be used to avoid having bone graft in communication with a lamina not involved in the planned fusion. Cancellous bone chips are packed into the decorticated facet joints. Once bone grafting is completed, the muscle and fascial layers are approximated tightly with absorbable suture, often over a deep self-suction surgical drain. The subcutaneous layers are well approximated to avoid dead space, and the skin is closed.

Posterolateral or Intertransverse Process Fusion Technique

Successful surgical exposure of the posterolateral gutters requires strategic placement of deep retractors. Cobb elevators are placed bilaterally directly on the posterior surface of the most cephalad transverse processes to sweep the deep tissues laterally (Fig. 19-15A). While retracting these tissues, the blades of the deep self-retaining retractor (we use a Gelpi-type retractor to avoid excessive tissue pressure) are placed along the transverse processes; simultaneously, the elevators are gently brought out posteriorly as the self-retaining retractor is engaged and spread. The same technique is repeated over the caudal transverse process so that a Gelpi retractor is placed at both ends of the wound (Fig. 19-15B). It should be noted that the use of different types of retractors for deep exposure may require the use of different techniques to apply the retractor and complete the exposure.

After exposure, the lateral gutter is inspected to ensure thorough soft tissue debridement from the transverse processes, the facet joint, and the pars interarticularis. Decortication of these structures is performed with a high-speed burr. The facet joints involved in the fusion are also denuded of cartilage and decorticated using the burr. Local bone graft (spinous process, laminar fragments), if available, and harvested iliac crest bone graft is placed over the intertransverse ligament to bridge the transverse processes. Cancellous bone is also placed into the facet joints and packed with a bone tamp and mallet. Once bone grafting is completed, the routine closure proceeds as previously described previously.

POSTERIOR ILIAC CREST BONE GRAFTING

Bone grafting is performed to provide a bridging scaffold of osteoconductive and possibly osteoinductive material to accelerate or augment the normal healing process of bone. Autologous bone graft has an osteoinductive capacity not found in allograft bone and provides for a significantly higher rate of successful bone fusion. However, harvesting autologous bone can add significant morbidity to a spinal fusion.

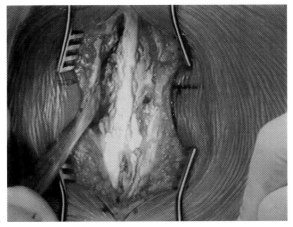
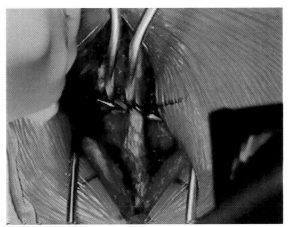

A   B

FIGURE 19-15. A: Cobb elevator is used to sweep deep tissues laterally off of the transverse processes. **B:** Gelpi retractors.

The most common forms of autologous bone graft include iliac crest bone, generally harvested from posterior iliac crest, and local bone graft obtained from the surgical site (spinous process and laminae).

The posterior iliac crest can be reached through subcutaneous dissection of the inferior aspect of the primary surgical incision or through a separate incision centered over the posterior superior iliac spine (PSIS). There are advantages and disadvantages to either approach. Performing a subcutaneous dissection through the primary surgical incision obviates the need for an additional incision. However, hematoma formation from the iliac crest can result in wound complications that would affect both the primary surgical site and the iliac crest site. Also, a secure closure of the dissected fascia overlying the iliac crest may be more difficult to achieve through this approach. Alternatively, using a second skin incision over the iliac crest avoids the previously mentioned complication. Although a second surgical incision leaves the patient with two surgical scars, the benefit obtained from a separate iliac crest incision may outweigh cosmetic results.

Technique

The iliac crest can be accessed either through a separate parasagittal incision or through an extension of the operative midline incision. For a parasagittal incision, a longitudinal line, approximately 6 to 8 cm in length, is drawn centered just lateral to the PSIS (Fig. 19-10). Two thirds of the incision should be above the PSIS. **Placement of the incision further laterally places the cluneal nerves at risk. Placement directly over the PSIS may make the patient prone to more postoperative pain from direct pressure, especially for thin patients.** After the skin is incised, electrocautery may be used to continue the subcutaneous dissection while controlling hemostasis. Alternatively, the iliac crest can be reached through the same midline skin incision used for the spinal fusion. This requires further caudal extension of the incision. With this approach, dissection is carried out laterally above the fascia toward the PSIS.

With either approach, the dissection at this point is the same. Once the iliac crest is encountered, the electrocautery is used to incise the fascia along the curvature of the crest (Fig. 19-16). The gluteus musculature is elevated in a subperiosteal fashion from the lateral surface of the ilium with the use of a Cobb elevator. A Taylor retractor is then placed deep into the wound and secured into the lateral wall of the ilium. ◼ An osteotome is used along the lateral wall of the ilium to score the outer table, creating strips of cortical bone. ◼ A curved osteotome is used along the base of the exposure and along the upper aspect of the lateral wall of the crest, driven between the inner and outer table to release cortical strips. ◼ Special care should be taken to maintain the posterior cap of the iliac crest intact unless needed for additional bone. At this point curettes and/or gouges are used to harvest cancellous bone.

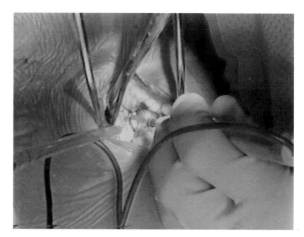

FIGURE 19-16. Incising iliac crest fascia with cautery.

<u>Maintaining posterior cap intact minimizes postoperative pain when sitting or laying supine, especially with thin patients.</u> ◼ **The sciatic notch must be avoided during bone graft harvesting; inadvertent injury to this region can lead to a sciatic nerve injury or a significant bleeding problem from injury to the superior gluteal artery.** After harvesting of the available cancellous bone, the wound is irrigated copiously and bone wax or Gelfoam are applied to the bleeding cancellous surfaces for hemostasis. ◼ The fascial layer is closed with heavy absorbable suture. If necessary, a deep or subcutaneous wound drain can be placed.

TRANSPEDICULAR SCREW INSTRUMENTATION

Transpedicular screw fixation represents a major advancement in spinal implants and the ability to control and stabilize vertebrae from a posterior approach. Pedicle screws are placed through the pedicle of lumbar vertebrae from a posterior to anterior direction. Unlike hooks, secure fixation of the screws does not depend on the presence of an intact posterior bony arch, making screw fixation the implants of choice in patients with a previous or concurrent laminectomy. Pedicle screws provide a great resistance to various loads because of their bone purchase into the vertebral body. By obtaining fixation into the anterior column, greater rotational control is achieved. There are many pedicle screw systems available on the market today. A list of Food and Drug Administration (FDA) approved pedicle screw systems is available from the North American Spine Society.

Screw Insertion Technique

Although many pedicle screw systems exist, they all share a similar screw insertion technique. Pedicles screw insertion is technically demanding, requiring an excellent knowledge of the regional anatomy and pathoanatomy of the lumbar spine. Malpositioning of a screw can result in neurologic injury, violation of a normal adjacent intervertebral disc space, and failure of fixation. This description of screw insertion is not meant as a sole source of instruction for a surgeon; it is an adjunct approach. Pedicle screw placement should only be attempted by a qualified spinal surgeon following fellowship training or during a direct apprenticeship.

Intraoperative fluoroscopy using anteroposterior and lateral images may be of significant value to identify the direction of the pedicles. Oblique imaging can be helpful to follow insertion directly along the axis of the pedicle. Surgical exposure of the base of the transverse process is mandatory for pedicle screw insertion. This can be accomplished using the midline posterior spinal approach described previously or a paraspinal approach, avoiding muscle dissection in the midline. The accessory process, pars interarticularis, and the transverse process are important landmarks for the screw insertion point that must be visualized (Fig. 19-10). There are several anatomic relationships that may be helpful in identifying the location of the pedicle. The use of a lumbar spine

model is instrumental in gaining an appreciation and understanding of the posterior arch and the pedicular anatomy.

First, a line drawn longitudinally along the lateral border of the pars intersects with the medial border of the pedicle in all lumbar pedicles except L5 (Fig. 19-17). At L5 the opposite is true, a longitudinal line drawn along the lateral border of the L5 pars intersects with the lateral border of the L5 pedicle. This occurs because there is an increase in the medial angulation of the central axis of each pedicle as one progresses through the lumbar spine from L1 to L5. Second, the intersection of a longitudinal line through the facet joint and a horizontal line (Fig. 19-17) through the middle of the transverse process marks the location of the pedicle deep to these structures. Finally, it is generally accepted that the medial angulation of the pedicle cortical tube progresses by 5 degrees between L1 and S1. For example, medial pedicle angulation at L1 is 5 degrees and L5 is 25 degrees. These anatomic landmarks are meant to be rough approximations only.

The starting point for a pedicle screw is found by bisecting the base of the transverse process horizontally, proceeding medially up against the lateral border of the facet joint.

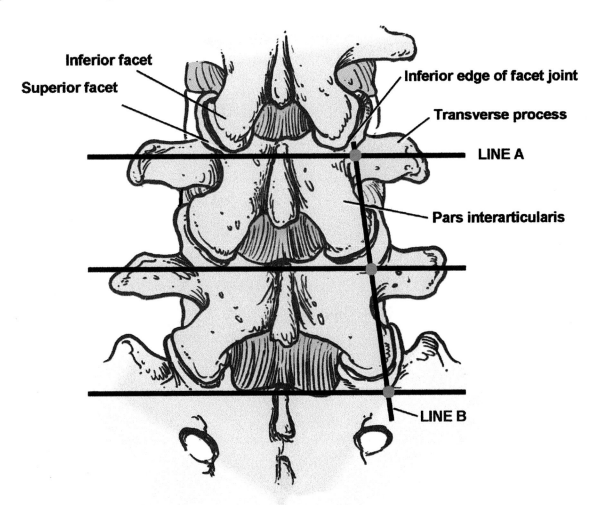

FIGURE 19-17. Starting point for pedicle screw: cross-section of line *A* bisection of transverse processes and *B* lateral border of the pars interarticularis.

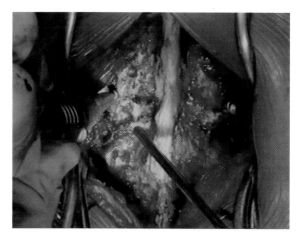

FIGURE 19-18. High-speed burr; decortication of mamillary process exposing entrance to pedicle.

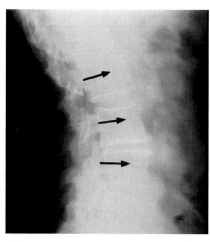

FIGURE 19-20. Preoperative lateral x-ray film. L3-4 disc space collapse (note position of pedicle and orientation for insertion of pedicle screws).

This usually places the starting point directly over the accessory process when it is present. Next, a 3-mm ball-tip high-speed burr or awl is aimed in an anteromedial direction and is used to make a starting hole along the lateral aspect of the facet (Fig. 19-18). ◗ The orientation of the pedicle in both the transverse and sagittal planes must be kept in mind at this point. It is necessary to refer to the intraoperative lateral radiograph to determine the sagittal orientation of the pedicle (i.e., cephalad, caudal, or perpendicular to the floor) (Figs. 19-19 and 19-20). A straight or curved blunt-tipped

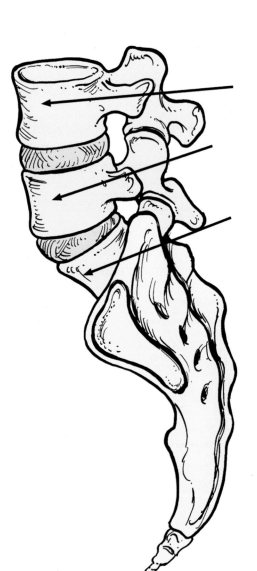

FIGURE 19-19. Pedicle screws parallel to endplates or with slight superior angulation to penetrate denser bone near endplate.

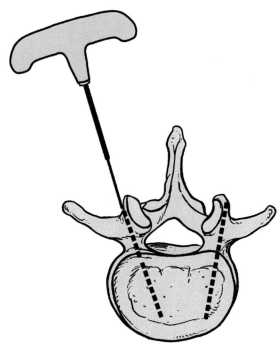

FIGURE 19-21. Probe is at pedicle entrance and angled at correct superior/inferior and medial/lateral orientation to create pedicle track.

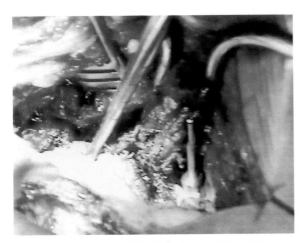

FIGURE 19-22. Pedicle finder in right L3 pedicle.

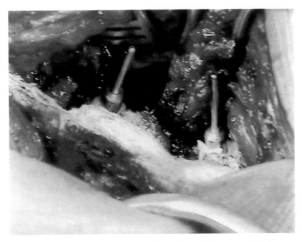

FIGURE 19-24. Radiopaque marker placed into pedicle to assess pedicle orientation.

pedicle-finder is placed into the starting hole and directed anteromedially in the transverse plane, as indicated by the level, and also in the sagittal plane, as indicated by the pedicle direction on the intraoperative lateral radiograph (Figs. 19-21 and 19-22). 'O◀ The probe is advanced to a depth of approximately 40 to 45 mm only if it passes with relative ease. If there is uncertainty about the position of the probe, a marker can be placed into the created hole and radiographic evaluation is done before continuing (Fig. 19-23). Next, a flexible ball-tipped probe is placed into the pedicle and all four walls (superior, inferior, medial, and lateral) are examined for continuity of bony surface. 'O◀ Depth of the created screw tract is also assessed, being sure of a bony deep endpoint. Radiopaque marker pins can be placed into the pedicle holes and an intraoperative radiograph or fluoroscopic image can be obtained to confirm intrapedicular positioning of the markers (Fig. 19-24). Following this, the pedicle hole may be tapped, and the screw inserted (Figs. 19-25 and 19-26). 'O◀ Once all screws are inserted, longi-

tudinal rods are connected and a cross-linking bar can be applied as well (Fig. 19-27). 'O◀ Standard wound closure over drains completes the procedure.

When screw fixation is used and posterolateral fusion is being done, it is recommended to obtain bone graft before placement of the screws. Then, after preparation of the screw hole, the lateral elements should be decorticated; 'O◀ and the bone graft placed in the lateral gutter before final insertion of the screws (Fig. 19-28). 'O◀ After screw insertion, visualization of the lateral gutter and bony elements may be quite limited, making complete decortication and proper grafting difficult if not impossible.

The preoperative MRI image of an individual with a symptomatic degenerative disc at L3-4 is seen in Figures 19-6 and 19-7. Notice the marked collapse of the disc space and

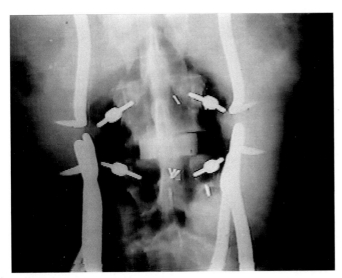

FIGURE 19-23. Intraoperative anteroposterior x-ray film with markers in pedicles of L3 and L4.

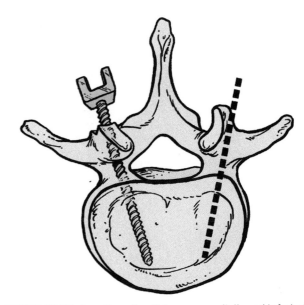

FIGURE 19-25. Insertion of pedicle screw medially and inferiorly close to the anterior cortex without penetrating it.

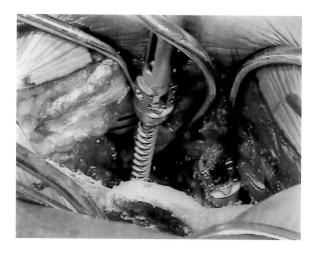

FIGURE 19-26. Insertion of pedicle screw.

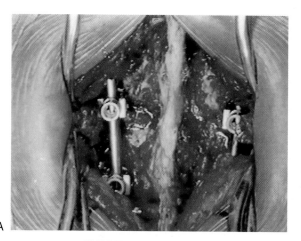

A

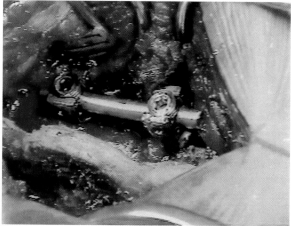

B

FIGURE 19-27. A: Rod and screw construct (see **B**, side view). **B:** Rod and screw construct.

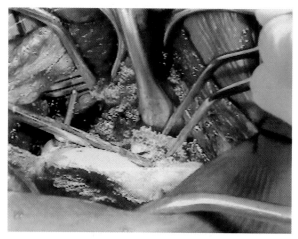

FIGURE 19-28. Placement of iliac crest bone graft into postero-lateral gutter.

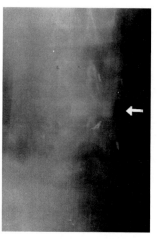

FIGURE 19-29. Anteroposterior x-ray film after anterior lumbar interbody fusion (ALIF) (*arrow* at femoral ring).

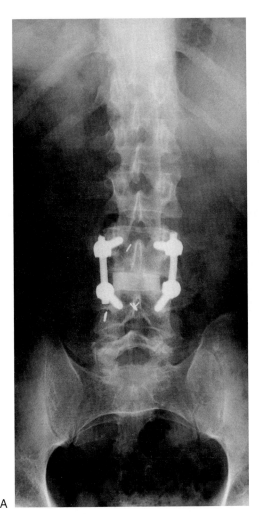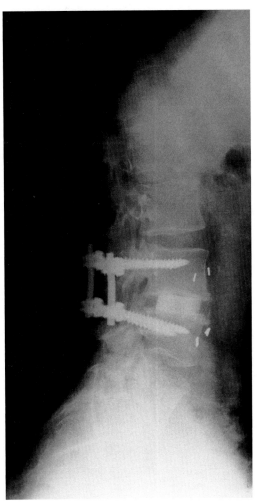

A   B

FIGURE 19-30. A: Anteroposterior x-ray film of final construct. **B:** Lateral x-ray film of final construct.

diminished signal on the T-2 weighted image indicating disc desiccation (Fig. 19-6). Plain radiographs, in the anteroposterior and lateral projection, of this individual demonstrate the loss of disc space height and early osteophytic changes (Figs. 19-4 and 19-5). Restoration of the disc space height was achieved with an ALIF using a femoral ring allograft as a structural support (Fig. 19-29). Postoperative radiographs demonstrate the final pedicle screw construct for a one level fusion (Fig. 19-30).

POSTOPERATIVE MANAGEMENT AND FOLLOW-UP

Immediate postoperatively management involves local wound care and mobilization of the patient. Generally the patient is fitted for a lumbosacral orthosis. Following discharge the patient is encouraged to increase activity gradually while maintaining lifting, bending, and squatting restrictions. Physical therapy is implemented on an outpatient basis to provide a structured exercise program. Part-time

sedentary work is allowed at 4 to 6 weeks. After 3 months the orthosis is discontinued and the patient is allowed to return to full time employment with light to moderate activity. Full heavy labor and vigorous activities may resume 6 months after surgery.

SUGGESTED READINGS

Frymoyer JW, Pope NH. Segmental instability. *Semin Spine Surg* 1991; 3: 109–118.
Herkowitz HN, Kurz LT. Degenerative spondylolisthesis with spinal stenosis: a prospective study comparing decompression with decompression and intertransverse process arthrodesis. *J Bone Joint Surg Am* 1991; 73A: 802.
Panjabi MM, Abumi K, Duranceau J, et al. Biomechanical evaluation of spinal fixation devices: I and II. *Spine* 1988; 13: 1129–1140.
White AA, Panjabi MM, Posner I, et al. Spinal stability: evaluation and treatment. *Instr Course Lect* 1981; 30: 457.
Wiltse LL, Bateman JG, Hutchinson RH, et al. Paraspinal sacrospinalis-splitting approach to the lumbar spine. *J Bone Joint Surg Am* 1968; 50: 919–926.

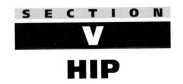

SECTION V
HIP

CHAPTER 20

HYBRID TOTAL HIP ARTHROPLASTY

WILLIAM L. JAFFE
CRAIG J. DELLA VALLE

Total hip arthroplasty has revolutionized the treatment of end-stage arthritis of the hip offering both patients and physicians a reliable treatment option that relieves pain and improves function. When compared with other medical and surgical interventions for common diseases, the cost of quality-adjusted life years associated with total hip arthroplasty is nearly unparalleled and it is felt to be among the most cost effective of all medical interventions available. It is estimated that more than 150,000 total hip arthroplasties are now performed annually in the United States. Given the aging of the population that is expected to occur over the next several decades, the number of patients requiring treatment of arthritis of the hip will increase greatly making an appropriate understanding of the surgical indications for and basic techniques of total hip arthroplasty imperative for orthopaedic surgeons. Hybrid total hip arthroplasty (insertion of a cementless acetabular component and a cemented femoral component) has emerged as a reliable method for prosthetic fixation and this chapter reviews in-depth the surgical technique for this procedure.

ANATOMY

The hip joint consists of the articulation between the cartilaginous surfaces of the femoral head and the pelvic acetabulum. The femoral neck forms an angle with the femoral shaft that ranges between 120 and 140 degrees with approximately 10 to 15 degrees of anteversion. The femur itself has an anterior and somewhat lateral bow that must be appreciated during femoral canal preparation. The acetabular surface is oriented approximately 45 degrees caudally and 15 degrees anteriorly. Two strong columns of bone (anterior and posterior) reinforce the acetabulum. Patients with a history of trauma or developmental hip disease may have altered anatomy outside of these ranges, and preoperative Judet views of the acetabulum or computed tomography (CT) scanning may be appropriate to accurately define a given patient's anatomy.

Important surgical landmarks within the acetabulum include the anterior and posterior walls and the sciatic notch, which can serve as guides to positioning the acetabular component. The base of the fovea is used as a guide to determine the appropriate depth for acetabular reaming. The transverse acetabular ligament marks the inferior margin of the acetabulum.

CLASSIFICATION

Classification is not applicable.

INDICATIONS

Total hip arthroplasty is indicated for patients with painful, end-stage arthritis of the hip who have failed nonoperative treatment (including the use of nonsteroidal antiinflammatory medications, the use of an assist device in the opposite hand, and activity modification) and for whom alternative reconstructive procedures are not deemed appropriate. Patients must also be willing to comply with the necessary precautions for avoiding dislocation and early mechanical failure of the prosthesis. When performed in the appropriate patient population, the cost to quality-adjusted life years ratio for total hip arthroplasty is unparalleled when compared with other medical interventions.

Patients should have a history of severe pain in the groin and/or proximal thigh along with corroborative physical examination and radiographic findings to confirm the presence of end-stage hip arthritis. The physical examination should include a thorough assessment of the lower back and other areas extrinsic to the hip to ensure that the hip pain experienced by the patient is not referred from a distant source. In cases in which the cause of the patient's pain is unclear (e.g., a patient with both hip and back pain as well as radiographic evidence of significant hip and lumbar spine arthrosis), we have successfully used an intraarticular lidocaine injection into the hip to confirm that the pain is arising from the hip joint. A clinical assessment for presence of a leg-length discrepancy is an integral portion of the physical examination. The presence of a significant hip flexion or adduction contracture is also important to note preoperatively so that these can be addressed at the time of surgery.

Options for patients with end-stage hip arthritis include arthrodesis, osteotomy, and arthroplasty. Arthrodesis of the hip is performed infrequently at our institution. It is reserved for young (<40 years old), usually male patients who have unilateral hip arthritis, and no history of pain in the lower back, spine, or contralateral hip. Patients who are unwilling or unable to comply with the lifestyle changes that are compatible with a successful arthroplasty (such as those who are manual laborers or have a history of recent intravenous drug abuse) are also considered for hip arthrodesis. Patients with inflammatory arthritis and nontraumatic osteonecrosis of the hip are poor candidates for arthrodesis given the high risk for involvement of the contralateral hip; in these patients, arthroplasty is a better option.

Osteotomy of the hip is reserved for patients who have a focal biomechanical derangement of the hip joint with an adjacent area of intact cartilage available for redirection into the weight-bearing portion of the joint. Osteotomy can be performed on either the femoral or the acetabular side of the joint. A congruous joint with good range of motion is a prerequisite. These procedures are most often used in younger patients with early degenerative arthritis secondary to the residua of developmental dysplasia of the hip or in those patients with early osteonecrosis (no evidence of acetabular degeneration) and a small area of femoral head involvement. Osteotomy is contraindicated in patients with inflammatory arthritis, given the typical concentric nature of the cartilaginous destruction in these patients and the expectation of further joint destruction.

Long-term follow-up studies of cemented total hip arthroplasty have shown survivorship of a cemented femoral component to be more than 90% at 20 years, with higher rates of both clinical and radiographic failure of the cemented acetabular component. This has lead to increased interest in the use of acetabular components inserted without cement to improve prosthetic longevity. Clinical studies demonstrate decreased rates of clinical and radiographic failure at intermediate term follow-up and support the use of these devices. The use of a cemented femoral component and an acetabular component inserted without cement (hybrid total hip arthroplasty) has met with excellent clinical success and is appropriate for most patients undergoing total hip arthroplasty. Although the use of femoral components inserted without cement has increased and midterm results appear promising, the excellent long-term results observed for femoral components inserted with modern cement techniques justify their continued widespread use.

Contraindications to total hip arthroplasty include patients with active joint sepsis and patients who are unwilling or unable to comply with the lifestyle changes compatible with a successful total hip arthroplasty. Relative contraindications are patients with severe medical comorbidities that make them poor surgical candidates and patients with paral-

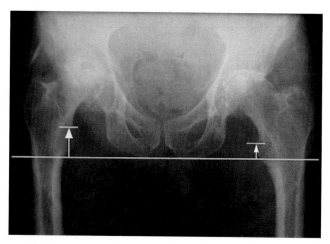

FIGURE 20-1. Leg-length determination on anteroposterior radiograph.

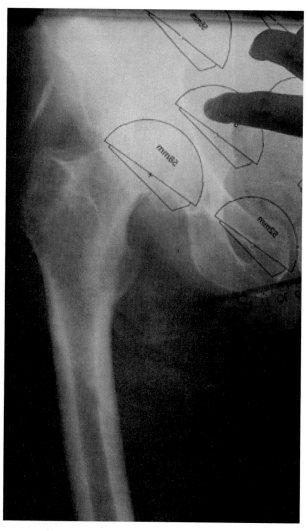

FIGURE 20-2. Acetabular component templating.

ysis of the abductor musculature that would make postoperative instability a great concern.

PREOPERATIVE PLANNING

Required radiographs for preoperative planning include an anteroposterior (AP) view of the pelvis, centered low to include the proximal half of the femur, as well as a lateral radiograph of the hip. A line drawn tangential to the bottom of the ischial tuberosities is used to determine the amount of preoperative leg-length discrepancy as the difference between this line and the top of the lesser trochanter bilaterally (Fig. 20-1). Clear overlay templates provided by the manufacturer are then used to approximate the level of the femoral neck cut and the size of the acetabular and femoral components to be used. The acetabular component should lie next to the acetabular teardrop medially (i.e., the outer table of the medial wall of the acetabulum), and the new center of rotation of the hip is marked on the radiograph (Fig. 20-2). The previously selected femoral component template is then placed over the radiograph and rotated around the new center of rotation of the hip until it lies within the femoral canal in both AP and lateral projections (Fig. 20-3A and B). A prosthesis of appropriate size and

neck length should be selected that will to re-create the patient's femoral offset (distance from the center of the femoral head to the central axis of the femoral shaft). The level of the femoral neck osteotomy is then estimated and marked with an appropriate compensation made to equalize leg lengths as determined on the AP radiograph of the pelvis.

A thorough preoperative medical assessment performed by a medical internist is mandatory to identify patients at high risk for perioperative morbidity and mortality who may benefit from preoperative medical optimization. Clinical issues that should be screened for and resolved before total hip arthroplasty include dental disorders, urinary tract disorders (outlet obstruction in men or recurrent infection in women), and any skin disorders or lesions; all of these may contribute to recurrent postoperative bacteremia. Patients with appropriate preoperative hemoglobin levels are encouraged to donate one unit of autologous blood preoperatively.

EQUIPMENT

General Equipment

- Large bone hook
- Mallet
- Cobb elevator

FIGURE 20-3. Femoral component templating. **A:** Anteroposterior. **B:** Lateral.

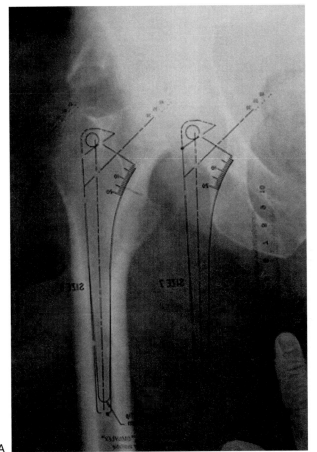

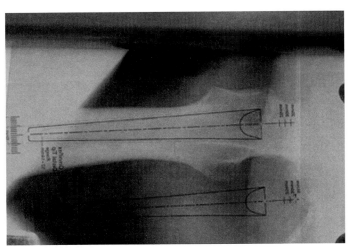

A

B

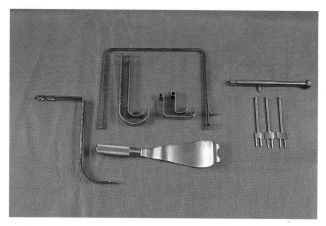

FIGURE 20-4. Retraction devices: anterior acetabular retractor *(left)*; Charnley incisional retractor with regular and deep blades *(middle top)*; broad femoral neck (jaws) retractor *(middle bottom)*; small, medium, and large double-prong wing retractors with insertion handle *(right)*.

- Standard and long knife handles
- Standard and long cautery blades

Retraction Devices (Fig. 20-4)

- Charnley incisional retractor with regular and deep blades
- Morris retractor
- Hohman retractors regular and bent
- Double-prong wing retractors with insertion handle; small, medium, and large
- Anterior acetabular retractor
- Broad femoral neck (jaws) retractor

Bony Preparation (Fig. 20-5 and 20-6)

- Blunt-tipped Charnley tapered reamer (canal finder)
- Harris curette
- Femoral reamers
- Femoral broach trial
- Femoral broach handle
- Acetabular reamers and trials
- Bone screw instruments

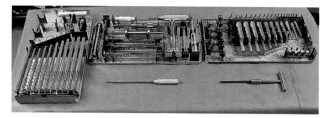

FIGURE 20-5. Bone preparation: Femoral reamers *(left tray)*; femoral broach handle *(middle tray, top)*; Harris curette (middle bottom); Femoral broach trial *(right tray, top)*; blunt-tipped Charnley tapered reamer (canal finder) *(bottom right)*.

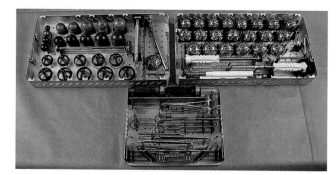

FIGURE 20-6. Acetabular reamers and trials *(top trays)*; bone screw instruments *(bottom tray)*.

Cement Equipment (Fig. 20-7)

- Cement gun kit with vacuum attachment
- Break-away nozzle
- Cement pressurizer
- Femoral brush
- Tampon for drying femoral canal
- Bucks cement restrictor

PATIENT POSITIONING AND PREPARATION

Care must be taken when positioning the patient for total hip arthroplasty to avoid iatrogenic injury and to ensure appropriate siting of anatomic landmarks for component positioning. We use a hip positioner that firmly secures the patient to the operating table in the lateral decubitus position. In markedly obese patients, the positioner is angled with the anterior portion more caudad, to allow for firm contact with the anterior superior iliac spine without undue soft tissue compression. The down leg has a foam pad placed beneath the knee at the fibular head (to protect the peroneal nerve) and beneath the lateral malleolus to prevent pressure-induced injury (Fig. 20-8A and B). The abdominal area must be well padded, particularly in obese patients. An axillary roll, made from carefully rolled sheets, is used on the up-

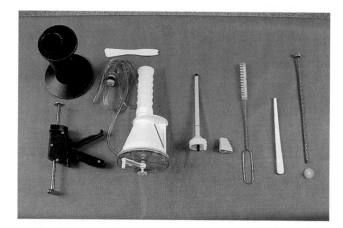

FIGURE 20-7. Cement equipment *(left to right)*: cement gun with vacuum attachment *(left)*; breakaway nozzle, cement pressurizer (yellow), femoral brush, tampon for drying femoral canal, Bucks cement restrictor.

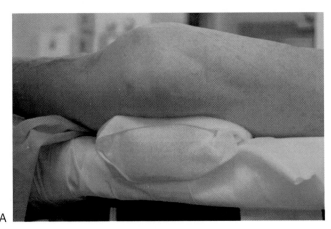

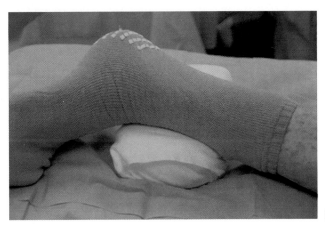

A   B

FIGURE 20-8. Patient preparation. **A:** Knee pad. **B:** Lateral malleolar pad.

per chest to protect the brachial plexus on the down side from injury. A pillow is placed between the legs to pad the down leg, and is taped into place. The operative table must be level with the floor and the pelvis should be perpendicular to the floor to allow for accurate positioning of the acetabular component (Fig. 20-9).

Before surgical prepping, the hip is taken through a range of motion to ensure that 90 degrees of flexion is possible with the patient firmly secured in the positioner. A first-generation cephalosporin (or clindamycin in patients with known allergies to penicillin or cephalosporins) is administered preoperatively. The entire extremity is then prepped from above the iliac crest to include the foot, sequentially using Betadine scrub and paint. The foot is covered with a glove and the extremity draped in a full-length stockinette. The area of the surgical incisions is covered with an iodinated nonpermeable adhesive. The surgical team wears body exhaust hoods during the procedure.

SURGICAL INCISION AND LANDMARKS

The principal landmark for planning the surgical incision is the greater trochanter, which is palpable beneath the skin.

The anterior superior iliac spine is another useful landmark for determining the most proximal extent of the incision; this is particularly useful in patients with a high developmental dislocation of the hip. The area of the greater trochanter is identified, as is the femoral shaft. Abduction of the leg can assist in identifying the tip of the greater trochanter. A 15-cm skin incision with a gentle posterior curve is planned. The incision is centered over the greater trochanter and in line with the femur with the hip held in approximately 30 degrees of flexion (Fig. 20-10).

APPROACH

After the skin is incised, the subcutaneous tissue is divided in the line of the incision until the deep fascia layer is identified (Fig. 20-11). Care is taken to confirm appropriate positioning inline with the femoral shaft during the dissection to prevent drifting either anterior or posterior to the femur, which will make subsequent exposure more difficult. Hemostasis is obtained with electrocautery and the deep fascia is divided, taking care not to damage the underlying muscle. Abduction of the hip during the incision of the fas-

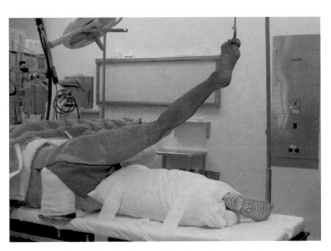

FIGURE 20-9. Patient positioning for surgical prep.

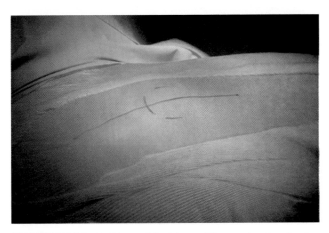

FIGURE 20-10. Outline of incision with greater trochanter marked.

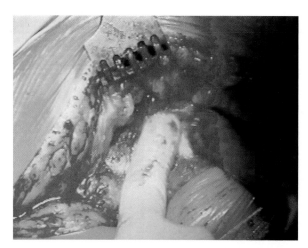

FIGURE 20-11. Subcutaneous tissue has been divided and the deep fascial layer is identified. The femur is palpated beneath this layer to ensure that the incision in the deep fascia layer is centered appropriately.

cia lessens the risk of injury to the underlying muscle. The deep fascia is then split in line with its fibers to expose the underlying bursae and short external rotators of the hip, and a Charnley type self-retaining retractor is placed into the wound. **The knee is maintained in flexion, and the hip is held extended to avoid placing undue tension on the sciatic nerve.**

The bursa on the posterior aspect of the hip joint is then incised and the short external rotators are identified. Great care is taken to identify and fully cauterize all vessels that lie on the surface of the short external rotators of the hip. The extremity is now placed into internal rotation to place tension on the short external rotators and a Homan retractor is placed over the piriformis tendon (Fig. 20-12). The short external rotators are then tenotomized, using the electrocautery to expose the underlying capsule (Fig. 20-13). Although usually unnecessary for routine total hip arthroplasty, the quadratus femoris muscle can be released from

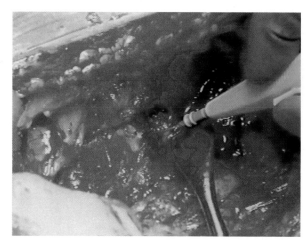

FIGURE 20-13. The short external rotators of the hip are tenotomized with an electrocautery to expose the underlying capsule.

the femur if needed. **If the quadratus femoris muscle is to be released, one must take care to identify and cauterize the large branch of the medial femoral circumflex artery that lies within the muscle belly.** If additional exposure is needed, up to half of the gluteus maximus insertion from the femoral shaft can also be released. An elliptically shaped capsulectomy is then performed, and the hip is carefully dislocated with the assistance of a large bone hook, using a combination of flexion, internal rotation, and adduction. **The hip should be dislocated with the use of traction by a large bone hook rather than forceful levering of the leg and femur by the second assistant. This avoids femoral shaft fractures in osteopenic patients.**

PROCEDURE

The appropriately sized trial prosthesis (chosen by preoperative templating) is aligned with the proximal femur so that

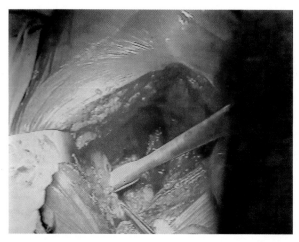

FIGURE 20-12. Homan retractor is placed over the piriformis tendon.

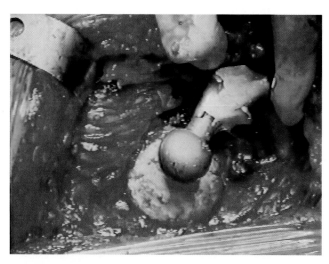

FIGURE 20-14. Planning of femoral neck osteotomy with trial prosthesis.

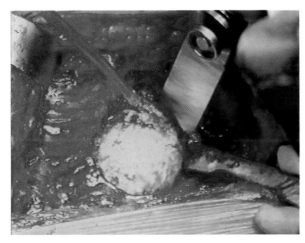

FIGURE 20-15. Femoral neck osteotomy with oscillating saw.

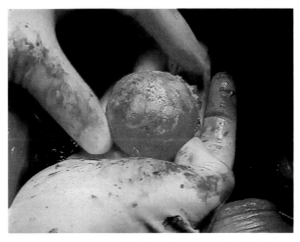

FIGURE 20-17. Femoral head after removal, showing osteoarthritic changes.

the center of the prosthetic head (with a plus 5-mm neck length) is aligned with the center of the native femoral head (Fig. 20-14). A plus 5-mm neck is used so that a shorter or longer neck size is available if changes are necessary at the time of trial reduction. The level and inclination of the femoral neck osteotomy are then marked using the electrocautery. The osteotomy is performed with an oscillating saw (Fig. 20-15), while the assistant on the other side of the table holds the extremity with the thigh parallel to the floor and the knee flexed, so that the lower leg is perpendicular to the floor. An osteotome can be used to complete the superior portion of the femoral neck osteotomy if necessary (Figs. 20-16 and 20-17). ◨ The proximal femur is then lifted superiorly with a large bone hook by the assistant on the other side of the table, and with the electrocautery a rent is made in the anterior hip capsule for placement of the anterior acetabular retractor (Fig. 20-18). An anterior retractor is then used to keep the proximal femur out of the way during acetabular preparation. **Great care must be taken to keep the tip of the anterior acetabular retractor from straying too**

far medially to avoid damage to the femoral neurovascular bundle.

Wing retractors are then impacted into the iliac wing superiorly and ischium posteriorly to provide circumferential acetabular exposure (Figs. 20-19 and 20-20). ◨ The remaining labrum and associated soft tissues are then carefully resected using the electrocautery. **Great care is exercised when resecting the soft tissue in the inferior aspect of the acetabulum and pulvinar. Specifically, no tension is placed on the soft tissues inferiorly while they are being resected; this is to avoid injury to a branch of the obturator vessels that can then retract and cause profuse bleeding.** After removal of the pulvinar, the medial wall of the acetabulum is visualized and acetabular reaming is then performed directly medially until the acetabular floor is identified. Sequential reaming is then performed with the reamer held in approximately 40 degrees of cup abduction and 10 degrees of anteversion until subchondral bone is identified and a perfect hemisphere has been created (Fig. 20-21). ◨ An acetabular trial that is the same size as the final reamer used is then

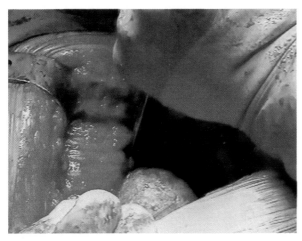

FIGURE 20-16. Completion of femoral neck osteotomy with osteotome.

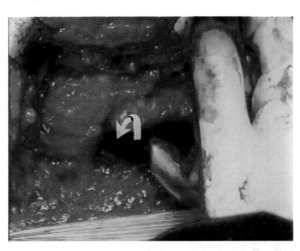

FIGURE 20-18. Placement of anterior acetabular retractor.

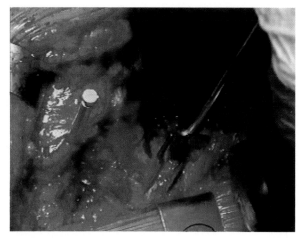

FIGURE 20-19. Placement of posterior wing retractor for acetabular exposure.

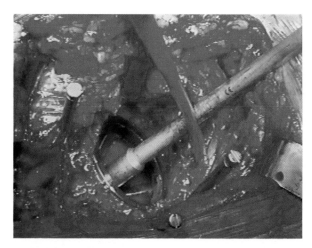

FIGURE 20-22. Trial acetabular component in place.

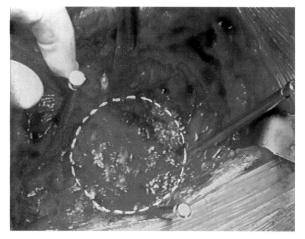

FIGURE 20-20. Circumferential acetabular exposure obtained.

inserted and tested for size and fit (Fig. 20-22). A reamer 2 mm smaller than the last used is then placed into reverse and used to impact morselized bone from the resected femoral head into the acetabulum (Fig. 20-23). The acetabular component selected is next impacted into place in 40 degree of cup abduction and 10 degrees of anteversion (Figs. 20-24 and 20-25). The component we use is approximately 0.75 mm larger in diameter than labeled because of macro-texturing, resulting in increased interference fit. Two screws placed into the posterior-superior quadrant (as described by Wasielewski) are then used to augment initial stability (rarely longer than 25 mm, because longer screws may exit the pelvis and endanger surrounding neurovascular structures) (Figs. 20-26 and 20-27). ◼ This system divides the acetabulum into halves from the anterior superior iliac spine caudally and then bisects this line to form four quadrants (Fig. 20-28). In their anatomic study of cadavers, Wasielewski et al. found that the posterior-superior quadrant offered the greatest margin of safety and the highest quality bone for adjunctive screw fixation. We routinely use

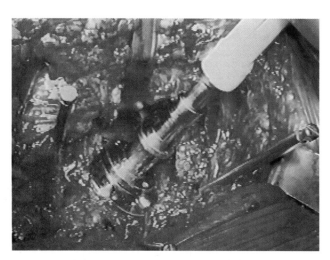

FIGURE 20-21. Reamer in acetabulum.

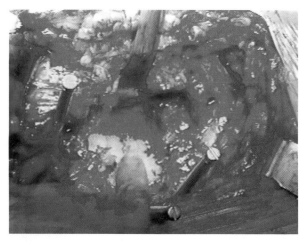

FIGURE 20-23. Placement of morselized bone graft into the acetabulum.

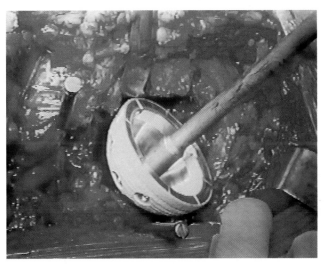

FIGURE 20-24. Component before final seating.

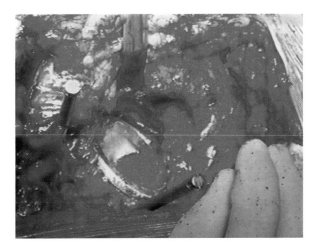

FIGURE 20-25. Final appearance of inserted acetabular component.

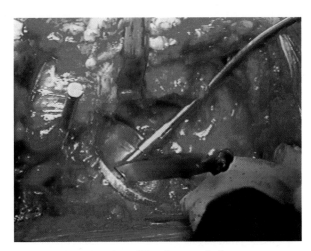

FIGURE 20-26. Drilling for acetabular screws.

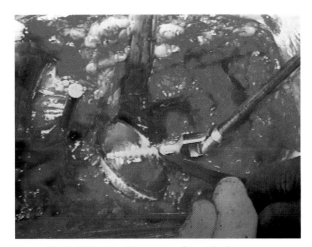

FIGURE 20-27. Placement of acetabular screw.

a 10-degree elevated rim liner that is placed in the posterior-superior portion of the component (Fig. 20-29). Polyethylene thickness is maintained at a minimum of 8 mm. The acetabulum is protected with a lap sponge, and femoral preparation is begun after removal of the acetabular retractors.

A broad flat retractor is placed under the proximal femur to aid with exposure (Fig. 20-30). Any remaining soft tissue is removed from the base of the femoral neck. A blunt T-handle reamer is used to identify the central portion of the femoral canal followed by sequential reaming until cortical bone is reached (Figs. 20-31 and 20-32). Great care is taken to avoid eccentric reaming of the canal. A Harris curette can

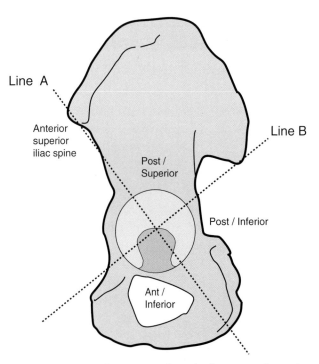

FIGURE 20-28. Quadrant system for safe placement of acetabular screws.

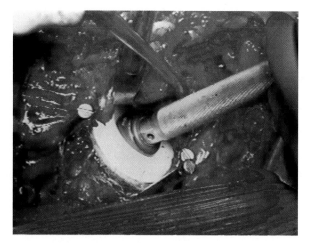

FIGURE 20-29. Insertion of polyethylene liner.

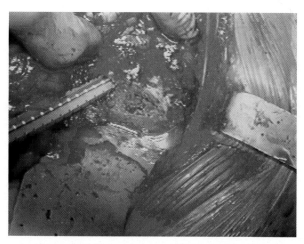

FIGURE 20-32. Insertion of femoral reamer.

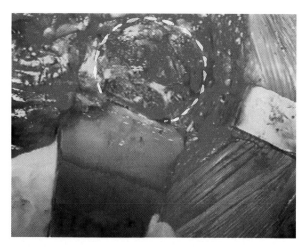

FIGURE 20-30. Exposure of proximal femur with retractor.

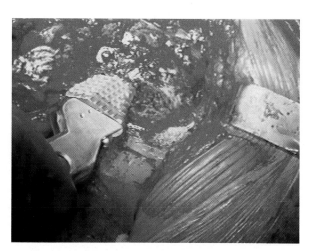

FIGURE 20-33. Femoral broach in place.

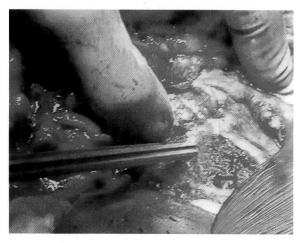

FIGURE 20-31. Insertion of blunt T-handled reamer.

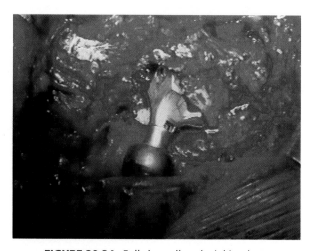

FIGURE 20-34. Full-size collared trial in place.

then be used to confirm that sufficient reaming has been performed so that cortical bone is present circumferentially in the distal canal. For cement application, a reamer two sizes larger than the component is used to create a cement mantle of appropriate thickness. <u>The lower extremity is then positioned with the leg held perpendicular to the ground for appropriate estimation of femoral version during broaching.</u> Broaching is then carefully performed, starting with the smallest broach, until adequate fit and fill are achieved with the broach held in approximately 15 degrees of anteversion (Fig. 20-33). ◼ Care is taken to avoid varus positioning of the broach by maintaining the broach handle in a lateral position, hugging the base of the greater trochanter during insertion. **Broaching is carried out by allowing the mallet to fall onto the top of the insertion handle but not with undue force. If the broach fails to advance, the next smallest sized broach is reinserted and advanced, and then the larger size is attempted again to avoid causing a fracture.** The appropriate-sized femoral head with a plus 5-mm neck (as was used initially to intraoperatively template the level of the femoral neck cut) is then placed onto a full-sized collared trial component (Fig. 20-34) in preparation for the trial reduction. The hip is reduced with the assistance of a bone hook and brought through a range of motion after the Charnley retractor is loosened to assess stability. **If the hip is trialed while the Charnley retractor is tight, the surgeon may overestimate stability secondary to the soft tissue tension provided by the retractor, leading to problems with postoperative dislocation.** If trial reduction reveals inadequate or excessive soft tissue tension, a longer or shorter neck length is trialed before final component selection. <u>In general, the center of the prosthetic femoral head should lie at the level of the greater trochanter if leg-length equalization has been carried out.</u> A lap pad is placed beneath the trial head before it is removed from the wound to ensure that it is easily retrievable if it becomes dislodged from the femoral stem. If inadequate stability is observed, the surgeon must search for sources of bony or prosthetic impingement

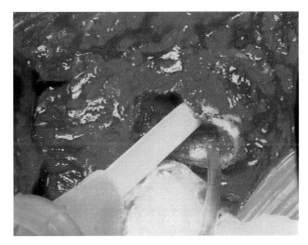

FIGURE 20-36. Insertion of cement into femoral canal.

or adjust the version of the femoral or acetabular components as needed.

Once the appropriate-sized components have been selected the femoral canal is prepared. A cement restrictor is inserted to a depth of at least 1 cm deeper than the tip of the prosthesis (Fig. 20-35). For optimal cement technique to be achieved, the femoral canal is irrigated and dried to remove all blood, marrow contents, and debris. Two packages of cement are then mixed under suction and inserted into the femoral canal in a retrograde manner, using a cement gun once the cement has reached a doughy consistency (Fig. 20-36). After insertion into the canal, the cement is pressurized to maximize the quality of the cement mantle (Fig. 20-37). We do not use a proximal or distal centralizer on the femoral stem, because we are concerned that these devices can create imperfections within the cement mantle. In addition, it is our experience centralizers do not improve component positioning or cement technique. The stem is inserted in the same version as the trial components, taking care to hold the lower leg perpendicular to the floor throughout cementation (Fig. 20-38). ◼ Any extruding cement is

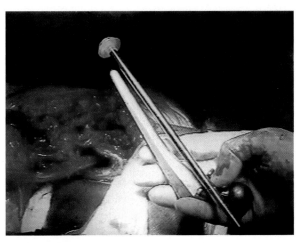

FIGURE 20-35. Estimation for depth of cement restrictor.

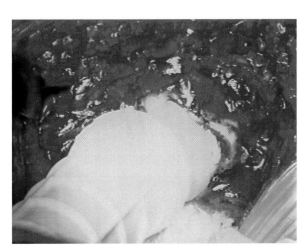

FIGURE 20-37. Pressurization of cement.

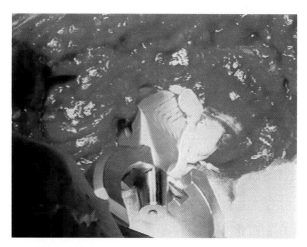

FIGURE 20-38. Insertion of femoral component.

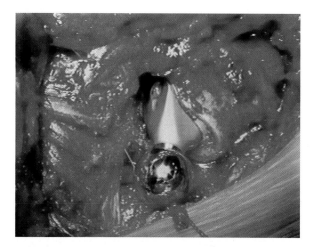

FIGURE 20-39. Femoral component with modular head in place.

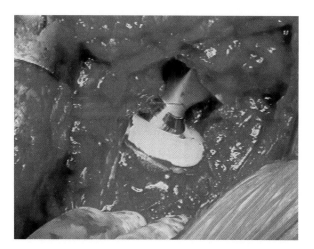

FIGURE 20-40. Final reduction of components.

trimmed. ▶ The hip is then trialed a second time after the cement has fully hardened to confirm neck length for optimal stability. The Morse taper is now cleaned and dried, and the modular femoral head is gently impacted onto the Morse taper (Fig. 20-39).

Following final reduction of the hip (Fig. 20-40), the wound is copiously irrigated with sterile saline, and a large Hemovac is placed into the wound exiting distally and in a nondependent position (anterior to the incision). The deep fascia is closed with an absorbable, nonbraided heavy suture, followed by closure of the subcutaneous tissues with inverted absorbable sutures and skin staples. A postoperative radiograph of the hip is obtained to confirm appropriate component position.

POSTOPERATIVE PROTOCOL

Prophylactic intravenous antibiotics are continued for 24 hours postoperatively. A first-generation cephalosporin or clindamycin in patients with a penicillin allergy is used. The surgical drains are removed on the morning after surgery. We use 325 mg of aspirin daily, in conjunction with elastic compression stockings and mechanical foot pumps for thromboembolic prophylaxis. A pillow is kept between the patient's legs at all times, and patients may lie on the operative side while sleeping if desired.

Patients are mobilized on the first postoperative day with a physical therapist and are weight bearing as tolerated on the operative extremity initially with the use of a walker. Patients are first out of bed to a hip chair and are then instructed in progressive ambulation as tolerated. Physical and occupational therapy includes instruction in total hip precautions with avoidance of hip flexion of greater than 90 degrees and any degree of internal rotation or adduction. Patients are discharged with Lofstrand crutches and are advanced to the use of a cane in the contralateral hand at the discretion of a home physical therapist (usually at 3 weeks). The occupational therapy department arranges for the use of an elevated toilet seat and additional devices, such as reachers, sock-aides, long shoe horns, elastic shoe laces (for conversion of a laced shoe to a slip on), and shower seats, as indicated. Patients use an assist-device for the first month, which is discontinued later at the discretion of the surgeon.

FOLLOW-UP

Patients should be examined and have radiographs performed at 1, 6, and 12 months and then annually. Follow-up is important to make early determination of failure mechanisms such as osteolysis and component wear and loosening that can be addressed before major bone compromise has occurred.

SUGGESTED READINGS

Callaghan JJ, Albright JC, Goetz DD, et al. Charnley total hip arthroplasty with cement. Minimum twenty-five-year follow-up. *J Bone Joint Surg Am* 2000;82:487–497.

Callaghan JJ, Brand RA, Pedersen DR. Hip arthrodesis. A long-term follow-up. *J Bone Joint Surg Am* 1985;67:1328–1335.

Charnley J. *Low friction arthroplasty of the hip. Theory and practice.* New York: Springer-Verlag, 1979.

Jaffe WL, Hawkins CA. Normalized and proportionalized cemented femoral stem survivorship at 15 years. *J Arthroplasty* 1999;14:708–713.

Jazrawi LM, Adler EM, Jazrawi AJ, et al. Radiographic comparison of grit-blasted hydroxyapatite and arc-deposited hydroxyapatite acetabular components. A four-year follow-up study. *Bull Hosp Joint Dis* 2000;59(3):144–148.

Laupacis A, Bourne R, Rorabeck C, et al. The effect of elective total hip replacement on health-related quality of life. *J Bone Joint Surg Am* 1993;75:1619–1626.

Madey SM, Callaghan JJ, Olejniczak JP, et al. Charnley total hip arthroplasty with use of improved techniques of cementing. The results after a minimum of fifteen years of follow-up. *J Bone Joint Surg Am* 1997;79:53–64.

Millis MB, Murphy SB, Poss R. Osteotomies about the hip for the prevention and treatment of osteoarthrosis. *Instr Course Lect* 1996;45:209–226.

National Center for Health Statistics, 1998, 1999, 2000 National Hospital Discharge Survey. Data extracted and analyzed by AAOS Department of Research and Scientific Affairs. Available at http://www.aaos.org/wordhtml/research/arthropl.htm.

Smith SE, Harris WH. Total hip arthroplasty performed with insertion of the femoral component with cement and the acetabular component without cement. Ten to thirteen-year results. *J Bone Joint Surg Am* 1997;79:1827–1833.

Smith SW, Estok DM, Harris WH. Total hip arthroplasty with use of second-generation cementing techniques. An eighteen-year-average follow-up study. *J Bone Joint Surg Am* 1998;80: 1632–1640.

Wasielewski RC, Cooperstein LA, Kruger MP, et al. Acetabular anatomy and the transacetabular fixation of screws in total hip arthroplasty. *J Bone Joint Surg Am* 1990;72:501–508.

CHAPTER 21

FEMORAL NECK FRACTURE: CLOSED REDUCTION AND INTERNAL FIXATION

KENNETH J. KOVAL

Hip fractures are a common and often devastating injury in the geriatric population with an impact that extends far beyond the obvious orthopaedic injury into the domains of medicine, rehabilitation, psychiatry, social work, and medical economics. Despite improvements in patient care, including advances in operative technique and implant technology, fractures of the proximal femur continue to consume a major portion of national health care resources. The increasing number of hip fractures that occur each year has made it difficult to keep pace with this growing health care problem. With the aging of the U.S. population, the annual number of hip fractures is projected to double by the year 2050. This chapter describes closed reduction and internal fixation of a displaced femoral neck fracture.

ANATOMY

The *femoral neck* comprises the region between the base of the femoral head and the intertrochanteric line anteriorly and the intertrochanteric crest posteriorly (Fig. 23-1). The femoral neck forms an angle with the femoral shaft ranging from 125 to 140 degrees in the anteroposterior plane and 10 to 15 degrees (anteversion) in the lateral plane. The cancellous bone of the femoral neck is characterized by trabeculae organized into medial and lateral systems. The medial trabecular system forms in response to the joint reaction force on the femoral head; the epiphyseal plates are perpendicular to the medial trabecular system. The lateral trabecular system resists the compressive force on the femoral head resulting from contraction of the abductor muscles (Fig. 21-1).

CLASSIFICATION

Several systems for classifying femoral neck fractures have been proposed. One such scheme is anatomically based and divides the femoral neck into three regions: subcapital, transcervical, and basocervical (Fig. 21-2). Most femoral neck

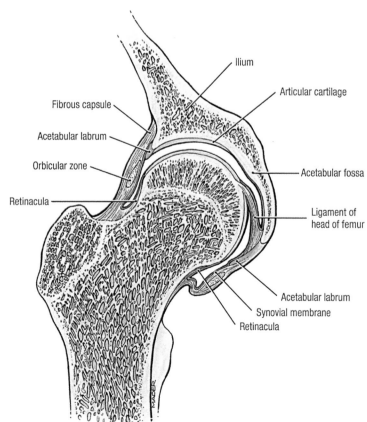

FIGURE 21-1. Hip joint, coronal section. (From Agur AMR, Lee MJ. *Grant's atlas of anatomy,* 10th ed. Philadelphia: Lippincott Williams & Wilkins, 1999, with permission.)

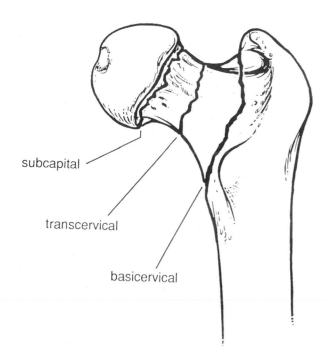

FIGURE 21-2. The femoral neck region can be divided into three regions: subcapital, transcervical, and basocervical.

fractures are subcapital; transcervical femoral neck fractures are usually the result of repetitive stresses. Because the subcapital and transcervical regions are entirely intracapsular, fractures in these regions exhibit different characteristics from those in the basocervical region, which is extracapsular. Fractures that are entirely intracapsular are at increased risk for osteonecrosis and nonunion, sequelae that are uncommon after extracapsular fracture.

The classification system proposed by Pauwels is based on the angle of inclination of the fracture line (Fig. 21-3):

Type I: fracture line 30 degrees from the horizontal
Type II: fracture line 50 degrees from the horizontal
Type III: fracture line 70 degrees from the horizontal

The most popular femoral neck fracture classification system, introduced by Garden in 1961, has four types based on the degree of fracture displacement on the anteroposterior radiograph (Fig. 21-4):

Type I: incomplete or impacted fracture in which the bony trabeculae of the inferior portion of the femoral neck remains intact; includes "valgus-impacted" fractures
Type II: complete fracture without displacement of the fracture fragments
Type III: complete fracture with partial displacement of the fracture fragments
Type IV: complete fracture with total displacement of the fracture fragments, allowing the femoral head to rotate back to an anatomic position; radiographically, the bony trabeculae of the femoral head line up with the bony trabeculae of the acetabulum

Perhaps the simplest—and in many situations the best—approach is to classify femoral neck fractures as nondisplaced (Garden types I and II) or displaced (Garden types III and IV). Further differentiation can be difficult to establish radiographically and has been shown to be subject to wide variability. The nondisplaced/displaced scheme, which has the virtue of grouping together fractures with similar treatment alternatives and similar prognoses, is my preference for classifying femoral neck fractures.

INDICATIONS

There is general agreement that surgical management is the treatment of choice for almost all hip fractures, including those involving the femoral neck. Impacted and nondisplaced femoral neck fractures should undergo *in situ* internal fixation using multiple cancellous lag screws. Whereas virtually all patients with a nondisplaced femoral neck fracture should be treated by internal fixation, such is not the case for displaced femoral neck fractures.

The choice of internal fixation over prosthetic replacement may be difficult. Although different investigators have provided indications for primary prosthetic replacement based on various criteria, I do not believe that specific indications

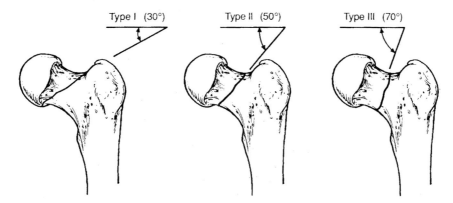

FIGURE 21-3. The classification system proposed by Pauwels is based on the angle of inclination of the fracture line: type I, fracture line 30 degrees from the horizontal; type II, fracture line 50 degrees from the horizontal; and type III, fracture line 70 degrees from the horizontal.

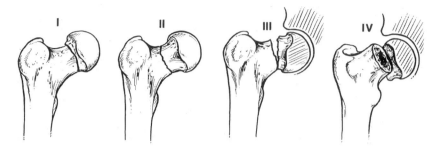

FIGURE 21-4. The Garden classification is based on the degree of fracture displacement on the anteroposterior radiograph: type I, incomplete or impacted fracture in which the bony trabeculae of the inferior portion of the femoral neck remains intact (this category includes "valgus-impacted" fractures); type II, complete fracture without displacement of the fracture fragments; type III, complete fracture with partial displacement of the fracture fragments; and type IV, complete fracture with total displacement of the fracture fragments, allowing the femoral head to rotate back to an anatomic position.

based solely on patient care or fracture type is preferable or even possible. Rather, each clinical situation should be assessed individually, with careful consideration of patient factors (e.g., physiologic patient age, associated medical problems) and fracture factors (e.g., bone quality, amount of comminution, interval form injury to surgical treatment) to arrive at a treatment decision. If successful, fracture reduction (i.e., closed or open) and internal fixation provide the best and most durable result after displaced femoral neck fracture.

I feel that elderly individuals who have sustained a displaced femoral neck fracture and are relatively healthy, have minimal fracture comminution, and can undergo surgery within 24 to 48 hours of injury should have an attempt at fracture reduction and internal fixation; hemiarthroplasty is restricted to older, less healthy, low-demand individuals. **Elderly patients with a displaced femoral neck fracture and multiple medical comorbidities are best served by a single operation that is associated with a low failure rate (i.e., prosthetic replacement)—particularly when the presence of posterior femoral neck comminution substantially increases the risk for healing complications.**

At the Hospital for Joint Diseases in New York, the strategy for treating displaced femoral neck fractures involves internal fixation using multiple cannulated cancellous screws after closed or open reduction for most patients with adequate bone density. I treat this fracture as an urgent situation, with rapid medical stabilization and surgical treatment within 24 hours of admission whenever possible. Prosthetic replacement is reserved for those physiologically older individuals in whom internal fixation is unlikely to succeed: those with marked osteopenia or fracture comminution, or both. Such patients tend to be older and have lower functional demands. They may be unable to ambulate without assistive devices, and associated medical problems often limit their life expectancy.

PREOPERATIVE PLANNING

A standard radiographic examination of the hip consists of the following elements:

- Anteroposterior view of the pelvis (Fig. 21-5)
- Anteroposterior and cross-table lateral view of the involved proximal femur (Figs. 21-6 and 21-7).

The lateral radiograph can help to assess posterior comminution of the proximal femur; a cross-table lateral view is preferred to a frog lateral view because the latter requires abduction, flexion, and external rotation of the affected lower extremity and involves a risk of fracture displacement.

Internally rotating the involved femur 10 to 15 degrees offsets the anteversion of the femoral neck and provides a true anteroposterior view of the proximal femur. A second anteroposterior view of the contralateral side can be used for preoperative planning.

A displaced femoral neck fracture in which the femoral head is posterior to the femoral shaft and the distal fragment is externally rotated can be misinterpreted as an intertrochanteric fracture. If the fracture pattern is misinterpreted, the femoral neck fracture may be properly diagnosed only after the anesthetized patient is placed on a fracture table and traction and internal rotation have been applied. If prosthetic replacement is the preferred procedure, the patient would have to be moved from the fracture table to a flat table. This pitfall can be avoided by

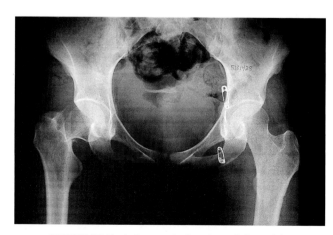

FIGURE 21-5. Anteroposterior view of the pelvis.

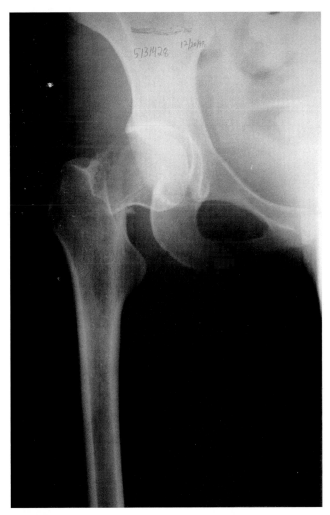

FIGURE 21-6. Anteroposterior view of the involved proximal femur.

the use of anteroposterior and cross-table lateral radiographs when evaluating proximal femur fractures. If these radiographs do not clarify the nature of the fracture pattern, a radiograph taken with the extremity internally rotated should be taken.

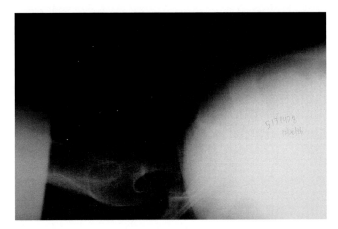

FIGURE 21-7. Cross-table lateral view of the involved proximal femur.

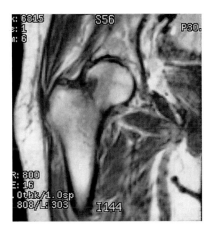

FIGURE 21-8. Magnetic resonance image shows a nondisplaced, right femoral neck fracture.

Magnetic resonance imaging (MRI) is useful when a hip fracture is suspected but not apparent on standard radiographs (Fig. 21-8). MRI has been shown to be at least as accurate as bone scanning in identification of occult fractures of the hip and can be performed within 24 hours of injury. MRI within 48 hours of fracture does not, however, appear to be useful for assessing femoral head viability or vascularity or predicting the development of osteonecrosis or healing complications.

EQUIPMENT

The basic instruments necessary for open reduction and internal fixation of a displaced femoral neck fracture using multiple cannulated cancellous screws include the following items (Fig. 21-9):

■ Fracture table that can be converted into a flat operating table if closed reduction is unsuccessful and prosthetic replacement becomes necessary

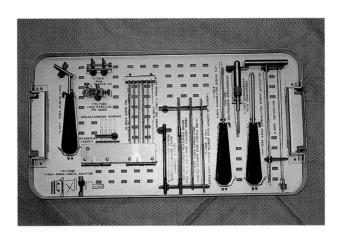

FIGURE 21-9. The cannulated screw instruments *(left to right, selected mention)*: 4.0-mm drill sleeve, two 1.3-mm sleeves, parallel pin guide, pin guides, cannulated screw sleeve measuring gauge, direct measuring gauge, cannulated cortex reamer, 4.0-mm cannulated screw tap, self-holding screw driver, screwdriver with countersink, cannulated screw extractor, and obturator.

- Guide wires
- Guide wire insertion device
- Cannulated depth gauge
- Cannulated reamer
- Cannulated screwdriver
- 6.5-mm cannulated screws

PATIENT POSITIONING AND FRACTURE REDUCTION

The patient is positioned supine on a fracture table that can be converted into a flat operating table if closed reduction is unsuccessful and prosthetic replacement becomes necessary. Fracture reduction involves 90 degrees of flexion of the injured hip with external rotation to disengage the fracture fragments (Fig. 21-10). ◉ Traction is applied as the leg is internally rotated and brought into full extension (Fig. 21-11). The maximum internal rotation of the injured lower extremity is then compared with the uninjured leg (Fig. 21-12); if the two do not match, a successful reduction has most probably not been obtained. The image intensifier, however, should be used for anteroposterior and lateral assessment of the adequacy of the fracture reduction.

To properly assess the fracture reduction and guide implant insertion, the surgeon must obtain unobstructed anteroposterior and cross-table lateral radiographic images of the entire proximal femur (including the hip joint) before making the skin incision. ◉ Without visualization of the entire proximal femur, it is difficult to assess the guide wire position as it is advanced into the femoral head. Inappropriate screw length or location may result from inadequate radiographic visualization. It may be necessary to alter the positioning of the patient or image intensifier to obtain an unobstructed cross-table lateral radiograph. In men, placement of the scrotum away from the image beam

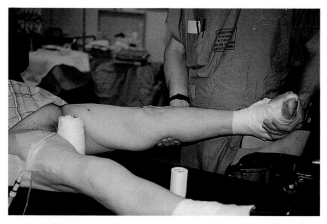

FIGURE 21-11. Traction is applied as the leg is internally rotated and brought into full extension.

can help delineate the femoral head on the lateral radiographic view.

An adequate reduction is probably the most important factor affecting the incidence of nonunion and osteonecrosis. To determine the quality of fracture reduction, I measure the angle of the femoral head on the true anteroposterior and cross-table lateral radiographs. An acceptable reduction may have up to 15 degrees of valgus angulation and less than 10 degrees of anterior or posterior angulation. Some variation is acceptable, particularly when a valgus reduction is obtained.

If the fracture reduction is acceptable, the patient's lower extremities are placed in foot holders. A padded perineal post is placed in the ipsilateral groin; care must be taken that there is no impingement of the labia or scrotum. **It is imperative that the genital area be inspected before fracture reduction to verify that the scrotum is not incarcerated against the fracture post and that the mucosa of the labia is not placed against—or even directed toward—the fracture post, which can result in labial slough.** The uninvolved leg is then flexed, abducted, and externally rotated to allow positioning of the image intensifier for a lateral view (Fig. 21-13). Alternatively, the contralateral extremity can be abducted with the hip and knee extended (Fig. 21-14); this maneuver, however, places greater pressure from the fracture post on the perineum.

Before preparing the lower extremity, the surgeon must ensure that the fracture has remained reduced and that nonobstructive biplanar radiographic visualization of the entire proximal femur, including the hip joint, is obtainable (Fig. 21-15). The lower extremity, from the pelvis to the lower thigh, is then prepared and draped. For this purpose, I prefer an isolation screen.

APPROACH

Although the screws can be inserted percutaneously, I prefer a limited open technique to facilitate screw insertion. A

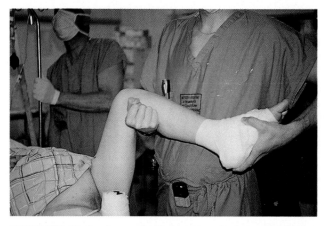

FIGURE 21-10. Fracture reduction involves 90 degrees of flexion of the injured hip with external rotation to disengage the fracture fragments.

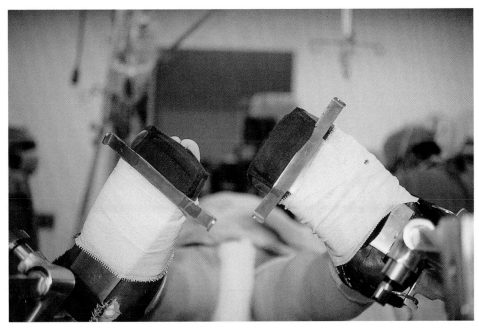

FIGURE 21-12. The maximum internal rotation of the injured lower extremity is then compared with the uninjured leg; if the two do not match, a successful reduction has probably not been obtained.

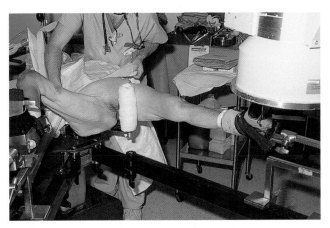

FIGURE 21-13. The uninvolved leg is then flexed, abducted, and externally rotated to allow positioning of the image intensifier for a lateral view.

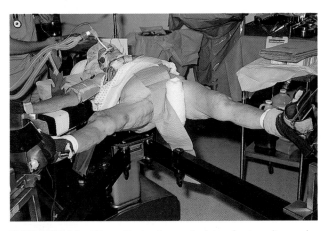

FIGURE 21-14. Alternatively, the contralateral extremity can be abducted with the hip and knee extended.

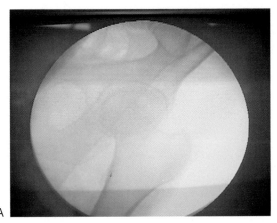

A

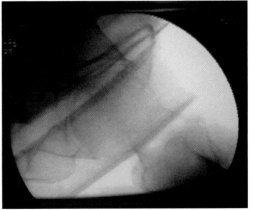

B

FIGURE 21-15. AP **(A)** and lateral **(B)** radiographic confirmation that nonobstructive biplanar radiographic visualization of the entire proximal femur, including the hip joint, is obtainable.

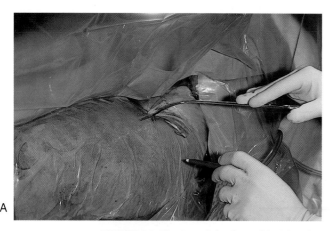
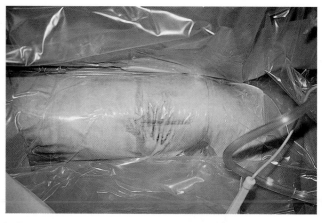

A

B

FIGURE 21-16. A straight, lateral incision is made from the base of the greater trochanter **(A)** and extends 2 to 3 inches down the thigh **(B)**.

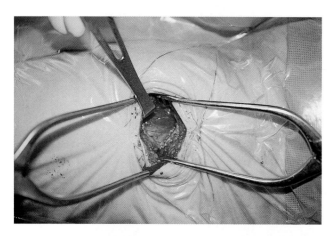

FIGURE 21-17. The iliotibial band is divided longitudinally, with care taken to ensure that the deep dissection remains posterior to the tensor fasciae latae muscle proximally.

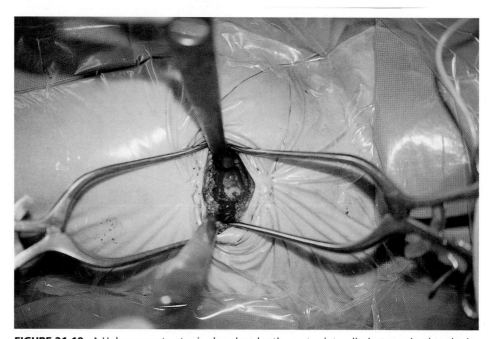

FIGURE 21-18. A Hohmann retractor is placed under the vastus lateralis, just proximal to the insertion of the gluteus maximus. The vastus lateralis is then elevated from the lateral femur in a posterior-to-anterior direction, with care taken to identify and ligate the perforating branches of the profunda femoral artery.

straight lateral incision is made from the base of the greater trochanter, extending 2 to 3 inches down the thigh (Fig. 21-16). After incision of the skin and subcutaneous tissue, the iliotibial band is divided longitudinally, with care taken to ensure that the deep dissection remains posterior to the tensor fasciae latae muscle proximally (Fig. 21-17). ◧ The vastus lateralis fascia is divided longitudinally to expose its muscle fibers and the posterior portion of the fascia elevated off the underlying muscle down to the linea aspera. A Hohmann retractor is placed under the vastus lateralis, just proximal to the insertion of the gluteus maximus (Fig. 21-18). ◧ The vastus lateralis is then elevated from the lateral femur in a posterior-to-anterior direction, with care taken to identify and ligate the perforating branches of the profunda femoral artery.

PROCEDURE

Three guide wires are inserted into the femoral neck and head under image intensification. A guide wire can be placed anterior to the femoral neck to estimate femoral neck anteversion, but I find this is unnecessary. The guide wires should all be parallel and oriented in an inverted triangular configuration, with one wire inferior and two wires superior; this orientation provides the most mechanically secure fracture fixation (Fig. 21-19). The guide wires can be inserted using an insertion apparatus or a freehand technique; I prefer a freehand technique. The inferior wire is placed adjacent to the inferior neck cortex to resist varus displacement, ◧ while one of the two superior wires is adjacent to the posterior femoral cortex to resist posterior displacement. ◧ These guide wires should be spaced apart to maximize fixation stability and inserted into the dense subchondral bone. **A common pitfall during cancellous lag screw insertion is to place the first guide wire or screw in the middle of the femoral**

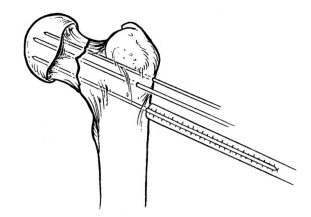

FIGURE 21-20. After the guide wire positions have been set, the screw lengths are determined.

neck and head, making it difficult to insert the remaining screws; this may result in a mechanically weaker configuration in which the screws are too close to one another.

The surgeon should avoid cancellous screw insertion through the cortical subtrochanteric region; this creates a stress riser effect, increasing the risk for subsequent fracture. To minimize the stress riser effect, the cancellous screws should be inserted proximal to the lesser trochanter in the cancellous bone of the metaphyseal region.

After the guide wire positions have been set, the screw lengths are determined (Fig. 21-20). ◧ The screws should lie in the dense subchondral bone for optimal fixation, and the threads should completely cross the fracture site. The outer cortex of the proximal femur is then reamed and the screws inserted (Fig. 21-21). ◧ There is no need to ream the entire screw tract; this can result in loss of the guide wire during reamer removal. Good-quality radiographs are necessary to confirm proper placement of the screws, including rotation of the proximal femur under fluoroscopy to detect possible intraarticular screw penetration. After screw insertion, any traction is released and the screws retightened. ◧

Because capsular distention with increased intracapsular pressure has been implicated as a possible cause of posttrau-

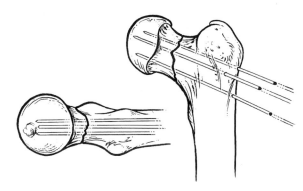

FIGURE 21-19. Three guide wires are inserted into the femoral neck and head under image intensification. The guide wires should all be parallel and oriented in an inverted triangular configuration, with one wire inferior and two wires superior. This orientation provides the most mechanically secure fracture fixation.

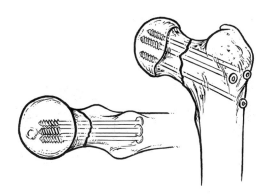

FIGURE 21-21. The outer cortex of the proximal femur is then reamed and the screws inserted.

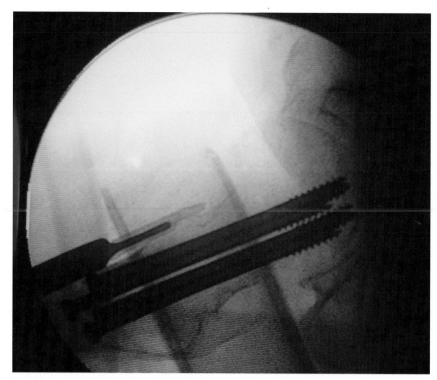

FIGURE 21-22. Because capsular distention with increased intracapsular pressure has been implicated as a possible cause of posttraumatic osteonecrosis, I usually perform a capsulotomy at surgery. The capsulotomy is performed under image intensification using a scalpel directed along the anterior femoral neck.

matic osteonecrosis, I usually perform a capsulotomy at surgery; the capsulotomy is performed under image intensification using a scalpel directed along the anterior femoral neck (Fig. 21-22). The wound is closed in layers over suction drains.

The screw position must be fluoroscopically assessed before wound closure. It has been demonstrated that femoral head penetration can be missed on anteroposterior and cross-table lateral radiographic evaluation. Accurate evaluation of screw position involves rotating the radio-

graphic beam under fluoroscopy. This continuous fluoroscopic evaluation while the beam is passed from an anteroposterior to lateral position is helpful to detect femoral head penetration.

POSTOPERATIVE PROTOCOL

The Hospital for Joint Diseases rehabilitation protocol is outlined in Table 21-1.

TABLE 21-1. HOSPITAL FOR JOINT DISEASES REHABILITATION PROTOCOL

Period	Rehabilitation Protocol
Day 1	Dangle legs from bed Out of bed to chair Ambulation training with walker for 15 feet (weight bearing as tolerated)
Day 2	Ambulation training for 20 feet
Day 3	Ambulation training for 40 feet
Day 4	Stair climbing
Day 5+	Progression of ambulation and stair climbing for endurance and distance with gradual decrease of assistance from the therapist for the following: 1. Daily occupational therapy for instruction in activities of daily living 2. Daily strengthening exercises in supine, sitting, and standing positions 3. Daily range of motion exercises for patients who had internal fixation; patients who had prosthetic replacement are limited to 90 degrees of flexion for 6 weeks

SUGGESTED READINGS

Blair BJ, Koval KJ, Kummer F, et al. A biomechanical comparison of multiple cancellous screws to the sliding hip screw for the treatment of basocervical fractures. *Clin Orthop* 1994;306:256–263.

Cobb AG, Gibson PH. Screw fixation of subcapital fractures of the femur: a better method of treatment. *Injury* 1986;17:259–264.

Crawford EJP, Emery RJH, Hansell DM, et al. Capsular distention and intracapsular pressure in subcapital fractures of the femur. *J Bone Joint Surg Br* 1988;70:195–198.

Frandsen PA, Andersen E, Madsen F, et al. Garden's classification of femoral neck fractures: an assessment of inter-observer variation. *J Bone Joint Surg Br* 1988;70:588–590.

Garden RS. Malreduction and avascular necrosis in subcapital fractures of the femur. *J Bone Joint Surg Br* 1971;53:183–197.

Lu-Yao GL, Keller RB, Littenberg B, et al. Outcomes after displaced fractures of the femoral neck: a meta-analysis of one hundred and six published reports. *J Bone Joint Surg Br* 1994;76:15–25.

Madsen F, Linde F, Anderson E, et al. Fixation of displaced femoral fractures: a comparison between sliding screw plate and four cancellous bone screws. *Acta Orthop Scand* 1987;58:212–216.

Speer KP, Spritzer CE, Harrelson JM, et al. Magnetic resonance imaging of the femoral head after acute intracapsular fracture of the femoral neck. *J Bone Joint Surg Am* 1990;72:98–103.

Stromqvist B, Nilsson LT, Egund N, et al. Intracapsular pressure in undisplaced fractures of the femoral neck. *J Bone Joint Surg Br* 1988;70:192–194.

CHAPTER 22

HEMIARTHROPLASTY OF THE FEMORAL NECK

KENNETH J. KOVAL

Hip fractures are a common and often devastating injury in the geriatric population, with an impact that extends far beyond the obvious orthopaedic injury into the domains of medicine, rehabilitation, psychiatry, social work, and medical economics. Despite improvements in patient care, including advances in operative technique and implant technology, fractures of the proximal femur continue to consume a major portion of national health care resources. The increasing number of hip fractures that occur each year has made it difficult to keep pace with this growing health care problem. With the aging of the U.S. population, the annual number of hip fractures is projected to double by the year 2050. This chapter describes hemiarthroplasty of a displaced femoral neck fracture.

ANATOMY

The *femoral neck* comprises the region between the base of the femoral head and the intertrochanteric line anteriorly and the intertrochanteric crest posteriorly (see Fig. 23-1). The femoral neck forms an angle with the femoral shaft ranging from 125 to 140 degrees in the anteroposterior plane and 10 to 15 degrees (anteversion) in the lateral plane. The cancellous bone of the femoral neck is characterized by trabeculae organized into medial and lateral systems. The medial trabecular system forms in response to the joint reaction force on the femoral head; the epiphyseal plates are perpendicular to the medial trabecular system. The lateral trabecular system resists the compressive force on the femoral head resulting from contraction of the abductor muscles (see Fig. 21-1).

CLASSIFICATION

Several different systems for classifying femoral neck fractures have been proposed. One such scheme is anatomically based and divides the femoral neck into three regions: subcapital, transcervical, and basocervical (see Fig. 21-2). Most femoral neck fractures are subcapital; transcervical femoral neck fractures are usually the result of repetitive stresses. Because the subcapital and transcervical regions are entirely intracapsular, fractures in these regions exhibit different characteristics from those in the basocervical region, which is extracapsular. Fractures that are entirely intracapsular are at increased risk for osteonecrosis and nonunion, sequelae that are uncommon after extracapsular fracture.

The classification system proposed by Pauwels is based on the angle of inclination of the fracture line (Fig. 22-1):

Type I: fracture line 30 degrees from the horizontal
Type II: fracture line 50 degrees from the horizontal
Type III: fracture line 70 degrees from the horizontal

The most popular femoral neck fracture classification system, introduced by Garden in 1961, has four types based on the degree of fracture displacement on the anteroposterior radiograph (Fig. 22-2):

Type I: incomplete or impacted fracture in which the bony trabeculae of the inferior portion of the femoral neck remains intact (including "valgus-impacted" fractures)
Type II: complete fracture without displacement of the fracture fragments
Type III: complete fracture with partial displacement of the fracture fragments

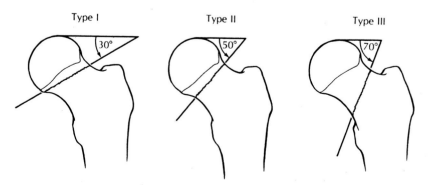

FIGURE 22-1. The Pauwels classification of femoral neck fractures. From Rockwood CA, Jr., Green DP, Bucholz RW, Heckman JO, eds. *Rockwood and Green's fractures in adults,* 4th ed; vol. 2. Philadelphia: Lippincott-Raven, 1996: 1670, with permission.

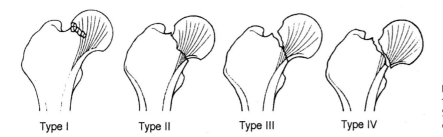

Type I Type II Type III Type IV

FIGURE 22-2. The Garden classification of femoral neck fractures. From Hansen S, Swiontkowski M, *Orthopedic trauma protocols.* New York: Raven Press, 1993:238.

Type IV: complete fracture with total displacement of the fracture fragments, allowing the femoral head to rotate back to an anatomical position (radiographically, the bony trabeculae of the femoral head line up with the bony trabeculae of the acetabulum)

Perhaps the simplest—and in many situations the best—approach is to classify femoral neck fractures as nondisplaced (Garden types I and II) or displaced (Garden types III and IV). Further differentiation can be difficult to establish radiographically and has been shown to be subject to wide variability. The nondisplaced/displaced scheme, which has the virtue of grouping together fractures with similar treatment alternatives and similar prognoses, is my preference for classifying femoral neck fractures.

INDICATIONS FOR HEMIARTHROPLASTY AFTER FEMORAL NECK FRACTURE

Hemiarthroplasty should be restricted to older, less healthy, low-demand individuals who have sustained a displaced femoral neck fracture. Factors favoring prosthetic replacement over internal fixation include pathologic bone, comminution of the posterior femoral neck, severe chronic illness (especially rheumatoid arthritis and chronic renal failure), and a limited life expectancy. Inactive elderly patients are candidates for modular or Austin-Moore–type unipolar hemiarthroplasty. Those with displaced femoral

neck fractures who can ambulate functionally outside the home (i.e., community ambulators) and whose likelihood of success with internal fixation is low should receive a modular unipolar or bipolar hemiarthroplasty—with the awareness that revision may be required in the future because of loosening of the femoral component or acetabular degenerative changes, including protrusion. The risk of these problems is greater in younger, more active individuals.

PREOPERATIVE PLANNING

A standard radiographic examination of the hip consists of the following views:

- Anteroposterior view of the pelvis (Fig. 22-3)
- Anteroposterior and cross-table lateral view of the involved proximal femur (Fig. 22-4)

TEMPLATING

Before proceeding to hemiarthroplasty, it is important to perform preoperative templating to determine the approximate femoral stem and unipolar or bipolar head size. In most patients, the normal hip is used as a template to duplicate normal leg length and hip offset. Proper hip offset helps maintain proper soft tissue tension, which is critical to the stability and biomechanics of the hip.

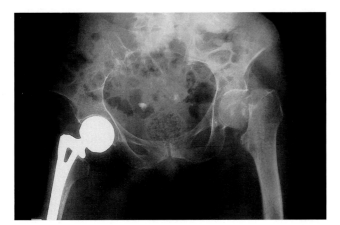

FIGURE 22-3. Anteroposterior radiograph of the pelvis demonstrates a displaced, left femoral neck fracture.

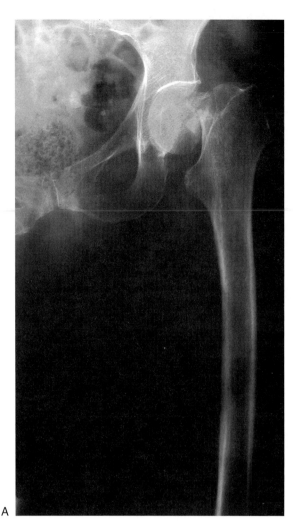

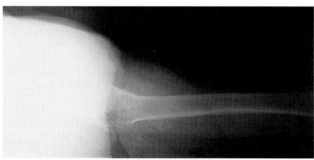

FIGURE 22-4. Anteroposterior **(A)** and lateral cross-table **(B)** views of the left hip demonstrate a displaced femoral neck fracture.

A

B

Templating begins with an anteroposterior view of the pelvis that includes as much of the proximal femur as possible. The pelvis should not be rotated, and it is helpful if the noninjured leg is rotated internally 15 degrees to get a true profile view of the proximal femur (this eliminates the normal anteversion). It is not necessary to obtain this view of the injured extremity. On the anteroposterior view, the center of the head is marked on the noninjured hip. The center can be determined by using a ruler to calculate the diameter of the head and then identifying the midpoint. A line is then drawn down the center of the femoral shaft. The distance from this line to the center of the femoral head is the hip offset.

Using templates, magnified to account for radiographic magnification, a stem of appropriate size is chosen. It is important to check that the stem also matches both anteroposterior and lateral views of the injured hip before templating on the normal hip. For cemented insertion, adequate space must be maintained around the stem to accommodate the cement mantle (usually 2 mm). This calls for a smaller stem than for noncemented, press-fit insertion. For nonce-

mented, press-fit insertion, the best fit is chosen to achieve intimate bony contact, which may be metaphyseal or diaphyseal depending on type of implant chosen.

The template is placed over the anteroposterior pelvis film, directly in line with the femoral canal (Fig. 22-5). It is then slid down the canal until one of the neck length markings matches the offset of the normal hip. The distance from this marking down to the lesser trochanter is measured using the magnified ruler markings on the template. This distance is recorded and later measured intraoperatively to mark the level of the desired neck cut. The distance from the lesser trochanter to the center of the femoral head is also measured to recreate this distance intraoperatively. The neck length marking on the template that most closely matches the offset of the normal hip is the neck length that will be used first when performing an intraoperative trial and—assuming intraoperative stability—for the prosthesis itself.

Some patients have hips with a larger offset than available on the templates. These patients usually need a prosthesis with a high-offset geometry. If a high-offset stem is not used, the soft tissue tension of the hip abductors will be sub-

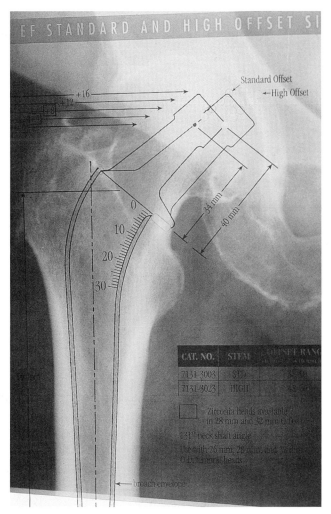

FIGURE 22-5. Use of a template to determine the optimal femoral stem size.

normal; these muscles may function suboptimally, and hip stability may be compromised.

EQUIPMENT

Instruments for cemented unipolar hemiarthroplasty of the hip after femoral neck fracture include femoral head and

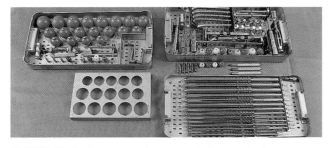

FIGURE 22-6. Equipment for cemented unipolar hemiarthroplasty for a femoral neck fracture: femoral head and neck trials *(left tray, top)*; femoral head sizers *(left tray, bottom)*; broaches *(right tray, top)*; and reamer set *(right tray, bottom)*.

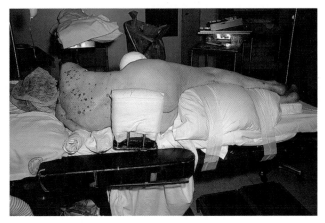

FIGURE 22-7. Use of a lateral position to hold the patient in a lateral decubitus position.

neck trials, femoral head sizers, broaches, and a reamer set (Fig. 22-6).

PATIENT POSITIONING

When performing hemiarthroplasty of the hip after femoral neck fracture, I most commonly use a posterior approach, with the patient in the lateral decubitus position. A lateral positioner is used to maintain this position, and a soft axillary roll is placed under the upper thorax to protect the brachial plexus (Fig. 22-7). The ankle and the knee of the noninjured leg are padded to prevent iatrogenic nerve injury, and a pillow is placed between the legs to help abduct the operative extremity and facilitate the exposure. Before preparing the operative site, the hip is flexed to 90 degrees to ensure that the lateral positioner is not blocking the range of hip motion. The entire injured extremity is then prepared and draped up to and including the iliac crest.

APPROACH

A slightly curved incision is made in line with the femur, centered over the greater trochanter with the hip flexed approximately 30 degrees (Fig. 22-8). The incision begins approximately 5 to 6 cm proximal to the greater trochanter and continues the same distance distal to the greater trochanter. The subcutaneous tissues are divided in line with the incision and the fascia lata is identified. A periosteal elevator is used to clear the fascia lata, which is then incised in line with the femur. At the proximal aspect of the incision, the muscle fibers of the gluteus maximus are visible as the fascia lata thins out superficial to the maximus. The gluteus maximus fibers are bluntly split in an anterior-to-posterior direction, and a Charnley retractor is inserted deep to the fascia lata for exposure (Fig. 22-9). Care is taken to palpate the sciatic nerve and ensure that it is not trapped in the blades of the retractor.

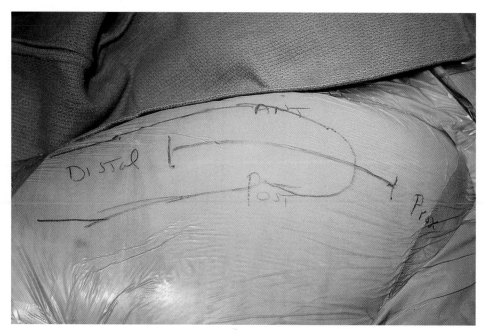

FIGURE 22-8. The skin incision for a posterior approach to the hip.

The trochanteric bursa is reflected posteriorly. The hip is maintained in extension during the posterior dissection; this relieves the sciatic nerve of any unnecessary strain and assists the exposure as the short external rotators are released. The sciatic nerve is again palpated—it is not necessary to expose it—before beginning the posterior exposure to ensure that it is not in danger of injury. A blunt retractor is passed above the superior border of the piriformis, deep to the gluteus minimus but superficial to the superior capsule, to assist the exposure. The hip is internally rotated to place the short external rotators under tension. Electrocautery is used to release the short rotators and the underlying capsule directly off bone along the posterior border of the proximal femur. The quadratus femoris is partially released, as necessary. Perforating vessels are identified and cauterized; there is

usually a large branch of the medial femoral circumflex within the body of the quadratus femoris. The short external rotators can be reflected separately or in conjunction with the posterior hip capsule. I prefer releasing the external rotators and capsule together. It is helpful to make a T-type incision in the capsule below the piriformis so that two sleeves of tissue overlay the posterior hip joint; a suture is passed through each of these sleeves. These sutures are helpful for retraction during reduction of the prosthetic hip and for later capsular reattachment. The capsulotomy is extended superiorly and inferiorly to enhance visualization of the acetabulum.

PROCEDURE

The femur is flexed and internally rotated to expose the femoral neck. A femoral neck osteotomy is performed using an oscillating saw, with the extremity positioned so the foot is superior, pointing toward the ceiling, and the leg perpendicular to the floor (Fig. 22-10). ◉ The location of the cut with respect to the lesser trochanter is determined by preoperative templating, and the angle of the cut is matched to a trial or broach. **Shortening of the limb by excessive femoral neck resection and placement of a short femoral neck component may increase the risk for prosthetic dislocation because of soft tissue laxity—specifically the gluteus medius. Lengthening of the affected limb is poorly tolerated by patients and may result in increased pressure on the acetabular cartilage, increasing the risk of acetabular erosion. As a general rule, the femoral neck should be osteotomized approximately 1 cm proximal to the lesser trochanter.**

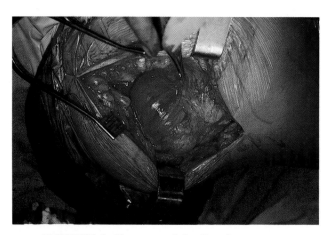

FIGURE 22-9. Placement of the Charnley retractor.

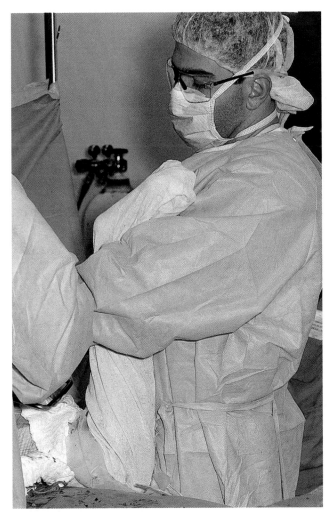

FIGURE 22-10. Positioning of the extremity with the foot superior, pointing toward the ceiling, and the leg perpendicular to the floor.

Osteotomy of the femoral neck before removal of the femoral head enhances the exposure. The femoral head is extracted using a cork screw and a skid ; it may be necessary to incise the ligamentum teres. ◖ If exposure is difficult, a bone hook is passed under the femoral neck and used to retract the femur. If exposure remains a problem and the gluteus maximus is tight, the proximal portion (1 to 1.5 cm) of the gluteus maximus insertion can be released off the linea aspera of the femur using electrocautery. Care must be taken not to release too far distally to minimize bleeding from perforating vessels.

After the femoral head is extracted, it is sized using a caliper or precut templates (Fig. 22-11). ◖ The acetabulum is visually inspected to evaluate the condition of the cartilage. If the pulvinar is excessively large, it is trimmed using a cautery. Trial heads of appropriate size are tested in the acetabulum for a good suction fit, and the largest head that seats fully in the acetabulum is selected. ◖ **Placement of a prosthetic femoral head that is smaller in diameter than**

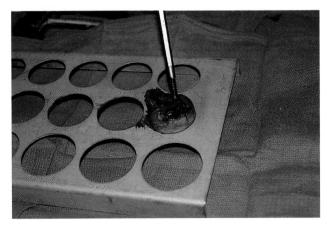

FIGURE 22-11. Sizing of the femoral head using precut templates.

that removed at surgery will result in asymmetric loads within the acetabulum and an increased risk of acetabular wear and subsequent protrusio; use of a larger-diameter prosthetic femoral head than that removed at surgery may not fully seat within the acetabulum, increasing the risk of prosthetic dislocation.

The femoral canal is exposed by passing a broad, flat retractor under the proximal femur. Remaining soft tissue is excised from the posterior and lateral aspect of the femoral neck to the lesser trochanter. A box osteotome is used to open the proximal femur (Fig. 22-12). ◖ If the greater trochanter overhangs the femoral canal, a small notch of bone is removed from the greater trochanter to prevent reaming and broaching in varus. A blunt T-handled starting reamer is placed down the femoral canal in line with femur, directed toward the knee (Fig. 22-13). The femoral canal is reamed using hand or power reamers ◖, increasing in size incrementally until the appropriate-size reamer is reached; the final reaming size depends on the size of the canal and on the type of prosthesis selected.

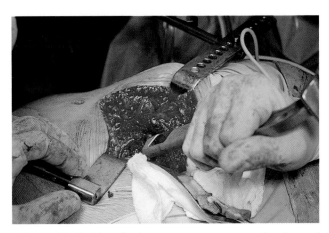

FIGURE 22-12. Use of a box osteotome to open the femoral canal.

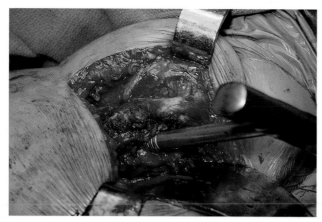

FIGURE 22-13. Placement of a blunt T-handled starting reamer down the femoral canal in line with femur, directed toward the knee.

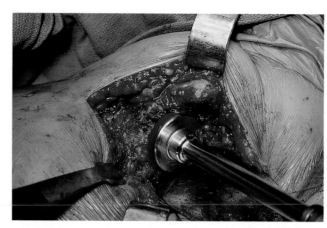

FIGURE 22-15. Use of a calcar planar to even out the femoral neck.

Broaching is then performed using a broach at least two sizes smaller than the templated size of the femur (Fig. 22-14). The broach handle is held in the appropriate amount of anteversion (approximately 15 degrees). With the leg positioned perpendicular to the floor, it is easier to appreciate the amount of anteversion of the broach. **Excessive anteversion results in an internal rotation deformity and increases the risk of anterior hip dislocation; retroversion creates an external rotation deformity and increases the risk of posterior dislocation. Inappropriate femoral version can be avoided by careful observation of the distal femoral axis during the femoral neck osteotomy, preparation of the femoral canal, and insertion of the femoral prosthesis.** When broaching and reaming, it is important to resist the tendency to fall into varus by providing a laterally directed force as the broaches and reamers are advanced. The broach is periodically advanced and removed rather than simply hammered straight down the canal; this technique reduces the risk of iatrogenic femur fracture and helps avoid incarcerating the broach in the femur. After the broach is fully seated to the level of the femoral neck cut, the next size of broach is used, and the process is repeated until the appropriate-size broach is fully impacted. The final broach size is selected based on preoperative templating and, more importantly, on the ease of insertion. A broach that advances too easily is probably too small, and one that requires excessive force of insertion increases the risk of femoral fracture. In cemented applications, it is less important to achieve a tight interlock of the broach with the femur, and there is no need to broach with excessive force.

After broaching is completed, a calcar planer is used to even out the femoral neck cut (Fig. 22-15). With the broach in place, a trial head with the appropriate neck length can be used to assess hip stability through a range of motion.

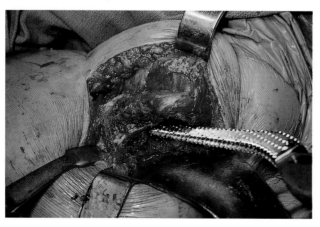

FIGURE 22-14. Broaching of the femoral canal.

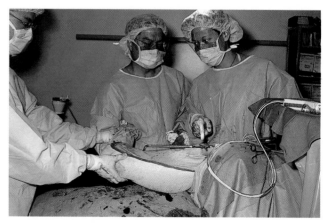

FIGURE 22-16. Checking stability in response to external rotation with the hip in full extension.

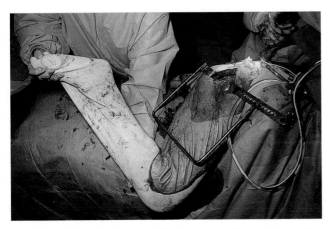

FIGURE 22-17. Checking stability in the position of sleep (i.e., flexion and adduction).

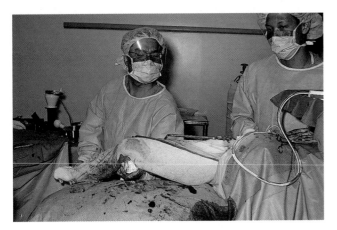

FIGURE 22-18. With the hip in neutral position, the amount of laxity to straight-pull from the foot is tested.

Stability in response to external rotation with the hip in full extension is assessed (Fig. 22-16), as well as stability of the hip in the position of sleep (i.e., flexion and adduction) (Fig. 22-17). In the flexed position, the hip should be internally rotated to determine the point at which the hip begins to lift out of the joint (an angle of more than 30 degrees is preferred). With the hip in neutral position, the amount of laxity to straight pull from the foot should be tested (Fig. 22-18). Although this is probably less important than other tests of stability, the push-pull laxity should be minimal if an appropriate femoral neck length and suction fit have been achieved. The distance from the level of the lesser trochanter to the center of the head is measured with a ruler and compared with the preoperative template. The center of the head should also lie at roughly the level of the top of the trochanter. Various neck lengths should be tested until stability is achieved.

After measurements are made and stability testing completed, the hip is dislocated, the broach and trial head are removed, and the canal is brushed and irrigated (Fig. 22-19). If the prosthesis is to be cemented, the canal is packed with a sponge while the cement is prepared. A cement plug is inserted to the appropriate depth before cement insertion (Fig. 22-20). The cement is vacuum mixed and inserted in retrograde fashion using a cement gun and good pressurization technique (Figs. 22-21 and 22-22). Alternatively, the cement can be hand packed into the femoral canal. In some systems, a distal centralizer can be attached to the tip of the prosthesis before insertion, which helps to prevent varus positioning. Selection of the centralizer size is based on intraoperative measurement of canal di-

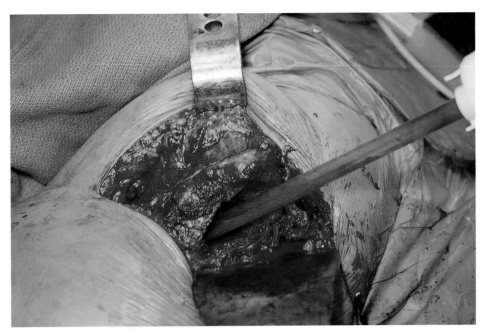

FIGURE 22-19. Irrigation of the femoral canal.

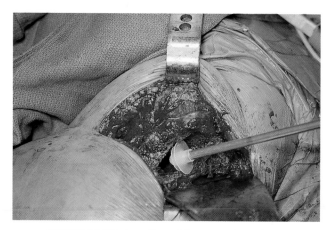

FIGURE 22-20. Insertion of the cement restrictor.

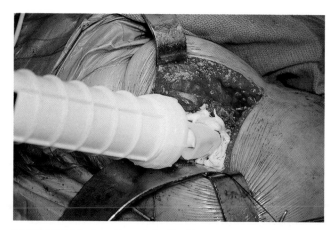

FIGURE 22-22. Insertion of the liquid cement down the femoral canal using a cement gun.

ameter. The prosthesis is inserted using manual force and light taps with a mallet as it is fully seated to the level of the calcar cut (Fig. 22-23). 🎥 The position of the prosthesis should be maintained until the cement hardens; any excess cement is removed using a curette before hardening. Stability is then reassessed using head and neck trials. The final prosthetic head with the appropriate neck length is lightly impacted onto the clean and dry trunnion, and the hip is reduced after clearing all soft tissue from the opening of the acetabulum. Hip stability is once more assessed before wound closure. The short external rotators and underlying capsule are reattached through drill holes to the greater trochanter. The fascia lata is closed using interrupted sutures, followed by skin closure. A Hemovac drain placed deep to the fascia lata is preferred.

POSTOPERATIVE PROTOCOL

The Hospital for Joint Diseases rehabilitation protocol is outlined in Table 22-1.

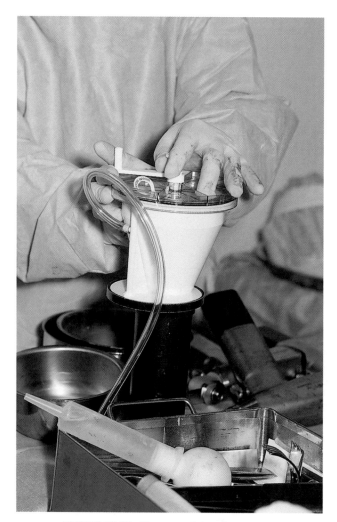

FIGURE 22-21. Vacuum mixing the cement.

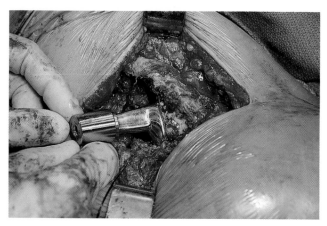

FIGURE 22-23. Insertion of the prosthesis.

TABLE 22-1. HOSPITAL FOR JOINT DISEASES REHABILITATION PROTOCOL

Period	Rehabilitation Protocol
Day 1	Dangle legs from bed Out of bed to chair Ambulation training with walker for 15 feet (weight bearing as tolerated)
Day 2	Ambulation training for 20 feet
Day 3	Ambulation training for 40 feet
Day 4	Stair climbing
Day 5+	Progression of ambulation and stair climbing for endurance and distance with gradual decrease of assistance from the therapist for the following: 1. Daily occupational therapy for instruction in activities of daily living 2. Daily strengthening exercises in supine, sitting, and standing positions 3. Daily range of motion exercises for patients who had internal fixation; patients who had prosthetic replacement are limited to 90 degrees of flexion for 6 weeks

SUGGESTED READINGS

Beckenbaugh RD, Tressler HA, Johnson EW. Results after hemiarthroplasty of the hip using a cemented femoral prosthesis: a review of 109 cases with an average follow-up of 36 months. *Mayo Clin Proc* 1977;52:349–353.

Bochner RM, Pellicci PM, Lyden JP. Bipolar hemiarthroplasty for fracture of the femoral neck: Clinical review with special emphasis on prosthetic motion. *J Bone Joint Surg Am* 1988;70:1001–1010.

Chan RNW, Hoskinson J. Thompson prosthesis for fractured neck of the femur: a comparison of surgical approaches. *J Bone Joint Surg Br* 1975;57:437–443.

Eiskjaer S, Gelineck J, Soballe K. Fractures of the femoral neck treated with cemented bipolar hemiarthroplasty. *Orthopedics* 1989;12:1545–1550.

Follacci FM, Charnley J. A comparison of the results of femoral head prosthesis with and without cement. *Clin Orthop* 1969;62:156–161.

Hunter GA. Should we abandon primary prosthetic replacement for fresh displaced fractures of the neck of the femur? *Clin Orthop* 1980;152:158–161.

Lausten GS, Vedel P, Nielsen PM. Fractures of the femoral neck treated with a bipolar endoprosthesis. *Clin Orthop* 1987;218:63–67.

Lu-Yao GL, Keller RB, Littenberg B, et al. Outcomes after displaced fractures of the femoral neck: a meta-analysis of one hundred and six published reports. *J Bone Joint Surg Br* 1994;76:15–25.

Phillips TW. The Bateman bipolar femoral head replacement: a fluoroscopic study of movement over a four-year period. *J Bone Joint Surg Br* 1987;69:761–764.

Sikorski JM, Barrington R. Internal fixation versus hemiarthroplasty for the displaced subcapital fracture of the femur: a prospective randomized study. *J Bone Joint Surg Br* 1981;63:357–361.

Soreide O, Lerner AP, Thunold J. Primary prosthetic replacement in acute femoral neck fracture. *Injury* 1975;6:286–293.

Wathne RA, Koval KJ, Aharonoff GB, et al. Modular unipolar versus bipolar prosthesis: a prospective evaluation of functional outcome after femoral neck fracture. *J Orthop Trauma* 1995;9:298–302.

Yamagata M, Chao EY, Illstrup DM, et al. Fixed-head and bipolar hip endoprosthesis. *J Arthroplasty* 1987;2:327–341.

INTERTROCHANTERIC FRACTURES: SLIDING HIP SCREW

KENNETH J. KOVAL

Hip fractures are one of the most devastating injuries in the elderly. These injuries impact far beyond the obvious orthopaedic injury into the domains of medicine, rehabilitation, psychiatry, social work, and medical economics. The significance of hip fractures in the elderly becomes even more important as the number of geriatric hip fractures occurring each year increases in the face of increasing pressure for health care cost containment at all levels of our health care system. This chapter discusses the use of a sliding hip screw for stabilization of an intertrochanteric hip fracture.

ANATOMY

Fractures in the region between the greater and lesser trochanters are characterized as *extracapsular fractures* because they are located distal to the anatomic limits of the hip joint capsule (Fig. 23-1). The cancellous bone in this intertrochanteric region is well vascularized. Surgeons rarely encounter the problems of nonunion and osteonecrosis that can complicate intracapsular fractures.

CLASSIFICATION

Classification is based on the status of the posteromedial cortex:

In stable fracture patterns (Fig. 23-2), the posteromedial cortex remains intact or has minimal comminution, making it possible to obtain a stable reduction.

Unstable fracture patterns are characterized by greater comminution of the posteromedial cortex (Fig. 23-3). Unstable fracture patterns also include intertrochanteric fractures with subtrochanteric extension and those with a reverse obliquity pattern.

INDICATIONS

Virtually all intertrochanteric hip fractures require surgery. Nonoperative management is appropriate only in selected patients who are nonambulatory and who experience minimal discomfort from their injury, or patients who are medically too sick to undergo surgery.

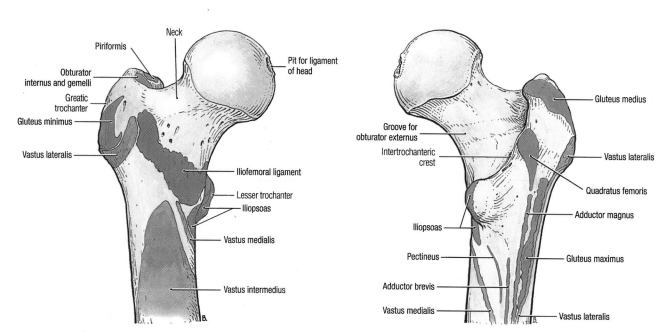

FIGURE 23-1. Muscle attachments of the proximal femur. **(A)** Proximal femur, anterior view. **(B)** Proximal femur, posterior view. (From Agur AMR, Lee MJ. *Grant's atlas of anatomy,* 10th ed. Philadelphia: Lippincott Williams & Wilkins, 1999, with permission.)

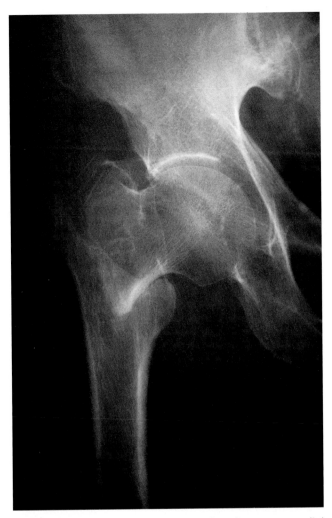

FIGURE 23-2. Stable fracture. Notice that the posteromedial cortex remains intact.

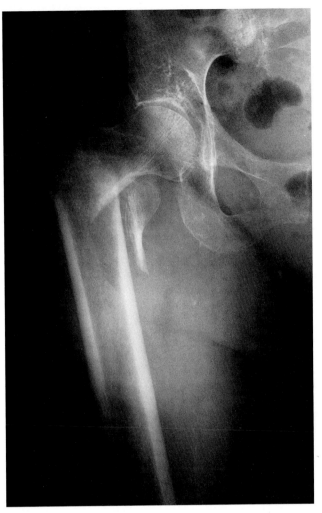

FIGURE 23-3. Unstable fracture. Notice the greater comminution of the posteromedial cortex.

PREOPERATIVE PLANNING

A standard radiographic examination of the hip consists of the following views:

- Anteroposterior view of the pelvis (Fig. 23-4)
- Anteroposterior and cross-table lateral view of the involved proximal femur (Figs. 23-5 and 23-6).

The lateral radiograph can help to assess posterior comminution of the proximal femur; a cross-table lateral is preferred to a frog lateral view because the latter requires abduction, flexion, and external rotation of the affected lower extremity and involves a risk of fracture displacement.

Internally rotating the involved femur 10 to 15 degrees offsets the anteversion of the femoral neck and provides a true anteroposterior of the proximal femur. A second anteroposterior view of the contralateral side can be used for preoperative planning.

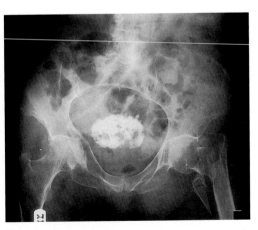

FIGURE 23-4. Standard radiographic view: anteroposterior view of the pelvis, showing a left intertrochantene hip fracture.

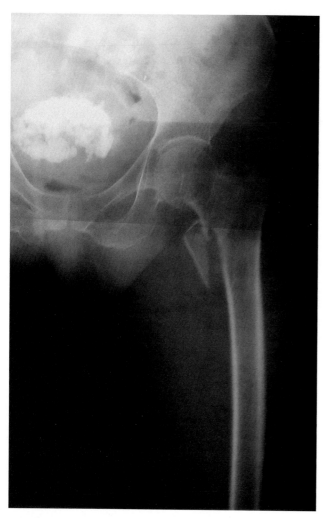

FIGURE 23-5. Standard radiographic view: anteroposterior view of the involved proximal femur.

Magnetic resonance imaging (MRI) is useful when a hip fracture is suspected but not apparent on standard radiographs. MRI has been shown to be at least as accurate as bone scanning in identification of occult fractures of the hip

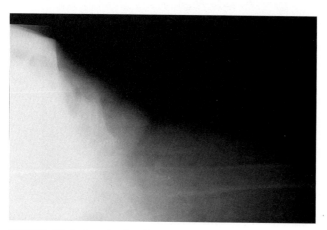

FIGURE 23-6. Standard radiographic view: cross-table lateral view of the involved proximal femur.

and can be performed within 24 hours of injury. MRI within 48 hours of fracture does not, however, appear to be useful for assessing femoral head viability or vascularity or for predicting the development of osteonecrosis or healing complications.

EQUIPMENT

The basic instruments necessary for insertion of a sliding hip screw (Fig. 23-7):

- Guide pins
- Angle guides
- Depth gauge
- Adjustable reamer
- Guide wire repositioner
- Tap
- Lag screw extenders
- Insertion handle
- 3.5-mm drill
- Drill guide
- Screwdriver

PATIENT POSITIONING AND FRACTURE REDUCTION

The patient is positioned supine on a fracture table with both lower extremities resting in padded foot holders. A padded perineal post is placed in the ipsilateral groin, with care taken that there is no impingement of the labia or scrotum. In female patients, it is important to verify that the mucosa of the labia is not everted against the perineal post.

The fracture is then reduced. Intertrochanteric hip fractures can be reduced using gentle longitudinal traction with the leg externally rotated followed by internal rotation. The uninvolved leg is then flexed, abducted, and externally rotated to allow positioning of the image intensifier for a lateral view (Fig. 23-8). Alternatively, the contralateral extremity can be abducted with the hip and knee extended; this maneuver, however, places greater post pressure on the perineum.

The fracture reduction must be assessed before preparing the patient, and the surgeon must be certain that nonobstructive biplanar radiographic visualization of the entire proximal femur, including the hip joint, is obtainable. **Inadequate visualization of the entire proximal femur can result in inappropriate lag screw length or positioning. The surgeon must be prepared to deal with residual varus angulation, posterior sag, or malrotation. Fracture reduction with varus angulation or posterior sag results in difficulty centering the lag screw in the femoral neck and head. Varus angulation can usually be corrected by placing additional traction on the lower extremity to disengage the**

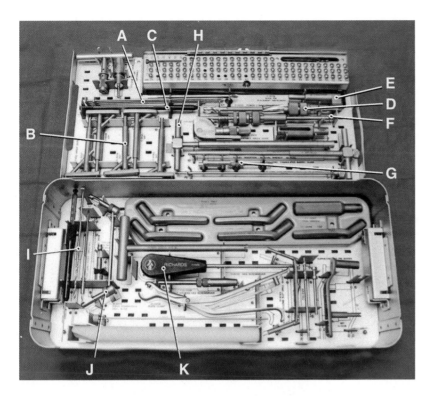

FIGURE 23-7. The basic instruments necessary for insertion of a sliding hip screw: guide pins *(A)*, angle guides *(B)*, depth gauge *(C)*, adjustable reamer *(D)*, guide wire repositioner *(E)*, tap *(F)*, lag screw extenders *(G)*, insertion handle *(H)*, 3.5-mm drill *(I)*, drill guide *(J)*, and screwdriver *(K)*.

fracture fragments, followed by repeat fracture reduction. Occasionally, the lower extremity must be abducted to correct a varus malreduction. If residual varus remains, the surgeon should check the position of the fracture fragments on the lateral radiographic view, because posterior sag may prevent adequate fracture reduction. In this situation, traction should be released and the fracture manipulated to disengage the fragments. Posterior sag requires manual correction using a crutch, bone hook, or periosteal elevator. If unrecognized, posterior sag results in guide pin positioning in the anterior femoral neck and posterior femoral head. I rotate the lower extremity under fluoro-

scopic control to determine whether the fracture fragments move as a single unit. In patients in whom the femoral shaft moves independently from the proximal fragment, excessive internal rotation of the leg is avoided. Instead, the lower extremity is placed in neutral or slight external rotation.

APPROACH

A straight, 8- to 10-cm lateral incision is made, starting at the base of the greater trochanter and extending distally (Fig. 23-9). The incision is deepened through the subcutaneous tis-

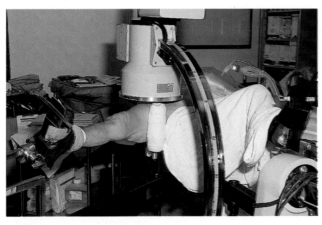

FIGURE 23-8. Patient positioning. The uninvolved leg is flexed, abducted, and externally rotated to allow positioning of the image intensifier.

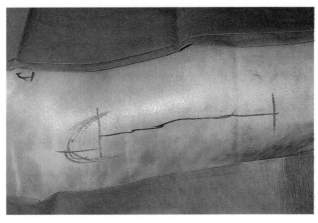

FIGURE 23-9. In this approach, a straight, 8- to 10-cm, lateral incision starts at the base of the greater trochanter and extends distally.

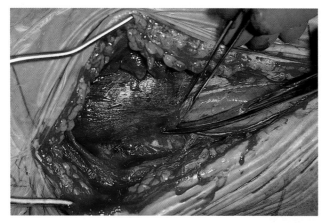

FIGURE 23-10. The incision is deepened through subcutaneous tissue, and the iliotibial band is incised in line with its fibers, with care taken to remain posterior to the tensor fasciae latae muscle.

sue, and the iliotibial band is incised in line with its fibers, with care taken to remain posterior to the tensor fasciae latae muscle (Fig. 23-10). This exposes the vastus lateralis and its covering fascia. Rather than using a muscle-splitting approach through the vastus lateralis, I prefer to incise the fascia of the vastus lateralis and reflect the muscle from the intermuscular septum. ◧ Care should be taken to identify and ligate the perforators from the profunda femoral artery (Fig. 23-11) ◧ ; if cut, they may retract posteriorly through the intermuscular septum, making them difficult to control. The lateral aspect of the proximal femur is cleared of soft tissue using a periosteal elevator, and the vastus lateralis is retracted anterior with a Hohmann retractor. ◧

PROCEDURE

Stable Fractures

Using image intensification, a starting point is identified on the lateral cortex of the proximal femur. This is usually

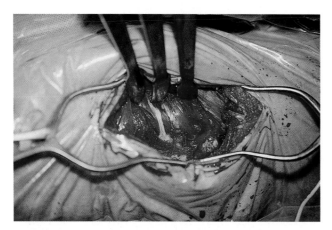

FIGURE 23-11. Care should be taken to identify and ligate the perforators from the profunda femoral artery.

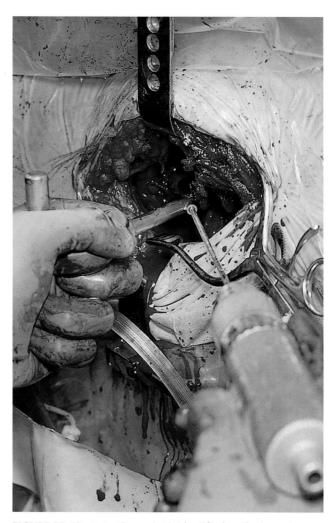

FIGURE 23-12. A starting point is identified on the lateral cortex of the proximal femur, usually at the level of the lesser trochanter, centered between the anterior and posterior cortical margins. A drill hole is made and a guide pin inserted into the femoral neck and head under image intensification using the 135-degree guide.

at the level of the lesser trochanter, centered between the anterior and posterior cortical margins. A drill hole is made and a guide pin inserted into the femoral neck and head under image intensification using the 135-degree guide (Fig. 23-12). A guide pin can be placed anterior to the femoral neck to estimate femoral neck anteversion, although I find this unnecessary. The position of the guide pin is adjusted until it lies in the center of the femoral head and neck on the anteroposterior and lateral planes. ◧

Baumgaertner et al. devised the concept of tip-apex distance (TAD) to determine lag screw position within the femoral head. This measurement, expressed in millimeters, is the sum of the distances from the tip of the lag screw to the apex of the femoral head on the anteroposterior and lateral radiographic views (after controlling for radiographic

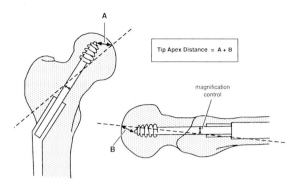

FIGURE 23-13. The tip-apex distance (TAD) is used to determine lag screw position within the femoral head.

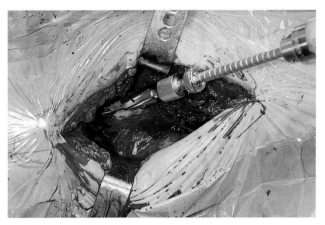

FIGURE 23-15. Reaming of the femoral neck and head over the guide pin is performed to the desired final position of the lag screw.

magnification). Peripheral malposition of the lag screw is not differentiated from shallow lag screw positioning; only the actual distance from the tip of the lag screw to the apex of the femoral head is considered. Based on evaluation of a series of patients, he recommended that, if guide pin location yields a TAD of more than 25 mm, the surgeon should reassess the fracture reduction and reposition the guide pin (Fig. 23-13).

If the guide pin cannot be positioned appropriately in the femoral head and neck, the fracture reduction and plate angle should be reassessed, particularly for residual varus and posterior sag. Occasionally, a 130- or 140-degree insertion is needed to optimize lag screw position. When the guide pin is confirmed to be in the desired position, it is advanced to the level of the subchondral bone, and the length of the lag screw is determined (Fig. 23-14). ◘ In stable intertrochanteric fractures, significant fracture impaction is not anticipated, and a screw length is chosen that maximizes screw-barrel engagement, allows for about 5 mm of impaction, and lies within 1 cm of the subchondral bone. For example, if the guide pin measures

100 mm to the subchondral bone, a 90-mm-long lag screw may be selected; once fully seated 5 mm from the subchondral bone, the lag screw would be inset 5 mm into the plate barrel.

Reaming of the femoral neck and head over the guide pin is performed under image intensification to the desired final position of the lag screw (Fig. 23-15). **The position of the guide pin during reaming must be monitored to detect possible binding of the guide pin within the reamer, which may result in guide pin advancement and femoral head penetration. The position of the guide pin may be lost during reamer removal; the guide pin can be replaced using a guide pin repositioner available in many sliding hip screw sets or by a free lag screw inserted backward into the reaming channel.** ◘ The reamed tract is tapped, even in elderly patients, to prevent femoral head rotation during lag screw insertion. The lag

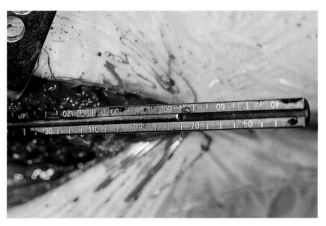

FIGURE 23-14. When the guide pin is in the desired position, it is advanced to the level of the subchondral bone, and the length of the lag screw is determined.

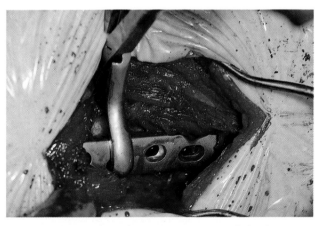

FIGURE 23-16. When the proper position of the lag screw within the femoral head has ben confirmed, a three- or four-hole, 135-degree side plate is placed over the screw.

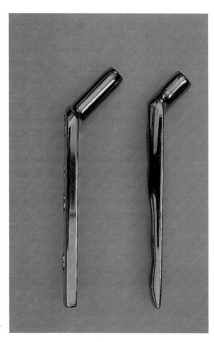

FIGURE 23-17. A standard (long-barrel) plate is used for most intertrochanteric fractures.

screw is then inserted to within 1 cm of the subchondral bone. ◉

When the proper position of the lag screw within the femoral head has been confirmed, a three- or four-hole, 135-degree side plate is placed over the screw (Fig. 23-16). ◉ I routinely use a three-hole plate for fixation of stable and unstable intertrochanteric fractures. I prefer the use of a "keyed" sliding hip screw system. In a keyed system, the lag screw is captured within the plate barrel such that the screw can slide along the barrel but cannot rotate. Use of a keyed sliding hip screw system requires that the lag screw be oriented so that the plate can be properly positioned along the femoral shaft.

A standard (long-barrel) plate is used for most intertrochanteric fractures (Fig. 23-17). The longer barrel maximizes the amount of screw-barrel engagement and minimizes the likelihood of the lag screw "jamming" within the plate barrel. However, a short-barrel plate is used if a lag screw of less than 85 mm has been inserted. This helps to prevent postoperative impaction that exceeds the sliding capacity of the device. The minimum amount of available screw-barrel slide necessary to reduce the risk of fixation failure with use of a sliding hip screw has been estimated to be 10 mm.

The plate is loosely clamped to the femoral shaft and the fracture impacted by releasing the traction on the extremity and gently displacing the femoral shaft toward the proximal fragment. The plate clamp is then tightened, and the fracture position is reassessed. This impaction

maneuver enhances fracture stability and helps prevent fracture distraction that may result in excessive postoperative screw-barrel slide. ◉ The plate-holding screws are then inserted. ◉ The need for a compression screw is determined by direct visualization of the lag screw within the plate barrel (Fig. 23-18); a compression screw is inserted if there is risk of postoperative screw-barrel disengagement.

The compression screw is not used to achieve fracture impaction. A compression screw is not used routinely because it is an added expense and because the compression screw often loosens (even during uneventful fracture healing) and can become a source of lateral thigh pain.

The wound is closed in layers over suction drains.

Unstable Fractures

The most frequently encountered unstable intertrochanteric fractures are characterized by loss of the posteromedial buttress. Another type of unstable intertrochanteric fracture is the reverse obliquity pattern, which begins just proximal to the lesser trochanter and extends laterally and distally with an oblique orientation.

The general treatment approach for fractures with posteromedial comminution is similar to that described for stable fracture patterns in the preceding section: anatomic fracture alignment followed by internal fixation using a sliding hip screw. In older patients, the posteromedial fragment is

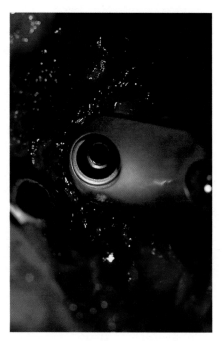

FIGURE 23-18. Insertion of the plate-holding screws. The need for compression is determined by direct visualization of the lag screw within the plate barrel.

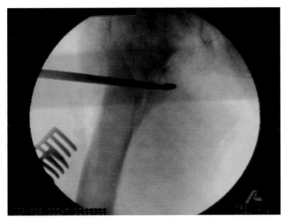

FIGURE 23-19. In this procedure for treating unstable fractures, the posteromedial fragment can be reduced using a bone hook and can be provisionally stabilized using a Verbrugge or standard reduction clamp.

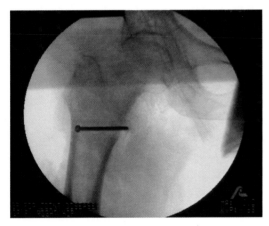

FIGURE 23-20. Definitive fracture fixation involves the use of one or more cerclage wires or one or more lag screws directed from anterolateral to posteromedial aspects.

usually ignored. In younger patients, an attempt should be made to stabilize large posteromedial fragments in a near-anatomic position to prevent excessive screw-barrel slide, which would result in limb shortening. <u>Reduction and stabilization of the posteromedial fragment can be performed before or after lag screw and side plate application. I prefer the former, because this method facilitates anatomic fracture reduction of the posteromedial fragment. If the main fracture fragments are reduced and stabilized primarily, it may be impossible to reduce the posteromedial fragment anatomically.</u>

To mobilize and reduce the posteromedial fragment, there should be no traction on the lower extremity; because the iliopsoas is attached to the lesser trochanter, traction results in proximal migration of the posteromedial fragment. The extremity is externally rotated to better expose the posteromedial area of the femoral shaft. The posteromedial fragment can be reduced using a bone hook and provisionally stabilized using a Verbrugge or standard reduction clamp (Fig. 23-19). Definitive fracture fixation involves use of one or more cerclage wires or one or more lag screws directed from anterolateral to posteromedial aspects (Fig. 23-20). These screws cannot be inserted through the proximal hole of the plate. Proper angulation cannot be achieved because of the limitations of the screw hole and its position distal to the involved area. After the posteromedial fragment is stabilized, traction is placed on the lower extremity, and the head and neck fragment reduced. The sliding hip screw is then inserted as previously described.

POSTOPERATIVE PROTOCOL

The Hospital for Joint Diseases rehabilitation protocol is outlined in Table 23-1.

TABLE 23-1. HOSPITAL FOR JOINT DISEASES REHABILITATION PROTOCOL

Period	Rehabilitation Protocol
Day 1	Dangle legs from bed Out of bed to chair Ambulation training with walker for 15 feet (weight bearing as tolerated)
Day 2	Ambulation training for 20 feet
Day 3	Ambulation training for 40 feet
Day 4	Stair climbing
Day 5+	Progression of ambulation and stair climbing for endurance and distance with gradual decrease of assistance from the therapist for the following: 1. Daily occupational therapy for instruction in activities of daily living 2. Daily strengthening exercises in supine, sitting, and standing positions 3. Daily range of motion exercises for patients who had internal fixation; patients who had prosthetic replacement are limited to 90 degrees of flexion for 6 weeks

SUGGESTED READINGS

Aune AK, Ekeland A, Odegaard B, et al. Gamma nail vs compression screw for trochanteric femoral fractures: 15 reoperations in a prospective, randomized study of 378 patients. *Acta Orthop Scand* 1994;65:127–130.

Baumgaertner MR, Curtin SL, Lindskog DM, et al. The value of the tip-apex distance in predicting failure of fixation of peritrochanteric fractures of the hip. *J Bone Joint Surg Am* 1995;77:1058–1064.

Blair BJ, Koval KJ, Kummer F, et al. A biomechanical comparison of multiple cancellous screws to the sliding hip screw for the treatment of basocervical fractures. *Clin Orthop* 1994;306:256–263.

Desjardins AL, Roy A, Paiement G, et al. Unstable intertrochanteric fracture of the femur: a prospective randomized study comparing anatomical reduction and medial displacement osteotomy. *J Bone Joint Surg Br* 1993;75:445–447.

Gehrchen PM, Nielsen JO, Olesen B. Poor reproducibility of Evans' classification of the trochanteric fracture. *Acta Orthop Scand* 1993;64:71–72.

Gundle R, Gargan MF, Simpson AH. How to minimize failures of fixation of unstable intertrochanteric fractures. *Injury* 1995;26:611–614.

Leung KS, So WS, Shen WY, et al. Gamma nails and dynamic hip screws for pertrochanteric fractures. *J Bone Joint Surg Br* 1992;74:345–351.

Lunsjo K, Ceder L, Stiggson L, et al. Two-way compression along the shaft and the neck of the femur with the Medoff sliding plate. *J Bone Joint Surg Br* 1996;78:387–390.

Stappaerts KH, Deldycke J, Broos PLO, et al. Treatment of unstable peritrochanteric fractures in elderly patients with a compression hip screw or with the Vandeputte (VDP) endoprosthesis: a prospective randomized study. *J Orthop Trauma* 1995;9:292–297.

CHAPTER 24

SLIPPED CAPITAL FEMORAL EPIPHYSIS

GAIL S. CHORNEY

Slipped capital femoral epiphysis is the most common hip disorder in adolescents. It is characterized by the anterior and superior migration of the femoral neck. Although this shift in location gives the femoral head the appearance of lying posteriorly and inferiorly, it actually remains stable in the acetabulum. The average age at presentation is 12 years for girls and 14 years for boys. The slip occurs during the preadolescent hormonal changes of puberty. Children with a vertical capital physis are more prone to developing a slip. There is also an association with obesity. Most of the patients are in the 99th percentile for weight. Patients may present with pain for several days or many weeks, but pain is not necessarily an indication of slip severity. The current classification used is based on the stability of the physis. Children who have an effusion and are unable to bear weight have an unstable slip. The children who are bearing weight at the time of presentation have a stable slip.

ANATOMY

By definition, a slipped capital femoral epiphysis can occur only in skeletally immature patients. The timing of the slip generally coincides with the beginning of puberty. The theory is that the physis is weaker at that physiologic point, because the columnar architecture becomes disorganized when the physis begins to fuse. The histology of the capital physis in patients with slipped capital femoral epiphysis shows almost total loss of the columns and is similar to the histology of the proximal tibial physis in patients with Blount disease. Because both types of histology have a high association with obesity, the obesity is thought to play a role in the weakening of the physis. In patients with known collagen problems, such as those with Down syndrome, the fibrous septa between the columns is unable to support the architecture.

The orientation of the physis in affected patients is often more vertical than normally observed. Calculating the stresses across the physis in obese patients reveals a considerable increase in the forces, and it is therefore not a surprise that these patients are more susceptible to slips. There has also been reported in the literature an association between the occurrence of slips and increased retroversion of the femoral head. However, these studies are often performed after the slip, and it is not clear whether the retroversion is cause or effect.

It is the femoral neck that migrates rather than the femoral head, as the name of the disorder implies. The femoral neck drifts anteriorly and superiorly. On radiographs, the femoral head is located inferiorly and posteriorly. There is a rare variation known as the valgus slip, in which the migration of the femoral neck is in the opposite direction so that the femoral head rests more anteriorly and superiorly. The reason for the difference in position is not known.

CLASSIFICATION

Slipped capital femoral epiphyses were formerly classified as acute, subacute, or chronic. The classification was based solely on the amount of time symptoms were present at the time of the initial evaluation. The timing was determined by patient history. This classification proved not to be useful in determining outcome. Slipped capital femoral epiphyses are now classified by the amount or degree of the slip. This classification is beneficial in a prognostic manner. It does not affect the decision to operate or the technique.

Slips are stable or unstable. Unstable hips are those in which the patients are unable to bear weight. Patients who walk into the doctor's office complaining of thigh or hip pain have a stable slip. Stable hips have virtually no risk of avascular necrosis. Unstable hips have a high incidence of avascular necrosis. Fortunately, there are far more stable slips than unstable ones.

The physis is considered to be divided in thirds. The amount of slip is graded as I, II, or III or as a complete slip. If the slip is only a few millimeters or in the first third starting from the lateral side, the slip is a mild or Grade I slip. In a complete slip, there is no continuity between the femoral head and the femoral neck. (Fig. 24-1). The worse the slip, the greater the residual deformity will be. With greater deformity, there is an increased risk of osteoarthritis. Complete slips are associated with instability and carry a high risk of avascular necrosis. All grades of slipped femoral capital epiphysis are treated with *in situ* pinning.

INDICATIONS FOR SURGERY

Stable and unstable slips may continue to progress, but there is more urgency to stabilize an unstable slip. These patients are admitted immediately and scheduled for surgical stabilization as soon as possible. Stable slips can be scheduled over the next several days if it is more convenient for the surgeon and patient.

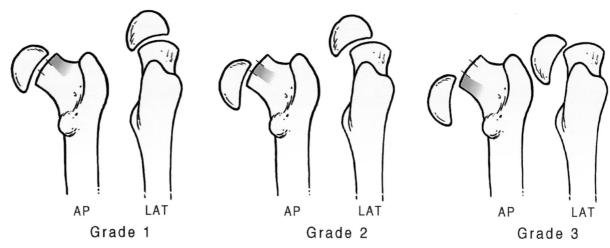

FIGURE 24-1. The classification of a slipped capital femoral epiphysis is based on the degree of slip: Grade I, first third; Grade II, second third; Grade III, last third.

The goal of surgery is to stabilize the physis so that it does not slip further. The preferred method is to percutaneously pin the hip with a single implant. The femoral head is pinned *in situ*. This technique is associated with minimal morbidity, a shortened hospital stay, and a decreased incidence of complications. The presence of a slip on radiographs of a patient that is skeletally mature does not indicate surgical intervention, because there is no risk of further slippage when the physis is fused.

PREOPERATIVE PLANNING

There is an association of slipped capital femoral epiphysis with certain metabolic disorders. The more common of these disorders are hypothyroidism, growth hormone insufficiency, and renal disorders. Other syndromes with known collagen deficiencies such as Down syndrome also have an increased incidence of slipped capital femoral epiphysis. Concomitant disorders have generally been diagnosed before the time of presentation of a slipped epiphysis. Although it is suspected through research that patients with slipped capital femoral epiphysis have an unknown type of endocrine disorder, a workup is not cost effective for each patient. A careful history and physical examination is all that is needed. If the patient falls out of the usual age range for slips, an endocrine workup is indicated. Patients younger than 10 or older than 16 years of age would meet that criteria.

Each patient should have an anteroposterior and lateral radiograph of the unaffected hip to check for bilateral slip presentation. If radiographs reveal a second slip, both hips may undergo *in situ* pinning at the same time.

EQUIPMENT

Percutaneous pinning is done best on a fracture table. The image intensifier is a necessity. A 6.5 mm cannulated hip pin is used to stabilize the physis. A 7.3 mm cannulated pin may also be used. Generally, only one pin is placed. However, in unstable slips, it may be desirable to place two pins. In those cases, if there is not enough room in the femoral head to place two 7.3 mm pins, 6.5 mm cannulated pins are indicated.

PATIENT POSITIONING AND PREPARATION

After the patient is anesthetized, the patient is positioned on the fracture table (Fig. 24-2). The operative leg is positioned with the hip extended, abducted, and internally rotated. This position generally produces a gentle reduction. A gentle reduction in this manner does not increase the incidence of avascular necrosis.

The nonoperative leg is positioned with the hip extended and abducted or with the foot in a stirrup and the hip and knee flexed. The position of the nonoperative leg is not im-

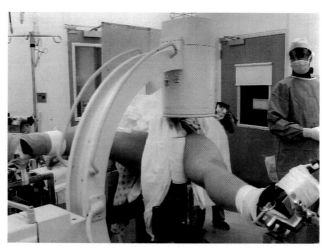

FIGURE 24-2. Patient position on the table.

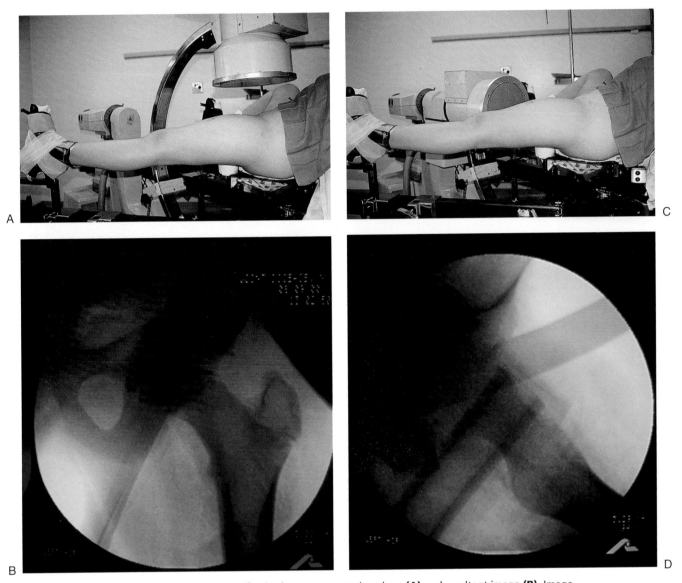

FIGURE 24-3. Image intensifier in the anteroposterior plane **(A)** and resultant image **(B)**. Image intensifier in the lateral plane **(C)** and the image obtained **(D)**.

portant as long as it does not impede the position of the image intensifier.

It is imperative that the image intensifier be positioned and images taken before proceeding with the surgery. Good images of the hip are needed in the anteroposterior and lateral planes. The physis and outline of the femoral head must be distinctly visualized to place the pin properly and avoid penetration of the joint. It should be possible to obtain views in both planes by rotating the arm of the image intensifier (Fig. 24-3). 📹

The patient is prepared for surgery from the umbilicus to the lateral groin and the thigh. A "shower curtain" draping is generally used. Most starting points for the percutaneous pinning are anterior. **Care should be taken to ensure that the draping does not prevent an anterior entrance point.**

SURGICAL INCISION LANDMARKS

Stabilization of slipped capital femoral epiphyses is achieved by a percutaneous procedure. After the correct entrance point is achieved at the beginning of the case, the remainder of the case is then straightforward. The entrance point is determined by understanding the correct position for the pin. The head of the pin should be in the center of the femoral head and perpendicular to the physis in the anteroposterior and lateral planes. **Because the femoral head is no longer in an anatomic position, concentrating on the point where the pin enters the femoral neck will result in failure.**

With the image intensifier in the anteroposterior plane, a guide wire or any other type of straight edge is placed on the anterior groin. The guide wire is adjusted until an image is obtained that shows the guide wire perpendicular to the ph-

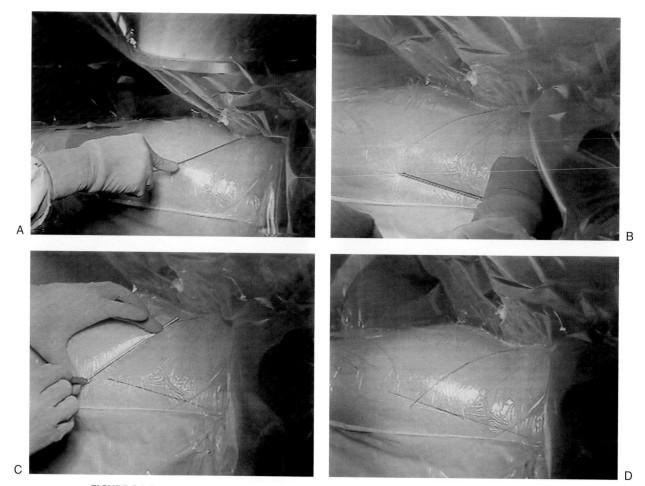

FIGURE 24-4. A: An anteroposterior line is drawn on the skin. **B:** A lateral line is drawn on the skin. **C:** Anteroposterior and lateral lines are extended until they intersect. **D:** The entrance point for the pin is the intersection of lines.

ysis. A skin marking pen is then used to draw a line on the skin along the straight edge. The same maneuver is used with the image intensifier in the lateral plane. A straight line is drawn on the skin. The intersection of these two lines is the entrance point. The more severe the slip, the more anterior the entrance point will be (Fig. 24-4).

PROCEDURE

The guide wire is placed percutaneously on the femoral neck by penetrating the skin at the predetermined entrance point (Fig. 24-5). ◙ The wire is advanced onto the femoral neck a short distance (2.5 cm). Its position is examined in the anteroposterior and lateral planes. ◙ The surgeon looks at where the pin will be located in the femoral head, not where it is entering the femoral neck. If the position is satisfactory, the wire is advanced in the femoral head. The surgeon usually feels a small amount of resistance as the guide wire crosses the physis. Only a few threads of the pin need to pass the physis. The pin should not go to the edge of the joint (Fig. 24-6).

After the guide wire is placed, a 1-cm incision is made in the skin (Fig. 24-7). The incision is carried down through the fascia lata. A large hemostat is used to spread the soft tissue.

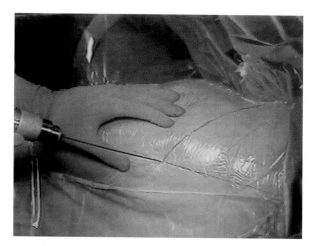

FIGURE 24-5. The guide wire enters the skin at the intersection of the drawn anteroposterior and lateral lines.

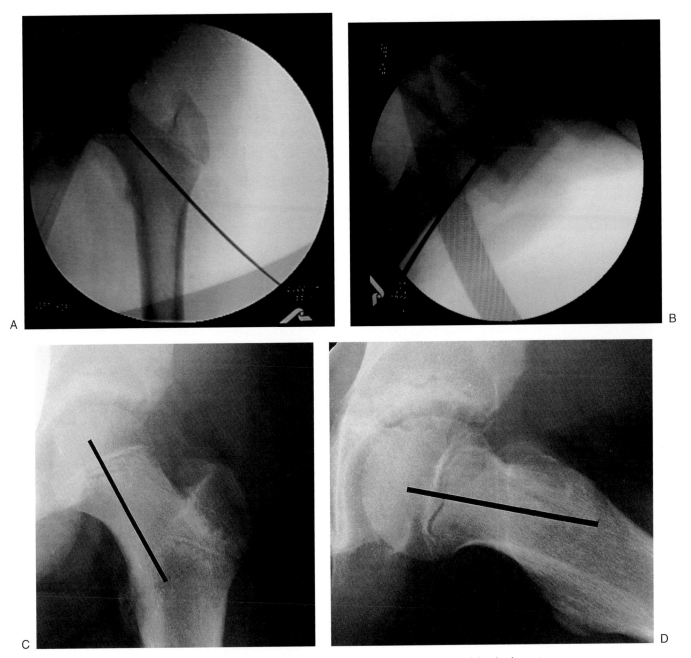

FIGURE 24-6. Image intensifier views of the guide wire in the correct position in the anteroposterior **(A)** and lateral **(B)** planes. The guide wire is perpendicular to the physis and in the center of the femoral head. Radiographs **(C, D)** with a drawn black bar simulating the proper position of the guide wire and therefore the correct position for the hip pin.

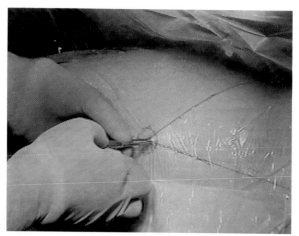

FIGURE 24-7. A 1-cm incision is made over the guide wire and continued through the fascia lata.

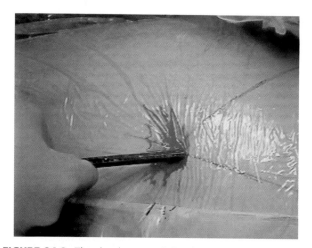

FIGURE 24-8. The depth gauge is in place over the guide wire and in contact with the femur.

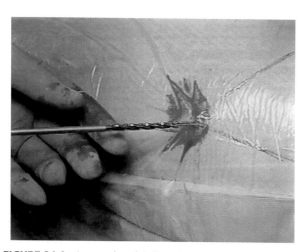

FIGURE 24-9. A cannulated drill is placed over the guide wire.

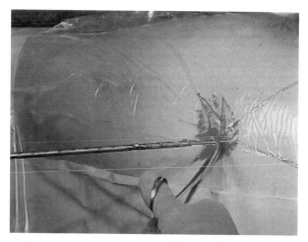

FIGURE 24-10. A hemostat is placed on the guide wire as the drill is withdrawn to ensure the guide wire remains in the bone.

The length of the pin to be inserted is determined by using the depth gauge supplied in the instrument set. The depth gauge is placed over the guide wire and pushed onto the bone (Fig. 24-8). The image intensifier is used to confirm that the depth gauge is on the bone. The pins come in 0.5-cm increments.

The cannulated drill is placed over the guide wire (Fig. 24-9). � The drilling is done under the visual control of the image intensifier. **If the guide wire catches in the drill, it may be advancing with the drill and cross the joint line.** This occurs when there may still debris in the drill from previous cases or if the guide wire becomes bent. The surgeon should drill just to the tip of the guide wire. The drill is then withdrawn. Care should be taken not to remove the guide wire with the drill. <u>It is helpful to use a hemostat to hold onto the guide wire as the drill is withdrawn from the incision</u> (Fig. 24-10).

The cannulated hip pin is placed over the guide wire and advanced with the T-handle wrench (Fig. 24-11). The final

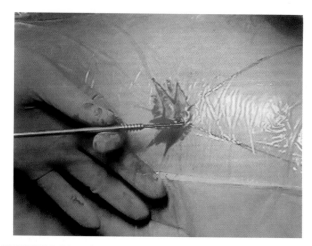

FIGURE 24-11. Advancement of the cannulated hip pin after positioning it over the guide wire.

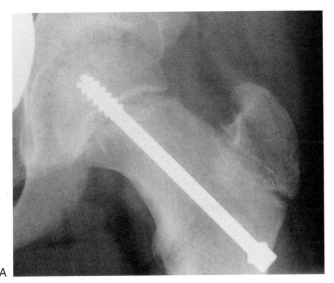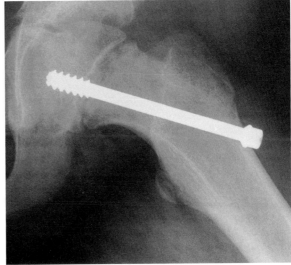

A

B

FIGURE 24-12. Anteroposterior **(A)** and lateral **(B)** radiographs show the pin in the correct position.

position of the pin is checked in the anteroposterior and lateral planes. The cannulated drill is placed over the guide wire, and drilling is started. As the drill is withdrawn, a hemostat is placed on the guide wire so it does not come out of the wound. The hip pin is then placed over the guide wire and advanced with the T-handle wrench. ◼ If the position is satisfactory, the guide wire is withdrawn (Fig. 24-12). The small wound is then irrigated and closed. Only the subcutaneous and skin layers need closure. A small dressing is then applied (Fig. 24-13). ◼

FOLLOW-UP

Many patients are able to be discharged on the day of surgery. A criteria for discharge is independent ambulation

on crutches. Partial weight bearing is allowed. Because the pain relief is significant postoperatively, most patients are able to ambulate with crutches without difficulty. Patients can be weaned off their crutches as their pain diminishes.

Any unusual increases in pain should be evaluated. Avascular necrosis and chondrolysis are the two most serious complications. The use of a single implant decreases the incidence of both complications.

Approximately one third of patients have a bilateral slip. One half of these cases have both hips involved at the time of the initial presentation. The remaining patients present over the next 18 to 24 months while the physis is closing. Patients should be followed until the capital physis fuses. Ordering an anteroposterior and frog lateral radiograph rather than views of just the operative side allows both hips to be evaluated.

The implant does not have to be removed routinely. If avascular necrosis occurs and the pin is not penetrating into the joint, the pin should be removed. Because the implant is placed percutaneously, removal of the pin often results in a larger incision and increased morbidity. If the pin does have to be removed, it can often be accomplished by feeding the guide wire through the pin.

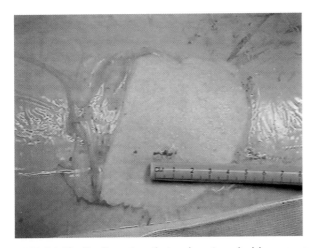

FIGURE 24-13. Confirmation that only a 1-cm incision was required.

SUGGESTED READINGS

Aronsson DD, Loder RT. Treatment of the unstable (acute) slipped capital femoral epiphysis. *Clin Orthop* 1996;322:99–110.

Aronson J, Tursky EA. The torsional basis for slipped capital femoral epiphysis. *Clin Orthop* 1996;322:37–42.

Herman MJ, Dormans JP, Davidson RS, et al. Screw fixation of grade III slipped capital femoral epiphysis. *Clin Orthop* 1996;322:77–85.

Jago ER, Hindley CJ, Jago RD. The removal of metalwork in children. [Erratum appears in *Injury* 1998;29:736.] *Injury* 1998;29:439–441.

Jerre R, Karlsson J, Romanus B, et al. Does a single device prevent further slipping of the epiphysis in children with slipped capital femoral epiphysis?. *Arch Orthop Trauma Surg* 1997;116:348–351.

Kallio PE, Mah ET, Foster BK, et al. Slipped capital femoral epiphysis: incidence and clinical assessment of physeal instability. *J Bone Joint Surg Br* 1995;77:752–755.

Loder RT, Wittenberg B, DeSilva G. Slipped capital femoral epiphysis associated with endocrine disorders. *J Pediatr Orthop* 1995;15:349–356.

McAfee PC, Cady RB. Endocrinologic and metabolic factors in atypical presentations of slipped capital femoral epiphysis: report of four cases and review of the literature. *Clin Orthop* 1983;180:188–197.

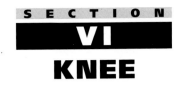

CHAPTER 25

DIAGNOSTIC ARTHROSCOPY OF THE KNEE

BIREN V. CHOKSHI
JEFFREY E. ROSEN

The knee is the largest joint in the human body and one of the most frequently injured. The knee and its supporting structures are subjected to high-energy forces, especially during sporting activities. The lower extremities act as a large moment arm, through which the weight of the body imparts these high forces onto the knee. The surgeon undertaking diagnostic and operative arthroscopy of the knee should be able to identify all of the structures of the knee that can be visualized and are accessible with an arthroscope.

Although office arthroscopy has been reported in the literature, we believe the procedure is best performed under sterile conditions in an operating room setting. Diagnostic arthroscopy can be performed under local, regional, or general anesthesia. The advantages of local anesthesia include low morbidity when compared with the potential complications associated with a regional or general anesthetic. Local anesthesia may be best suited for experienced surgeons performing diagnostic and uncomplicated arthroscopic procedures only. The disadvantages of local anesthesia include the possibility of patient discomfort during more involved procedures or those during which a tourniquet is used. Regional anesthesia and general anesthesia keep the patient more comfortable if a procedure runs longer than expected or the use of a tourniquet is required. Regional anesthesia has the added advantage of better postoperative pain control.

ANATOMY

The knee is a compound joint composed of three articulations: two condyloid joints, which are the medial and lateral articulations of the distal femur and proximal tibia, and one sellar joint, which is formed by the articulation of the patella with the anterior aspect of the distal femur (Fig. 25-1). The surfaces of all three compartments of the knee joint are covered with articular cartilage.

The two meniscal cartilages, medial and lateral, sit between the articular surfaces of each compartment and are connected anteriorly by the transverse intermeniscal ligament. These crescent, or C-shaped, fibrocartilaginous structures deepen the concavity of the proximal tibia, have a role in nutrition and lubrication of the joint, and aid in protecting the articular surfaces. The peripheral one third of the meniscus is vascular, has the potential for healing, and can be considered for meniscal repair. The inner two thirds of the meniscal cartilage is nourished by synovial fluid. The medial meniscus is a more C-shaped structure, whereas the lateral meniscus is more circular. Both meniscal cartilages are triangular in cross section and can be palpated during arthroscopy on their inferior and superior surfaces.

Four main ligaments contribute to the stability of the knee, which is further enhanced by a complex arrangement of additional ligaments, tendons, and capsular tissue. The medial and lateral collateral ligaments resist valgus and varus angulation, respectively, and are palpable at the joint line. The anterior and posterior cruciate ligaments resist anterior and posterior displacement of the tibia on the femur, respectively, and can be visualized and palpated within the intercondylar notch. The popliteus tendon originates from the lateral femoral condyle and inserts on the proximal tibia. It can be seen traversing the posterior aspect of the lateral compartment by looking into the hiatus behind the posterior horn of the meniscus.

INDICATIONS

Arthroscopy of the knee can be used as a diagnostic and operative tool. As an adjunctive tool, the arthroscope is used to obtain or confirm a variety of diagnoses and should be used in conjunction with a complete history, thorough physical examination, and appropriate imaging studies. Diagnostic arthroscopy provides direct visualization and tactile information about the intraarticular structures of the knee. Damage to these structures can be assessed and the information then used to develop a treatment strategy. Meniscal and articular cartilage lesions, synovial lesions, and ligament

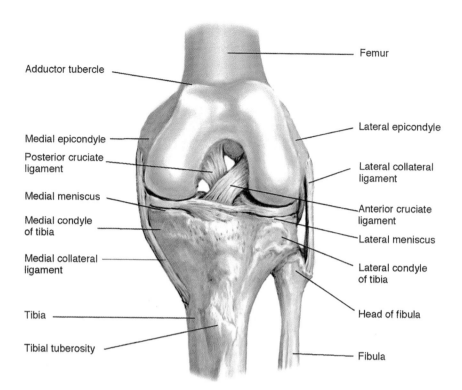

Adductor tubercle

Femur

Medial epicondyle

Posterior cruciate
ligament

Medial meniscus

Medial condyle
of tibia

Medial collateral
ligament

Tibia

Tibial tuberosity

Lateral epicondyle

Lateral collateral
ligament

Anterior cruciate
ligament

Lateral meniscus

Lateral condyle
of tibia

Head of fibula

Fibula

FIGURE 25-1. Anterior aspect of bony structures of the knee. From Bickley LS, *Bates' guide to physical examination and history taking,* 8th ed. Philadelphia: Lippincott Williams & Wilkins, 2003.

injuries are pathologic conditions that can be addressed with an arthroscopic examination of the knee.

When assessing damage to the meniscal cartilage, the morphology, size, stability, and location of the tear should be described. The meniscus is divided into thirds: anterior horn, body, and posterior horn. Basic patterns of meniscal tears include longitudinal, horizontal, oblique, radial, and degenerative. The stability of the tear should also be documented. Articular cartilage damage is classified based on the location, size, and depth of involvement. The cruciate ligaments are examined for intrasubstance damage or avulsion from their insertion sites. Tears are classified as partial or complete. Synovial lesions are classified by their location, color, and morphology. Tissue can be obtained for specimen and sent for histologic examination.

After the surgeon is comfortable with the use of the arthroscope and is confident in his or her ability to manipulate instruments through a number of different portals, progression to operative arthroscopy can gradually be made. Basic arthroscopic procedures should be mastered before attempting complex surgeries:

■ Synovial biopsy
■ Synovectomy
■ Débridement of cartilage lesions
■ Removal of loose bodies
■ Partial meniscectomy

As the skill of the arthroscopic surgeon increases, more complex procedures can be undertaken:

■ Lateral release
■ Saucerization of discoid lateral meniscus

■ Meniscal repair
■ Arthroscopic drilling and treatment of cartilage lesions
■ Arthroscopic assisted cruciate ligament reconstructions

PREOPERATIVE PLANNING

Preoperative planning should include a thorough physical examination and a complete standard radiographic examination. The physical examination consists of the following elements:

■ Assessment of passive and active range of motion and of overall alignment
■ Tests for anterior-posterior, varus-valgus, and rotational instability (e.g., Lachman, drawer, pivot shift)
■ Palpation for focal areas of tenderness
■ Provocative tests for meniscal pathology (flexion-rotation)
■ Testing for patella tracking and instability
■ Assessment of gait

Radiographic examination should include the following elements:

■ Anteroposterior, weight-bearing view of both knees
■ Anteroposterior and lateral views of the involved knee
■ Patella view

Magnetic resonance imaging (MRI) may be useful when the physical examination does not clearly point to a cause for the patient's symptoms and may help to delineate the exact nature and extent of ligament and cartilage pathology.

MRI is particularly useful for identifying lesions of the subchondral bone, nondisplaced fractures, tumors, synovial lesions, and extraarticular soft tissue lesions.

EQUIPMENT

The following instruments are needed for diagnostic and basic operative arthroscopy of the knee (Fig. 25-2):

- Arthroscopic video camera and monitor
- Fiberoptic light source
- 4.5-mm, 30-degree arthroscope
- Sheath for arthroscope
- Trocar for arthroscope
- 4.5-mm, 70-degree arthroscope
- Arthroscopic infusion pump or gravity inflow setup
- Multiple 3-L bags of arthroscopic fluid
- Suction setup
- Manual probe
- Manual meniscal cutters or biters
- Grasping forceps
- Motorized arthroscopic shaver system and an assortment of shaver blades

- Suture material for portal closure
- Tourniquet
- Lateral post or leg holder

PATIENT POSITIONING AND PREPARATION

All surgical procedures should begin with a complete, systematic examination under anesthesia. ◼ Range of motion in all planes is assessed and recorded. Patella mobility should be compared with the nonoperative extremity and documented. Next, the knee is assessed for any varus or valgus laxity, rotational laxity, or anterior or posterior instability. Pivot shift testing should be performed and compared with the uninvolved knee.

The procedure is performed with the patient placed supine on the operating room table. A tourniquet is positioned over padding that is placed on the upper most aspect of the patient's thigh. Some surgeons prefer to place the lower extremity into a leg holder and to drop the foot of the table. Other surgeons choose to leave the lower extremity flat on the table and use a lateral side post for counterpressure with application of a valgus stress to the knee. A leg holder is useful when the surgical assistant is not available to

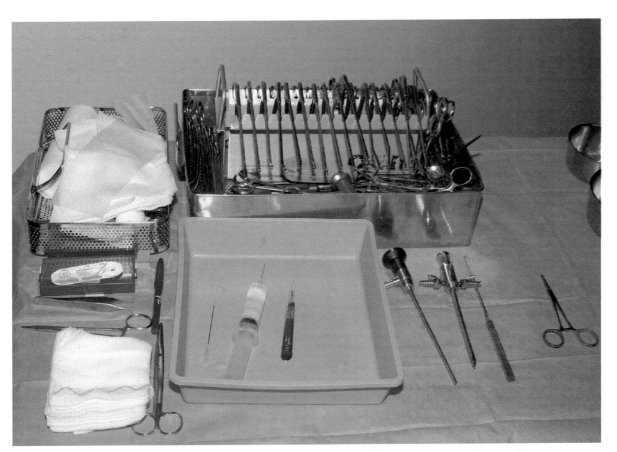

FIGURE 25-2. Instruments for diagnostic and basic operative arthroscopy: dressings, sutures, forceps, needle driver, marker, suture scissors *(left column)*; graspers and biters *(top tray)*; spinal needle, syringe (normal saline), no. 11 scalpel *(bottom tray)*; arthroscope, arthroscopic cannula and blunt trocar, probe, straight clamp *(far right)*.

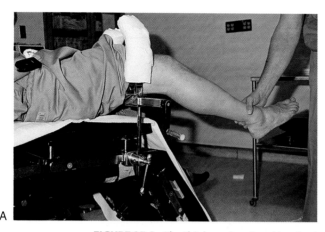
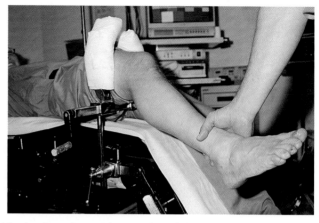

A   B

FIGURE 25-3. The thigh can be placed in a leg holder for the arthroscopic procedure. **(A)** The foot of the bed is dropped, and the leg can hang free or be manipulated. **(B)** Valgus or varus stress can be applied to the knee by using the leg holding device for counter traction.

help support the leg and provide a valgus stress; however, the holder may impede access to the lateral compartment and patellofemoral compartments through superior portals (Fig. 25-3). The leg holder also limits the ability to manipulate the leg to place the knee into a figure-of-four position. Alternatively, the surgeon can lever the leg against a lateral post to open up the medial compartment of the knee (Fig. 25-4). The post does not confine or restrict the knee from being positioned or fully flexed. **Excessive stress applied to the knee while the leg is placed in a confining leg holder can result in periarticular fractures or tearing of the collateral ligaments. Care must be taken to avoid these complications, especially in patients who may be at increased risk (i.e., arthroscopic procedures in the older patient or those with disuse osteoporosis).**

The extremity is then prepared and draped from the ankle to the tourniquet. Many commercially available draping systems are easily applied and provide access to the knee and lower extremity. After preparing and draping the patient, all arthroscopic tubing and equipment should be connected in an organized manner so they will not become tangled during the procedure and interfere with the surgery (Fig. 25-5).

SURGICAL INCISION LANDMARKS AND PORTAL PLACEMENT

Precise placement of arthroscopic portals is key to the success of the procedure. Improper placement of viewing and working portals will make it difficult to visualize parts of the knee joint and hinder the ability to maneuver instruments.

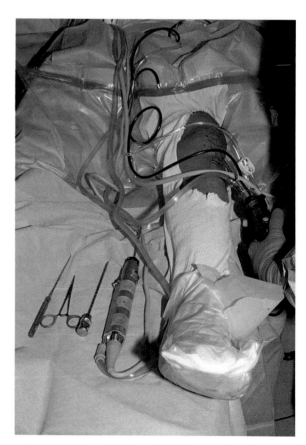

FIGURE 25-5. Organization of tubing and equipment for arthroscopy: probe, straight clamp, blunt trocar, power shaver *(lower left)*; arthroscope and camera in surgeon's hand *(far right).*

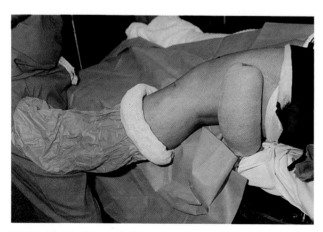

FIGURE 25-4. Alternatively, arthroscopy can be performed on a flat table using a lateral post for countertraction.

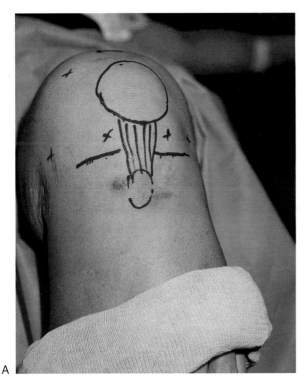 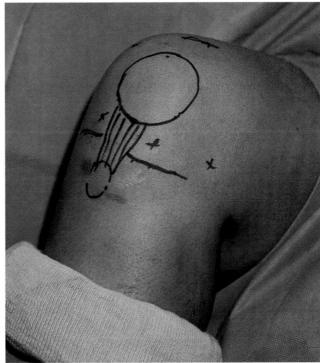

A   B

FIGURE 25-6. A, B: The skin is marked to outline the knee anatomy before inflation with arthroscopic fluid. The positions of standard and accessory portals should be marked in case they are needed.

Poorly placed portals also increase the risk of injury to the chondral surfaces and may result in articular scuffing. Correct portal site placement is best accomplished by preoperatively identifying all soft tissue and bony landmarks and then drawing the outline of these structures on the skin with a marking pen (Fig. 25-6). Markings should be made before distention of the knee joint, because this may become difficult after distention has occurred.

The following landmarks are useful for portal placement and should be outlined on the knee:

- Patella
- Patellar tendon
- Medial joint line
- Lateral joint line
- Posterior aspect of the medial and lateral femoral condyles

All standard and potential accessory portals should be marked on the skin. Two basic arthroscopic portals are used for diagnostic and operative arthroscopy: anterolateral and anteromedial (Fig. 25-7). The anterolateral portal is the standard viewing portal used by most arthroscopic surgeons and is located approximately 1 cm above the lateral joint line and 1 cm lateral to the edge of the patellar tendon. **If a portal is placed too inferiorly, the anterior horn of the lateral meniscus may be damaged. An anterolateral portal that is placed too high risks damage to the chondral surfaces of the lateral femoral condyle and may prevent viewing of and access to the posterior lateral joint structures. If the portal is placed** too close to the edge of the patellar tendon, the arthroscope will pass through the fat pad and make viewing and maneuvering within the joint difficult. When an anterior cruciate ligament reconstruction is planned, it may be helpful to place the portal closer to the edge of the patellar tendon to provide better access to the medial aspect of the lateral femoral condyle. This often requires partial débridement of the infrapatellar fat pad for better visualization.

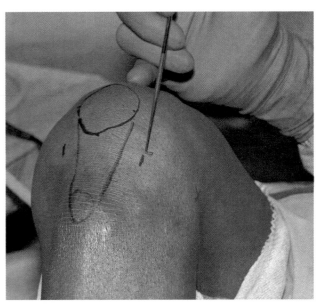

FIGURE 25-7. Anterolateral and anteromedial portals.

The anteromedial portal is the standard initial working portal for knee arthroscopy. This portal is located 1 cm above the medial joint line and approximately 1 cm medial to the edge of the patellar tendon. It can be created before extension of the joint with arthroscopy fluid, or it may be created after localization with a spinal needle while viewing from inside the knee. Our preference is to create the antero-medial portal after localization with a spinal needle. This allows small adjustments to be made before the portal is created and may ensure better access to the site of primary pathology. The arthroscopic surgeon should become adept at switching the working and viewing portals for more versatile access to all aspects of the knee joint. The anteromedial portal may also be used as a viewing portal by switching the arthroscope from the anterolateral portal. **If the portal is placed too inferiorly, the anterior horn of the medial meniscus may be damaged. A portal that is placed too high risks damage to the chondral surfaces and may not allow access to the posterior aspect of the medial compartment. If the portal is positioned too close to the edge of the patellar tendon, instruments may get caught in the infrapatellar fat pad, or they may not be able to access the posterior horn of the medial meniscus.**

The superolateral portal is an accessory portal site that may be used for inflow or outflow. It can also be used for placement of the arthroscope to visualize the tracking of the patella in the femoral groove. Instruments may be placed into this portal to perform arthroscopic procedures such as a lateral release or excision of a medial plica. The portal is located just lateral to the tendon of the quadriceps muscle and approximately 2 to 3 cm above the superolateral corner of the patella (Fig. 25-8). Newer arthroscopic surgery systems allow inflow and outflow through the arthroscopic camera sheath and may be used without an accessory inflow or outflow portal (i.e., two-incision technique) (Fig. 25-9). The

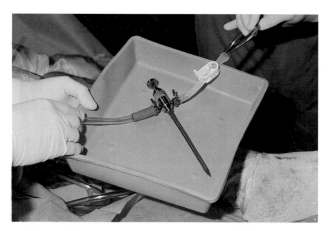

FIGURE 25-9. Arthroscopic cannula with inflow and outflow.

superomedial portal may be established as an accessory inflow or outflow cannula instead of the superolateral portal. The site for this portal is approximately 2 to 3 cm above the superomedial corner of the patella. The cannula or instruments should be passed underneath the medial edge of the vastus medialis muscle.

The posteromedial portal is an accessory portal that provides access to the structures of the posteromedial compartment. This portal can be located by palpating the soft spot at the posteromedial corner of the knee. The portal is placed in the triangular soft spot formed by the posteromedial edges of the femoral condyle and proximal tibia. It is best identified by marking the landmarks and the site of portal placement on the skin before distension of the knee. It is located 1 cm above the posteromedial joint line at the posterior edge of the femoral condyle (Fig. 25-10). The knee should be flexed to 90 degrees, and the joint should be fully distended before creation of the portal. If a 70-degree arthroscope is placed through the intercondylar notch, this portal site can be created under direct visualization from within the knee. Palpation of the soft spot can be seen as an indentation of the capsule, and a spinal needle can be used

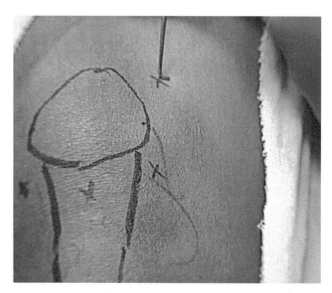

FIGURE 25-8. Superolateral portal.

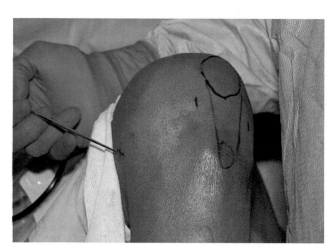

FIGURE 25-10. Posteromedial portal.

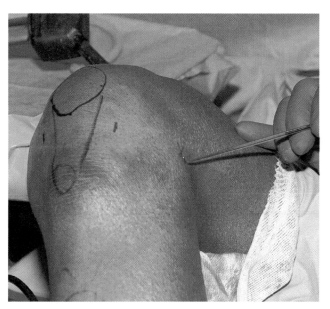

FIGURE 25-11. Posterolateral portal.

for localization and confirmation before establishing the portal. The posterolateral portal is an accessory portal that provides access to the posterolateral corner of the knee. It is established in a fashion similar to the posteromedial portal. Its location is at the posterolateral soft spot, which is found at the posterior edge of the iliotibial band and anterior edge of the biceps femoris tendon, approximately 2 cm above the joint line, at the posterolateral corner of the knee (Fig. 25-11). This portal can also be created under direct visualization with a 70-degree arthroscope passed through the intercondylar notch. **If a trocar or instrument is passed posteriorly and penetrates the capsule, there is a risk of injury to the neurovascular structures in the popliteal space.**

An anterior central portal has been described that accesses the knee by passing through the patellar tendon. This

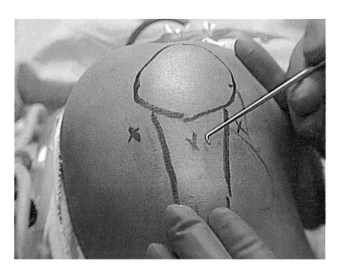

FIGURE 25-12. Anterior central portal.

portal site is located approximately 1 cm below the inferior pole of the patella at the midline (Fig. 25-12). The patellar tendon is split, and the arthroscope is passed through this split into the knee. The arthroscope should first be passed into the superomedial aspect of the knee, which is in 45 degrees of flexion. This allows the arthroscope to pass into the knee above the infrapatellar fat pad. When this portal is used for visualization, it allows the anteromedial and anterolateral portals to be used for instrumentation.

SURGICAL APPROACH AND PROCEDURE

After preparing and draping are complete and all surgical landmarks have been outlined on the skin, the knee is flexed to between 70 and 90 degrees. If a tourniquet is not routinely going to be used during the procedure, the portal sites can be infiltrated with 5 mL of a local anesthetic mixed with epinephrine. This helps control bleeding at the portal sites. **Care must be taken not to infiltrate the sites with excessive fluid, because this may distend the infrapatellar fat pad and interfere with visualization.** Next, the thumb is placed on the lateral tibial condyle and rolled up into the soft spot 1 cm above the lateral joint line. This helps to confirm that the portal site is just above the level of the meniscus. Using a no. 11 scalpel, a 4- to 5-mm incision is made through the skin and subcutaneous tissue and then extended down through the capsule. The knife edge should be facing up to avoid inadvertent laceration of the meniscus. Caution must be used so that the knife is not plunged too deeply, because this may cut the chondral surface of the lateral femoral condyle.

An arthroscopic sheath with a blunt trocar is introduced through the portal and directed into the intercondylar notch. The trocar and sheath are then retracted slightly and advanced into the suprapatellar pouch as the knee is brought into full extension. At this point, the trocar is removed from the sheath; any fluid from inside the knee can be collected in a basin and sent as a specimen for analysis, if so desired. The arthroscope is then inserted into the sheath, and the knee joint is inflated with fluid. Any difficulty accomplishing this maneuver may indicate that the sheath is caught in the patellar tendon or the ligamentum mucosa. If this occurs, the sheath should be removed and reintroduced into the joint.

Successful arthroscopy requires a systematic and careful examination of all parts of the knee joint. The arthroscopic surgeon should develop a consistent method of moving from one portion of the knee to the next and then perform the examination in the same manner for all arthroscopic knee cases.

Our preferred order of examination is as follows:

- Suprapatellar pouch
- Patella
- Patellofemoral articulation

- Lateral gutter
- Medial gutter
- Medial femoral condyle
- Medial meniscus and the medial compartment
- Intercondylar notch
- Anterior cruciate ligament
- Posterior cruciate ligament
- Lateral femoral condyle
- Lateral meniscus and the lateral compartment

In each part of the knee, the surgeon carefully visualizes all structures and uses a probe for manual palpation. All visual and tactile information (i.e., chondral softness) should be recorded. The suprapatellar pouch and medial and lateral gutters are inspected for the presence of loose bodies and for the condition of the synovial lining. Samples of the synovial tissue can be obtained and sent for analysis, if needed. The articular surface of the patella and femoral groove is carefully examined for chondral damage. ◤ The arthroscopic surgeon can visualize all portions of the knee by using a combination of movements of the arthroscopic sheath and by changing the direction of orientation of the arthroscopic lens. For observation of patellofemoral congruity and tracking, the arthroscope is best positioned in the superolateral portal with the lens pointing medially. A medial plica may be encountered on attempting to move the sheath to the medial gutter. If the sheath is caught in a thickened medial plica, it should be retracted slightly so that it disengages and can then be freely advanced into the medial gutter.

After inspection of the medial gutter is completed, the lens is directed medially while the scope is brought into the anteromedial aspect of the knee. If the anteromedial portal has not yet been established, the lens is directed laterally, and the portal is created after localization with a spinal needle (Fig. 25-13). This helps to ensure proper placement of the portal and adequate access to the involved portion of the knee. With the lens pointing superiorly, the medial femoral condyle is inspected as the knee is placed through a range of

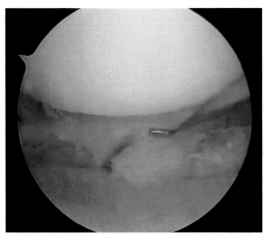

FIGURE 25-14. Visualization of the posterior horn of the medial meniscus, demonstrating a tear.

motion, and a probe is used to palpate the chondral surfaces. ◤ Next, the knee is placed in approximately 30 degrees of flexion, and a valgus force is applied. The arthroscope is carefully placed between the articulating surfaces, taking care not to cause any chondral damage. The scope should be retracted from between the chondral surfaces before the valgus stress is released. This can prevent inadvertent damage. The lens is then rotated to allow visualization of the anterior horn, body, and posterior horn of the medial meniscus (Figs. 25-14 and 25-15). Under direct visualization, a probe is used to manually palpate the superior and inferior surface of the meniscal tissue. ◤ The posterior horn is best viewed with the knee in 30 degrees of flexion and by externally rotating the tibia. The periphery of the posterior horn can be visualized by placing the arthroscope through the intercondylar notch (Fig. 25-16). The scope is advanced underneath the posterior cruciate ligament and

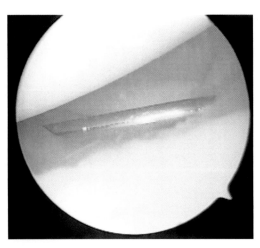

FIGURE 25-13. A spinal needle can be used to localize precise portal placement.

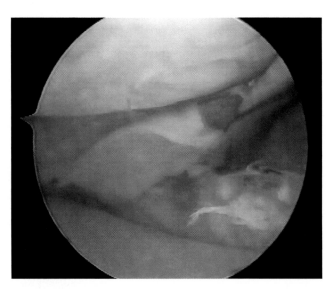

FIGURE 25-15. Visualization of the body of the medial meniscus, demonstrating a tear.

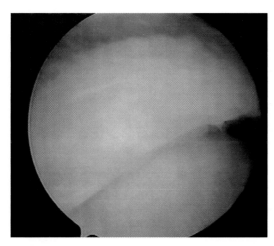

FIGURE 25-16. Visualization of the posterior horn of the medial meniscus with the arthroscope placed through the intercondylar notch.

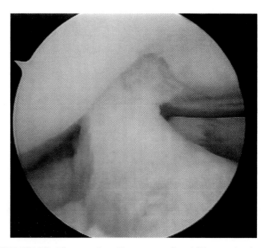

FIGURE 25-18. The cruciate ligaments should be probed as part of the inspection.

along the medial wall of the intercondylar notch. The knee is placed between 80 and 90 degrees of flexion as the sheath is advanced. After the scope enters the posteromedial compartment, the lens can be directed between 4:30- and 7:30-o'clock positions to visualize the posterior horn of the medial meniscus and the posterior cruciate ligament. Additional structures can be visualized by changing the 30-degree scope to a 70-degree scope.

With the lens directed medially, the arthroscope is brought into the intercondylar notch. Viewing may be obscured by the presence of the ligamentum mucosa or a thick septum dividing the medial and lateral compartments. The arthroscope should be used to follow the roof of the intercondylar notch from medial to lateral aspects until the lateral side of the ligamentum is reached. Dropping the scope down to the lateral side of the ligamentum mucosa allows an unobstructed view of the anterior and posterior cruciate ligaments (Fig. 25-17). ◉ To completely visualize the intercondylar notch, a thickened infrapatellar fat pad or ligamentum mucosa sometimes must be débrided. Both

ligaments are manually probed and inspected for any signs of disruption or hemorrhage (Fig. 25-18). ◉ Instability testing can be performed while observing the ligaments to help determine if they are functioning properly.

With the arthroscope above the anterior horn of the lateral meniscus, the knee is placed in a figure-of-four position to gain access to the lateral compartment (Fig. 25-19). The arthroscopic camera should be rotated in conjunction with the knee as it is placed into this position. Downward pressure on the thigh helps to open the lateral compartment. The lateral meniscus is inspected and palpated throughout its entire length (Fig. 25-20). ◉ The popliteus hiatus is visualized behind the posterior horn of the lateral meniscus and should be inspected for the presence of loose bodies. Manual pressure on the posterolateral aspect of the knee may help identify loose bodies as they are displaced into the joint. The posterolateral compartment can be viewed or accessed by means of a posterolateral portal or by the use of a 70-degree arthroscope placed through the intercondylar notch, as described previously.

After diagnostic or operative arthroscopy is completed, the knee is irrigated with copious amounts of fluid and suctioned dry to remove debris from the joint. All portal sites are closed with simple nylon suture. Local anesthetic with epinephrine may be injected into the knee to help with postoperative pain control and hemostasis.

POSTOPERATIVE PROTOCOL

At the end of surgery, the knee is covered with a dry, sterile dressing and wrapped with an elastic bandage. If the surgeon has performed diagnostic or basic operative arthroscopy, such as an uncomplicated partial meniscectomy or chondral shaving (Fig. 25-21), the patient is instructed to ambulate with a cane or crutches, as needed, and to fully bear weight as tolerated, with no limitation on the range of motion. If

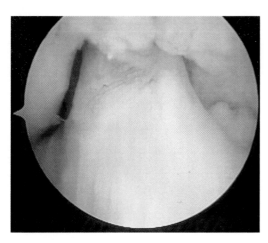

FIGURE 25-17. Anterior cruciate ligament.

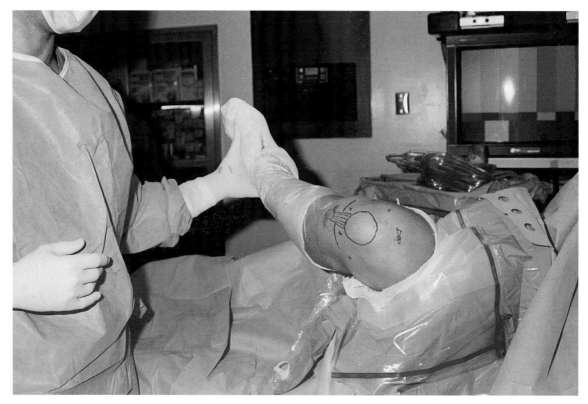

FIGURE 25-19. The leg is placed into a figure-of-four position to gain access to the lateral compartment of the knee.

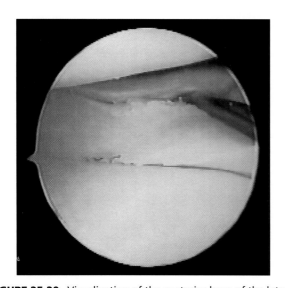

FIGURE 25-20. Visualization of the posterior horn of the lateral meniscus, demonstrating a tear. The probe is placed in the superior surface of the tear.

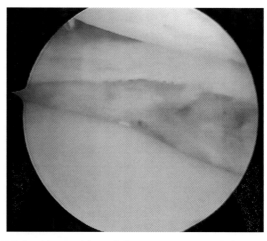

FIGURE 25-21. Partial medial meniscectomy and débridement has been completed.

subchondral drilling, meniscal repair, or other more complex arthroscopic procedures are performed, the postoperative protocol, including the weight-bearing status, varies according to the procedure performed and the surgeon's preference. Home exercises may be started immediately, as symptoms allow. These exercises can include active range of motion, quadriceps sets, straight leg raises, and partial wall squats.

Instructions are given for keeping the wounds dry and for icing the knee for 15 to 20 minutes every hour. Patients are instructed to contact the surgeon for any persistent drainage or increasing pain with range of motion, which may suggest a postoperative infection.

FOLLOW-UP

Patients are instructed to return for a follow-up visit at 7 to 10 days after surgery for suture removal. Bandages may be removed after 24 hours, and incisions covered with Band-Aids. The incisions should be kept dry for 48 hours. The range of motion, amount of swelling, and gait are assessed. If patients are progressing well with home exercises, they may be instructed on advancing their home program and on quadriceps strengthening. If a patient returns to the office with poor range of motion and fails to progress with a home therapy program, she or he should be sent for formal physical therapy with the goals of achieving full range of motion and increasing quadriceps control and strength. Most patients are usually able to return to work within a few days of surgery. A return to sporting activity is possible 3 to 6 weeks after diagnostic arthroscopy or basic operative arthroscopic procedures.

SUGGESTED READINGS

Curran WP, Woodward EP. Arthroscopy: its role in diagnosis and treatment of athletic knee injuries. *Am J Sports Med* 1980;8:415–418.

Dandy DJ. Basic technique: the standard approach. In: McGinty JB, ed. *Operative arthroscopy.* Philadelphia: Lippincott-Raven, 1996.

DeHaven KE. Principles of triangulation for arthroscopic surgery. *Orthop Clin North Am* 1982;13:329–336.

Johnson LL. *Arthroscopic surgery: principles and practice,* 3rd ed. St. Louis: Mosby–Year Book, 1986.

Johnson LL. *Comprehensive arthroscopic examination of the knee.* St. Louis: CV Mosby, 1981.

Keene GCR, Paterson RS, Teague DC. Advances in arthroscopic surgery. *Clin Orthop* 1987;224:64.

Metcalf RW. *Instructional manual of arthroscopic surgery.* Salt Lake City, UT: Press Publishing, 1980.

Watanabe M, Takeda S, Ikeuchi H. *Atlas of arthroscopy.* Tokyo: Igaku Shoin, 1969.

CHAPTER 26

ANTERIOR CRUCIATE LIGAMENT: ENDOSCOPIC RECONSTRUCTION

YOUNG HO OH
MARK I. PITMAN

Anterior cruciate ligament (ACL) injuries are common. They commonly result from contact and noncontact types of sporting activities. These injuries often result in instability of the knee and may prevent individuals from participating in cutting- and pivoting-type sporting activities. ACL injuries may make the individual susceptible to additional injuries of the knee, such as meniscal tears and osteochondral defects, and to premature arthrosis of the knee. Reconstruction of the ACL is recommended for individuals who have symptomatic instability during sports or activities of daily living.

The results of ACL reconstruction have been excellent. The success rate has been reported to be more than 95% in terms of patient satisfaction, with most individuals returning to their preinjury level of activity.

ANATOMY

The ACL originates from the posterior medial surface aspect of the lateral femoral condyle, crosses anteriorly and medially to the posterior cruciate ligament (PCL), and inserts widely on the anteromedial tibial plateau between the tibial eminences. The average length is 31 to 38 mm, and the average width is 11 mm. It is an intraarticular and intrasynovial ligament, which consists of an anteromedial bundle (i.e., taut in flexion and lax in extension) and a posterolateral bundle (i.e., taut in extension and lax in flexion). The ACL acts as the primary restraint to anterior translation of the knee (Fig. 26-1).

INDICATIONS

An isolated rupture of the ACL is an extremely common injury and most commonly results in instability of the knee. For an active, healthy person who wishes to return to some level of athletic activity, reconstruction of the ACL is recommended. A minimum range of motion (ROM) of 5 to 90 degrees (with minimal residual inflammation) is usually desired and should be achieved before surgical intervention.

PREOPERATIVE PLANNING

A thorough history is obtained and physical examination performed. A positive Lachman's test result (Fig. 26-2) and

a present pivot shift (Fig. 26-3), which should always be compared with the contralateral knee, are usually diagnostic of an ACL injury. Possible concomitant injuries, such as those of the meniscus, medial collateral ligament, posterolateral corner, and PCL, should also be ascertained during the examination.

Radiographs, which include anteroposterior, lateral, and merchant views of the knee, are necessary to rule out any fractures, degenerative changes, and malalignment. Magnetic resonance imaging may be helpful to rule out other possible associated injuries, especially meniscal tears, and to confirm an ACL injury.

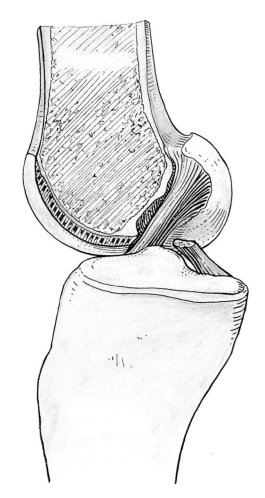

FIGURE 26-1. Anterior cruciate ligament, medial view.

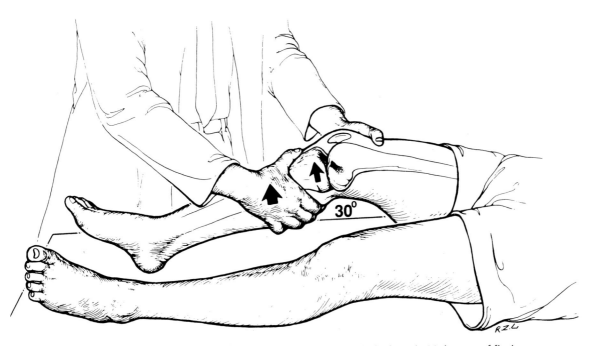

FIGURE 26-2. The Lachman test is an anterior drawer test with the knee in 30 degrees of flexion. It tests anterior cruciate ligament integrity, with an emphasis on the posterolateral bundle. Reprinted from Tria AJ, Jr, Hosea TM. Diagnosis of knee ligament injuries. In: WN Scott (ed.), *Ligament and extensor mechanism injuries of the knee: diagnosis and treatment.* St. Louis: Mosby Year-Book, p. 94. © 1991, Mosby Year-Book, with permission from Elsevier.

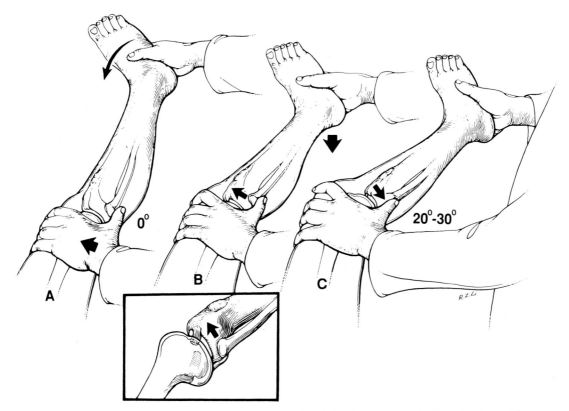

FIGURE 26-3. The pivot shift of Galway and MacIntosh begins with knee in full extension, with internal rotation of tibia and valgus stress. The thumb subluxates the tibia forward, and a "clunk" of reduction is felt in the first 20 to 30 degrees of flexion, which correlates with anterior cruciate ligament disruption. Reprinted from Tria AJ, Jr, Hosea TM. Diagnosis of knee ligament injuries. In: WN Scott (ed.), *Ligament and extensor mechanism injuries of the knee: diagnosis and treatment.* St. Louis: Mosby Year-Book, p. 95. © 1991, Mosby Year-Book, with permission from Elsevier.

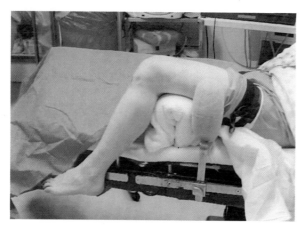

FIGURE 26-4. Position of the patient.

EQUIPMENT

An arthroscopic system is required: pump, light source, scope, camera, and hand and motorized instruments. ArthroWands (ArthroCare, Sunnyvale, CA) may also be helpful. The Arthrex (Naples, FL) transtibial ACL reconstruction system is used for instrumentation throughout the illustrated procedure in this chapter. The following is a list of necessary equipment, most of which is included in the system:

- Oscillating saw
- Adapteur drill guide C-ring with the target PCL-oriented marking hook
- 2.4-mm drill tip guide pins
- Cannulated headed reamers (usually 10 mm)
- Transtibial femoral ACL drill guide (usually 7-mm-offset tip)
- Extra-long 2.4-mm guide pin with suture eye (Beath-type guide pin)
- Sizing block

- Workstation for the bone–patella tendon–bone graft
- Cannulated, titanium interference screws
- Tunnel notcher
- 2-mm pin lock guide pin
- Pin lock cannulated screwdriver set

PATIENT POSITIONING

The patient is positioned supine on the operating table. The procedure can be done under general or regional anesthesia. The appropriate extremity is then examined under anesthesia, and the findings recorded in the operative report. A tourniquet is applied high on the upper thigh. If necessary, the knee is shaved. As is done for routine knee arthroscopy, a removable post is placed adjacent to the thigh, or the extremity is placed in a leg holder (Fig. 26-4). The entire extremity is prepared up to the tourniquet and then sterilely draped. A preoperative antibiotic (usually a first-generation cephalosporin such as intravenous piggyback administration of 1 g of cefazolin) is given before any incision is made.

INCISION

A single incision for endoscopic-assisted ACL reconstruction a with bone–patella tendon–bone autograft is illustrated. In clear instances of an ACL rupture, the graft is harvested first. If there is any doubt about the diagnosis, diagnostic arthroscopy may be performed initially. Landmarks are drawn out with an indelible surgical marker: the four borders of the patella, the tibial tubercle, and the patella tendon. The incision is straight and just medial to the tubercle, extending from the inferior border of the patella to 2 cm distal to the tubercle (Fig. 26-5). Before the

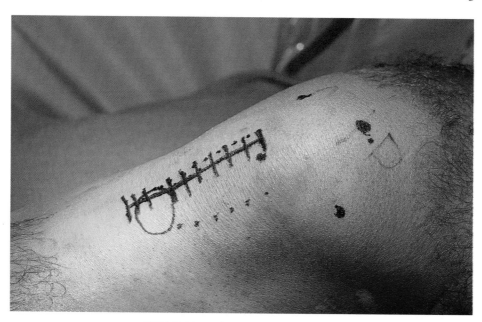

FIGURE 26-5. Placement of the incision.

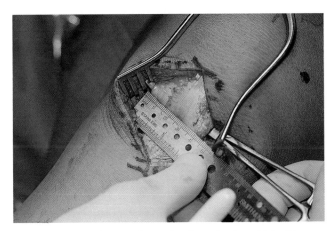

FIGURE 26-6. The patella tendon is cut in the middle 10 cm.

incision is made, an Esmarch bandage is used as a tourniquet to exsanguinate the extremity. With the knee flexed, the tourniquet is inflated to approximately 300 mm Hg (approximately 150 mm Hg above the systolic blood pressure).

GRAFT HARVEST AND PREPARATION

Graft Harvest

With the knee at 30 to 45 degrees of flexion, the incision is carried though skin and subcutaneous tissue down to the level of the paratenon. Hemostasis is achieved with Bovie cautery. The paratenon is sharply incised on the patella tendon and then completely incised as far proximally (up to the middle patella) and distally (2 to 3 cm distal to the tubercle) with Metzenbaum scissors. The edges of the tendon are identified, and the width of the tendon is measured. The middle 10 cm of the tendon is marked along the tendon (Fig. 26-6). With a 10-mm-wide, parallel, double-blade scalpel, the tendon is completely incised parallel along its fibers in the middle portion of the tendon, extending from the distal pole of the patella to the tibial tu-

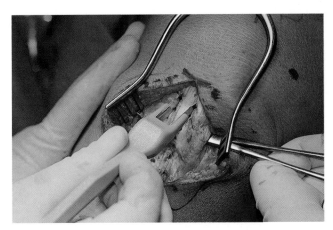

FIGURE 26-7. The patella tendon is cut using a 10-mm, double-blade scalpel.

bercle (Fig. 26-7). A ruler is used to mark a length of 25 mm distal to the insertion of the tendon on the tubercle. Keeping the same 10 mm width of the incised tendon, an outline of the osteotomy cut (10 × 25 mm) is made with a scalpel. An oscillating saw with a 7-mm-deep stop blade (Arthrex) is used to cut the bone plug from the tibia in a rectangular fashion (Fig. 26-8). A 0.25-inch, curved osteotome is used to carefully lift the bone plug out on each side (Fig. 26-9). **Care should be taken not to lift it from the distal end because the bone plug may fracture from levering.** The tibial plug is put back in its place as attention is directed toward the patella bone plug. A graft-harvesting patella retractor makes exposure of the entire patella easier. A ruler is used to mark a length of 20 cm proximal to the origin of the patella tendon in the middle patella. Keeping the same 10 mm width of the incised tendon, an outline of the osteotomy cut (10 × 20 mm) is made with a scalpel. The oscillating saw is again used, and the bone plug from the patella is cut in a triangular fashion—which is done to minimize the potential stress riser left in the patella after harvesting—by angling the saw blade 45 degrees to the cortex on each side and on the proximal cross-cut end. (Fig. 26-10). A 0.25-inch, curved osteotome is used to carefully lift the bone plug on each side in a similar fashion to the tibial bone plug. The graft is then clamped at each end and carefully dissected free from its remaining soft tissue attachments (Fig. 26-11). The graft is then carefully taken to a separate table for preparation. The tourniquet may be let down at this point after harvesting, unless intraarticular bleeding impedes optimal arthroscopic visualization.

Graft Preparation

The excess soft tissue and fat pad are carefully removed from the graft with Metzenbaum scissors. The length of the tendinous portion of the graft is measured and recorded (in this case, 45 mm long), because this determines the angle at which the Adapteur drill guide C-ring is set and minimizes graft-tunnel mismatch. The length of each bone plug is also measured, verified, and recorded. We usually use the patella bone plug (10 × 20 mm) in the femoral tunnel and the tibial bone plug (10 × 25 mm) in the tibial tunnel. The bone plugs are then shaped and contoured with a bone cutter, a small rongeur, and a 10 × 10 mm crimper. The bone fragments that are removed are saved for later bone grafting of the patella. **The bone plugs should be trimmed until the plug can be fit easily into the 10-mm sizing block (Arthrex) but not into the 9-mm sizing block (Fig. 26-12).** If this step is not done adequately, the graft will not fit into the tunnels created. The cancellous side of the tendon is labeled with an indelible marker at the tendo-osseous junction at the patella bone plug end (i.e., the bone plug to be inserted into the femoral tunnel). The graft is then placed on the graft

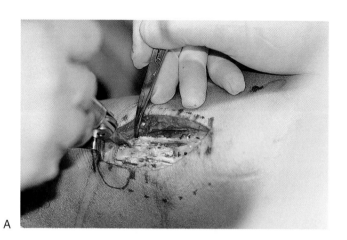

A

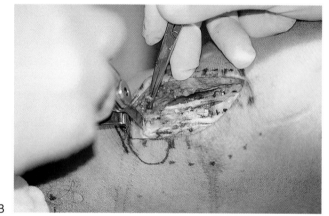

B

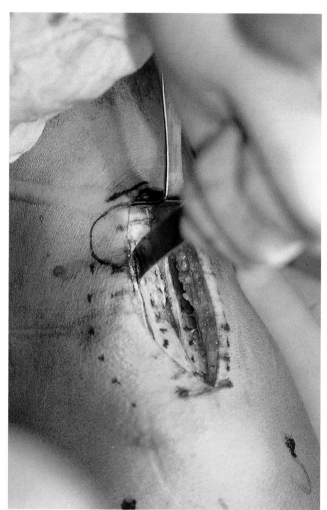

C

FIGURE 26-8. A to C: An oscillating saw is used to cut a tibial bone plug.

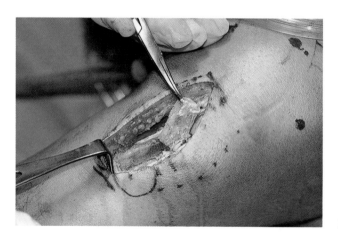

FIGURE 26-9. Procurement of the tibial bone plug.

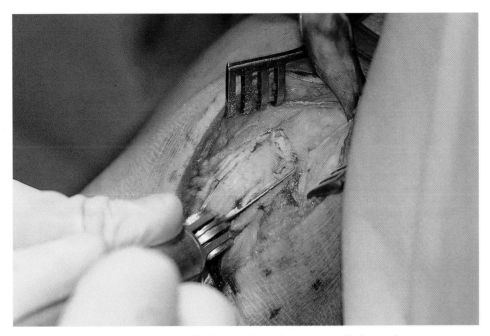

FIGURE 26-10. An oscillating saw is used to cut a patella bone plug.

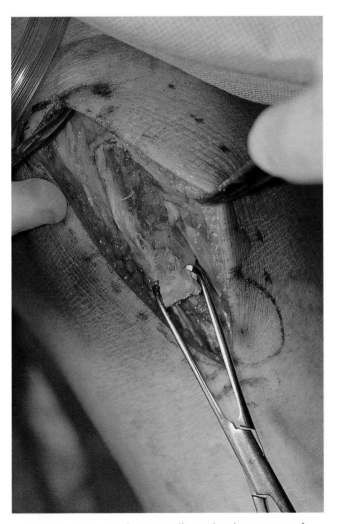

FIGURE 26-11. Free bone–patella tendon–bone autograft.

workstation (Arthrex) (Fig. 26-13). Two holes spaced 5 mm apart are drilled with a 1.5-mm drill bit in the patella bone plug in an anterior-to-posterior, cancellous-to-cortical direction. Two holes spaced 5 mm apart are also drilled with a 1.5-mm drill bit in the tibial bone plug perpendicular to each other: one in a side-side direction proximally and one in an anterior-to-posterior, cancellous-to-cortical direction distally. The no. 5 Ethibond (Ethicon, Inc., Somerville, NJ) sutures are then passed with a free, straight needle into each of the holes drilled. The sutures are clamped at each end and then set aside in a moist lap pad (Fig. 26-14).

ARTHROSCOPIC PROCEDURE

An inferolateral portal is established through the operative incision just adjacent to the patella tendon. The arthroscope is inserted through this portal, and inflow is set at a level above the systolic blood pressure. A superomedial portal is made for outflow, which is placed to gravity. Diagnostic arthroscopy is then performed, evaluating the suprapatellar pouch, patellofemoral joint, medial compartment, intercondylar notch, and lateral compartment. ◻◄ Any chondral injuries or chondromalacia should be documented (Fig. 26-15). An inferomedial portal is established through the operative incision as a working portal. Both menisci should be carefully examined and probed for any tears. Unstable meniscal tears should be repaired or resected, depending on the type and location of the tear.

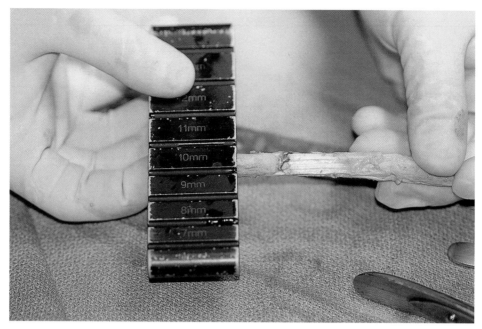

FIGURE 26-12. Bone plug sizing using a sizing block.

Notch Preparation

The remnants of the native ACL are carefully removed with a motorized, 5.5-mm, full-radius, aggressive shaver. ◙ Ligamentum mucosum and some patellar fat pad, both of which may impede visualization, usually require débridement. Soft tissues remaining on the notch laterally and posteriorly are also débrided until the over-the-top position (i.e., the junction of the roof of the intercondylar notch and the back wall of posterior cortex of the lateral femoral condyle) can be recognized. ◙ ArthroWands, such as the LoPro 90° or TurboVac 90 (ArthroCare, Sunnyvale, CA), can be used for hemostasis and further débridement of soft tissues. ◙ Throughout the procedure, special care is taken not to damage the native PCL.

A 5.5-mm, round burr is used to complete the notchplasty after an adequate soft tissue débridement has been done. The minimum amount of bone is removed from the medial aspect of the lateral femoral condyle from an anterior-to-posterior direction and from an apex-to-inferior direction to visualize the over-the-top position and to prevent impingement of the graft. ◙ **Special attention should be given not to misinterpret a vertical ridge (i.e., resident's ridge), usually located two thirds of the way posteriorly, as the over-the-top position; this ridge should be removed smoothly until the true back wall is clearly identified. An arthroscopic probe is used to verify that this position has been clearly reached. This part of the procedure is crucial, because it determines the correct isometric position of the femoral tunnel.**

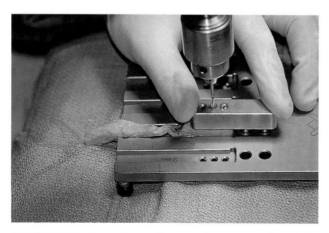

FIGURE 26-13. Bone plug graft preparation on a graft workstation.

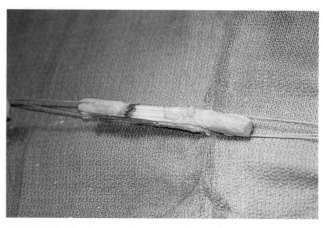

FIGURE 26-14. Prepared bone–patella tendon–bone autograft.

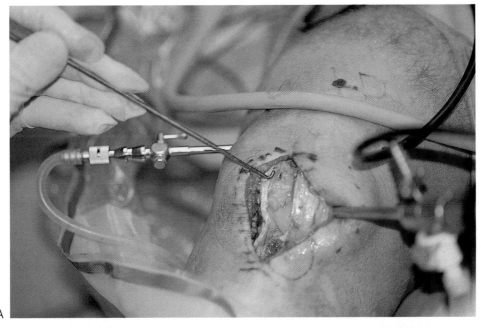

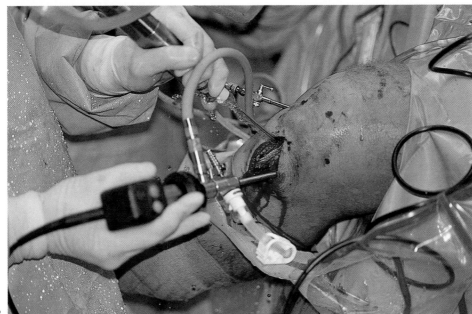

FIGURE 26-15. A and B: Arthroscopy of knee after the graft is harvested.

At this point, the tentative position of the femoral tunnel can be manually marked with an ArthroCare wand. The mark should be placed 7 mm anterior to the back wall (to leave a 2-mm wall of posterior cortex when reaming a 10-mm [5-mm-radius] tunnel) — and at the 1-o'clock position in the left knee and the 11-o'clock position in the right knee. ■◖ Because it is the left knee in the illustrated case, the 1-o'clock position is used (Fig. 26-16). The proper position of the femoral tunnel is later confirmed with the 7-mm-offset transtibial femoral guide after the tibial tunnel has been made.

Tibial Tunnel

The adapter drill guide C-ring with the appropriate targeting hook (Arthrex) is used to create the tibial tunnel. The N ± 7 rule is employed to determine the setting on the guide, whereby 7 degrees is added to the length of the tendinous

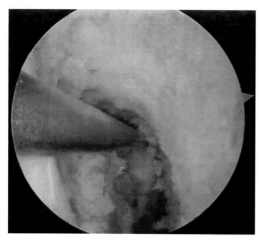

FIGURE 26-16. Over-the-top position at 1 o'clock in the left knee.

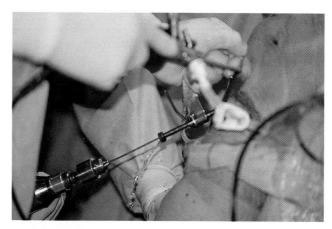

FIGURE 26-18. Tibial tunnel guide wire drilling with the use of a tibial drill guide.

portion of the graft. In our case, 7 is added to 45 for a total of 52; therefore, the guide is set at 52. Using this method minimizes the possibility of graft-tunnel mismatch.

The tip of the guide is then placed through the anteromedial portal. For proper placement of the guide pin, several parameters are used: the posterior one half of the ACL stump footprint, the posterior edge of the anterior horn of the lateral meniscus, the anterolateral aspect of the medial tibial eminence, and 7 mm anterior to the PCL (Fig. 26-17). After the proper position for the guide pin has been established, the cannulated, calibrated guide pin sleeve is advanced through the C-ring up to the anteromedial aspect of the tibia by retracting the incision inferiorly. The sleeve should be placed on the tibial cortex halfway between the tibial tubercle and the posteromedial border of the tibia. With the arm of the target marking hook kept parallel to the slope of the tibial plateau, the sleeve is advanced and secured against the tibia (usually positioning it approximately 1 cm above the pes anserinus and 1.5 cm medial to the tibial tubercle). **The guide pin sleeve should not be overtightened,**

nor should excessive torque be placed on the C-ring. The 2.4-mm drill-tip guide pin is placed in the sleeve and drilled through the tibia under direct arthroscopic visualization until the tip of the pin is seen just penetrating intraarticularly (Fig. 26-18). The sleeve is released, and the C-ring is removed.

After the proper placement of the guide pin is verified, a curved curette is placed intraarticularly over the guide pin to prevent it from further advancement during drilling, and a 10-mm, cannulated-headed reamer is used to precisely drill the tibial tunnel over the guide pin (Fig. 26-19). The reamer and guide wire are removed. With a notchplasty-tunnel rasp (Arthrex) placed through the tibial tunnel, the posterior edge of intraarticular end of the tunnel is smoothed down. With an aggressive shaver, the excess soft tissue, cartilage, and bone are removed from the intraarticular end of the tunnel. **The excess soft tissue, which can impede graft passage, is also removed from the tunnel entrance with sharp dissection.** A tibial tunnel cannula (Arthrex) is placed in the tibial tunnel to prevent fluid extravasation.

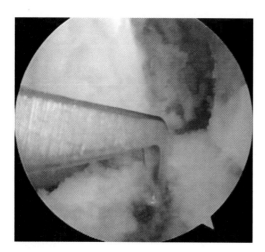

FIGURE 26-17. Intraarticular placement of the tibial guide.

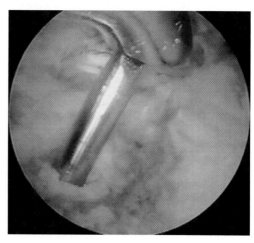

FIGURE 26-19. Tibial tunnel reaming over a guide pin.

Femoral Tunnel

A 7-mm-offset transtibial femoral guide (Arthrex) is advanced through the tibial tunnel and placed over the posterior edge of the back wall at the 1-o'clock position (11 o'clock for the right knee). With the knee flexed at 70 to 90 degrees, an extra-long guide pin with suture eye (Arthrex) is placed through the femoral offset guide (Fig. 26-20). If the tip of the guide pin is not close to the mark previously made to approximate the femoral tunnel, the proper position of the femoral tunnel should be reassessed. After the proper position of the femoral tunnel is confirmed, the guide pin is drilled into the femur through the cortex and out the anterolateral thigh. A 10-mm, cannulated-headed reamer is carefully advanced through the tibial tunnel and past the PCL over the guide wire. **The femoral tunnel is then carefully drilled under arthroscopic visualization in line with the guide wire and with the knee flexed at the same angle the guide wire was inserted.** The integrity of the posterior wall is periodically checked during the initial drilling. The femoral tunnel is drilled for a length of 25 mm (5 mm longer than the 20 mm patella bone plug that is to be used in the femoral tunnel) by using the calibrated laser lines on the reamer. The reamer is then carefully removed past the PCL and out through the tibial tunnel. The integrity of the posterior wall is again checked by arthroscopic visualization, and 2 mm of posterior cortex should be remaining.

Graft Passage

Manual control of the graft must be maintained at all times. All the free ends of the sutures from the patella bone plug are fed through the suture eye of the guide pin. A vise-grip or pin puller is placed on the proximal end of the guide pin, and the guide pin is carefully malleted out. The cancellous portion of the graft should be oriented anteriorly and should be passed through the tunnels in this orientation. **The sutures retrieved proximally at the anterolateral thigh are clamped, and the**

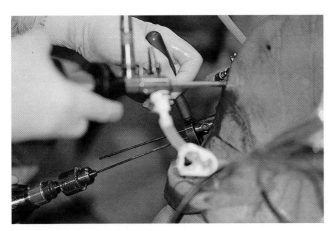

FIGURE 26-20. Femoral tunnel guide wire drilling with the use of a femoral offset guide.

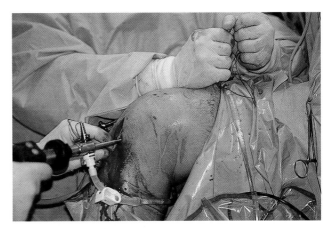

FIGURE 26-21. Passage of the graft using sutures.

graft is passed with these sutures (Fig. 26-21). Gentle traction is applied to the sutures from the tibial bone plug to keep a minimal amount of tension needed for graft passage. After the patella bone plug reaches the femoral tunnel entrance, a probe may be needed to tease the graft through the femoral tunnel. The previous mark made with an indelible marker on the cancellous side on the tendo-osseus junction is helpful in keeping the correct orientation while the graft is intraarticular. **The graft should pass with relative ease; otherwise, the bone plugs may not have been sized correctly or soft tissue at the tunnel site (especially at the entrance of the tibial tunnel) may be impeding smooth passage.**

Graft Fixation

A tunnel notcher (Arthrex) is placed in the anteromedial portal, and a keyhole notch is placed at the entrance of the femoral tunnel. With the knee hyperflexed at 100 to 110 degrees (this amount flexion limits screw divergence), a 2-mm Nitinol guide pin (Arthrex) is placed through a separate, more inferior, anteromedial portal into the femoral tunnel through the notch between the anterior aspect of the femoral tunnel and cancellous portion of the bone plug until the guide pin is seeded about 20 mm (Fig. 26-22). With the knee in the same position and the bone plug flush with the femoral tunnel entrance, a 7 × 20 mm metal interference screw (Arthrex) is screwed over the guide pin with a 3.5-mm, hex-head, cannulated screwdriver (Arthrex) through the soft tissues into the femoral tunnel (Fig. 26-23). As the screw is advanced in the femoral tunnel, increasing resistance should be felt, and grinding should be heard as interference fixation is achieved. The head of the screw should be advanced until the head of the screw is flush with the femoral tunnel entrance. The screwdriver and guide pin are removed.

With the graft fixed at the femoral end, graft impingement against the roof of the intercondylar notch is evaluated. Isometry of the graft can also be checked at this time as well. With constant tension on the tibial bone plug, the graft is cycled by flexing and extending the knee 15 to 20 times.

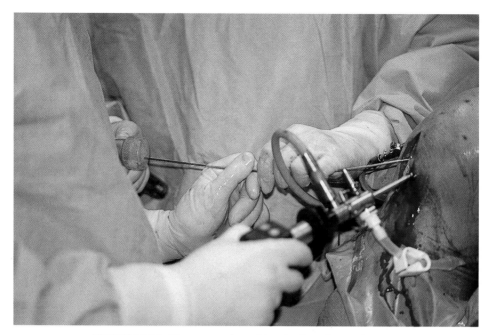

FIGURE 26-22. Placement of a guide wire for a femoral screw.

The arthroscope is removed, and attention is directed toward the fixation in the tibial tunnel. **With direct visualization of the entrance of the tibial tunnel, the cancellous side of the tibial bone plug should be oriented anteriorly** (Fig. 26-24). A tunnel notcher (Arthrex) is used to place a keyhole notch in the anterior aspect of the entrance of the tibial tunnel. With the knee as close to full extension as possible, a 2-mm Nitinol guide pin (Arthrex) is placed in the notch between the anterior aspect of the tibial tunnel and cancellous portion of the bone plug until the guide pin is seeded about 20 mm. With constant tension on the sutures from the tibial bone plug, a 9 × 25 mm metal interference screw (Arthrex) is screwed over the guide pin with the cannulated screwdriver. As the screw is advanced through the tibial tunnel, increasing resistance should be felt, and grinding should be heard as interference fixation is

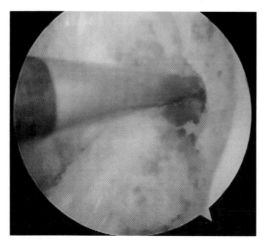

FIGURE 26-23. Placement of a screw in the femoral tunnel.

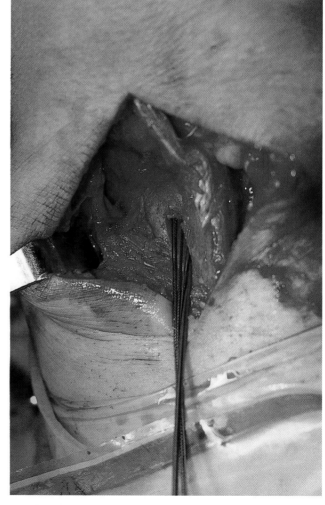

FIGURE 26-24. A bone–patella tendon–bone graft in the tibial tunnel.

achieved. The head of the screw should be advanced until the head of the screw is flush with the tibial tunnel entrance. The screwdriver and guide pin are removed. If less than 5 to 10 mm of tibial bone plug is protruding out the tibial tunnel, the excess bone can be carefully burred to the level of the tibial tunnel. If more than 10 mm of bone is protruding, alternative means of fixation should be considered.

After fixation is completed, a Lachman's test and pivot shift are repeated to assess stability of the reconstruction. If satisfactory, the sutures from each end of the bone plugs are removed. Otherwise, the sutures may be used for additional fixation.

Closure

The excess bone removed from the preparation of the graft is used to bone graft the patella. If additional bone graft is needed, this can be obtained from the tibial bone plug donor site. The paratenon is closed over the patella with 0 Vicryl sutures. The patella tendon is not reapproximated, but the overlying paratenon is closed with 0 Vicryl sutures in a running fashion. The subcutaneous tissue is closed with undyed 2-0 Vicryl sutures in an interrupted fashion. The skin is closed with a 3-0 Monocryl suture in a running subcuticular fashion. The 0.5-inch Steri-strips are placed transversely over the incision for reinforcement. An injection of a mixture of 10 mL of 0.25% Marcaine with epinephrine and 5 mg of Duramorph is injected intraarticularly. The incision is covered with sterile dressings, Webril, and an Ace bandage. A drain in not routinely used. The extremity is placed in a hinged brace locked in full extension.

POSTOPERATIVE PROTOCOL

This procedure is done on an outpatient basis. The patient is allowed to bear weight as tolerated with the brace in full extension and with crutches. Ice or a cold therapy unit is used continuously for 3 to 5 days. The knee brace is worn for approximately 4 to 6 weeks during ambulation and sleep, and crutches are used until adequate control of quadriceps is regained, which is usually for 2 weeks. The patient is allowed to shower in 7 to 10 days after surgery. The patient is initially seen 5 to 7 days after surgery for a wound check and for immediate initiation of an accelerated rehabilitation program (Table 26-1) and then at 2 weeks, 6, weeks, 12 weeks, and 24 weeks.

TABLE 26-1. HOSPITAL FOR JOINT DISEASES GUIDELINES FOR REHABILITATION AFTER ANTERIOR CRUCIATE LIGAMENT RECONSTRUCTION WITH A PATELLA TENDON GRAFT

These are general guidelines for rehabilitation after anterior cruciate ligament reconstruction. Progression is based on criteria and is individualized for each patient. The therapist must continually evaluate for the following complications: flexion contracture, patella baja, arthrofibrosis, patella tendonitis, and increased joint laxity.

Phase I: 1 to 3 Weeks

Goals: full range of motion (ROM), emphasizing extension; normal patella mobility; normal gait pattern; control of edema and pain
Postoperative day 1: weight bearing as tolerated, ambulation in a brace at 0 degrees of extension with crutches; brace locked at 0 degrees at night; continuous passive motion at 0 to 90 degrees; towel roll under heel; Cryocuff
Postoperative day 2: continue continuous passive motion, towel roll, and Cryocuff; patella mobility exercises; prone hangs; quadriceps sets and straight leg raising and hip abduction in a brace at 0 degrees; active assisted knee flexion and passive extension with the opposite leg; gait training on stairs
Postoperative day 3 through 3 weeks: continue as above; hamstring stretching; electrical stimulation for quadriceps re-education; progressive resistance exercises for hip (e.g., Cybex Multi Hip); progressive resistance exercises for hamstrings (e.g., prone knee flexion, knee flexion with Thera-Band resistance while sitting); mini wall squats; calf raises; bilateral leg press at 90 to 40 degrees; short-crank bicycle (avoid hyperextension); Aquaciser (when incision is well healed)

Phase II: 3 to 9 Weeks

Entry criteria: full ROM and patella mobility; minimal edema; nonantalgic gait; good quadriceps set without extensor lag
Early: discontinue crutches (no limp); discontinue postoperative brace (good quadriceps control); StairMaster exercise (small steps); proprioception activities (e.g., biomechanical ankle platform system, single-limb-stance balance activities); Tigney exercises (e.g., cable column, Thera-Band resistance); unilateral leg press at 90 to 30 degrees

(continued)

TABLE 26–1. HOSPITAL FOR JOINT DISEASES GUIDELINES FOR REHABILITATION AFTER ANTERIOR CRUCIATE LIGAMENT RECONSTRUCTION WITH A PATELLA TENDON GRAFT (continued)

Intermediate: open chain quadriceps exercise at 90 to 30 degrees; cable column retrograde and forward walking; Smith press squats; retrograde and forward treadmill; forward and lateral step-up and step-down exercises
Late: isokinetic knee flexion and extension at 90 to 30 degrees; increase pace on treadmill

Phase III (Functional Phase): 9 to 15 Weeks

Entry criteria: pain free; no effusion; good eccentric and concentric quadriceps and hamstring control
Goal: master functional tasks of desired physical activity
Early: ProFitter balance board; simulated running with cable column; Euroglide; Aquaciser running program; bilateral jumps on a mini-trampoline
Intermediate: retrograde treadmill running; KT-1000 arthrometer testing; isokinetic testing
Late: forward treadmill running (usually at 3.5 to 4 months); bilateral jumping (e.g., box jumps, long and vertical jumps)

Phase IV (Return to Sports): 16 to 24 Weeks

Entry criteria: KT-1000 result of less than 3 mm; isokinetic and test values less than 20%; pain free and apprehension free; functional testing less than 10% of opposite leg
Early: advance running program; advance agility and lateral movements; full arc extension exercises; unilateral hopping and jumping
Intermediate: continue as above; shuttle runs; pivoting and cutting activities
Late: return to full sports activity (usually 6 months or more); use functional brace if KT-1000 result is more than 5 mm side to side or if there is pain with sports activity

SUGGESTED READINGS

Bach BR, Levy ME, Bojchuk J, et al. Single-incision endoscopic anterior cruciate ligament reconstruction using patella tendon autograft: minimum two-year follow-up evaluation. *Am J Sports Med* 1998;26:30–40.

Jackson DW, Gasser SI. Tibial tunnel placement in ACL reconstruction. *Arthroscopy* 1994;10:124–131.

Jackson DW, Jennings LD. Arthroscopically assisted reconstruction of the anterior cruciate ligament using a patella tendon–bone autograft. *Clin Sports Med* 1988;7:785–800.

Johnson DL, Fu FH. Anterior cruciate ligament reconstruction: why do failures occur? *Instr Course Lect* 1995;44:391–404.

Kurosaka M, Yoshiya A, Andrish JT. A biomechanical comparison of different surgical techniques of graft fixation in anterior cruciate ligament reconstruction. *Am J Sports Med* 1987;5:225–229.

Miller MD, Hinkin DT. The "N + 7" rule for tibial tunnel placement in endoscopic anterior cruciate ligament reconstruction. *Arthroscopy* 1996;12:124–126.

Noyes FR, Butler DL, Grood ES, et al. Biomechanical analysis of human ligament grafts used in knee ligament repairs and reconstructions. *J Bone Joint Surg Am* 1984;66:344–352.

Paulos LE, Cherf J, Rosenberg TD, et al. Anterior cruciate ligament reconstruction with autografts. *Clin Sports Med* 1991;10:469–485.

Shelbourne KD, Nitz P. Accelerated rehabilitation after anterior cruciate ligament reconstruction. *Am J Sports Med* 1992;18:292–299.

CHAPTER 27

HIGH TIBIAL OSTEOTOMY

PATRICK A. MEERE

The treatment of genu varum and gonarthrosis has been revolutionized by the advent of successful arthroplasty techniques. Because of this success, the role of the HTO has essentially been downgraded to a temporizing procedure. The estimated duration of pain relief and acceptable functional level after a HTO is on the order of 8 to 10 years. Most series report a greater than 50% conversion to knee arthroplasty or loss of symptomatic relief beyond 10 years. Relatively speaking, HTO is viewed as an optional delay before the more "definitive" total knee arthroplasty. The major advantage of the HTO is that, once healed, it allows for minimal restriction of activities postoperatively. As with any surgery, however, the postoperative outcome is strongly related to the preoperative severity of disease and level of function. Properly selected, physiologically younger patients should be allowed to return to vigorous activities, which would otherwise be prohibited after knee replacement arthroplasty.

The goal of the procedure is to restore the mechanical axis lateral to the midline of the knee joint to significantly reduce excessive joint forces across the worn medial tibiofemoral joint space and consequently retard the mechanical degenerative process. Long-term clinical studies have shown that age, weight, and degree of correction play a determinant role in the duration of pain relief and functional autonomy.

ANATOMY

A detailed knowledge of the local anatomy is critical in any periarticular surgery. In the case of a HTO, the surgeon must be mindful of the arterial branching pattern in the posterior high tibial area. The main arterial popliteal trunk divides at approximately the level of the base of the fibular head into the anterior and posterior arteries. The distal portion of the popliteal artery lies superficial to the popliteus and deep to the gastrosoleus complex (Fig. 27-1A). **Because of their immediate proximity to the proximal tibia, the posterior arteries are at risk of injury from blunt compression or sharp injury during surgical exposure.** With respect to the local nerve anatomy, the structure at greatest risk is the common peroneal nerve as it wraps posteroanteriorly, slightly lateral to the operated zone (Fig. 37-1B).

The osseous anatomy of the proximal tibia is asymmetric and must be well conceptualized in planning the closed wedge reduction and osteoclysis of the medial tibial hinge. Failure to appreciate the contours of the inverted metaphyseal flare may lead to incongruous osteotomy surfaces or dangerously deep penetration with sharp instruments (Fig. 27-1B). **Iatrogenic fracture of the medial cortical periosteal hinge causes irreversible loss of intrinsic stability.** On the anterior aspect of the tibial metaphysis lies the tibial tubercle with its sensitive patellar ligamentous insertion. Care must be taken to avoid injury to this structure because its disruption leads to disastrous mechanical consequences.

In most cases, the closed reduction causes sufficient axial compression so as to warrant a shortening fibular osteotomy or disruption of the proximal tibiofibular joint. Both of these procedures have the potential for a local peroneal direct or indirect lesion.

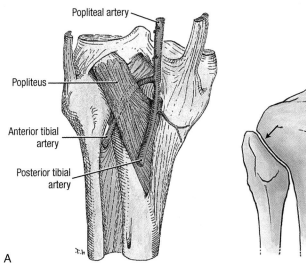

Popliteal artery

Popliteus

Anterior tibial artery

Posterior tibial artery

A

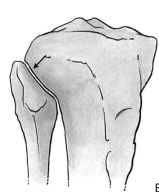

B

FIGURE 27-1. A: Division of the popliteal artery. **B:** Anterolateral view of the proximal tibiofibular joint *(arrow)*.

CLASSIFICATION

From a historical perspective, the procedure was popularized and defined in its modern form by M.B. Coventry. The standard procedure consists of a laterally based, closing wedge osteotomy proximal to the tibial tubercle. The method has since undergone variations based on the instrumentation and fixation methods. It remains, nonetheless, an established standard. In severe corrections, it may yield a slight loss of length and potential joint obliquity. An alternate technique, the semicircular (dome) osteotomy, was subsequently developed and gained popularity abroad. Although it offers theoretical advantages, it is technically more difficult, because it requires a hemispherical supratubercular osteotomy.

With the development of superior fixation devices and advances in grafting methods, a pure opening wedge technique and a hybrid (closing and opening) technique have gained popularity in selected centers. The intended advantage of this method is the delivery of bone augmentation and restitution of joint alignment. Its champions also point to this being less invasive surgery on the safer, medial aspect of the tibial metaphysis. The downside lies in the need for bone augmentation, particularly autogenous harvesting with second-site morbidity or allograft with potentially delayed osseointegration. The use of either material source still requires rigid fixation and weight-bearing protection postoperatively. My preferred method is the classic closed wedge osteotomy. The rationale for this stems from its established record and my personal experience.

INDICATIONS

The indications for HTO can be summarized as follows:

- Isolated monocompartmental medial tibiofemoral osteoarthritis (mechanical, degenerative, noninflammatory arthritis)
- Physiologic age older than 65 years
- Absence of morbid obesity
- Minimum preoperative range of motion of 90 degrees of flexion
- Extension deficit of less than 15 degrees
- Passively correctable varus deformity of less than 15 degrees
- Lateral tibial subluxation less than 10 mm
- Absence of ligamentous instability

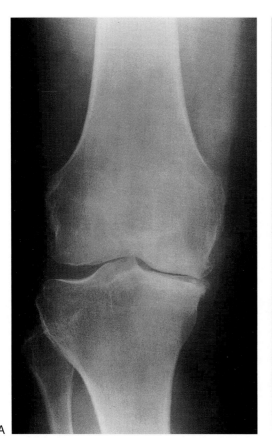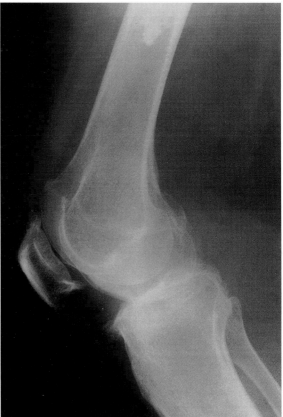

A   B

FIGURE 27-2. Preoperative weight-bearing radiographs demonstrate varus osteoarthritis: anteroposterior view **(A)** and lateral view **(B)**.

PREOPERATIVE PLANNING

The need for proper preoperative planning cannot be overstated in the case of upper tibial osteotomy. The exact angular correction must be determined with the use of a long leg alignment film series. The potential distortion attributable to fixed contractures must be eliminated through the use of weight-bearing views (Fig. 27-2). This minimizes the risk of overcorrection if the joint space asymmetry is amplified by spurious opening of the lateral space from a medial joint contracture in an unloaded situation. The goal of the procedure is to restore the valgus alignment of the leg. Numerous studies have demonstrated that one of the most reliable prognostic factors is a correction to a valgus alignment of at least 8 degrees. This implies a transfer of the mechanical axis to a point within the innermost portion of the lateral third of the joint line on the coronal anteroposterior projection.

Various methodologies have been devised to template the osteotomy. The point of reference remains the medial cortical hinge. The proximal level is set at a level allowing for a safe thickness of the proximal fragment to minimize the risk of iatrogenic fracture or intraarticular penetration of the fixation hardware. Based on this proximal reference, a triangular wedge is calculated to yield a resultant tibiofemoral axis of at least 8 degrees. The lateral height of the right-angle inverted triangle should not exceed 15 mm. Care must also be given to properly measure the posterior slope of the tibial joint line. Loss of flexion can result from inadvertent reduction of the anatomic slope. After successful radiographic templating is completed, many surgeons complete the preoperative planning by fashioning a metallic triangular template of the appropriate dimension for intraoperative assistance.

EQUIPMENT

A radiolucent table and fluoroscopic imaging are critical for the delineation and execution of the osteotomy. Rigid, medium-gage Kirschner wires (K-wires) are used as guide wires. Most commercially available HTO instrumentation sets include a cannulated protractor. Alternatively, a precut, customized metallic wedge template can be used for sizing the lateral height of the resected fragment. A cannulated large fragment set and a specially contoured tibial metaphyseal compression plate or blade plate are necessary for the instrumentation and fixation of the closed osteotomy. This method of fixation is more reliable than the traditional staples. The oscillating saw should be fitted with a rigid, long, and narrow blade. This minimizes the risk of inadvertent excursion into surrounding soft tissues. The osteotomy margins may require final adjustments and debridement of the medial hinge before the final closure and fixation. This is best achieved with sharp osteotomes and fine curettes.

Intraoperative radiographs are preferable before closure. Immobilization is usually provisional in the immediate postoperative period and is best achieved through a well-molded posterior long leg splint or a bivalved long leg cast made of plaster of Paris.

PATIENT POSITIONING AND PREPARATION

The patient is placed supine onto the operating table. After an adequate anesthesia level has been achieved, a tourniquet is applied to the affected proximal thigh. Intravenous antibiotics are then administered. A sandbag may be placed in order to assist in positioning during the procedure. A simple urethral catheterization may then be performed using standard protocol. The affected lower extremity is then prepared and draped in a standard sterile fashion. The draping should allow for a free extremity, i.e., full circumferential access distal to the mid-thigh area. Based on the surgeon's preference, the leg may then be exsanguinated and the tourniquet pressure applied. If a tourniquet is used, inflation should be performed with the knee in flexion, so as to minimize quadriceps tethering.

SURGICAL INCISION AND LANDMARKS

Two approaches are possible. These differ only in their cutaneous and subcutaneous routes and extent. The classic incision is a curved anterolateral incision. It originates at a point slightly distal to Gerdy's tubercle and tibial ridge to proceed first medially then veers inferiorly in a gentle curve to a point lateral and distal to the tibial tubercle. Due to the probable need for future conversion to a total knee arthroplasty, an alternate incision route is now commonly used, namely, the anterior midline approach (Fig. 27-3). The rationale of this approach is to minimize the risk of skin necrosis associated with intersecting scars at acute angles. The incision must be of sufficient length to allow for a subcutaneous deep exposure of the lateral tibial metaphysis up to Gerdy's tubercle. This then ensures proper visualization of the proximal insertion of the anterior lower leg extensor muscles.

APPROACH

After hemostasis of the subcutaneous layer, the proximal border of the extensor group is detached and reflected distally and laterally by subperiosteal elevation. Once completed, the full lateral anterior metaphyseal flare should be accessible for instrumentation. Hemostasis of the deep layer is then performed. The approach is subperiosteal, and no internervous planes are used. No major nerve or vessels are at risk in this relatively shallow anterolateral approach. The

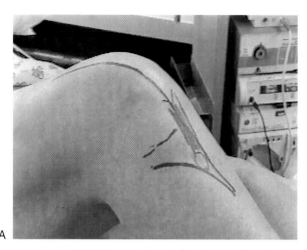

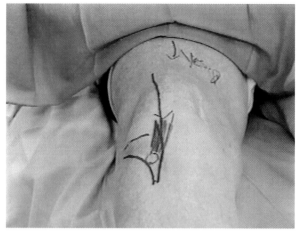

A   B

FIGURE 27-3. Surgical incision and landmarks: classic anterolateral incision **(A)** and anterior mid-line **(B)**.

surgical structures at risk are the major popliteal vessels and the peroneal nerve. The risk is incurred at the time of the osteotomy and closed reduction.

PROCEDURE

A K-wire is used to determine the exact position of the joint line in the coronal plane. This is done by laying a wire anterior to the surface of the knee and is confirmed by fluoroscopy (Fig. 27-4). The cutaneous landmarks are then marked with a surgical pen on the anterior tibial surface. A second K-wire is subsequently dragged distally in a parallel fashion so as to lie 5 to 10 mm below the margin of the tibial plateaus. Cutaneous landmarks are again drawn. This level represents the proximal fixation margin. Under fluoroscopic guidance, a K-wire is inserted at the selected level, aiming medially from the lateral side (Fig. 27-5). This wire serves as a guide wire for the instrumentation of the proxi-

mal fragment. The author's preferred method is a cannulated blade plate (Fig. 27-6). Instrumentation of the fixation blade slot is the next step. A third level is then determined by again dragging a wire distally by a minimum of 5 mm. This level represents the actual proximal osteotomy margin. **Insufficient thickness of the proximal tibial fragment may lead to intraarticular fracture at the time of instrumentation or potential cutting out of the proximal fixation hardware.** Under fluoroscopic guidance, one or two parallel K-wires are then inserted at the selected lower level, aiming medially from the lateral side (Fig. 27-7). If two wires are used, their points of insertion correspond to the anterior and posterior margins of the central third of the tibial metaphysis in the sagittal plane. It is of great importance to respect the slope of the tibial joint surface. Failure to do so may lead to unacceptable recurvatum or flexion deformity. After successful insertion of these wires, a cannulated protractor (Fig. 27-8) is used to determine the position and angle of the inferior border of the intended wedge. Alternatively, the lateral height of the anticipated wedge can be measured based on a preoperative template. **The maximal amount of resec-**

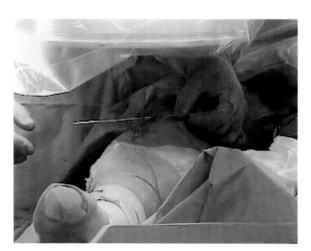

FIGURE 27-4. Fluoroscopic determination of proximal fixation level.

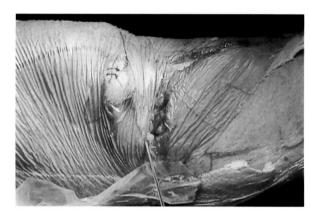

A

FIGURE 27-5. Position and insertion of proximal guide wire: clinical view **(A)**, anteroposterior fluoroscopy. *(continued)*

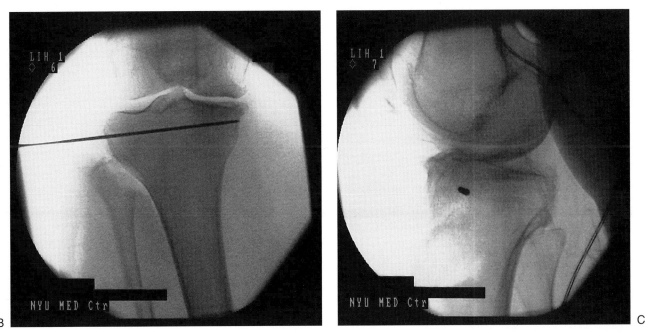

FIGURE 27-5. *Continued.* Anteroposterior fluoroscopy **(B)**, and lateral fluoroscopy **(C)**.

FIGURE 27-6. Creation of proximal blade slot: clinical view **(A)** and fluoroscopy view **(B)**.

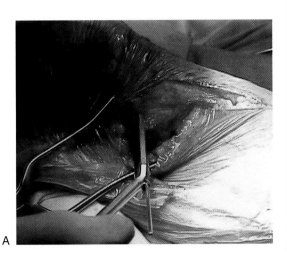

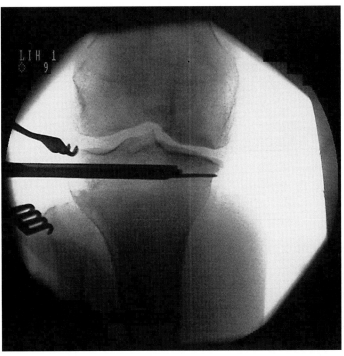

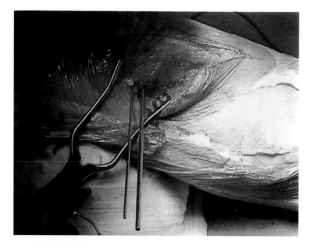

FIGURE 27-7. Insertion of proximal guide wires.

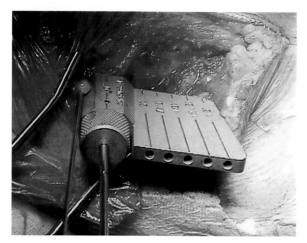

FIGURE 27-8. Close-up view of a cannulated protractor.

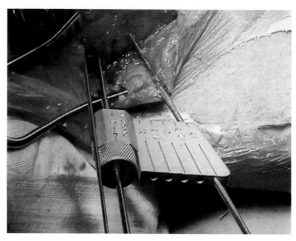

FIGURE 27-9. Insertion of a distal guide wire using a cannulated protractor.

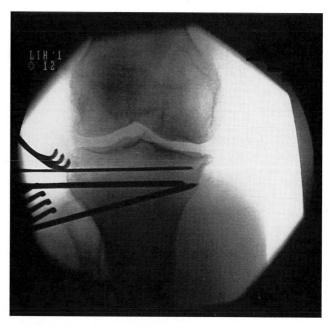

FIGURE 27-10. Fluoroscopic evaluation of proximal and distal guide wires.

tion should generally be less than 15 mm. This precaution minimizes the risk of lateral, peroneal nerve compression injury and overcorrection in valgus. After insertion of the inferior guide wire (Fig. 27-9), final fluoroscopic verification is made (Fig. 27-10). The wires should converge to a point immediately adjacent to the internal border of the medial cortex. **Transection of the cortical hinge has a potentially catastrophic effect on the stability of the closed osteotomy and should be avoided at all cost by careful positioning of the guide wires.** Before the osteotomy, release of the lateral column is necessary. Two methods are available: resection of a small segment of the fibula, or a dissociation of the proximal tibiofibular joint. The former method is the most widely used option.

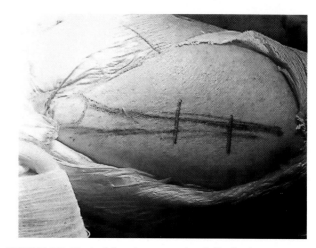

FIGURE 27-11. Incision for a proximal fibula-shortening osteotomy.

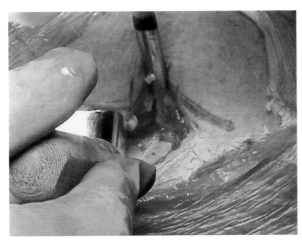

FIGURE 27-12. Exposure for a segmental shortening osteotomy of a proximal fibula.

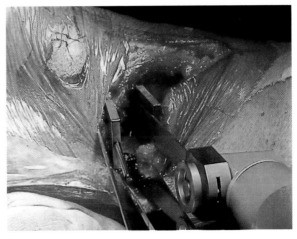

FIGURE 27-14. Distal osteotomy of a proximal tibia.

A separate incision is made along the lateral border of the proximal and mid-fibula (Fig. 27-11). The incision measures approximately 6 cm and is centered on a point corresponding to the junction of the proximal and central-third of the fibula. Any resection limited to the proximal third incurs an unacceptable risk of direct peroneal nerve injury. The subcutaneous dissection is carried along the intercompartmental septum down to the periosteum. Subperiosteal exposure of a 2.5-cm segment is then made. Using proper soft tissue protection this segment is osteotomized through parallel transverse osteotomies and then resected (Figs. 27-12 and 27-13). ◧ Some surgeons have described an alternative method consisting of a beveled oblique osteotomy without bone resection. This method carries a theoretical risk of local tissue excessive compression and injury.

After the lateral column shortening has been completed, the closing wedge osteotomy can resume. The proximal cut is made first. ◧ The position of the oscillating saw is confirmed by fluoroscopy in both planes. The saw-blade is guided by the inferior margin of the inserted K-wires. The osteotomy stops short of perforating the medial cortex.

After completion of the proximal osteotomy, the position is confirmed by fluoroscopy. The distal angulated osteotomy is then made in the same anteroposterior plane. The blade uses the superior portion of the inclined wire as a guide. As discussed above, it is of paramount importance to avoid transgression of the medial cortex. After completion of the second cut, the wedge fragment is extracted. An osteotome and fine curettes are routinely used to refine the deep portion of the osteotomy (Figs. 27-14 to 27-16). ◧ The wedge osteotomy is then closed under vigilant fluoroscopic visualization (Fig. 27-17) ◧ After closure of the wedge, the new lateral metaphyseal contour may require trimming and smoothening to facilitate insertion of the fixation hardware.

Historically, some authors have favored fixation by means of external cast immobilization. This technique offers the advantage of postoperative adjustment but the disadvantage associated with cast immobilization. External fixa-

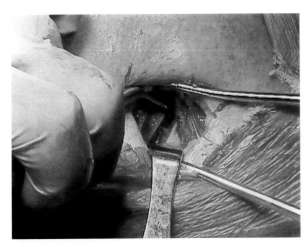

FIGURE 27-13. Excision of a segment during a shortening osteotomy of a proximal fibula.

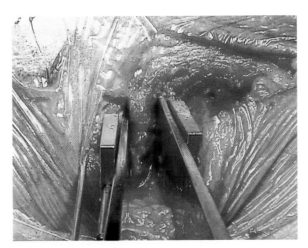

FIGURE 27-15. Completion of a proximal tibial osteotomy with an osteotome.

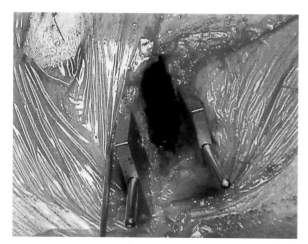

FIGURE 27-16. Completed wedge resection before closed reduction.

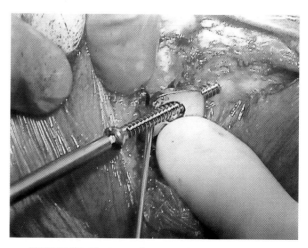

FIGURE 27-19. Screw fixation of a distal fragment.

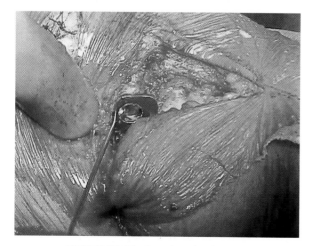

FIGURE 27-17. Completed reduction.

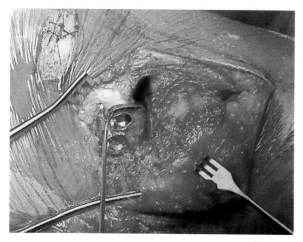

FIGURE 27-18. Completed osteotomy before closed reduction.

tion by special fixators such as the Ilizarov apparatus have also been described. Olive wires carry, however, a higher risk of nerve and soft tissue complications.

My preferred technique is the use of a compression blade plate applied to the lateral tibial metaphyseal border (Fig. 27-18). Distal fixation is achieved by standard bicortical fixation technique (Fig. 27-19). Final fluoroscopic verification is important to allow for any screw length adjustment (Fig. 27-20). After fixation has been accepted, closure is initiated over a deep drain. The deep layers are closed with resorbable multifilament braided interrupted sutures. The skin and subcutaneous tissues are closed according to the surgeon's preference. A final examination of the angular correction is then made before the application of a sterile dressing. Final radiographs are then obtained. A provisional cast splint is recommended to allow coronal plane stabilization. In the event of a medial cortical transsection and displacement with failure of the medial hinge, a full circumferential cast is fashioned with provisional bivalve division to allow for postoperative swelling.

POSTOPERATIVE PROTOCOL

The drain should be maintained until cessation of active bleeding. It typically can be removed on the first postoperative day. The use of a hinged long leg brace is preferred to ensure proper healing and avoid accidental displacement. The selected brace should include a double upright hinge system with customized valgus alignment. The range of motion need not be restricted if stable fixation was achieved.

Partial weight bearing may be authorized based on the stability of the completed fixation. In uncertain cases, the initial loading should be limited to weight of the leg with a gradual increase over a 6-week period. The use of an assistive device is strongly recommended in the initial postoperative period.

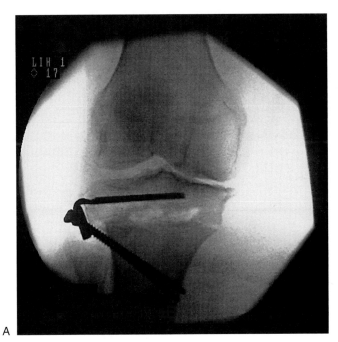
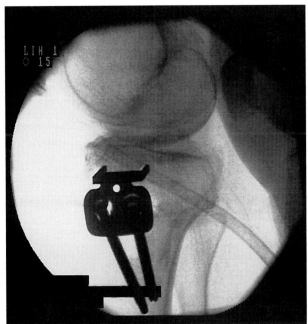

A

B

FIGURE 27-20. Postoperative anteroposterior **(A)** and lateral **(B)** fluoroscopy of a completed high tibial osteotomy.

Active range of motion may be initiated early with unloaded heel slide exercises. Loaded open chain knee exercises are to be avoided. Isometric strengthening program is favored until osseous consolidation has been confirmed.

COMPLICATIONS

With imprecise positioning of the superior wires or with an incomplete proximal osteotomy, an undesired fracture may be sustained at the time of the controlled osteoclysis of the medial cortex (closing of the wedge). Ideally, the medial cortex should retain an intact periosteal hinge to avoid destabilization. If the hinge is disrupted but undisplaced, protective bracing may be sufficient. However, in cases of associated translation and unacceptable shifting of the proximal fragment further internal fixation is recommended.

Another potential fracture results from intraarticular transgression of the lowest plateau. This complication definitely requires an open arthrotomy with restoration of the articular surface and subchondral internal fixation.

In cases of excessive shortening or inadequate lateral columnar (fibular) release, a nerve palsy may ensue. This lesion, if unrecognized immediately postoperatively, may lead to a complete loss of peroneal innervation. If recognized early, surgical intervention may be indicated to allow for nerve exploration and possible decompression neurolysis. Any residual deficit is treated supportively with an ankle foot orthosis (AFO) and follow-up electromyographic testing at 6 weeks.

In addition to the specific complications discussed above, the postoperative period naturally also entails continued vigilance and treatment of standard complications. These include bleeding, superficial nerve lesions, infection, thromboembolic events, among others.

FOLLOW-UP

The patient should be evaluated on a daily basis for the first three to five days to control for any potential complication. If discharge took place within days, a wound check is recommended at the 7 to 10 day mark. Routine verbal contact with the physiotherapist or rehabilitation specialist is favored until the next office visit. This typically takes place 4 to 6 weeks after surgery. A radiograph is done at that time to ensure early consolidation and absence of displacement or collapse of the osteotomy. Outpatient therapy is subsequently prescribed with gradual weight bearing and resistance for the next 6 weeks. At this 3-month visit, the patient should have regained autonomous, unassisted ambulation. Further follow-up visits are then scheduled on a 3-month interval basis until 1 year postoperatively and on a yearly basis thereafter.

SUGGESTED READINGS

Amendola A, Rorabeck CH, Bourne RB, et al. Total knee arthroplasty following high tibial osteotomy for osteoarthritis. *J Arthroplasty* 1989;4[Suppl]:S11–S7.

Bauer GC, Insall J, Koshino T. Tibial osteotomy in gonarthrosis (osteoarthritis of the knee). *J Bone Joint Surg Am* 1969;51:1545–1563.

Berman AT, Bosacco SJ, Kirshner S, et al. Factors influencing long-term results in high tibial osteotomy. *Clin Orthop* 1991;272:192–198.

Billings A, Scott DF, Camargo MP, et al. High tibial osteotomy with a calibrated osteotomy guide, rigid internal fixation, and early motion: long-term follow-up. *J Bone Joint Surg Am* 2000;82:70–79.

Coventry MB. Osteotomy of the upper portion of the tibia for degenerative arthritis of the knee: a preliminary report, 1965. *Clin Orthop* 1989;248:4–8.

Coventry MB, Ilstrup DM, Wallrichs SL. Proximal tibial osteotomy: a critical long-term study of eighty-seven cases. *J Bone Joint Surg Am* 1993;75:196–201.

Haddad FS, Bentley G. Total knee arthroplasty after high tibial osteotomy: a medium-term review. *J Arthroplasty* 2000;15:597–603.

Hofmann AA, Wyatt RW, Beck SW. High tibial osteotomy: use of an osteotomy jig, rigid fixation, and early motion versus conventional surgical technique and cast immobilization. *Clin Orthop* 1991;271:212–217.

Hutchison CR, Cho B, Wong N, et al. Proximal valgus tibial osteotomy for osteoarthritis of the knee. *Instr Course Lect* 1999;48:131–134.

Insall JN. High tibial osteotomy in the treatment of osteoarthritis of the knee. *Surg Annu* 1975;7:347–359.

Insall JN, Joseph DM, Msika C. High tibial osteotomy for varus gonarthrosis: a long-term follow-up study. *J Bone Joint Surg Am* 1984;66:1040–1048.

Mont MA, Alexander N, Krackow KA, et al. Total knee arthroplasty after failed high tibial osteotomy. *Orthop Clin North Am* 1994;25:515–525.

Naudie D, Bourne RB, Rorabeck CH, et al. The Install Award. Survivorship of the high tibial valgus osteotomy: a 10- to -22-year followup study. *Clin Orthop* 1999;367:18–27.

CHAPTER 28

TOTAL KNEE ARTHROPLASTY

PAUL E. DI CESARE

More than 200,000 total knee arthroplasties are performed annually in the United States for patients with disabling knee pain or impairment of knee function and in whom conservative treatment was not successful. A variety of implant designs are available for total knee arthroplasty. Classification considers the amount of constraint on the implant and the surgical approach taken to the posterior cruciate ligament (i.e., sacrificed, retained, or substituted). Implant selection for more or less constrained implants is based on the patient's needs, taking into consideration the function of the knee ligaments, deformity, host bone quality, and any bone loss.

When total knee arthroplasty is performed, most surgeons fix the implant to the host bone using cement and resurface the femoral, tibial, and patellar components. Whenever possible, the least constrained implants should be applied, because they are considered to have the best longevity due to decreased loosening forces. Fully constrained implants have been reported to have increased rates of infection, tibial loosening, and wear.

ANATOMY

The knee is a large synovial joint consisting of three intraarticular compartments: *medial,* the articulation between the medial femoral condyle and medial tibial plateau; *lateral,* the articulation between the lateral femoral condyle and lateral tibial plateau; and *patellofemoral,* the articulation between the patella and femoral intercondylar groove. Between the medial and lateral tibial plateaus is the nonarticular intercondylar region, which provides attachment sites for the anterior and posterior cruciate ligaments, and the medial and lateral menisci. The anterior and posterior cruciate ligaments are considered to be extraarticular because they are enclosed by synovium. Within the intercondylar region are two intercondylar eminences, or spines, medial (anterior) and lateral (posterior); neither serve as attachment sites for the cruciate ligaments.

All the neurovascular structures of the leg are posterior to the knee joint, and as a result, the posterior approach is reserved for procedures involving those structures. The patella is the largest sesamoid bone and functions to protect the knee joint, to facilitate knee joint lubrication, and to increase the lever arm of the knee extensor mechanism. Deep to the patella tendon is the fat pad. The knee also contains the medial and lateral menisci; each is attached to the tibia by the coronary ligament. The menisci increase joint stability by increasing the joint concavity, act as shock absorbers

to more evenly distribute forces across the knee, contribute to joint lubrication, and aid in knee rotation. The menisci structure is divided into an avascular red zone (i.e., peripheral one third) and a vascular white zone (i.e., inner third).

The knee is stabilized by a complex array of ligaments, tendons, and soft tissues (Fig. 28-1). The ligaments on the medial side of the knee often merge with each other, making identification of each layer difficult. The medial side of the knee consists of three layers: outer, middle, and deep. The outer, or most superficial, layer is the deep fascia of the thigh, whose fibers enclose the muscles and tendons of the pes anserinus before they insert into the tibia. The middle layer of the medial knee is the superficial medial collateral ligament that extends from just distal to the adductor tubercle to insert as a quadrangular ligament approximately 6 cm below the joint line into the subcutaneous border of the tibia. The superficial medial collateral ligament lies slightly posterior to the knee axis of rotation. Proximal and anterior to the insertion of the superficial medial ligament, a fibrous tissue band extends from the middle layer to the medial side of the patella as the medial patellofemoral ligament. The semimembranosus tendon continues posteriorly across the popliteal fossa and inserts into the posterior portion of the tibial medial condyle. The deep layer of the medial knee consists of the joint capsule; the deep medial collateral ligament, which extends from the medial epicondyle of the femur to the medial meniscus; and the coronary ligament, which anchors the medial meniscus to the tibia. Each of the three muscles that insert into the pes anserinus on the anteromedial tibia—the sartorius (i.e., femoral nerve), the semitendinosus (i.e., sciatic nerve), and the gracilis (i.e., obturator nerve)—has a different nerve supply. Because all three muscles originate from widely separated positions on the pelvis (i.e., the sartorius from the anterior superior iliac spine, the semitendinosus from the ischial tuberosity, and the gracilis from the inferior pubic ramus), they function in a powerful manner to stabilize the pelvis on the leg, to flex the knee, and internally to rotate the tibia.

The lateral side of the knee also contains three layers: the outer, middle, and deep. The outer layer consists of the deep fascia of the thigh, the iliotibial band (which inserts into the area of the lateral tibial condyle known as Gerdy's tubercle), the biceps femoris, and the lateral patellar retinaculum. The middle layer consists of the superficial lateral collateral ligament and the lateral inferior genicular vessels. The deep layer consists of the knee joint capsule, the popliteus muscle and tendon, and the deep lateral collateral ligament (which extends from the lateral femoral condyle to the fibular head).

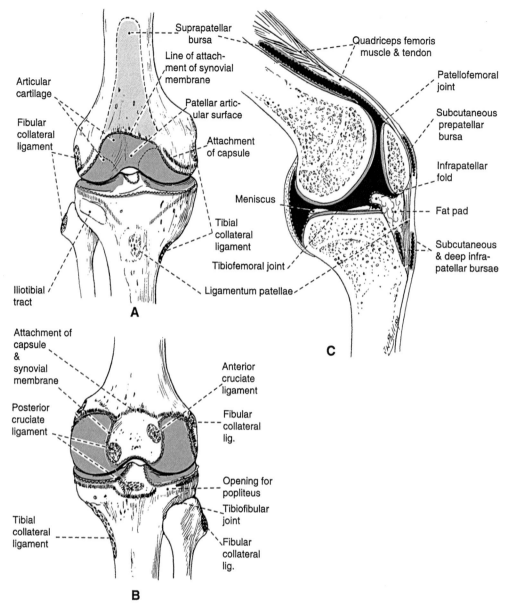

FIGURE 28-1. The anatomy of the knee joint, showing the attachments of the capsule, synovial membrane, ligaments, and menisci: anterior view **(A)**, posterior view **(B)**, and sagittal section cut to one side of the midline **(C)**. The attachment of the capsule is indicated with a *dashed black line* and that of the synovial membrane with a *red line*. Cavities filled with synovial fluid are shown in *black* in **C**.

The popliteal fossa is a diamond-shaped area that is formed inferiorly by the gap between the two heads of the gastrocnemius, by the semimembranosus and semitendinosus medially, and by the biceps femoris laterally. Its inferior boundaries are the two heads of the gastrocnemius.

The tibial nerve (i.e., terminal branch of the sciatic nerve) runs lateral to the popliteal artery as it enters the popliteal fossa, crosses the artery at the midpoint to run medial to it, and then exits the fossa between the two heads of the gastrocnemius. The tibial nerve supplies motor branches to the plantaris, gastrocnemius, soleus, and popliteus muscles, and

it has a single sensory branch, the sural nerve. The common peroneal nerve diverges laterally to the medial side of the biceps tendon and enters the peroneus longus muscle before winding around the fibula. The common peroneal nerve divides into deep and superficial peroneal nerves within peroneus longus muscle. The popliteal artery divides into its terminal branches, the posterior tibial, anterior tibial, and peroneal arteries, behind the gastrocnemius.

The popliteus is unusual in that its origin is distal to its insertion. The popliteus functions to unlock the knee from its fully extended screw-home position. This is accomplished by shifting the lateral femoral condyle behind the tibia and drawing the lateral meniscus posteriorly, preventing it from being trapped between the tibia and femur.

INDICATIONS

Total knee arthroplasty is indicated for patients who experience disabling knee pain, for those whose radiographs exhibit significant joint degeneration, and those for whom nonoperative treatment (e.g., oral medications, weight reduction and exercise programs, assistive ambulatory devices) has failed. Candidates considered for total knee arthroplasty must not be patients who would be more appropriately treated by another surgical procedure such as realignment osteotomy. Absolute contraindications include a lack of a functioning extensor mechanism, absence of neuromuscular control, active sepsis, a well-functioning knee arthrodesis, or a neuropathic joint (controversial). Relative contraindications include a history of knee sepsis or ipsilateral osteomyelitis, significant peripheral vascular disease, or an extended period of nonambulatory status. A patient with previous tuberculosis arthritis can be successfully implanted with total knee implants if she or he is given preoperative and postoperative chemotherapy and the infection is not active.

PREOPERATIVE PLANNING

Routinely, a standing, anteroposterior radiograph of both knees (Fig. 28-2A); a lateral view (Fig. 28-2B); and a sunrise view of the affected knee are obtained. A long, standing, anteroposterior radiograph showing the center of the femoral head, the knee, and as much of the tibia as possible (preferably including the ankle) can also be obtained. This type of radiograph is especially useful in patients with suspected abnormal femoral or tibial geometry, in which the mechanical axis may be difficult to determine. If long x-ray films are not available, an anteroposterior radiograph (14 × 17 inch x-ray film) of the entire femur permits similar calculations. To determine the angle between the mechanical and anatomic axes, the surgeon draws two lines to the center of the distal femur at the knee: one from the center of the femoral head and the second from the center of the femoral shaft, simulating the position of the intramedullary alignment rod that will be used during surgery. The resultant angle is usually 5 to 7 degrees. It may be less than 5 degrees in patients who have a more valgus femoral neck (e.g., in patients with previous total hip arthroplasty with a femoral component in valgus or in patients with coxa valga). Less commonly, the angle between the mechanical and anatomic axis is greater than 7 degrees (e.g., in patients with significant coxa vara or a broad pelvis with long femoral necks).

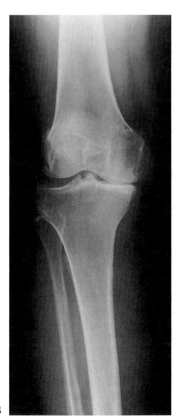 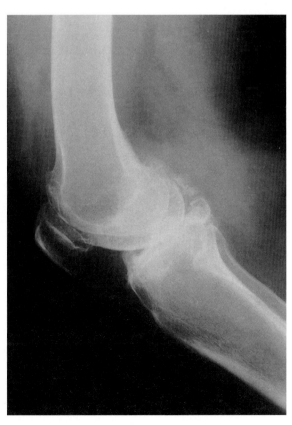

FIGURE 28-2. Anteroposterior standing (weight bearing) **(A)** and lateral **(B)** preoperative radiographs of the knee.

A, B

Most total knee systems include a femoral intramedullary alignment guide to help reestablish the anatomic axis. Typically, the surgeon dials in the desired distal femoral resection based on the intramedullary alignment rod placed into the center of the femur. As a general rule, the implant should be positioned such that, when the patient is standing, the joint is parallel to the ground, precluding shear forces across the joint. The distal femoral cut should be planned for the predetermined angle (usually 5 to 7 degrees) to be perpendicular to the anatomic axis that will then be perpendicular to the mechanical axis, thereby reestablishing normal alignment. **A special case is the patient with large thigh muscle or soft tissue; in this case, less valgus (e.g., 5 degrees) should be used to prevent the thighs from rubbing together during gait.** In patients with marked valgus or varus deformities, it is often easier to balance the total knee if less correction is planned (i.e., 7-degree cut for patients with valgus knee or a 5-degree cut for patients with marked varus knees).

Because the center of the proximal tibia and the center of the ankle are readily visualized during surgery, no preoperative calculations for the tibia are necessary. If an extramedullary tibia-cutting guide is used, it is applied directly to these key locations, and the proximal tibia is cut perpendicular to this line or with a slight (3- to 5-degree) posterior slope.

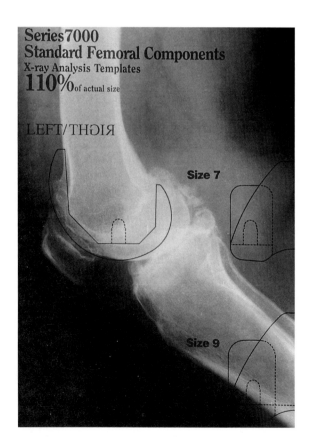

FIGURE 28-3. A preoperative template in the lateral projection is used to estimate the implant's size.

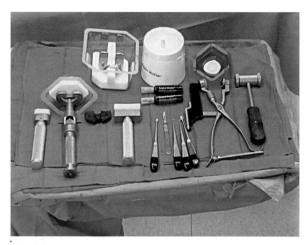

FIGURE 28-4. General instruments. *Top:* Femoral component, polymethylmethacrylate and mixing bowl, and the patella component. *Bottom:* Tibial component impactor, tibial component on a handle, femoral impactor, curettes and no. 10 blade scalpel, patella clamp, and mallet.

Preoperative templates in the anteroposterior and lateral projections should be used to estimate implant size (Fig. 28-3). Preoperative examination should note the knee range of motion and ligamentous stability. If these are altered, the surgeon may need to use special implants or anticipate alterations in surgical technique to accommodate these problems. **Hip range of motion is also important, because if the hip does not adequately flex, there may be problems in achieving the desired knee flexion.**

EQUIPMENT

Several manufacturers market total knee systems. After choosing a specific make and model, the surgeon should become familiar with its brand-specific surgical techniques. General instruments are shown in Figure 28-4. The following generic remarks are intended to review surgical techniques common to many total knee systems.

PATIENT POSITIONING AND PREPARATION

The patient is placed supine on the operating room table after anesthesia has been administered. A tourniquet is applied to the thigh. The patient's foot is moved to the end of the operating table to give the surgeon easy access from the side and the end of the table. The operative limb needs to be fixed in the flexed position during the operation; this is facilitated by using a leg-holding device or sandbag secured on the table at the level of the knee crease in the popliteal fossae. Bulky drapes should avoided on the distal tibia, ankle, and foot, because they can interfere with locating the center of the ankle and can displace the extramedullary tibial cutting guide and result in inaccurate cuts.

After sterile preparation of the limb, a sterile glove is placed over the foot and a stockinet placed from the foot to the middle of the thigh. The anterior aspect of the knee is exposed and draped with a clear, sterile, adhesive dressing. A small section (2 inches wide) of sterile, clear, adhesive dressing is wrapped around the ankle at the level of the malleoli.

SURGICAL INCISIONS AND LANDMARKS

The risk of surgical wound complications in knee arthroplasty patients is higher among those who have previously undergone knee surgery. In these patients, the blood supply to the anterior knee skin is tenuous because of the lack of an underlying muscular pedicle. The knee replacement surgical incision should incorporate previous incisions; if possible, the new incision should intersect the prior incision by an angle of at least a 60 degrees. When a parallel incision is required, the skin bridge should be at least 7 cm. Key anatomic landmarks are the patella and the tibial tubercle, both of which are easily palpated (Fig. 28-5).

APPROACH

In patients with no previous knee surgery, an anterior midline skin incision is followed by an anteromedial capsulotomy and a longitudinal incision in the quadriceps tendon. 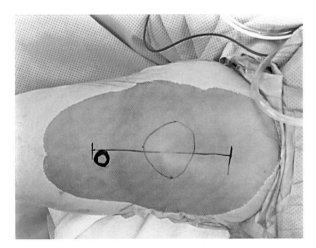 Alternative approaches include the subvastus or midvastus approach; they generally are used in patients who are not obese and exhibit minimal deformity, good preoperative range of motion (>90 degrees), and lack a significant flexion contracture (<15 degrees). The subvastus approach (i.e., Southern approach) and midvastus approach (in which the vastus medialis is reflected laterally or split in its midportion, with the superior portion reflected laterally) preserve the extensor mechanism, theoretically resulting in

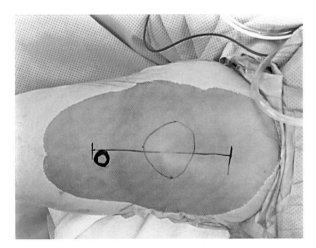

FIGURE 28-5. Key anatomic landmarks for the incision are the tibial tubercle and patella

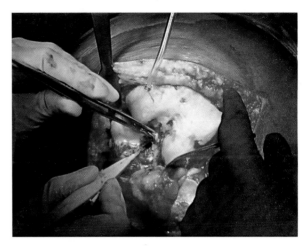

FIGURE 28-6. Removal of the anterior cruciate ligaments and the soft tissue on the anterior distal femur to expose the distal femur.

faster rehabilitation and preservation of the blood supply to the patella. In cases with marked valgus deformity, an anterolateral capsulotomy is another alternative, although difficulties in everting the patella may be encountered.

After a straight anterior skin incision is made, extending approximately 2 to 4 cm above the superior pole of the patella to just medial of the tibial tubercle, a standard medial parapatellar arthrotomy is performed. Lateral retinacular release can be performed—because it has been planned or because marked difficulty everting the patella is encountered. The patella is everted, the foot externally rotated, and the knee flexed to more than 90 degrees. The anterior cruciate ligaments (Fig. 28-6) and the soft tissue on the anterior distal femur are removed to expose the bone for later referencing for the femoral cut. If significant preoperative soft tissue contracture exists, a preliminary soft tissue release should be performed to aid exposure. If the knee has severe fixed varus or valgus deformity, releases will be required.

Although some total knee systems require interdependent preparation of the femur and tibia, they are typically prepared independently. Either the tibia or femur can be prepared first; most surgeons prepare the femur first, because resection of the posterior femoral condyles permits greater exposure of the upper tibia and facilitates its preparation. Fine tuning of minor varus or valgus imbalances should be performed after all bone cuts with provisional (trial) components are in place.

PROCEDURE

The bone preparations for total knee replacement can be broken down into three major steps: femoral, tibial, and patella preparation. Alignment of components in the coronal, sagittal, and transverse planes is critical for a long-term successful clinical outcome, because it has been demon-

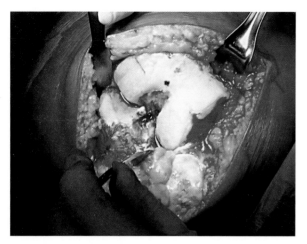

FIGURE 28-7. With the knee flexed, a site 1 cm anterior to the origin of the posterior cruciate ligament is identified as the insertion point for the femoral intramedullary alignment rod.

strated that malalignment is associated with an increased incidence of component loosening.

Femoral Preparation

Preparation of the femur consists of six steps: (1) drilling a hole in the distal femur and inserting the intramedullary femoral alignment guide; (2) cutting the distal femur; (3) measuring the anteroposterior dimension of the distal femur; (4) measuring to ensure no anterior femoral notching; (5) making the final anterior, posterior, and chamfer femoral cuts; and (6) preparing the trochlear groove or intercondylar notch, or both, for posteriorly stabilized substituting of femoral components.

With the knee flexed, a site 1 cm anterior to the origin of the posterior cruciate ligament is identified as the insertion point for the femoral intramedullary alignment rod (Fig.

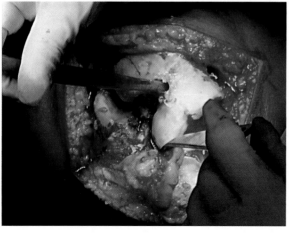
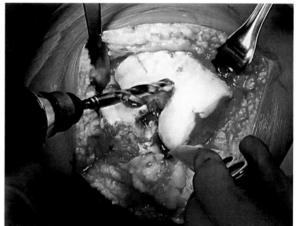

A   B

FIGURE 28-8. The intramedullary canal of the distal femur is opened using a blunt-tipped canal-finding tool **(A)** or a reamer **(B)**.

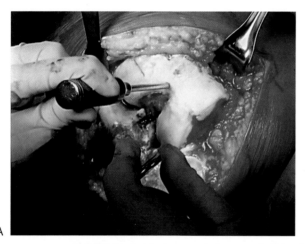
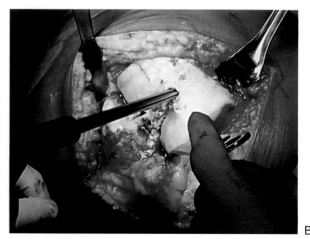

A   B

FIGURE 28-9. After suctioning of the canal **(A)**, a slotted or hollow intramedullary rod is inserted to prevent intramedullary fat pressurization **(B)**.

28-7). This places the drill hole just anterior to the distal femur intercondylar notch. This line must be parallel to the femoral shaft in both the anteroposterior and lateral projections. **The surgeon should be certain that only the cancellous bone of the distal femur is drilled to avoid potential femoral perforation. For this purpose, a blunt-tipped, canal-finding tool (Fig. 28-8A) or reamer (Fig. 28-8B) is used, because the hollow diaphysis provides little resistance. After the canal is thoroughly suctioned (Fig. 28-9A), a slotted or hollow intramedullary rod is inserted that prevents intramedullary fat pressurization (Fig. 28-9B).**

Most systems provide intramedullary alignment rods in multiple lengths. The standard rod typically extends to the proximal femur and provides the most accurate reproduction of the anatomic axis. **If the femoral anatomy is altered (by previous fracture malunion or in the case of a femur with a long-stem total hip femoral component), a shorter rod should be used.** In the rare case in which there is no access to the medullary canal (e.g., a retained femoral nail), an extramedullary alignment system should be used. Whenever possible, the longest intramedullary rod should be used to most accurately replicate the anatomic axis.

After insertion of the intramedullary alignment guide into the femur, it may be necessary to control rotation of the distal cutting block. In many systems, anatomic external rotation is built into the sizing block; in others, it is built into the implant. Rotational alignment must be correct for subsequent cuts, proper component orientation, and proper patella tracking. Proper orientation is along a transverse line drawn between the medial and lateral epicondyles; this line is often parallel to the posterior femoral condyles if no bone loss has occurred.

The distal femoral cutting block is attached to the femoral intramedullary alignment rod and set to the desired angular cut to the anatomic femoral axis (Fig. 28-10). Typically, this block is pinned into place, and the distal femoral resection is performed with an oscillating saw through a slotted cutting block (Fig. 28-11). The amount of bone removed in routine cases is identical to the amount that will be replaced by the femoral component. **Correct bone resection thickness is accomplished only if the distal femoral block is flush against the distal femoral condyles.** In cases of marked flexion contracture, the surgeon may wish to resect more femoral bone at the outset. After distal femoral resection, the pinholes are marked with methylene blue to facilitate repeat pin placement if further distal femoral resection is desired after trial components have been introduced and range-of-motion testing performed.

Accurate determination of the anteroposterior size of the distal femur is crucial for ensuring that the correct size of component is used; this can be accomplished using anterior or posterior referencing instruments. In anterior referencing, a preliminary anterior femoral cut is made flush with the anterior cortex of the femur. This should reduce the possibility of notching the anterior surface of the femoral cortex. In posterior referencing, the distance from the posterior

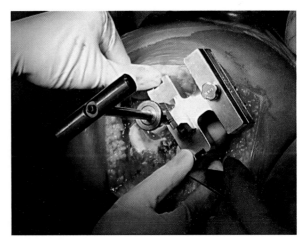

FIGURE 28-10. The distal femoral cutting block is attached to the femoral intramedullary alignment rod. The block is set to the planned angular cut relative to the anatomic femoral axis.

condyles to the anterior cortex is determined. There is no consensus about which referencing technique is better. Proponents of anterior referencing cite the lack of femoral notching as an advantage and accept the possibility of a flexion-extension mismatch (i.e., more looseness in flexion) if between sizes. Proponents of posterior referencing also site the lack of femoral notching, but acknowledge it is at greater risk of occurrence than anterior referencing. They also site as an advantage a balanced flexion-extension gap and accept the possibility of overstuffing the patellofemoral joint if a mismatch occurs between sizes. The femoral anteroposterior measuring guide should be placed flat against the cut distal femur; hyperflexion of the knee often assists in positioning the feet of the guide against the posterior condyles (Fig. 28-12). Uncommonly, the proximal tibia may have to be resected first to facilitate proper positioning of the sizing guide. With the feet of the guide on the cartilage of the pos-

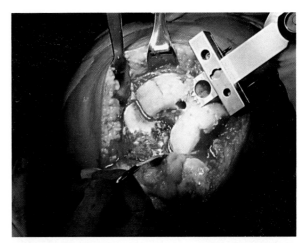

FIGURE 28-11. With the block pinned into position, the distal femoral resection is performed with an oscillating saw through the slotted cutting block.

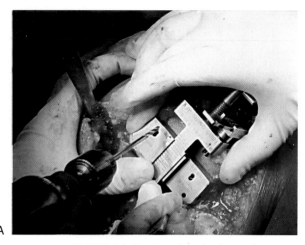
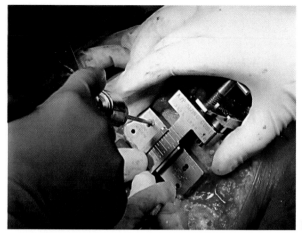

FIGURE 28-12. A and B: The femoral anteroposterior measuring guide is positioned flat against the cut distal femur with the feet of the guide against the posterior condyles. Holes for the anterior, posterior, and chamfer cuts are drilled.

terior condyles, a mobile gauge is moved until it rests on the anterior femoral surface. The guide displays the proper size of the femoral implant to be used. When using anterior referencing, if femur size falls between two standard implant sizes, the surgeon should use the smaller implant to avoid overstuffing the flexion gap; when using posterior referencing, it is better to use the larger implant to avoid notching the anterior surface of the femoral cortex.

After implant size is determined, the femoral cutting block is placed on the distal femur and secured with augmented fixation (Fig. 28-13). Care should be taken to ensure that the anterior femoral cut will not notch the anterior femoral cortex (Fig. 28-14). The surgeon should cut anterior (Fig. 28-15) or posterior condyles first, followed by the chamfers; performing cuts in this sequence ensures that the guide will maintain optimal stability during bone resection. Preparation of the distal femur concludes with placement of the appropriate trochlear groove or inter-

condylar notch resection guide and cutting tools (set the guide in the desired final mediolateral position of the femoral component) (Fig. 28-16). The femoral component should be placed as far laterally as possible to facilitate patella tracking (Fig. 28-17).

Proximal Tibia Preparation

The tibial cut can be performed using intramedullary or extramedullary (Fig. 28-18) alignment instrumentation. To optimize exposure of the proximal tibia, it can be subluxated anteriorly using an appropriate posterior retractor. The posterior cruciate ligament can be removed or recessed, if desired at this time.

The slotted cutting guide should be placed on the bone in the center of the proximal tibia (Fig. 28-19) and the distal aspect of the guide centered over the middle third of the ankle. For use of an intramedullary alignment guide, a pilot

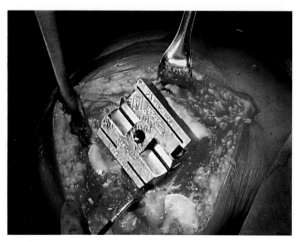

FIGURE 28-13. The femoral cutting block is positioned on the distal femur and secured.

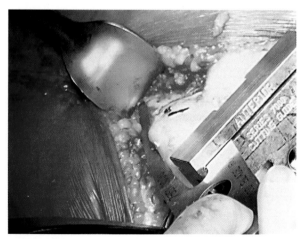

FIGURE 28-14. Guides should be used to avoid notching the anterior femoral cortex by the anterior femoral cut.

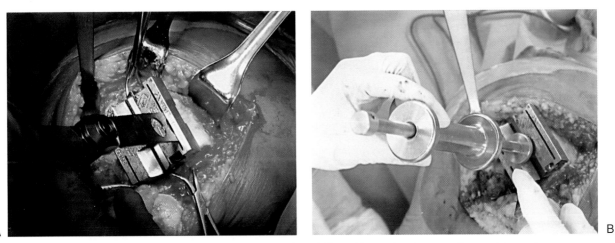

FIGURE 28-15. **A:** Cutting the anterior condyles is followed by cutting the posterior condyles and then the chamfers; the sequence supports optimal stability during bone resection. **B:** After the cuts are completed, the cutting block is removed with its extractor.

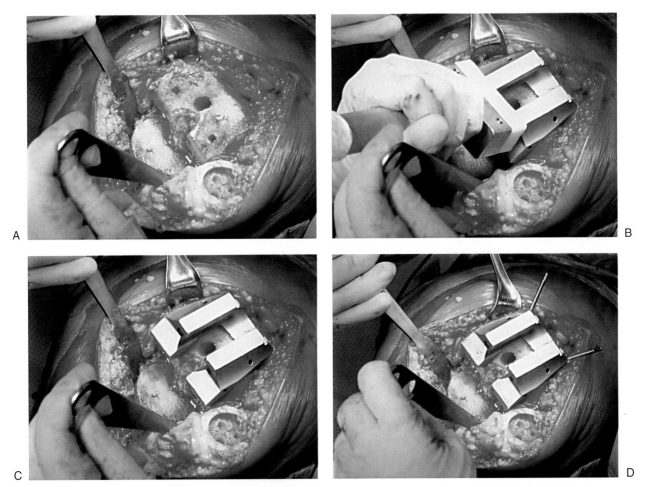

FIGURE 28-16. **A to F:** Preparation of the distal femur. Placement of the appropriate trochlear groove and intercondylar notch resection guide. Removal of bone is accomplished with the appropriate guides and cutting tools. Notice the final mediolateral position of the femoral component. *(continued)*

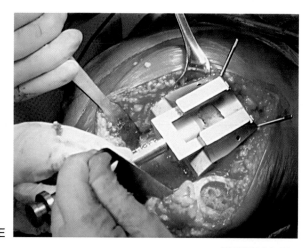
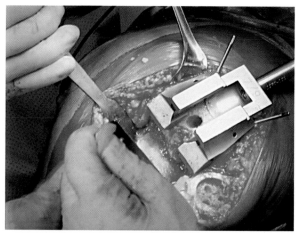

E F

FIGURE 28-16. A to F: *Continued.*

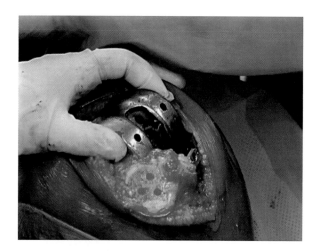

FIGURE 28-17. Placement of the femoral component as far lateral as possible to facilitate patella tracking.

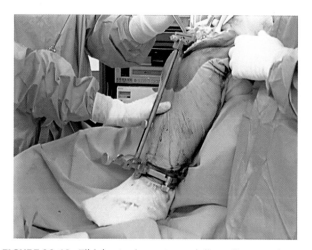

FIGURE 28-18. Tibial cut using extramedullary alignment instrumentation.

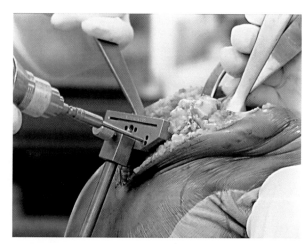

FIGURE 28-19. Placement of slotted cutting guide on the bone in the center of the proximal tibia. The distal aspect of the guide is centered over the middle third of the ankle.

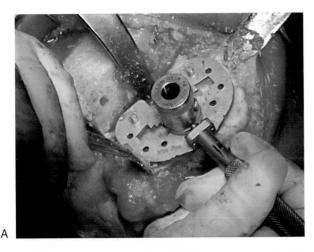

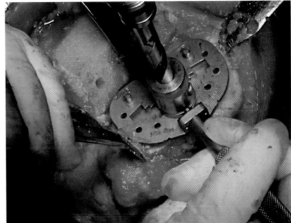

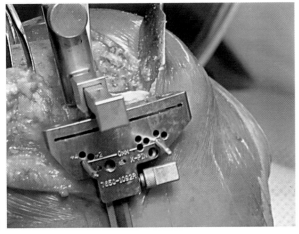

FIGURE 28-20. A to C: When using an intramedullary alignment guide, a pilot hole is drilled (centered on the proximal tibia) to gain access to the medullary canal.

hole is drilled (centered on the proximal tibia) to gain access to the medullary canal (Fig. 28-20). **It is important to center the guide over the proximal tibia in the mediolateral direction so that the guide is parallel to the mechanical axis of the tibia.** A similar cutting block, used with extramedullary alignment guides, is typically used to set the desired proximal tibial resection. The guide should be aligned to allow for 0 to 5 degrees of posterior slope and neutral varus-valgus alignment, and it should be set to remove the necessary amount of proximal tibia to be resurfaced (Fig. 28-21). Most systems include a tibial depth resection gauge to help determine the amount of bone to be resected. The cutting block is secured with pins and the proximal tibia resected with an oscillating saw (Fig. 28-22). In many cases, the tibial bone resection is below a tibial bone defect. If bone defects are excessive, alternative implants or augmentation wedges may be needed.

Next, the surgeon determines size and thickness of the tibial-articulating surface by using trial components with plastic inserts in a range of sizes. After appropriate implant size is determined, the keel guide is placed and rotated so that it is centered over the middle third of the tibial tubercle, and the keel is punched using appropriate instrumentation (Fig. 28-23).

Trial Reduction

Trial reduction and soft tissue balancing are performed next. The goal to obtain a balance of soft tissues so that stresses are evenly distributed throughout the components and to ensure

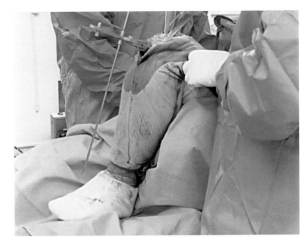

FIGURE 28-21. Alignment of the tibia cutting block should be checked with an extramedullary rod placed off of the tibial cutting block.

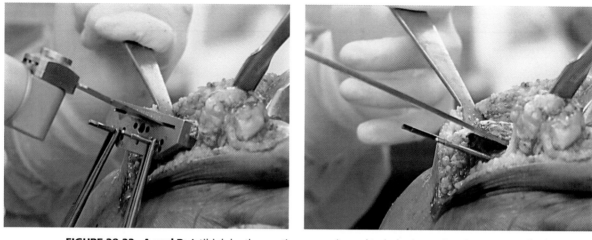

FIGURE 28-22. A and B: A tibial depth resection gauge is used to help determine the amount of bone to be resected. The cutting block is secured with pins and the proximal tibia resected with an oscillating saw.

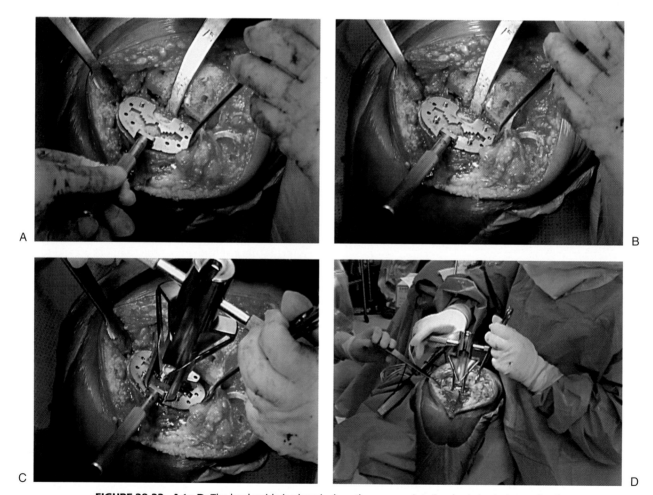

FIGURE 28-23. A to D: The keel guide is placed when the appropriate implant size is determined and rotated so that it is centered over the middle third of the tibial tubercle. The keel is punched using appropriate instrumentation.

a full and smooth arc of motion. With all trial components in place, the range of motion and ligament stability are assessed. The distal femur and proximal tibia should have been prepared so that a good fit of components exists along with a correct mechanical axis. The thickest tibial articulating surface should be used that still allows full flexion and full extension. Soft tissue tension in flexion and extension should be examined. Appropriate soft tissue releases are necessary if the medial or lateral side of the knee is disproportionately tight or if the flexion or extension gaps are not balanced. The surgeon should remove any osteophytes that can artificially tent or tighten a ligament and interfere with soft tissue balancing.

With trial components in place, varus and valgus stresses are applied with the knee in full extension and in slight flexion, because an intact posterior capsule can give a false impression of collateral stability in complete extension. If one side is tighter than the other, a soft tissue release is performed. These releases should be conducted in small stages (i.e., with partial release of one specific contracted element at a time), with reassessment of ligament balance after each release. Possible attendant deformities and their corresponding releases are summarized in the following sections.

Varus Deformity

Patients with a varus deformity may exhibit soft tissue contracture on the medial side of the knee. If soft tissue releases are necessary with the trial components in place, the surgeon should first elevate the superficial medial collateral ligament subperiosteally from the tibia, followed by the posteromedial corner of the capsule subperiosteally, the pes anserinus tendons subperiosteally, and the posterior cruciate ligament, if necessary, to achieve ligament balance.

Valgus Deformity

Patients with a valgus deformity may present with a soft tissue contracture on the lateral side of the knee. Frequently, these patients require a lateral patellar retinacular release. Although no consensus exists regarding proper sequence of releases, a sound approach is to sequentially release the popliteus tendon, posterior cruciate ligament, posterolateral capsule, iliotibial band (by Z-lengthening, cut on a diagonal or perforated with multiple small stab incisions through the superior portion of the medial parapatellar skin incision or through a separate incision on the lateral side of the distal femur), and lateral collateral ligament off of the distal femoral condyle. In cases with marked deformity, it may also be necessary to release the biceps femoris tendon by Z-lengthening through a separate incision because the tendon transverses with the peroneal nerve at the knee.

Flexion Deformity

Patients with a flexion deformity may present with a soft tissue contracture on the posterior side of the knee. This can usually be corrected by removing posterior osteophytes or resecting more of the distal femur. If these steps fail to achieve full extension, a subperiosteal release of the posterior cruciate ligament and posterior capsule from the femur should be performed. If full extension is still not achieved, the origin of the gastrocnemius tendons should be elevated from the posterior part of the femur. When resecting more distal femur, the surgeon should beware not to remove so much bone as to cause damage to the femoral attachments of the collateral ligament.

Patella Preparation

The patella can be prepared by using one of two methods: inset (Fig. 28-24) or resurfacing design. A caliper is used to measure the patella thickness. Typically, the exact amount of bone to be resurfaced is removed. **As a general rule, the patella should be made no thinner than 12 mm to avoid the risk of later patella fracture.** The patella should be sized, and for inset designed patellar components, the surgeon should ream to

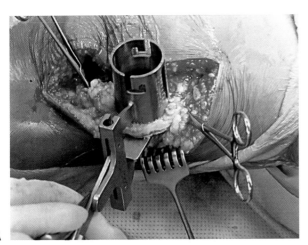
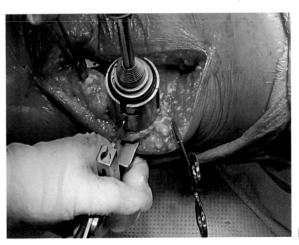

A   B

FIGURE 28-24. A to G: Preparation of the patella using an inset design. A caliper is used to measure the patella thickness. *(continued)*

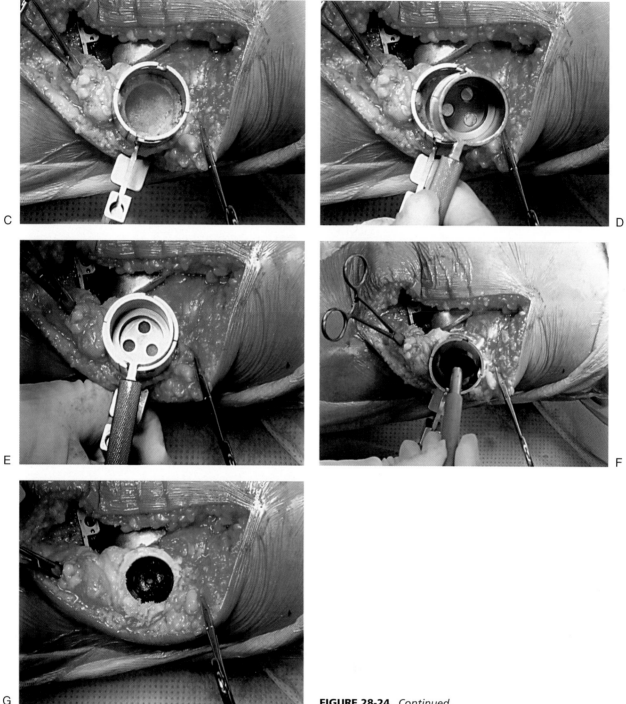

FIGURE 28-24. *Continued.*

remove the precise amount of bone to be resurfaced. When resurfacing the patella, it can be secured with sharp towel clips or manufacturer-supplied holding tools and cut flat with a saw. After cutting peg holes are drilled for the component, a trial component is placed and the thickness checked.

Patella Maltracking

Patellar subluxation or dislocation occurring during knee flexion is corrected by lateral retinacular release performed from inside the knee joint. If lateral retinacular release is performed, care must be taken to avoid the superolateral geniculate artery. A standard technique is to perform the release distal to the superior lateral geniculate artery and test tracking again; if the patella still does not track correctly, the release should be carried more proximally. **If a tourniquet is used, it should be released before closure to ensure that the vessel, if it is transected, is ligated; otherwise, a large postoperative hemarthrosis can occur.**

Implantation

Component cementing can be performed using one-step cement mixing or be done in stages. If one-step mixing is used,

the order of implantation is the tibia (Fig. 28-25), followed by the femoral component (Fig. 28-26), followed by the patella (Fig. 28-27). A trial plastic tibial insert (Fig. 28-28) is typically used during curing of the cement to permit later stability testing and to facilitate removal of any cement from the posterior aspect of the knee. Excess cement is removed during curing. After the cement hardens, the wound is checked for extruded cement, which should be removed. The final high-molecular-weight polyethylene tibial insert is locked into position on a clean and dry tibial base plate (Fig. 28-29).

Closure

Controversy surrounds the issue of whether the tourniquet should be deflated to establish hemostasis. If a lateral retinacular release is performed, the tourniquet should be deflated. A single drain is usually placed and the capsular repair performed (Fig. 28-30); range of motion and patella tracking should be checked again to ensure proper alignment and tracking. After skin closure, the incision is covered with a sterile dressing and wrapped with an elastic bandage from the toes to the groin. The patient is transferred from

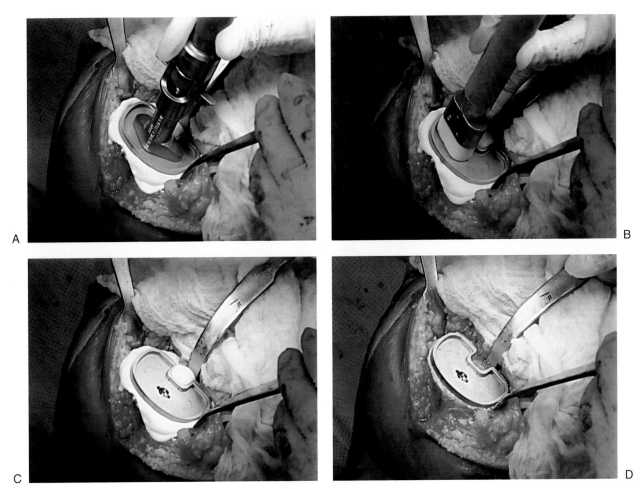

FIGURE 28-25. A to D: Tibial implantation.

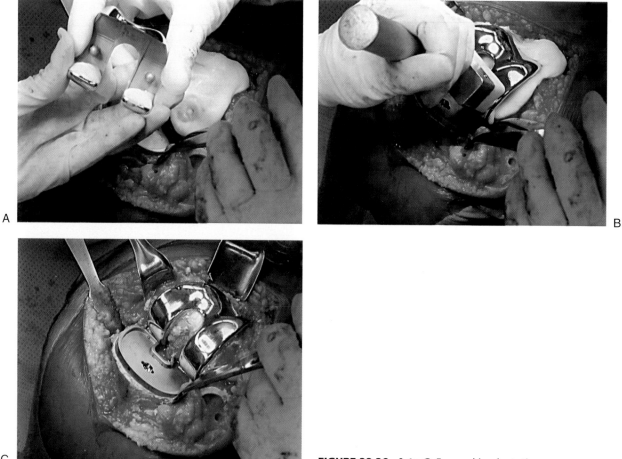

FIGURE 28-26. A to C: Femoral implantation.

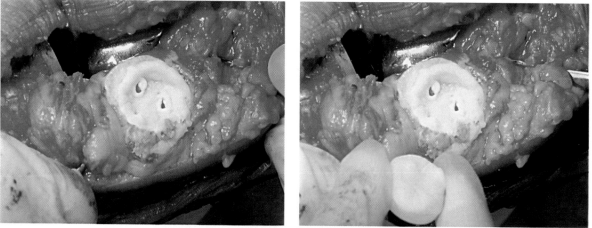

FIGURE 28-27. A to D: Patellar implantation. *(continued)*

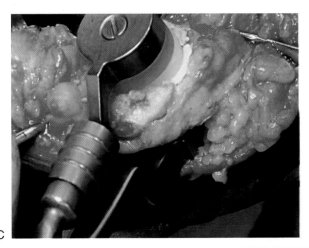

C

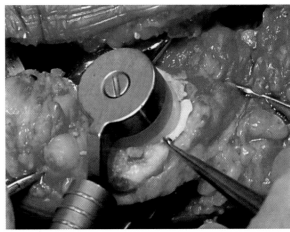

D

FIGURE 28-27. *Continued.*

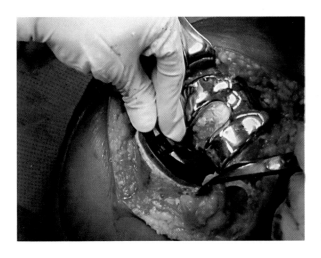

FIGURE 28-28. A trial plastic tibial insert is used during curing of the cement to permit later stability testing and to facilitate removal of any cement from the posterior aspect of the knee.

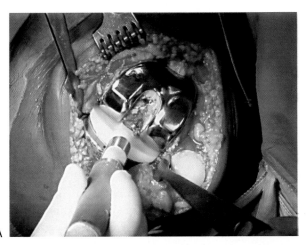

A

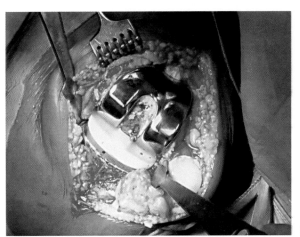

B

FIGURE 28-29. A and B: After the cement has hardened and any extruded cement has been removed, the final high-molecular-weight polyethylene tibial insert is locked into position on a clean and dry tibial base plate.

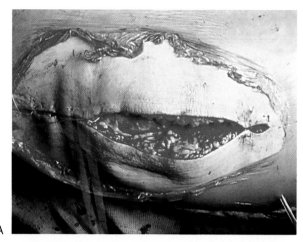

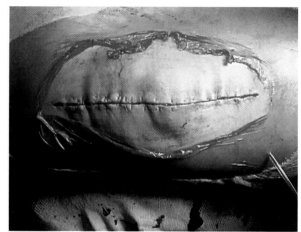

C

FIGURE 28-30. A to C: Closure. A single drain is placed before the capsular repair.

the operating room to the postanesthesia recovery room. In the recovery room, some surgeons elect to begin postoperative rehabilitation by placing the leg in a continuous passive motion (CPM) machine; others immobilize the knee to facilitate comfort and wound healing.

POSTOPERATIVE PROTOCOL

Total knee patients are hospitalized for approximately 3 to 5 days and then sent home or transported to a rehabilitation facility. All patients receive deep venous thrombosis prophylaxis (e.g., mechanical, pharmacologic) and begin physical therapy on the day after surgery. Prophylactic antibiotics are used until the drains are removed, usually 24 to 36 hours after surgery. Drains left in place for more than 48 hours have been associated with increased risk of infection.

During rehabilitation, range-of-motion exercises and gait training are emphasized. Patients may use a knee immobilizer for comfort; some use CPM as part of their rehabilitation protocol. The effect of CPM on outcomes after total knee arthroplasty remains equivocal. Potential advantages of CPM include improved early range of motion, decreased in-

cidence of deep vein thrombosis and pulmonary embolus, faster pain relief, and shorter duration of hospitalization. Potential disadvantages of CPM are increased wound complications and a lack of long-term benefits. To avoid wound problems with CPM, it is recommended to use a rate of one cycle per minute with 40 degrees of maximum flexion for the first 3 days. Surgical staples are removed on about postoperative day 14.

FOLLOW-UP

Final radiographs of the total knee arthroplasty are shown in Figure 28-31.Many factors influence the final range of knee motion after total knee arthroplasty. Most patients achieve a knee range of motion of approximately 110 degrees of flexion. Poor knee flexion (<90 degrees) may be improved by closed manipulation under spinal anesthesia. **This procedure should not be performed after 12 weeks from surgery because it holds an increased risk of periprosthetic fracture.** Most patients are in a structured physical therapy program for up to 3 months after surgery. After the patient has achieved the desired range of motion

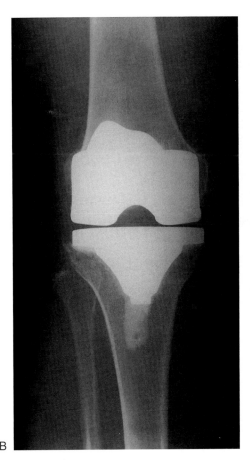
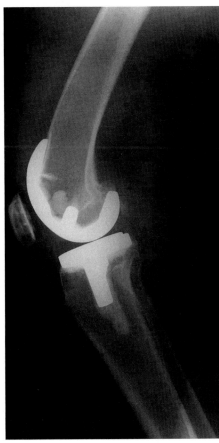

A, B

FIGURE 28-31. Postoperative anteroposterior **(A)** and lateral **(B)** radiographs of total knee arthroplasty.

and ambulates without aid, she or he is typically followed on a yearly basis.

SUGGESTED READINGS

Barrack RL, Wolfe MW. Patellar resurfacing in total knee arthroplasty. *J Am Acad Orthop Surg* 2000;8:75–82.

Barrack RL. Modularity of prosthetic implants. *J Am Acad Orthop Surg* 1994;2:16–25.

Bindelglass DF, Dorr LD. Current concepts review: symmetry versus asymmetry in the design of total knee femoral components—an unresolved controversy. *J Arthroplasty* 1998;13:939–944.

Callaghan JJ, Dennis DA, Paprosky WG, et al, eds. *Orthopaedic knowledge update: hip and knee reconstruction.* Rosemont, IL: American Academy of Orthopaedic Surgeons, 1995.

Chen B, Zimmerman JR, Soulen L, et al. Continuous passive motion after total knee arthroplasty: a prospective study. *Am J Phys Med Rehabil* 2000;79:421–426.

Chmell MJ, Moran MC, Scott RD. Periarticular fractures after total knee arthroplasty: principles of management. *J Am Acad Orthop Surg* 1996; 4:109–116.

Chmell MJ, Scott RD. Total knee arthroplasty in patients with rheumatoid arthritis: an overview. *Clin Orthop* 1999;366:54–60.

Cuckler JM. When it doesn't work: mechanisms of TKA failure. *Orthopedics* 1999;22:871–872.

Della Valle CJ, Steiger DJ, Di Cesare PE. Thromboembolism after hip and knee arthroplasty: diagnosis and treatment. *J Am Acad Orthop Surg* 1998;6:327–336.

Di Cesare PE. Adult reconstruction: knee. In: Spivak JM, Di Cesare PE, Feldman DS, et al, eds. *Orthopaedics: a study guide.* New York: McGraw-Hill, 1999:317.

Dieppe P, Basler HD, Chard J, et al. Knee replacement surgery for osteoarthritis: effectiveness, practice variations, indications and possible determinants of utilization. *Rheumatology (Oxford)* 1999;38:73–83. .

Ewald FC, Wright RJ, Poss R, et al. Kinematic total knee arthroplasty: a 10- to 14-year prospective follow-up review. *J Arthroplasty* 1999;14:473–480.

Harwin SF. Patellofemoral complications in symmetrical total knee arthroplasty. *J Arthroplasty* 1998;13:753–762.

Jacobs J, Shanbhag A, Glant TT, et al. Wear debris in total joint replacements. *J Am Acad Orthop Surg* 1994;2:212–220.

Krackow KA. *The technique of total knee arthroplasty.* St. Louis: CV Mosby; 1990.

Kuster MS, Horz S, Spalinger E, et al. The effects of conformity and load in total knee replacement. *Clin Orthop* 2000;375:302–312.

Lesh ML, Schneider DJ, Deol G, et al. The consequences of anterior femoral notching in total knee arthroplasty: a biomechanical study. *J Bone Joint Surg Am* 2000;82:1096–1101.

Li PL, Zamora J, Bentley G. The results at ten years of the Insall-Burstein II total knee replacement: clinical, radiological and survivorship studies. *J Bone Joint Surg Br* 1999;81:647–653.

Lonner JH, Lotke PA. Aseptic complications after total knee arthroplasty. *J Am Acad Orthop Surg* 1999;7:311–324.

Martin SD, Scott RD, Thornhill TS. Current concepts of total knee arthroplasty. *J Orthop Sports Phys Ther* 1998;28:252–261.

Moran CG, Horton TC. Total knee replacement: the joint of the decade. A successful operation, for which there's a large unmet need. *BMJ* 2000;320:820.

O'Driscoll SW, Giori NJ. Continuous passive motion (CPM): theory and principles of clinical application. *J Rehabil Res Dev* 2000;37:179–188.

Partington PF, Sawhney J, Rorabeck CH, et al. Joint line restoration after revision total knee arthroplasty. *Clin Orthop* 1999;367:165–171.

Rathjen KW. Surgical treatment: total knee arthroplasty. *Am J Knee Surg* 1998;11:58–63.

Robertson O, Dunbar M, Pehrsson T, et al. Patient satisfaction after knee arthroplasty: a report on 27,372 knees operated on between 1981 and 1995 in Sweden. *Acta Orthop Scand* 2000;71:262–267.

Scuderi GR, Insall JN, Scott N. Patellofemoral pain after total knee arthroplasty. *J Am Acad Orthop Surg* 1994;2:239–246.

Sethuraman V, McGuigan J, Hozack WJ, et al. Routine follow-up office visits after total joint replacement: do asymptomatic patients wish to comply? *J Arthroplasty* 2000;15:183–186.

Uvehammer J, Karrholm J, Brandsson S. In vivo kinematics of total knee arthroplasty: concave versus posterior-stabilized tibial joint surface. *J Bone Joint Surg Br* 2000;82:499–505

Windsor RE, Bono JV. Infected total knee replacements. *J Am Acad Orthop Surg* 1994;2:44–53.

CHAPTER 29

TENSION BAND WIRING OF THE PATELLA

KENNETH J. KOVAL

Fractures of the patella are relatively common, accounting for 1% of all fractures. Most of these fractures occur in patients between 20 and 50 years of age. The incidence in males is twice that for females. Although the treatment of minimally displaced patella fractures is relatively straightforward, the treatment of displaced patella fractures remains controversial. This chapter discusses open reduction and internal fixation (ORIF) of a displaced patella fracture using a tension-band wire construct.

ANATOMY

The patella is the largest sesamoid bone in the body; it lies deep to the tendinous fibers of the rectus femoris (Fig. 29-1). It is subcutaneous, covered only by a prepatellar bursa, a thin layer of subcutaneous tissue, and skin. It is oval with its apex distal. Most of the quadriceps aponeurosis inserts onto its proximal pole; its apex provides the origin for the patella tendon. Posteriorly, the proximal 75% of the patella is covered with articular cartilage that partially conforms to the articular surface of the distal femur. There are two major articular facets in the patella, the medial and lateral facets, separated by the major vertical ridge. There is a second vertical ridge near the medial border that isolates the odd facet from the medial facet. The lateral facet is generally the broadest of the three facets, occupying more than 50% of the articular surface.

CLASSIFICATION

Most fracture classifications for the patella are descriptive. Fractures are classified as nondisplaced or displaced. Generally accepted parameters for displacement are a greater than 3-mm fracture gap or 2-mm articular surface step-off. After the fracture is defined as nondisplaced or displaced, its pattern is categorized. There are three major categories of patella fractures: transverse, vertical, and stellate. Polar fractures are considered transverse fractures. The base or the apex fragments may be very small, however, and represent disruption of the quadriceps or patella tendon. Comminuted or stellate fractures are interchangeable terms, as are the terms vertical, longitudinal, and marginal fractures. There can be a combination of fracture patterns in a given injury.

SURGICAL INDICATIONS

Operative management is the treatment of choice for most displaced patellar fractures. Displacement more than 3 mm or articular incongruity of more than 2 mm is considered strong indication for surgical treatment. ORIF is indicated for displaced patellar fractures that have fragments large enough to be reduced and stably repaired and is the treatment of choice for most patellar fractures. Anterior tension banding is the fixation method most commonly used for patella fractures; this method converts the tension forces of the extensor mechanism to compressive forces at the articular surface during knee flexion. Partial patellectomy is indicated for cases that have severe comminution of the inferior or superior pole that is not amenable to ORIF techniques. Total patellectomy is generally indicated when the patellar is so severely comminuted that a well-reduced and stable construct cannot be achieved with ORIF.

PREOPERATIVE PLANNING

The standard radiographic evaluation for patella fractures includes anteroposterior and lateral views of the patella (Fig. 29-2). A supine anteroposterior radiograph is obtained, centered over the patella. Care should be taken to have the patella centered midline on the femur; this usually requires slight internal rotation of the extremity. **On the anteroposterior view, a bipartite or tripartite patella can be mistaken for an acute fracture; these forms represent a failure of fusion of the ossification centers. These normal variants usually manifest in the superolateral corner of the patella and are usually bilateral. Comparison views of the other knee should be taken when there is a question regarding the presence of a fracture or bipartite patella.**

The lateral radiograph can be taken as a cross-table lateral view, with the knee slightly flexed. The lateral view should include the proximal tibia to exclude tibial tubercle avulsion. The position of the patella with respect to the femur and the tibia should be evaluated. Patella baja may indicate a quadriceps tendon rupture, and patella alta may indicate a patella tendon rupture. The lateral view is most helpful in quantifying the amount of fracture displacement and articular incongruity.

For fractures of the patella, axial views can be helpful to diagnose longitudinal fractures and osteochondral defects. A tomogram or bone scan can be used to diagnose occult stress fractures. Computed tomography does not seem to add more information than conventional radiographs.

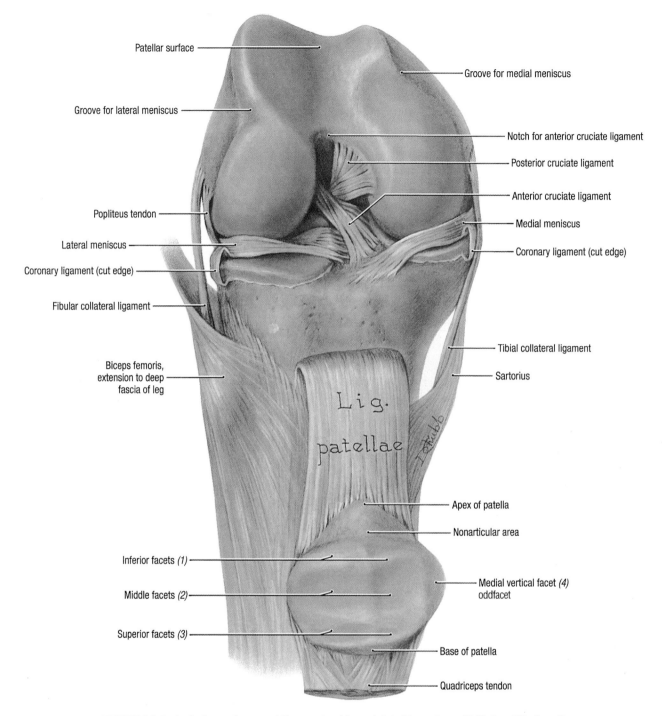

FIGURE 29-1. Articular surfaces and ligaments of knee joint. (From Agur AMR, Lee MJ. *Grant's atlas of anatomy,* 10th ed. Philadelphia: Lippincott Williams & Wilkins, 1999, with permission.)

EQUIPMENT

The equipment necessary for tension band wiring of the patella include the following items (Fig. 29-3):

- 0.062-inch Kirschner wires (K-wires)
- Wire driver
- Cerclage wire set
- 14-gauge angiocatheter

- Large and small, pointed reduction clamps
- Small fragment set

PATIENT POSITIONING

The patient is positioned supine on the operating table (Fig. 29-4). Because there is a tendency for the leg to externally to

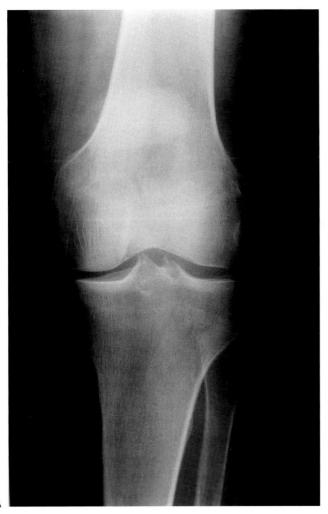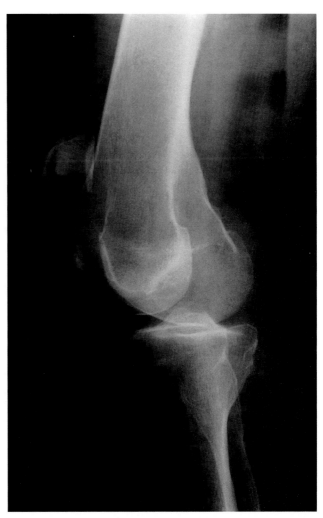

A   B

FIGURE 29-2. Anteroposterior **(A)** and lateral **(B)** radiographs show a displaced patella fracture.

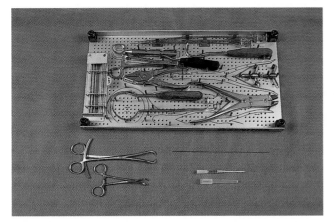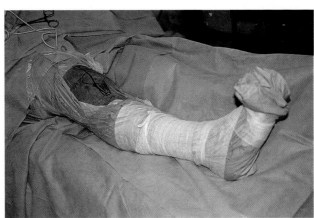

FIGURE 29-3. Equipment for tension band wiring of the patella: *top:* cerclage wire set; *bottom, left to right:* small and large pointed reduction clamps, 0.062-inch Kirschner wire, and 14-gauge angiocatheter.

FIGURE 29-4. Supine patient positioning for open reduction and internal fixation of the patella.

rotate, a small bump can be placed under the ipsilateral hip. The leg is draped free. Surgery is performed under tourniquet control. Before inflating the tourniquet, the quadriceps is pulled distally to ensure that it is not trapped under the tourniquet, which can displace the patella proximally, making reduction difficult.

SKIN INCISION

The skin incision can be transverse or longitudinal. I prefer a longitudinal midline incision, centered over the patella (Fig. 29-5).

APPROACH

The incision is carried down through the subcutaneous tissue and through the prepatellar bursa. The skin incision and approach are facilitated by slight knee flexion. A hematoma is usually encountered as soon as the bursa is

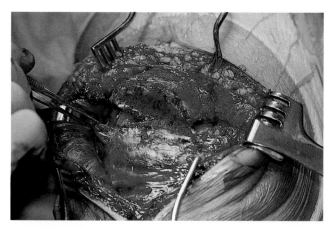

FIGURE 29-6. Exposure of the displaced fracture fragments.

opened and typically leads directly into the fracture site. ⬛️ Care should be taken to minimize direct dissection of the fracture fragments. The soft tissues surrounding the patella often hold nondisplaced fractures in place, and if this arrangement is disrupted, they may displace,

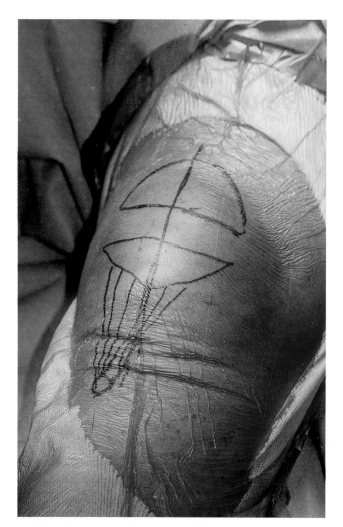

FIGURE 29-5. The longitudinal skin incision is centered over the patella.

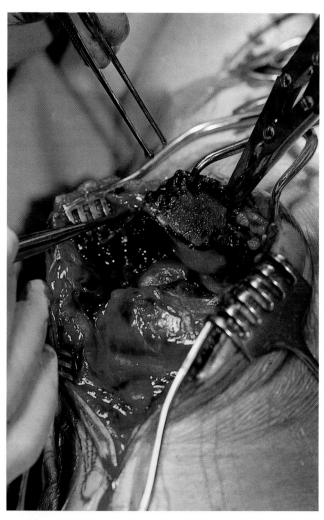

FIGURE 29-7. Identification of the medial and lateral retinacular tears.

creating a more complicated and unstable fracture pattern. The displaced fracture should be exposed (Fig. 29-6). 🎥 Clot should be removed with a combination of small curettes and the use of a small suction-tip device. 🎥 Irrigation should be used liberally to help remove the

hematoma and small inconsequential comminuted fragments. The extent of the medial and lateral retinacular injuries should be identified (Fig. 29-7). The undersurface of the patella, in addition to the patella groove, should be inspected for evidence of articular damage (Fig. 29-8). The

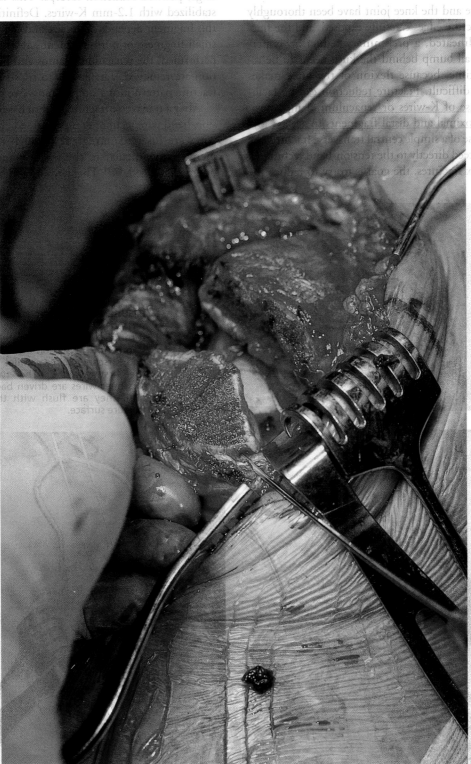

FIGURE 29-8. Exposure of the undersurface of the patella.

knee joint should be inspected and irrigated to remove any loose fragments.

PROCEDURE

After the fracture and the knee joint have been thoroughly irrigated, the fracture edges carefully exposed, and the fracture pattern delineated, a preliminary reduction is performed. The small bump behind the knee needs to be removed at this time, because flexion of the knee makes reduction more difficult. <u>Fracture reduction can be facilitated through use of K-wires or tenaculum clamps positioned in the proximal and distal fragments to act as "joysticks."</u> In the case of a simple central transverse fracture, the surgeon can proceed directly to the tension-band technique. In more complex fractures, the goal is to try to reduce the

fragments to create a transverse fracture pattern that can then be further stabilized with a tension-band technique. An example of this is a transverse fracture pattern that also has a vertical split through the proximal or distal fragments. The vertical split is first reduced and held temporarily with a large, pointed reduction forceps. This is then temporarily stabilized with 1.2-mm K-wires. Definitive stabilization of this fragment depends on its size and can be with K-wires or small-fragment or mini-fragment screws. After this has been performed, the tenaculum clamps and the provisional fixation are removed. The goal is to try to convert a complex fracture pattern into a simple transverse pattern.

After a transverse fracture pattern has been created, a tension-band wire technique is performed. Two 0.062-inch K-wires are inserted retrograde through the proximal fragment, perpendicular to the fracture and parallel to each other (Fig. 29-9). ■◄ The wires should be approximately 5

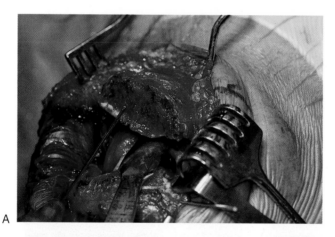

A

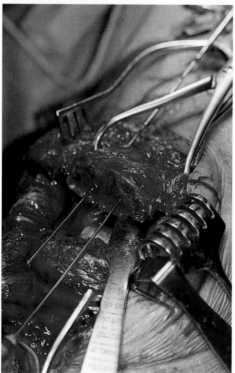

B

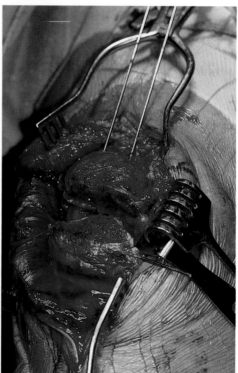

C

FIGURE 29-9. A: Retrograde insertion of a Kirschner wire through the proximal patella fragment. **B:** Insertion of a second Kirschner wire, parallel to the first wire. **C:** The two Kirschner wires are driven back until they are flush with the fracture surface.

mm from the anterior surface of the patella. Anterior placement of these wires allows a more effective tension band effect. The two fracture fragments are then reduced and held with a large, pointed reduction forceps (Fig. 29-10). Care should be taken to ensure that the articular surface is anatomically reduced by inspecting the anterior cortical and posterior articular surfaces. The articular surface can be inspected through the preexisting tears in the retinaculum. If there is no significant tear in the retinaculum, a small medial or lateral arthrotomy should be made to allow

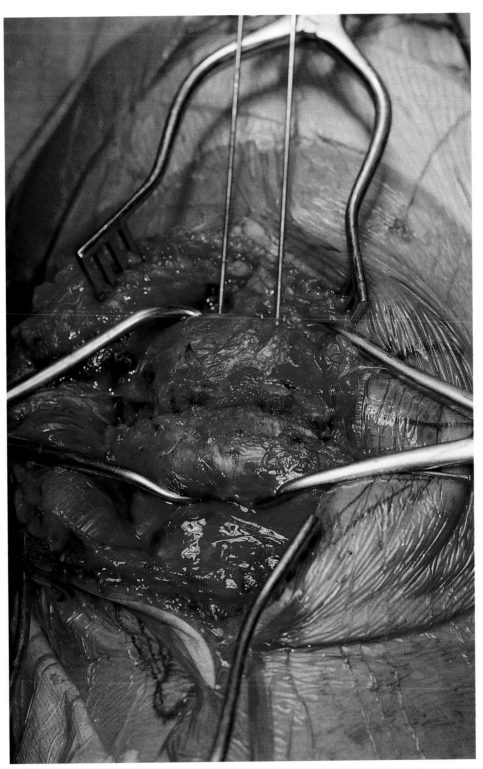

FIGURE 29-10. Fracture reduction and provisional fixation using a large, pointed reduction clamp.

inspection or palpation of the articular surface. The K-wires are then sequentially advanced through the distal fragment (Fig. 29-11). 📷 They should be advanced distally at least 1 cm beyond the inferior tip of the patella. The adequacy of the reduction should be checked clinically and radiographically (Fig. 29-12).

A 14-gauge angiocatheter is passed deep to the K-wires, hugging the proximal patella cortex (Fig. 29-13). 📷 A cerclage wire (usually 1.2 mm thick) is threaded through the catheter and used as a tension band (Fig. 29-14). **It is important that the cerclage wire contact the proximal and distal poles of the patella, without intervening soft tissue; otherwise, with knee motion, the fragments may slip apart on the K-wires until the tension band becomes taut.** The angiocatheter is then passed deep to the distal end of the K-wires, hugging the patella cortex (Fig. 29-15). The tension band is crossed anterior to the patella in figure-of-eight fashion and threaded through the distal angiocatheter. 📷 Two loops are made in the tension band wire, one on either side of the patella (Fig. 29-16). The tension band wire is then

tightened by a double knot technique with the knee in extension (Fig. 29-17). 📷 Before twisting, the wire should be tensioned by lifting up on the clamp. This ensures that both wires twist around each other rather than one wire wrapping around the other wire. The reduction should be checked periodically while the wire is being tightened (Fig. 29-18). The knots of the cerclage wire are cut, bent over, and impacted into the bone (Fig. 29-19). The proximal ends of the longitudinal wires are bent over, twisted to face posteriorly, and tapped into the cortex (Fig. 29-20) 📷; the distal ends are flared away from each other and cut below the edge of the patella tendon. 📷 If the K-wires are not buried deep to the quadriceps mechanism, they will cause soft tissue irritation and are at increased risk for wire backout. The distal aspect of the K-wires are flared away from each to minimize the risk for wire backout; they are not bent as much as the proximal aspect of the wires to facilitate hardware removal. An additional circumferential wire is used if there are associated longitudinal or stellate fracture lines.

After fracture stabilization, the knee is flexed to check

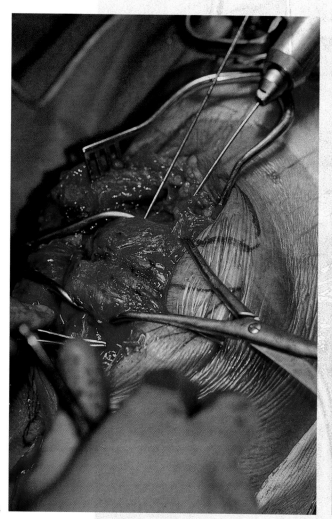
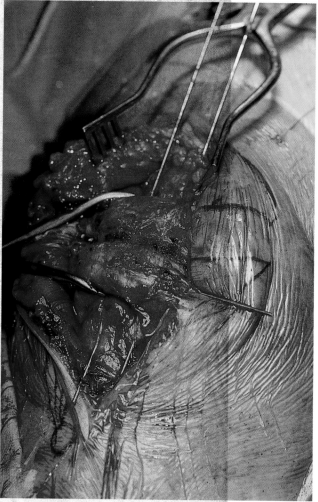

A   B

FIGURE 29-11. A and B: Advancement of the Kirschner wires across the fracture.

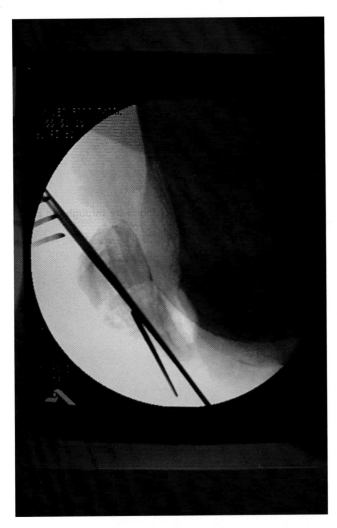

FIGURE 29-12. Lateral radiograph verifying fracture reduction and implant position. An additional Kirschner wire had been placed in the distal fragment because of a nondisplaced, longitudinal fracture fragment.

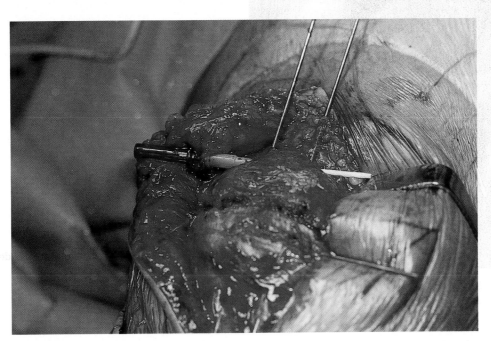

FIGURE 29-13. Passage of a 14-gauge angiocatheter deep to the Kirschner wires, hugging the proximal cortex of the patella.

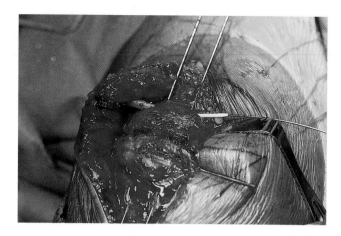

FIGURE 29-14. Insertion of a cerclage wire through the angio-catheter.

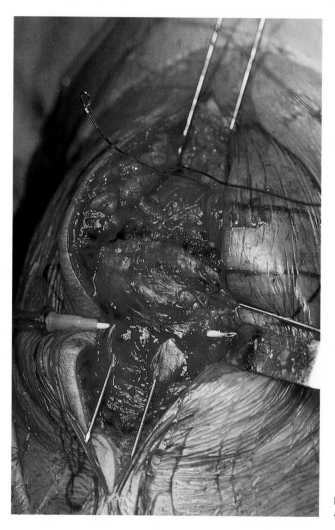

FIGURE 29-15. Passage of the angiocatheter deep to the distal aspect of the Kirschner wires.

the fixation stability, and the quality of reduction and implant position are verified radiographically (Fig. 29-21). The medial and lateral retinacular defects are repaired and the remainder of the incision closed in layers. Skin closure depends on the integrity of the skin. Subcuticular closure gives excellent cosmetic results but should be reserved for cases without skin injuries and minimal swelling. If there is concern regarding damage to the skin, nylon sutures should be used. A sterile dressing is applied consisting of fluffs, Webril, and an Ace wrap. The leg is placed into a knee immobilizer.

POSTOPERATIVE PROTOCOL

Postoperative care depends on the fracture type and the fixation stability. In patients with stable fixation, knee motion is initiated on postoperative day 1 with use of a continuous passive motion (CPM) machine. The patient is mobilized out of bed to ambulate while bearing weight as tolerated with the knee in full extension. Quadriceps strengthening is started in the early postoperative period. After there is radiographic evidence of healing, progressive weight-bearing and resistive exercises are started. The patient is progressively weaned from the brace, depending on the motion and strength. Full rehabilitation usually takes 4 to 6 months. If there are any symptoms or signs of loss of fixation during the postoperative period, range-of-motion exercises are stopped, and the patient is immobilized and followed closely.

In the case of unstable fracture fixation, early range of motion is not possible. The repair should be protected in a knee immobilizer or a knee brace with the hinges locked. The braces are removed only for wound checks and extremity cleaning. Quadriceps sets can be initiated, but the repair is protected until there are signs of healing. Range-of-motion activity is delayed for 3 to 6 weeks.

(text continues on page 318)

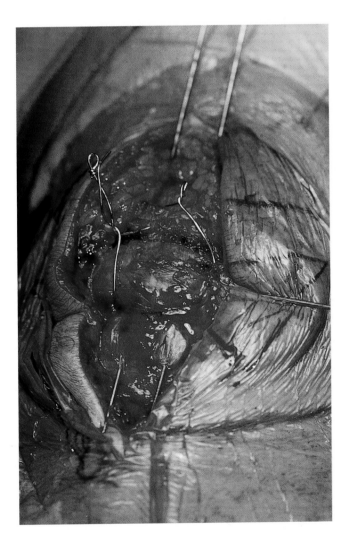

FIGURE 29-16. Placement of two loops in the tension band wire, one on either side of the patella.

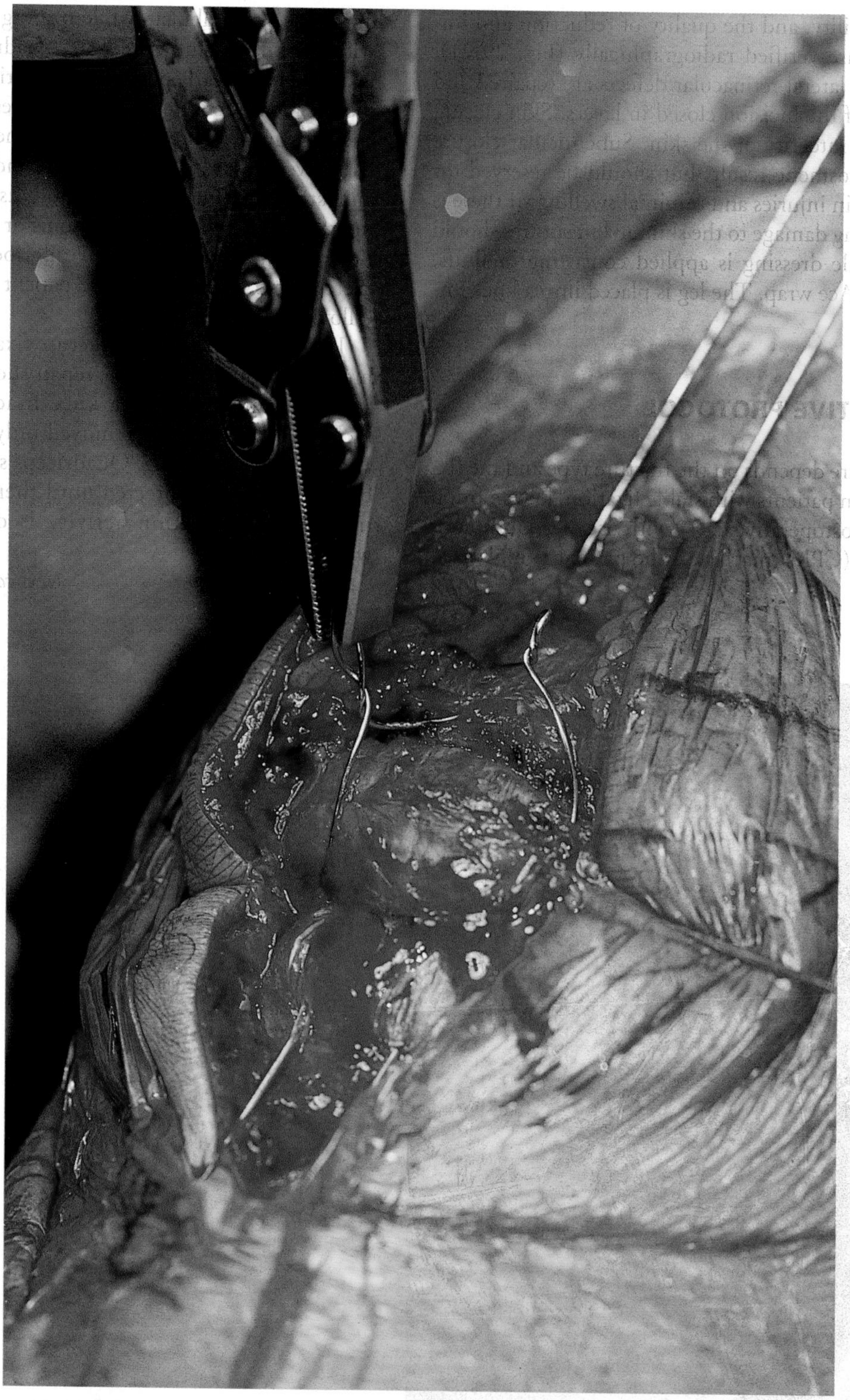

A

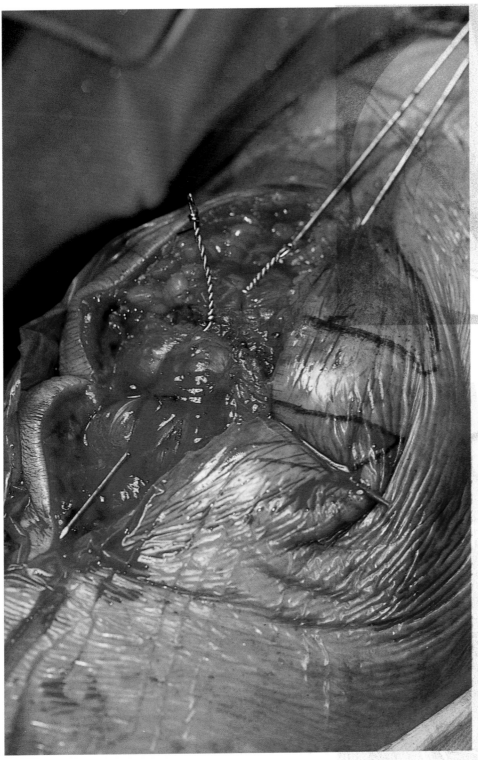

B

FIGURE 29-17. A and B: Tightening of the tension band wire with the knee in extension.

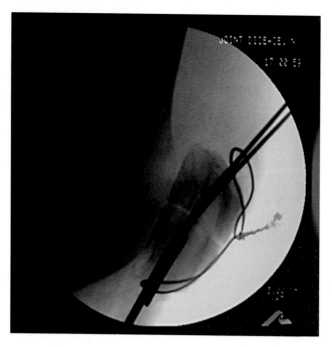

FIGURE 29-18. Lateral radiograph verifying fracture reduction and the implant's position.

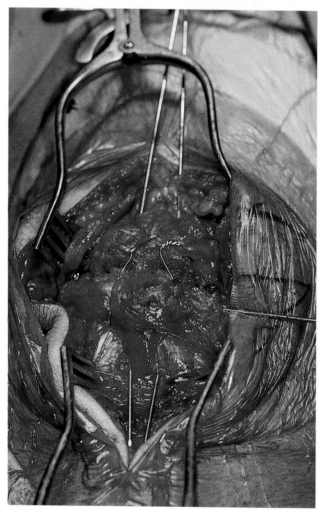

FIGURE 29-19. The cerclage wire knots have been cut, bent over, and impacted into the bone.

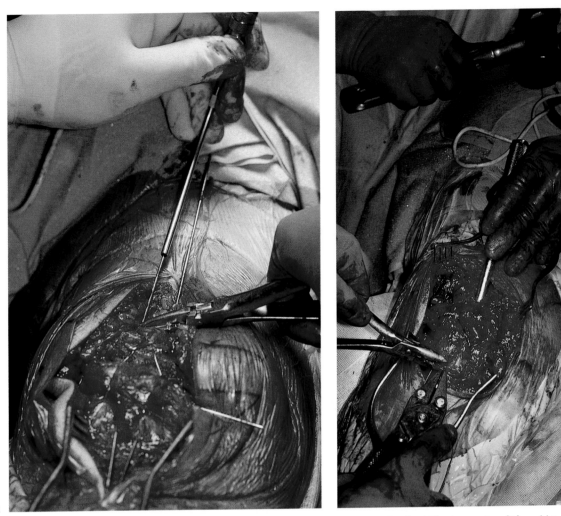

FIGURE 29-20. Bending of the proximal aspect of the longitudinal Kirschner wires **(A)** and impaction of the longitudinal Kirschner wires deep to the quadriceps **(B)**.

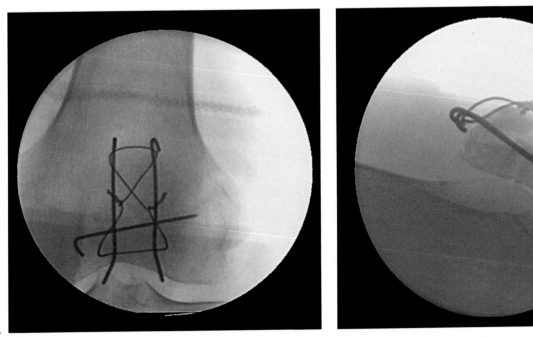

FIGURE 29-21. Final anteroposterior **(A)** and lateral **(B)** radiographs.

SUGGESTED READINGS

Benjamin J, Bried J, Dohn M, et al Biomechanical evaluation of various forms of fixation of transverse patellar fractures. *J Orthop Trauma* 1987;1:219–222.

Burvant JG, Thomas KA, Randan A, et al. Evaluation of methods of internal fixation of transverse patella fractures: a biomechanical study. *J Orthop Trauma* 1994;8:147–153.

Carpenter JE, Mathews LS. Fractures of the patella. *J Bone Joint Surg Am* 1993;75:1550–1561.

Johnson EE. Fractures of the knee, fractures of the patella. In: Rockwood CA, Green DP, Bucholz RW, et al, eds. *Rockwood and Green's fractures in adults,* vol 2, 3rd ed. Philadelphia: JB Lippincott, 1991:1762–1777.

Kaufer H. Mechanical function of the patella. *J Bone Joint Surg Am* 1971;53:1551–1560.

Levack B, Flanagan JP, Hobbs S. Results of surgical treatments of patella fractures. *J Bone Joint Surg Br* 1985;67:416–419.

Muller ME, Allgower M, Schneider R, et al. Manual of internal fixation, 2nd ed. New York: Springer, 1979:348–252.

Sanders R. Patella fractures and extensor mechanism injuries. In: Browner BD, Jupiter JB, Levine AM, et al, eds. *Skeletal trauma: fractures, dislocations, ligamentous injuries,* vol 2. Philadelphia: WB Saunders, 1992:1685–1716.

Weber MJ, Janecki CJ, McLeod P, et al. Efficacy of various forms of fixation of transverse fractures of the patella. *J Bone Joint Surg Am* 1980;62:215–220.

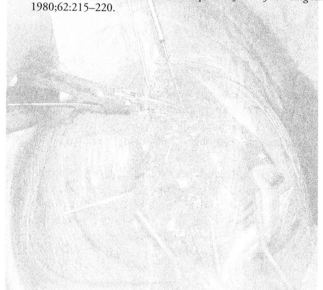

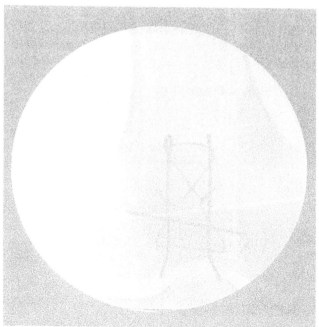

CHAPTER 30

LATERAL TIBIAL PLATEAU FRACTURE: OPEN REDUCTION AND INTERNAL FIXATION

KENNETH J. KOVAL

Tibial plateau fractures result from indirect coronal and from direct axial compressive forces. These forces drive the femoral condyle into the tibial plateau, producing a spectrum of fracture patterns. Fracture fragment size, location, and displacement are determined by the direction, magnitude, and location of the generated force, as well as by the bone quality and the degree of knee flexion at the moment of impact. The combination of compression and valgus produces a lateral plateau fracture, and compression coupled with varus results in a medial fracture pattern. The prevalence of lateral plateau fractures is related to the valgus inclination of the anatomic axis and the usual lateral direction of the applied force. This chapter discusses open reduction and internal fixation of the lateral tibial plateau.

ANATOMY

The tibial plateau is composed of medial and lateral articular surfaces (Fig. 30-1). The medial plateau is larger and is concave in the sagittal and coronal axes. The lateral plateau extends higher and is convex in the sagittal and coronal planes. The normal tibial plateau has a 10-degree posteroinferior slope. The two plateaus are separated from one another by the intercondylar eminence, which is nonarticular and serves as the tibial attachment of the cruciate ligaments.

CLASSIFICATION

The most widely accepted classification has been that proposed by Schatzker (Fig. 30-2). Type I is a wedge (split) fracture of the lateral tibial plateau. Type II is a split depression fracture of the lateral plateau; the femoral condyle first splits the condyle and then depresses the medial edge of the remaining plateau. Type III is a pure central depression fracture of the lateral plateau without an associated split. Type IV is a fracture of the medial tibial plateau that usually involves the entire condyle. Type V is a bicondylar fracture that typically consists of split fractures of the medial and lateral plateaus without articular depression. Type VI is a tibial plateau fracture with an associated proximal shaft fracture.

INDICATIONS

Controversy exists regarding the specific indications for open versus closed management of tibial plateau fractures. Some surgeons advocate nonoperative treatment for fractures with up to 1 cm of depression. Others accept only minimal displacement of the articular surface. However, there is general agreement that instability of more than 10 degrees (compared with the uninvolved knee) of the nearly extended knee is an indication for operative intervention. Open tibial plateau fractures or those associated with a compartment syndrome or vascular insult require emergent care.

The amount of articular displacement resulting in instability is unknown; it depends on the fracture type, location, and associated ligamentous disruption. Split fractures, in addition to disrupting the articular surface, involve the rim of the tibial plateau and are likely to be unstable in response to axial loading. Split depression fractures are at a higher risk for instability because of the depressed surface adjacent to the split component. Pure central depression fractures are usually stable unless the depression involves the entire plateau; the intact cortical rim provides varus-valgus stability. Plateau fractures that are associated with a tibial shaft fracture are usually not amenable to closed treatment, because traction often results in separation of the shaft components rather than reduction of the articular surface.

PREOPERATIVE PLANNING

Initial radiographs should include an anteroposterior, a lateral, and two oblique views and the 15-degree caudal plateau view (Fig. 30-3). These five radiographs are known as the *knee trauma series*. These films are analyzed for rim widening, articular depression, shaft extension, and bony avulsions. The amount of condylar depression can be measured from the remaining intact articular surface on the 10-degree caudal plateau or lateral radiographs.

Comparison radiographs of the contralateral extremity are useful for the preoperative plan. Tri-spiral and computed tomography coupled with sagittal reconstructions are helpful in evaluating the degree of articular displacement

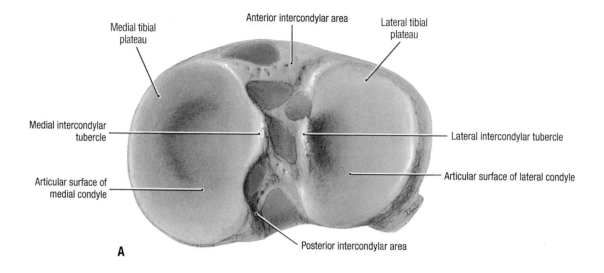

Medial tibial plateau

Anterior intercondylar area

Lateral tibial plateau

Medial intercondylar tubercle

Lateral intercondylar tubercle

Articular surface of medial condyle

Articular surface of lateral condyle

Posterior intercondylar area

A

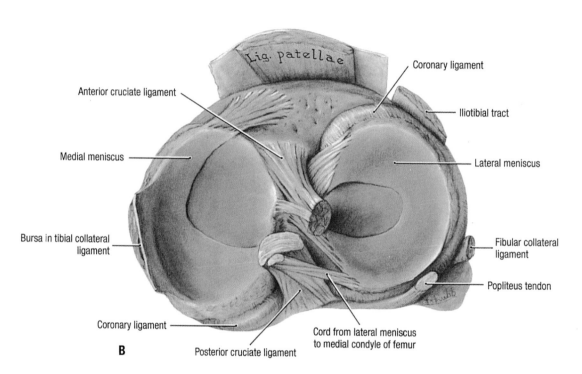

Lig. patellae

Anterior cruciate ligament

Coronary ligament

Iliotibial tract

Medial meniscus

Lateral meniscus

Bursa in tibial collateral ligament

Fibular collateral ligament

Popliteus tendon

Coronary ligament

Posterior cruciate ligament

Cord from lateral meniscus to medial condyle of femur

B

FIGURE 30-1. A and B: Right tibial plateau. (From Agur AMR, Lee MJ. *Grant's atlas of anatomy,* 10th ed. Philadelphia: Lippincott Williams & Wilkins, 1999, with permission.)

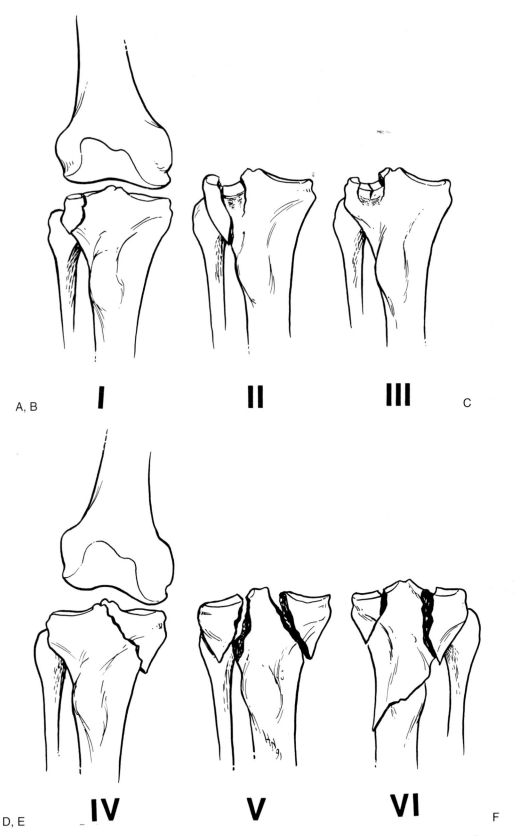

FIGURE 30-2. The Schatzker classification of tibial plateau fractures. **A:** Type I, split fracture of the lateral tibial plateau. **B:** Type II, split depression fracture of the lateral plateau. **C:** Type III, central depression fracture of the lateral plateau. **D:** Type IV, fracture of the medial tibial plateau. **E:** Type V, bicondylar tibial plateau fracture. **F:** Type VI, tibial plateau fracture with an associated proximal shaft fracture.

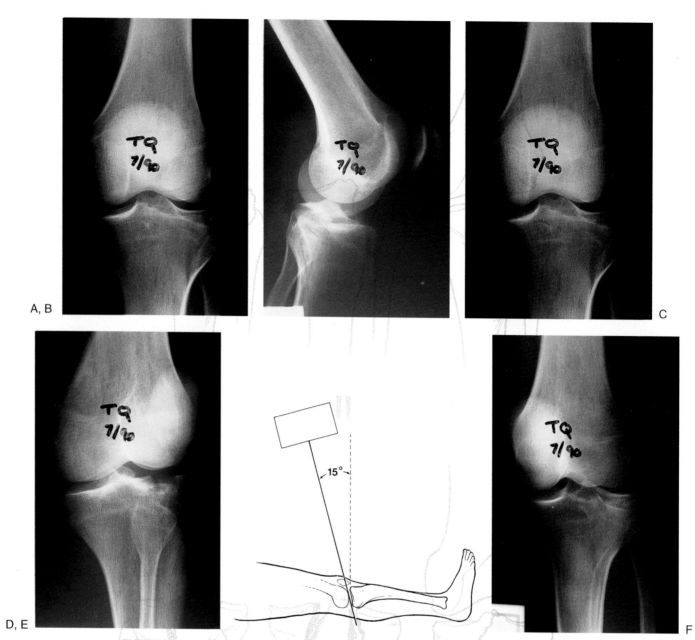

FIGURE 30-3. Radiographic evaluation of tibial plateau fractures should include an anteroposterior view **(A)**, a lateral view **(B)**, two oblique views **(C and D)**, and the 10-degree caudal plateau view **(E and F)**.

ture in the evaluation of meniscal and ligamentous injuries associated with these fractures.

The exact nature of the fracture should be understood before attempting any form of surgical intervention (Fig. 30-5). Although useful for simpler fractures, preoperative planning is critical for more complex injuries. This forces the surgeon to understand the "personality of the fracture" and mentally prepare an operative plan. All aspects of the reduction and fixation should be drawn out to help avoid technical pitfalls and ensure that all the needed equipment is available.

EQUIPMENT

Several basic instruments are necessary for open reduction and internal fixation of a tibial plateau fracture (Fig. 30-6):

- Small fragment plate and screws
- Large fragment plate and screws
- Large- and small-diameter cannulated screws
- Large and small pointed reduction clamps
- Femoral distractor with or without an external fixator set
- Tamp and gouge set

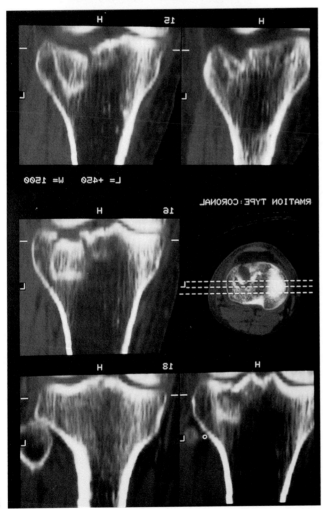

FIGURE 30-4. Computed tomographic scan **(A)** and sagittal reconstruction **(B)** of a tibial plateau fracture.

(Fig. 30-4). These studies are an excellent adjunct to plain x-ray films in the preoperative planning for lag screw placement, particularly when contemplating percutaneous fixation. Magnetic resonance imaging may play a role in the fu-

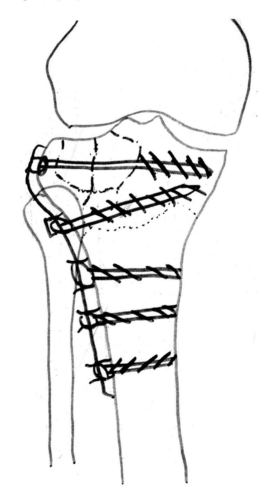

FIGURE 30-5. Preoperative plan for operative treatment of a lateral tibial plateau fracture.

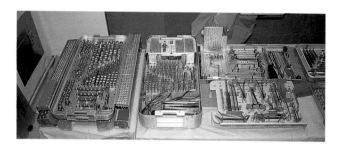

FIGURE 30-6. The instruments needed for open reduction and internal fixation of a lateral tibial plateau fracture: large fragment set and small fragment set *(left to right)*, cannulated screw set *(far right, top)*, second small fragment set *(far right, bottom)*.

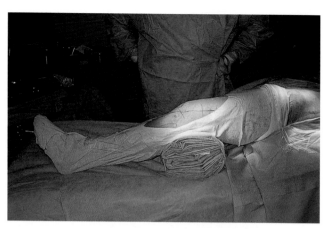

FIGURE 30-7. The patient is positioned supine with a bolster under the knee.

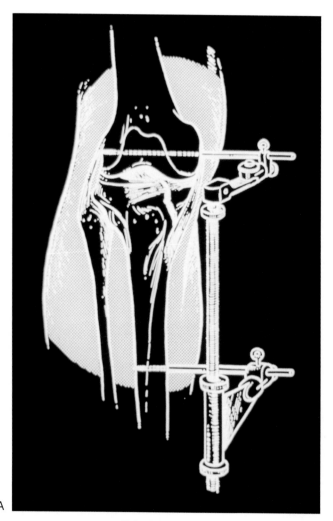

A

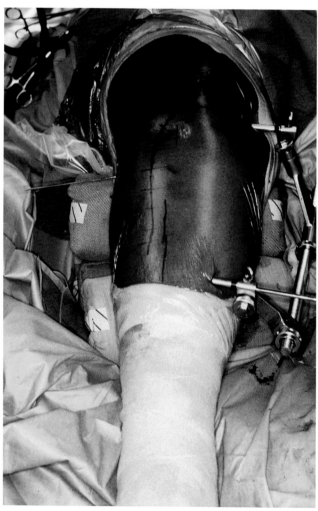

B

FIGURE 30-8. A and B: Use of a femoral distractor to reduce the lateral tibial plateau.

PATIENT POSITIONING AND FRACTURE REDUCTION

Patients should be positioned supine with a bolster under the knee or on a table that has the ability to flex the foot of the table (Fig. 30-7). The ipsilateral iliac crest should be prepared and draped if a need for autogenous bone graft is contemplated. The patient's position should take into account the need for intraoperative image intensification, with the ability to obtain anteroposterior, lateral, plateau, and oblique views. If arthroscopy is to be used, a well-padded leg holder or post should be available.

Fracture reduction can be aided by the use of ligamentotaxis using a femoral distractor. This instrument be placed on the ipsilateral side of the tibial plateau fracture, extending across the knee joint, with one pin in the femoral condyle and the other pin in the mid to distal tibia, well away from the anticipated distal end of the implant (Fig. 30-8). In the event of bicondylar or type VI fractures, bilateral femoral distractors may be required.

APPROACH

Before inflation of the tourniquet, the knee should be flexed to allow the quadriceps muscle to stretch distally. Exposure of the tibial plateau can be gained through a variety of approaches. The surgical approach should provide maximum visualization, combined with preservation of all vital structures and minimal soft tissue and osseous devitalization. Skin incisions for tibial plateau fractures should be longitudinal (Fig. 30-9). Midline skin incisions are favored in bicondylar fractures to allow access to both knee compartments and facilitate any future reconstructive procedures. Because most plateau fractures involve the lateral compartment, a lateral parapatellar incision and arthrotomy are often used. Medial fractures use a medial parapatellar approach. Flaps that are raised should be full thickness down

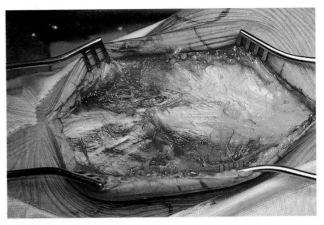

FIGURE 30-10. Exposure of the fascia and retinaculum through a full-thickness skin flap.

to the crural fascia and retinaculum and include the subcutaneous fat (Fig. 30-10). ■ **Excessive soft tissue dissection can result in osseous devascularization and increase the risk for soft tissue complications, including skin slough.**

After the level of the capsule has been reached, an arthrotomy is performed. The arthrotomy can be submeniscal (Fig. 30-11) ■ or vertical with division of the anterior horn of the lateral meniscus. When using a submeniscal arthrotomy, the surgeon should leave a soft tissue cuff on the proximal tibia for capsular reattachment or prepare to use Mitek anchors. With either approach, the split fracture component can be displaced open and depressed fracture fragments elevated. The joint must be examined for evidence of meniscal pathology, because meniscal tears have been reported in up to 50% of tibial plateau fractures. ■ Lesions that are not appropriate for repair should be excised at this time. Peripheral tears should have a suture repair at closure. Posteromedial fractures of the plateau can be approached through a separate incision between the medial gastrocnemius and semitendinosus and then between the medial collateral ligament and the posterior oblique ligament.

PROCEDURE

The split fracture line is identified (Fig. 30-12). Exposure of the depressed articular fragment is accomplished by opening the metaphysis like a book at the split fracture line and hinging the peripheral fragments outward, preserving their soft tissue attachments (Fig. 30-13). ■ Reduction of the depressed articular surface fragment should start by recognizing the area of uninvolved articular surface. Depressed articular fragments should be elevated *en mass* from below as large cancellous blocks to prevent articular surface fragmentation (Fig. 30-14). ■ This can be achieved with the use of a bone tamp or elevator working through the split component.

Once elevated, provisional stabilization of the articular fragments to the medial or lateral condyle using Kirschner

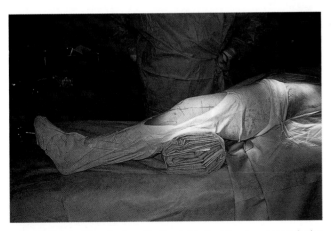

FIGURE 30-9. Use of a longitudinal skin incision to approach the lateral tibial plateau.

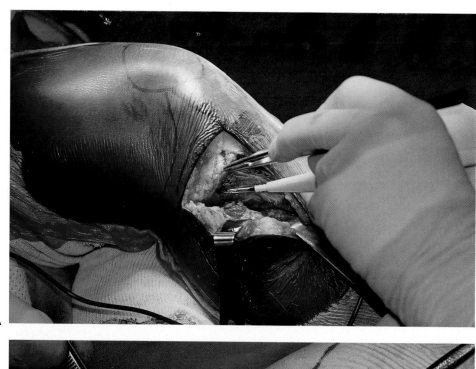

A

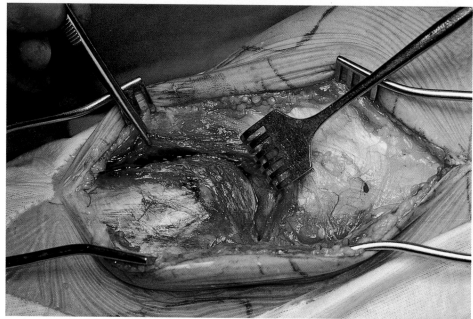

B

FIGURE 30-11. A and B: Use of submeniscal arthrotomy to approach the articular surface.

wires (K-wires) is performed (Fig. 30-15). ◲ These K-wires should be placed to avoid interfering with reduction of the split fragment. At this point, the metaphyseal defect should be bone grafted ◲ and the split fragment reduced ◲ and provisionally stabilized (Fig. 30-16).

Once satisfied with the fracture reduction, definitive stabilization is performed. Definitive stabilization requires the insertion of two 6.5- or 7.0-mm cancellous lag screws parallel to the joint (Fig. 30-17), followed by metaphyseal buttress plating (Fig. 30-18). This buttress must be located at the distal extent of the fracture line and serves to prevent

shear forces from causing late collapse. The choice of plates depends on the degree of cortical comminution and may be as simple as a washer (i.e., one-hole plate), two-hole plate, T- or L- buttress plate, or Burri plate. The surgeon should select that plate that offers stable fixation but minimizes bulk to prevent complications with wound closure.

After definitive fracture stabilization, the incision is irrigated and the wound closed. The coronary ligament of the knee capsule is reattached using sutures or Mitek anchors, or both (Fig. 30-19). Wound closure is performed over suction drains. **If the wound cannot be closed without tension, it is**

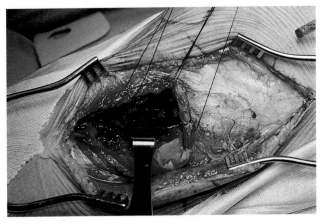

FIGURE 30-12. Identification of the split fracture component.

FIGURE 30-13. Working through the split fracture component to expose the area of articular depression.

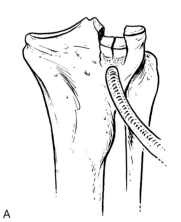

A

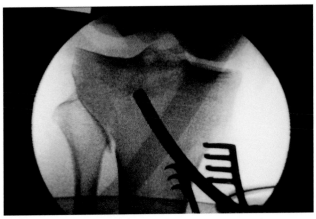

B

FIGURE 30-14. A and B: Use of a tamp to elevate depressed articular fragments *en mass* to prevent articular surface fragmentation.

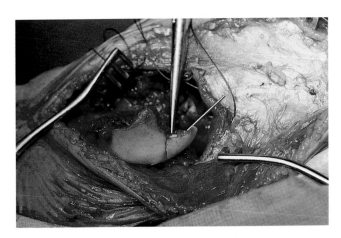

FIGURE 30-15. Reduction and provisional stabilization of the articular fragments using Kirschner wires.

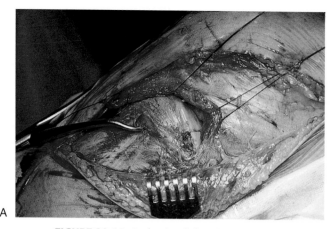
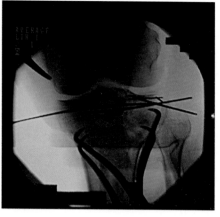

FIGURE 30-16. Reduction **(A)** and provisional stabilization **(B)** of the split fracture component.

preferable to leave the incision partially open and covered with a sterile dressing. Wound closure may then be performed at a later date.

POSTOPERATIVE PROTOCOL

Postoperatively, the knee should be protected in a hinged knee brace and started on continuous passive motion with a range of motion of 0 to 30 degrees and advanced as tolerated. The machine is kept on as much as possible during waking hours; early motion has been clearly demonstrated to promote cartilage healing. Physical therapy for active assisted range-of-motion exercises and touch-down weight bearing is initiated and continued until the patient is independent with ambulatory aids. Full weight bearing is permitted by 12 weeks based on radiographic evidence of consolidation.

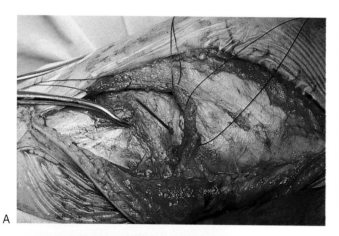
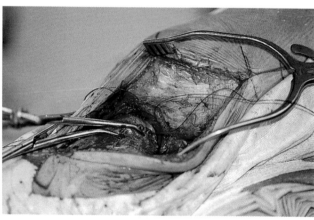
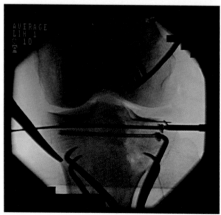

FIGURE 30-17. A to C: Placement of lag screws across the split fracture component.

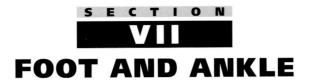

SECTION VII
FOOT AND ANKLE

CHAPTER 31

ARTHROSCOPY OF THE ANKLE

J. SERGE PARISIEN

Arthroscopy is a well-established procedure for the management of many synovial, chondral, and osteochondral lesions of the ankle. Mastering this challenging technique requires a good understanding of the regional anatomy and familiarity with the various arthroscopic portals. Many potential complications are associated with ankle arthroscopy. However, with proper indications and in the hands of an experienced surgeon, this technique usually yields a high percentage of excellent to good results, with the added advantages of minimal morbidity, shorter hospitalization, and rapid recovery time for the patient.

ANATOMY

Knowledge of the extraarticular anatomy and familiarity with the arthroscopic portals are two prerequisites for a successful ankle arthroscopic procedure. Three bones constitute the ankle joint: the tibia with its medial malleolus, the fibula with its lateral malleolus, and the talus. The tip of the medial malleolus is located approximately 2.0 cm distal to the joint line, and the tip of the lateral malleolus is placed approximately 2.0 cm distal and 2.0 cm posterior to the tip of the medial malleolus. The posterior margin of the joint is situated approximately 0.5 cm distal to the anterior articular margin (Fig. 31-1). The talar dome is wider anteriorly than posteriorly and has a convexity in the sagittal plane and a slight concavity in the coronal plane.

Three sensory nerves—the saphenous, superficial peroneal, and sural nerves—are present in the subcutaneous layer. The deep layer contains, anteriorly, the tibialis anticus tendon, the extensor hallucis longus, and the extensor digitorum longus. Between the extensor hallucis longus and the extensor digitorum longus lie the deep peroneal nerve and the dorsalis pedis artery. On the medial aspect of the joint, within the tarsal tunnel, are found the posterior tibial tendon, the flexor digitorum longus tendon, the posterior tibial artery and nerve, and the flexor hallucis longus tendon. Laterally, the peroneus brevis and peroneus longus lie behind the lateral malleolus and insert on the tuberosity of the

fifth metatarsal and onto the first metatarsal and medial cuneiform, respectively (Figs. 31-2 and 31-3). Medially, the deep and superficial fibers of the deltoid ligament give stability to the joint. The superficial, extraarticular layer runs from the anterior prominence of the medial malleolus and

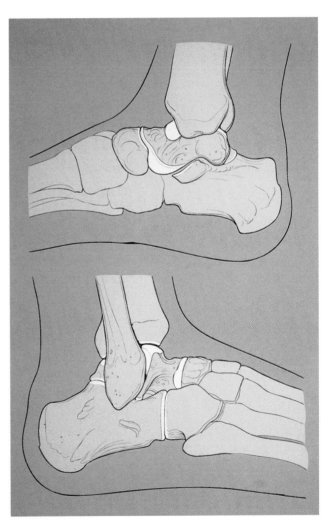

FIGURE 31-1. Bony components of the ankle joint.

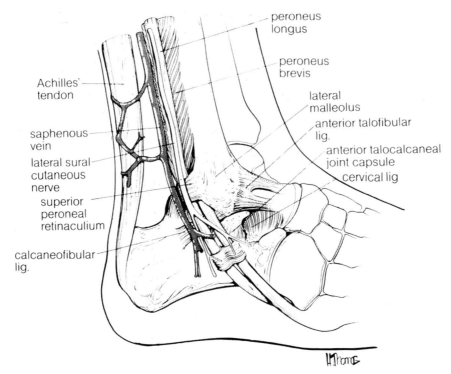

peroneus
longus

peroneus
brevis

Achilles'
tendon

lateral
malleolus

anterior talofibular
lig.

saphenous
vein

anterior talocalcaneal
joint capsule

lateral sural
cutaneous
nerve

cervical lig

superior
peroneal
retinaculium

calcaneofibular
lig.

FIGURE 31-2. Lateral aspect of the ankle joint. (From Parisien JS. Arthroscopic surgery of the ankle. In: *Arthroscopic surgery*. New York: McGraw-Hill, 1988:260, with permission.)

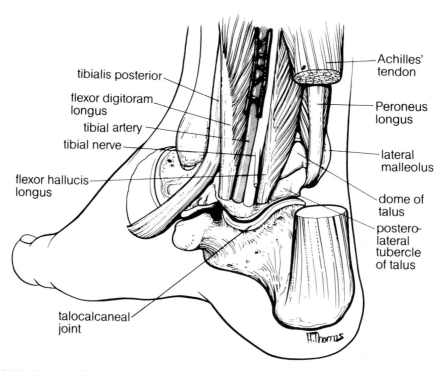

tibialis posterior

Achilles'
tendon

flexor digitoram
longus

Peroneus
longus

tibial artery

tibial nerve

lateral
malleolus

flexor hallucis
longus

dome of
talus

postero-
lateral
tubercle
of talus

talocalcaneal
joint

FIGURE 31-3. Medial aspect of the ankle joint. (From Parisien JS. Arthroscopic surgery of the ankle. In: *Arthroscopic surgery*. New York: McGraw-Hill, 1988:260, with permission.)

inserts onto the talus, calcaneus, spring ligament, and navicular. The deep, intraarticular layer originates from the posterior aspect of the medial malleolus and inserts on the posterior aspect of the talus. The lateral malleolus anteriorly gives rise to the anterior talofibular ligament and anteroinferior tibiofibular ligament and, more posteriorly, to the calcaneofibular ligament, posterior talofibular ligament, and posteroinferior tibiofibular ligament with its extension, the transverse tibiofibular ligament.

Arthroscopic Portals

Three primary portals are most commonly used in diagnostic and surgical arthroscopy of the ankle: the anteromedial, the anterolateral, and the posterolateral. Two accessory anterior portals can be used in addition to the primary portals. The anteromedial portal is developed medial to the tibialis anticus tendon at the joint line level. The saphenous vein and nerve are in proximity and located close to the anterior aspect of the medial malleolus. The anterolateral portal is located lateral to the peroneus tertius and extensor digitorum longus at or a little proximal to the joint line. This portal is in proximity to the terminal branches of the superficial peroneal nerve (Fig. 31-4). This nerve bifurcates approximately 6.5 cm proximal to the tip of the lateral malleolus into the medial dorsal and intermediate dorsal cutaneous branches. Whereas the medial sensory branches cross the anterior aspect of the ankle overlying the common extensor tendon,

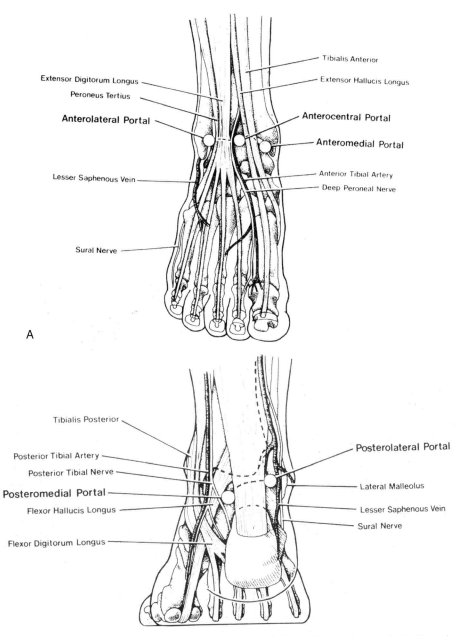

FIGURE 31-4. A: Anterior aspect of the ankle joint and the arthroscopic portals. **B:** Posterior aspect of the ankle joint and the arthroscopic portals. (From Parisien JS. Arthroscopic surgery of the ankle. In: *Arthroscopic surgery.* New York: McGraw-Hill, 1988:264–265, with permission.)

the intermediate dorsal, the most lateral sensory branch, crosses the anterolateral joint line over the common extensor tendon of the fourth and fifth toes, making it vulnerable to injury while placing the anterolateral portal.

The accessory anteromedial portal is placed approximately 1.0 cm inferior to the primary anteromedial portal. The accessory anterolateral portal is established approximately 1.0 cm anterior to the tip of the lateral malleolus. The anterocentral portal, located lateral to the extensor hallucis longus, is not recommended because of the potential injuries to the neurovascular bundle (i.e., deep peroneal nerve and anterior tibial artery).

The posterolateral portal is placed approximately 2.0 cm above the tip of the lateral malleolus, adjacent to the lateral border of the Achilles tendon, to avoid injury to the sural nerve.

The posteromedial portal is rarely used because of its proximity to the posterior neurovascular structures. It passes between the Achilles tendon and the posterior tibial neurovascular bundle. The lateral and medial coaxial portals, which have been described in hemophilic patients, are parallel to the bimalleolar axis of the ankle joint. They allow complete synovectomy of the posterior compartment of the ankle. Contrary to the conventional approaches, the coaxial posterolateral portal is established posterior to the peroneal tendon sheath, 1.5 cm to 2.0 cm proximal to the distal tip of the fibula. Using a blunt-tipped obturator through the posterolateral portal, the capsule is entered anterior to the

posterior tibial tendon and behind the posterior surface of the medial malleolus to develop the posteromedial portal.

Arthroscopic Anatomy

Several intraarticular structures are visible arthroscopically (Fig. 31-5). Medially, the medial malleolus articulates with the corresponding articular surface of the medial dome of the talus to form the medial talomalleolar space. The deep portion of the deltoid ligament is seen as it originates from the tip of the medial malleolus and runs vertically to insert onto the medial surface of the talus. The medial corner of the ankle, the area where the tibial plafond articulates with the medial dome of the talus, has a notch (i.e., notch of Harty). The anterior synovial recess is between the anterior tibial lip and the superior insertion of the capsule onto the distal tibia. Within the recess lies an irregular area of periosteum-covered bone that can be the site of the so-called impingement exostosis. Laterally, the anteroinferior tibiofibular ligament is seen along with the distal aspect of the lateral tibial plafond and the lateral aspect of the talus. Behind the anteroinferior tibiofibular ligament are located a synovial recess and the tibiofibular articulation. The space between the fibular and the lateral border of the talus forms the lateral talomalleolar space. It extends distally to the anterior talofibular ligament to form the lateral gutter. The anterior talofibular ligament is seen as a capsular reflection extending

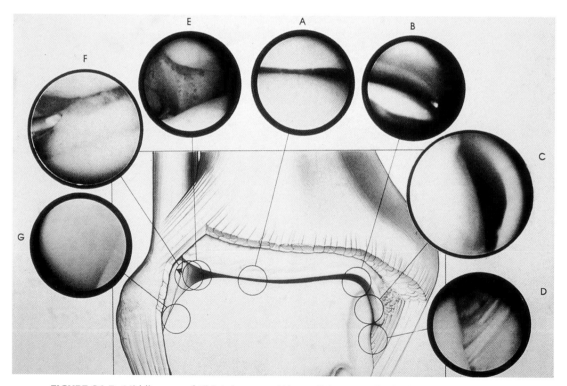

FIGURE 31-5. Middle area of tibiotalar space (A), medial aspect of talotibial space (B), medial talomalleolar space (C), intraarticular structures: deep portion of deltoid ligament (D), lateral aspect of tibiotalar space (E), lateral aspect of joint (F), and lateral talomalleolar space (G). (From Parisien JS. Arthroscopic surgery of the ankle. In: *Arthroscopic surgery.* New York: McGraw-Hill, 1988:261, with permission.)

from the tip of the lateral malleolus to the lateral aspect of the talus. The anterior gutter represents the reflection of the capsule as it attaches onto the neck of the talus anteriorly. It contains a synovial recess and a bare area of talar bone not covered by articular cartilage. With adequate distraction posteriorly, the posterior inferior tibiofibular ligament can be seen as a strong band running obliquely at a 45-degree angle from the tibia to the fibula. Inferior to this ligament is located the transverse tibiofibular ligament. With the arthroscope placed through the posterolateral portal, the posterior capsular pouch can be visualized that is smaller than its anterior counterpart. The posterior aspect of the deltoid ligament, the posterior aspect of the medial talus and tibial plafond, as well as the central and posterolateral aspects of the joint, can also be examined.

EQUIPMENT AND INSTRUMENTATION

Equipment includes 4.0- and 2.7-mm arthroscopes with 30-degree obliquity that can be used for ankle arthroscopy. The 70-degree arthroscope is also useful to visualize the posterior aspects of the gutters and better evaluate a posteriorly located osteochondral lesion of the talus. Small-joint instruments are necessary to cut, retrieve, and repair (Figs. 31-6 to 31-8).

The hand-maneuvered and motorized instruments include a small mosquito clamp, an 18-gauge spinal needle, a probe, a curved dissector, a grasping forceps, a small basket forceps, various surgical blades, small curettes, an osteotome, a rasp, and a small owl. Motorized instruments (i.e., full-radius resector, cartilage cutter, synovectomy blade, and small burrs) with various blades are available. Biodegradable pins are also available to reattach viable osteochondral lesions of the talus. An aiming device for adequate positioning of guide wires or screws is also available.

Some surgeons advocate the use of distraction devices to improve visualization of the joint. Two types of distraction technique are available: the invasive and the noninvasive.

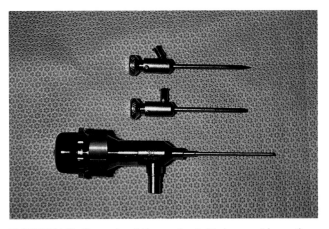

FIGURE 31-7. Shown is a 2.7-mm, short, 30-degree video arthroscope *(bottom)* with a trocar in the cannula *(top)*.

For the invasive technique, a 0.187-inch-diameter, threaded pin is drilled into the lateral aspect of the tibia approximately 2 inches proximal to the joint and behind the anterior tibial crest. A second pin is inserted distal to the joint into the lateral aspect of the os calcis, 0.5 inch anterior to its posterior border and 0.5 inch above its inferior border. The pins do not have to penetrate the medial cortex of the bones, and a pin cannula is used to protect the soft tissues while drilling. The distractor is secured with the locking thumb nuts, and distraction is applied until a joint space opening of 4 to 5 mm is obtained at the beginning. Distraction up to 8 mm can be achieved gradually. Distraction for more than 90 minutes is not recommended to avoid stretching the ligaments. Potential complications of the invasive technique are broken pins, pin tract problems, neurovascular damage, and stress fractures.

The noninvasive distraction can be achieved using a sterile ankle distractor and a foot strap. Many noninvasive sets are available on the market. Twenty-five pounds of traction for 1 hour are recommended. With increased distraction time and force, symptoms of paresthesia of the deep and superficial peroneal nerves may occur. The noninvasive mode

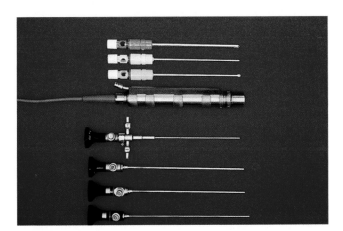

FIGURE 31-6. Shown are 4-mm, 30- and 70-degree arthroscopes *(bottom)* and motorized shaver with various blades *(top)*.

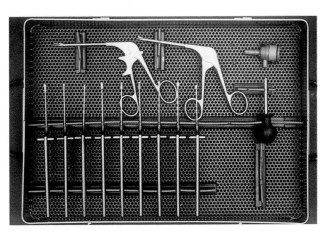

FIGURE 31-8. Set of hand instruments, including baskets, knives, and curettes.

is preferred to the invasive to avoid possible complications with the use of pins in the tibia and talus or calcaneus.

Gravity irrigation is usually used during arthroscopic surgery of the ankle. However, when an increased fluid pressure is desirable, an infusion pump can be used during the procedure. **Careful monitoring of the outflow system during the use of the pump is mandatory to avoid extravasation of fluid into the foot and lower leg.**

INDICATIONS AND CONTRAINDICATIONS

The indications for arthroscopic surgery of the ankle include soft tissue lesions and osteochondral lesions. The soft tissue lesions include localized or generalized posttraumatic synovitis; anterior or posterior soft tissue impingement from a chronic ankle sprain; syndesmotic impingement due to trauma; some rheumatologic disorders, such as rheumatoid arthritis; pigmented villonodular synovitis; hemophilia; syn-

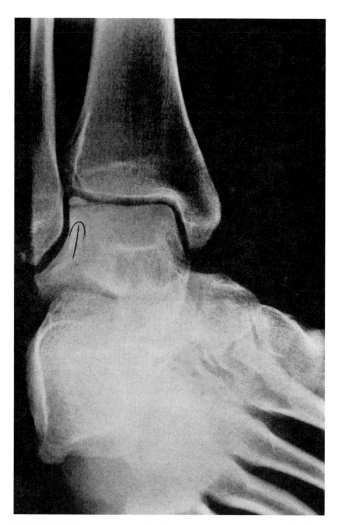

FIGURE 31-10. Osteochondral lesion on the lateral aspect of the talus.

ovial chondromatosis; some infectious synovitides; and some cases of arthrofibrosis.

Arthroscopy has been successfully used in the management of chondral and osteochondral lesions of the ankle (i.e., osteochondritis dissecans of the talus, impingement exostosis, and loose bodies (Figs. 31-9 to 31-12). Arthroscopy is being used in some centers for the management of acute ankle fractures to assess the articular surfaces, to obtain an anatomic reduction, and to remove loose articular fragments and debris from the joint. In chronic ankle fractures, arthroscopy has been very useful. It allows identification and removal of loose chondral or osteochondral loose fragments and the excision of scar tissue and proliferative synovium.

Arthroscopically assisted ankle arthrodesis, by minimizing the amount of soft tissue dissection, is an alternative to an open procedure, provided that there is no preexisting major varus or valgus deformity of the joint. The major benefits in the hands of the experienced arthroscopist seem to be a better tolerance by the patients, increased rate of fusion, and a low infection rate.

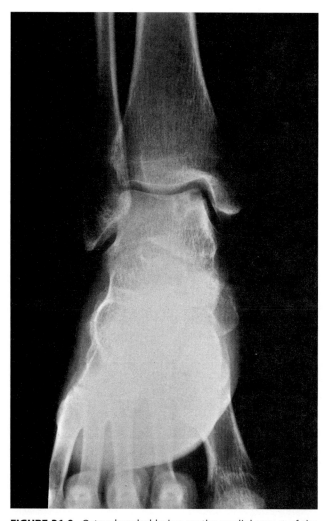

FIGURE 31-9. Osteochondral lesion on the medial aspect of the talus.

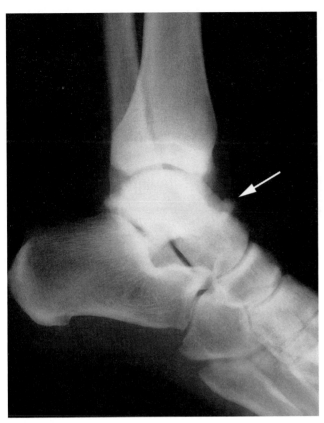

FIGURE 31-11. Impingement exostoses of the tibial plafond and talus.

scopic cannula is inserted into the anterior pouch of the ankle joint. From the anteromedial portal, the joint is visualized. The scope is then removed, and the blunt obturator is reinserted into the joint to develop the anterolateral portal lateral to the peroneus tertius and extensor tendons. This anterolateral portal is close to the intermediate branch of the superficial peroneal nerve. This nerve can be seen or palpated by placing the ankle in forced inversion. Visualization also can be achieved by means of transillumination. With the superficial peroneal nerve precisely localized and under constant observation, the skin is tented with the blunt obturator of the arthroscope. A vertical incision is made over the tip of the obturator for the placement of a small cannula into the joint through this newly created anterolateral incision (Fig. 31-14). The posterolateral portal may be used for inflow, if necessary. The 18-gauge needle can be used close

SURGICAL TECHNIQUES FOR SOFT TISSUE LESIONS

Anterior Lesions

The patient is placed in a supine position, with the ipsilateral buttock elevated on a folded sheet (Fig. 31-13). The leg is immobilized in a leg holder and the foot placed on a well-padded box or a roll of sheet. With this setup, the anterior and posterior aspects of the ankle are accessible with rotation of the leg. After preparing and draping the extremity in the standard fashion, the external landmarks are outlined with a marking pen: anterior tibialis, peroneus tertius tendons, joint line, medial and lateral malleoli, and superficial peroneal nerve branches.

The anterior portal is developed first by placing an 18-gauge needle medial to the tibialis anticus tendon. The joint is distended with normal saline solution. While palpating and retracting the tendon with the thumb of the opposite hand, a vertical skin incision is made with a no. 11 blade. A small mosquito clamp is used to dissect the subcutaneous tissue down to the capsule. The blunt trocar with the arthro-

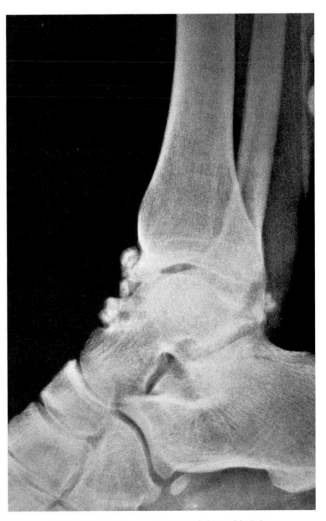

FIGURE 31-12. Loose bodies of the ankle joint.

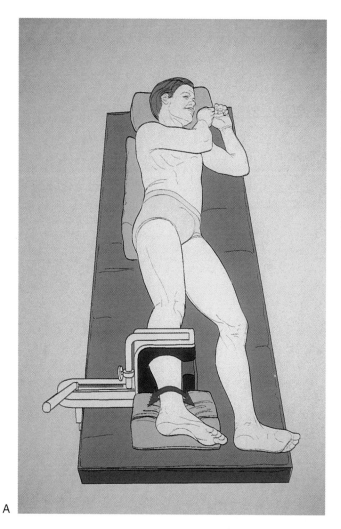

A

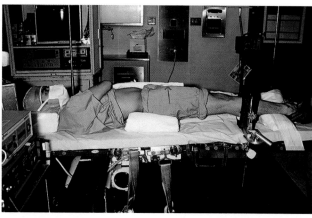

B

FIGURE 31-13. A: The illustration shows positioning for ankle arthroscopy. **B:** The photogaph shows positioning for ankle arthroscopy.

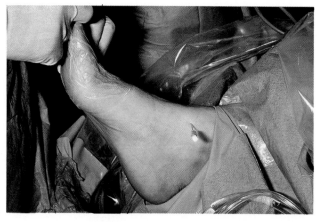

A

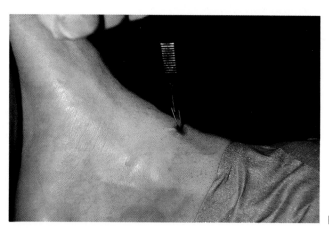

B

FIGURE 31-14. A: A spinal needle is placed medial to the tibialis anterior to distend joint capsule with normal saline. **B:** Vertical skin incision is made after removal of the needle. *(continued)*

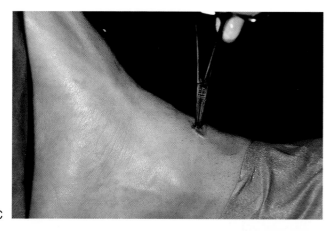

C

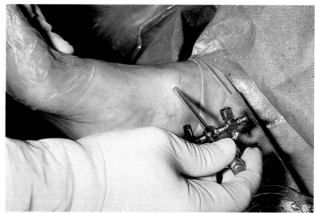

D

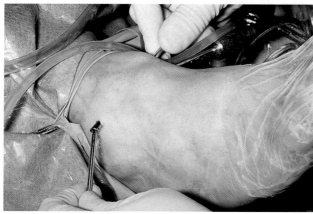

E

FIGURE 31-14. *Continued.* **C:** A small mosquito clamp is used to spread the soft tissue down to the capsule. **D:** An arthroscope is placed through the anteromedial portal. **E:** Development of the anterolateral portal.

to the Achilles tendon, 2.0 cm proximal to the tip of the lateral malleolus, to obtain a backflow before making a vertical skin incision and using the curved mosquito clamp to dissect the subcutaneous tissue.

Usually, the synovial pathology is located anteriorly, and soft tissue lesions can be addressed with the two anterior portals. Débridement of localized, nonspecific synovitis and excision of scar tissue can be done with a motorized shaver.

The anterolateral soft tissue impingement (which can be caused by the so-called meniscoid lesion or the presence of thick, inflamed synovial tissue in the lateral gutter or a separate fascicle from the anterior tibiofibular ligament) can be treated the same way (Figs. 31-15 to 31-17). Syndesmotic impingement due to scarring and inflammation in the area of the anterior tibiofibular ligament and distal tibiofibular joint can benefit from arthroscopic débridement. After clo-

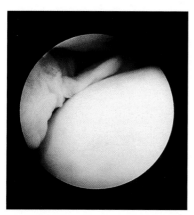

FIGURE 31-15. Synovial impingement in the anterolateral aspect of the right ankle.

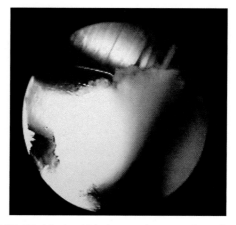

FIGURE 31-16. Meniscoid lesion on the anterolateral aspect of the ankle.

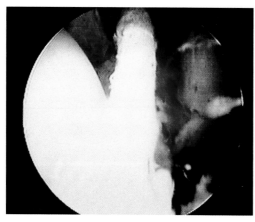

FIGURE 31-17. A fibrotic band on the anterior aspect of the ankle causing impingement.

sure of the portals with 3-0 nylon sutures, a compression dressing is applied for 2 to 3 days. Range-of-motion exercise is encouraged very early.

Posterior Soft Tissue Lesions

When the soft tissue lesion is posteriorly located or generalized with posterior involvement, distraction may be helpful to allow complete visualization. The use of the tourniquet with an infusion pump may speed the procedure. In general, if the ankle joint is tight and the pathology generalized or localized posteriorly, a noninvasive system can be used for the distraction before the start of the procedure (Fig. 31-18). The noninvasive clamp is attached to the table, and soft tissue distraction is obtained with the sterile strap over the dorsum of the foot and around the heel.

After complete synovectomy, the tourniquet is deflated

and a suction Hemovac is used before closure. A compression dressing is applied, and ambulation with crutches is advisable for the first 7 days.

SURGICAL TECHNIQUE FOR OSTEOCHONDRAL LESIONS

Posteromedial Lesions

Posteromedial lesions are more common and are located at the middle aspect of the dome of the talus, sometimes with posterior extension. They are managed with the scope placed in the anterolateral portal and the surgical instrument through the anteromedial portal. When removing a loose, degenerated, nonviable fragment, it is almost the rule that excision is achieved through the anteromedial portal. The following steps are usually necessary. The 70-degree scope is used through the anterolateral portal for visualization after a partial synovectomy is done with a small shaver. A sharp banana knife or smooth dissector is used through the medial portal to complete the dissection of the fragment. A small grasping forceps is used for the excision and a small curette to débride the base of the crater down to a bleeding bed (Figs. 31-19 and 31-20). Depending on the location of the lesion on the talar done, drilling can be done with 0.062-inch Kirschner wires (K-wires) through the medial malleolus (i.e., transmalleolar approach) or through the anteromedial portal. If the fragment is viable and is not too posterior, it can be fixated with absorbable pins or small, cannulated screws. When absorbable pins are used, stable fixation is achieved by using two or three pins. Stabilization of the lesion before drilling may be obtained through an accessory anteromedial portal with a small probe or a smooth K-wire. If the fragment is too posterior, fixation may be

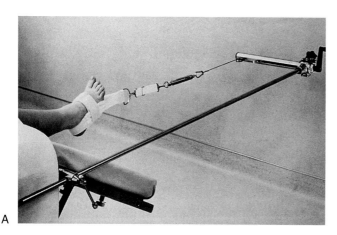

A

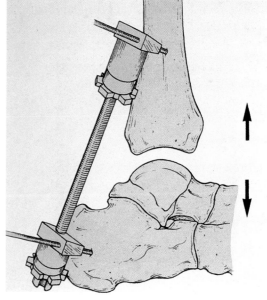

B

FIGURE 31-18. A: Noninvasive distraction. **B:** Invasive distraction

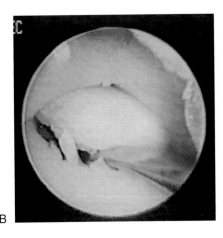
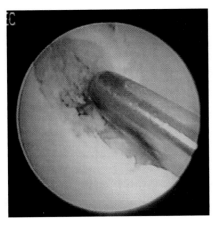

A, B

FIGURE 31-19. Excision of a posteromedial lesion of the talus in the right ankle. **A:** Manipulation of an osteochondral lesion of the talus. **B:** The defect is abraded with a motorized shaver.

achieved through an arthrotomy incision. Preoperative computed tomography or magnetic resonance imaging in the coronal and sagittal planes can be helpful in planning the procedure.

Anteromedial Lesions

Anteromedial lesions are unusual. They can be approached through the anteromedial portal with the scope placed laterally. Drilling, pinning, or excision can be achieved when indicated.

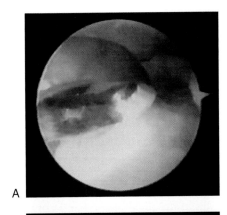

A

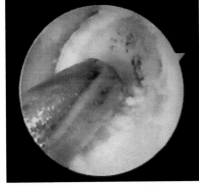

B

FIGURE 31-20. Excision of a posteromedial lesion of the talus in the left ankle. **A:** Curettage with a curette. **B:** Formal débridement with a motorized saw.

Anterolateral Lesions

Anterolateral lesions, because of their location, are easily accessible. They are approached with the scope placed medially and the surgical instrument laterally. A loose, viable articular fragment can be reduced and pinned. A degenerated fragment can be excised and the bed drilled with a small K-wire (Figs. 31-21 to 31-23).

Cystic Lesions

When a large cyst is present with normal overlying articular cartilage, bone grafting can be performed. Under fluoroscopy, a K-wire is placed into the osteochondral defect anteriorly through the anteromedial portal. A small window is removed with a core of subchondral bone. With the 70-degree scope placed laterally, the cyst can be curetted under direct vision with a long curette. If necessary, a small, 2.5-mm scope can be placed into the cyst to confirm the adequacy of the curettage. Bone graft is inserted into the cystic defect of the talus.

Posterolateral Lesions

Posterolateral lesions are uncommon. They can be visualized through the anteromedial portal using a 70-degree

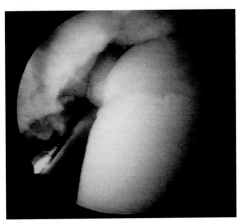

FIGURE 31-21. Arthroscopic view of an anterolateral lesion of the talus.

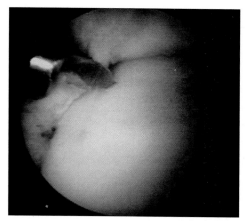

FIGURE 31-22. The lesion was drilled before fixation with a biodegradable pin.

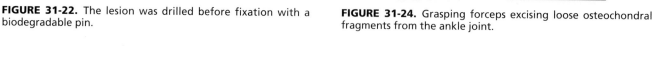

FIGURE 31-24. Grasping forceps excising loose osteochondral fragments from the ankle joint.

scope. Excision can be done through the anterolateral portal using the same steps described for the excision of postero-medial lesions. Drilling of the bed can be done through the posterolateral portal.

POSTOPERATIVE PROTOCOL

The wounds are closed with 3-0 nylon sutures, and a compression dressing is applied for 2 to 3 days. Range-of-motion exercise of the ankle is begun immediately. After removal of the dressing, ice applications are started. Weight bearing is allowed gradually, as tolerated by the patient, if the lesion is less then 1.0 cm in diameter. For larger lesions, non–weight-bearing ambulation is prescribed for 6 to 8 weeks. Rehabilitation is started under guidance of a physical therapist after complete healing of the wound and diminution of the swelling.

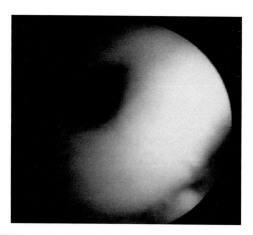

FIGURE 31-23. Biodegradable pin in a reduced fragment.

SURGICAL TECHNIQUE FOR LOOSE BODIES

Loose bodies can be chondral or osteochondral. They can be single or multiple, as seen in synovial osteochondromatosis (Fig. 31-24). When they are located in the anterior compartment, they can be removed through the two anterior portals. When placed posteriorly, visualization and extraction through the posterolateral portal are improved with some type of noninvasive distraction if the ankle is tight. After retrieval of the loose bodies, a careful assessment of the articular cartilage is done to rule out the presence of any chondral or osteochondral defect. In the latter situation, proper débridement should complete the procedure. Postoperatively, the patient is allowed to bear full weight, as tolerated.

SURGICAL TECHNIQUE FOR IMPINGEMENT EXOSTOSES

Exostoses of the ankle joint are most often present above the anterior lip of the tibial plafond and can be associated with a corresponding osteophyte on the opposing surface of the talus. They can also be found in the front of the malleoli, mostly the medial malleolus. This condition is common in runners, dancers, gymnasts, high jumpers, and football players. It may be caused by forced dorsiflexion injuries or capsular avulsion injuries after forced plantar flexion. Plain radiographs can demonstrate the presence of the lesions, and lateral radiographs in forced dorsiflexion can document the impingement when the two anterior spurs are present.

Although exostoses can be seen on x-ray films, they can be asymptomatic. When they are symptomatic and do not respond to conservative treatment, arthroscopic surgery is

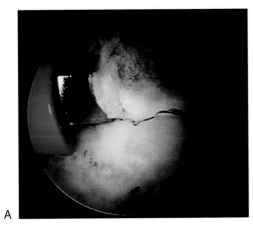 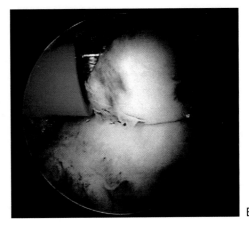

FIGURE 31-25. A: Exostosis on the anterior aspect of the tibial plafond. **B:** Exostosis being excised with an osteotome.

indicated for their removal. No distraction is necessary because the pathology is usually anterior. The standard anterolateral and anteromedial portals are used for the procedure. Partial synovectomy is very often necessary to improve visualization. The small shaver is then used to peel off the capsular insertion from the anterior aspect of the osteophyte. The osteophyte is removed with a small straight or curved osteotome (Fig. 31-25). The bone fragment is excised with a grasper. The remaining irregular surface can be smoothed off with a small burr or a rasp. An osteophyte on the talus can be removed with an abrader (Fig. 31-26). Before completion of the procedure, switching the scope between the anterior portals and intraoperative lateral radiographs can help to determine the adequacy of the anterior resection. Compression dressing is applied. After a short period of immobilization and ambulating with crutches, rehabilitation is started. Full return to sports activities or dancing may take 6 to 8 weeks.

SURGICAL TECHNIQUE FOR ARTHROSCOPICALLY ASSISTED ANKLE ARTHRODESIS

The patient is placed supine on the operating table, with noninvasive or invasive distraction attached to the ankle. To obtain the maximum visualization, the procedure is done under an image intensifier (Fig. 31-27). The three standard portals are used, the two anterior and the posterolateral portals. A motorized shaver is used to excise the adhesions with a synovectomy. The articular surfaces of the tibial plafond, talar dome, and medial and lateral malleolar spaces are excised with a combination of motorized shaver, curette, and rasps. The cancellous bone is exposed and small dimples are made on the opposing articular surfaces with the small burr. Anterior osteophytes, if present, are excised to achieve adequate reduction of the convex articular surface of the talus into the concave surface of the tibial plafond. Two guide

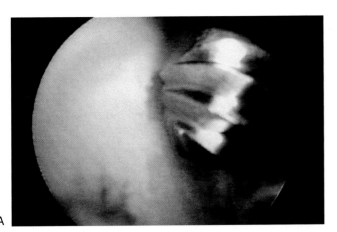 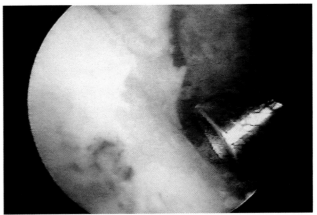

FIGURE 31-26. A: Exostoses, with the talar dome being removed with an abrader. **B:** After excision of the exostoses from the talar dome.

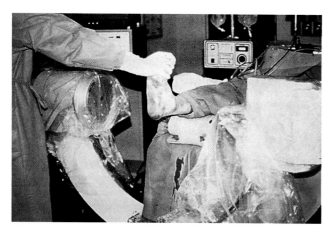

FIGURE 31-27. The procedure is done with image intensifier

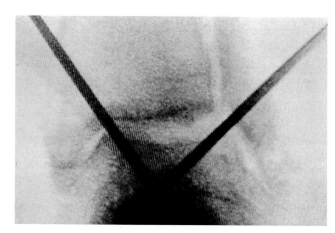

FIGURE 31-28. Guide pins are advanced into the talus.

pins are drilled from the malleoli and angled 45 degrees anteriorly and inferiorly. <u>After the tips of the pins are seen with the arthroscope, the distraction is released, and fluoroscopy is used to confirm the placement of the tibial and talar surfaces in a neutral position. The guide pins are then advanced distally into the talus</u> (Fig. 31-28), <u>and after determining the proper length of the screws to be used for fixation, two 6-5 mm cannulated screws are placed over the guide pins and advanced into the talus without violating the subtalar joint distally.</u> Permanent x-ray films are used to confirm the reduction and position of the fusion site and verify screw placement. The distraction apparatus is removed, and the arthroscopic portals are closed with 3-0 nylon sutures. The ankle is first placed in a posterior splint. After removal of the

stitches, a short leg cast is applied. Weight bearing is allowed in 2 to 3 weeks, as tolerated by the patient. The cast is removed in 6 to 8 weeks, when full union is seen on radiographs.

SUGGESTED READINGS

Acevedo J, Busch MT, Ganey TM, et al. Coaxial portals for posterior ankle arthroscopy: an anatomic study with clinical correlation on 29 patients. *Arthroscopy* 2000;16:836–842.

Ferkel R. *Arthroscopic surgery of the foot and ankle.* New York: Lippincott-Raven Publishers, 1996.

Guhl J. *Foot and ankle arthroscopy.* Thorofare, NJ: Slack,1993.

Parisien JS. *Techniques in therapeutic arthroscopy.* New York: Raven Press, 1993.

CHAPTER 32

ANKLE FUSION: CANNULATED SCREWS

KENNETH A. EGOL

Arthrosis involving the ankle and hindfoot results in pain, decreased range of ankle motion, and limited ambulatory ability. Ankle arthrodesis is the treatment of choice for patients suffering from disabling pain from osteoarthritis, posttraumatic arthritis, or rheumatoid arthritis. Numerous techniques have been reported in the literature to obtain successful union. These include screws, plates and screws, external fixation, and intramedullary devices. Each technique has been met with success and failure.

Often, there is an existing deformity in the hindfoot. Successful treatment of the underlying condition requires correction of any deformity at the time of arthrodesis to allow for optimal union rate and functional recovery.

The major problem with ankle arthrodesis is the rate of nonunion, which ranges from 0% to 40%. Risk factors for the development of a nonunion include diabetes, poor nutritional status, infection, nicotine use, and peripheral neuropathy.

ANATOMY

The ankle is a hinge joint. The bony anatomy of the ankle joint (tibiotalar) includes the distal tibia and fibula and the talar body (Fig. 32-1). As the tibial shaft flares in the supramalleolar region, the dense cortical bone changes to metaphyseal cancellous bone. The shape of the tibial articular surface is concave with distal extension of the anterior and posterior lips. This surface has been called the *tibial plafond,* which is a French word meaning *ceiling.* The wedge-shaped talar dome sits within the mortise and is wider anteriorly than posteriorly. When the ankle dorsiflexes, there is a compensatory external rotation of the fibula. This leads to abduction of the foot. The malleoli serve as pulleys for tendons reaching plantar surface of the foot from the posterior and lateral compartments of the leg.

The capsule is relatively weak anteriorly and posteriorly and is reinforced by collateral ligaments medially and laterally. On the medial side, the heavy deltoid ligament is attached above to the medial malleolus with its superficial fibers from the anterior colliculus and stronger deep fibers originating from the posterior colliculus. These fibers fan out to attach inferiorly to the talus and calcaneus. The anterior talofibular, calcaneofibular, and posterior talofibular ligaments are attached to the lateral malleolus. The syndesmotic ligament complex includes the anteroinferior and posteroinferior tibial-fibular ligaments, the interosseous ligament, and the transverse tibial-fibular ligament and functions to stabilize the distal fibula with the distal tibia.

INDICATIONS

The primary indication for any ankle arthrodesis is unremitting pain that interferes with activities of daily living that is not relieved by other treatment modalities such as nonsteroidal antiinflammatory medication, modification of shoe wear, bracing, or prior surgical débridement.

Frequently, pain is caused by degenerative arthritic changes. These degenerative changes may follow trauma such a severe ankle fracture or fracture-dislocation, pilon fracture, or unrecognized chondral injury. Rheumatoid arthritis or other collagen disease is a less common cause of ankle degeneration that may lead to complete loss of ankle joint function. Chronic sepsis of an ankle is an indication for fusion. Débridement performed first, followed by fusion, can be a successful way to salvage an extremity. The Charcot ankle may lead to progressive deformity and subsequent skin breakdown. Fusion about the ankle in the Charcot foot usually encompasses more than just the tibiotalar joint. Often, multiple hindfoot articulations must be fused to give the patient a stable, plantigrade foot. Severe deformity is a relative indication because equinus, varus, or valgus not amenable to surgical release can lead to difficulty walking. Ankle fusion may be the only option for a failed total ankle replacement if the limb is to be salvaged in a functional manner.

PREOPERATIVE PLANNING

The initial evaluation of the patient requiring ankle arthrodesis includes a careful assessment. A thorough history is essential specifically any preexisting medical conditions such as peripheral vascular disease or diabetes should be elicited. A careful physical examination, including assessment of any deformity, Achilles tightness, palpation of pulses, and sensory status, is mandatory. Peripheral neuropathy is a known cause of nonunion and its presence, although not an absolute contraindication, may lead to the use of adjunctive methods such as internal or external bone stimulation. Other areas of the hindfoot should be evaluated for presence of arthrosis. This can be done radiographically with use of computed tomography to assess the subtalar joint or selective lidocaine injection to rule out other areas of the "ankle" that may be the cause of persistent postoperative pain. If a subtalar arthrodesis will be required, it can be performed with only a slight extension of the surgical incision. Bone stock also must be assessed. If the indication is posttraumatic, there may be a need for bone grafting; if the fusion follows a failed total ankle replacement; major bone grafting usually is necessary. A standard radiographic ankle trauma series, including anteroposterior, lateral, and mortise views, is required to assess the joint (Fig. 32-2). Standing views may offer a better picture of the clinical situation.

Although numerous techniques are at the surgeon's disposal for performing this operation, I prefer a fusion of bony surfaces with compression provided by three cannulated, partially threaded screws. If bone stock does not suffice or if intraoperative complication leads to overresection of bony surfaces, an external fixator can be used to provide compression.

EQUIPMENT

The equipment needed to perform an ankle arthrodesis is similar to that needed to perform any surgery on the lower

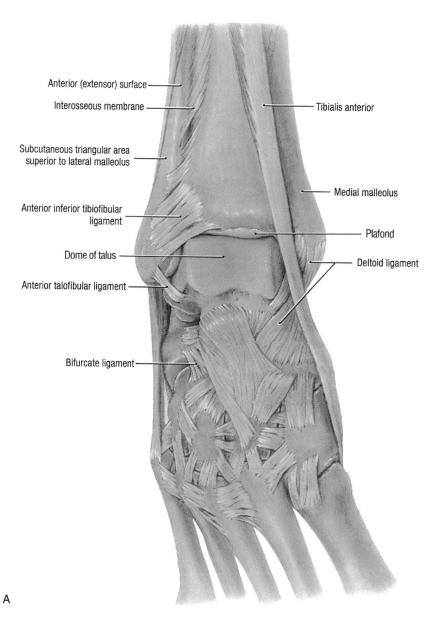

Anterior (extensor) surface

Interosseous membrane

Subcutaneous triangular area superior to lateral malleolus

Anterior inferior tibiofibular ligament

Dome of talus

Anterior talofibular ligament

Bifurcate ligament

Tibialis anterior

Medial malleolus

Plafond

Deltoid ligament

A

FIGURE 32-1. Ankle joint: anterior view **(A)** and posterior view **(B)**. (From Agur AMR, Lee MJ. *Grant's atlas of anatomy,* 10th ed. Philadelphia: Lippincott Williams & Wilkins, 1999, with permission.) *(continued)*

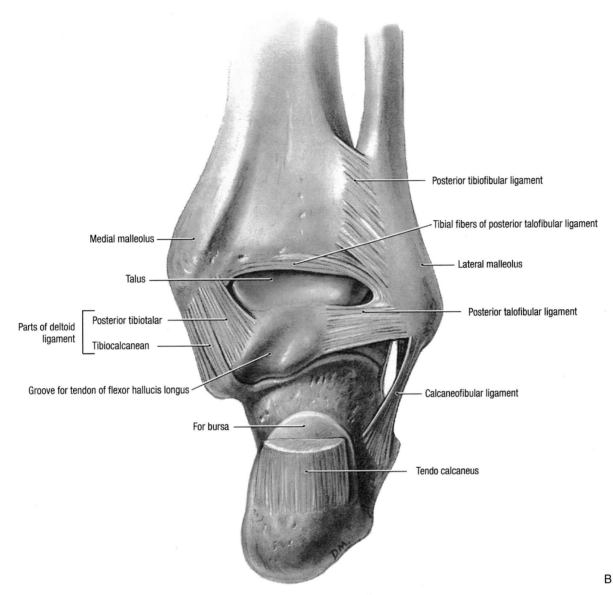

Medial malleolus

Talus

Parts of deltoid ligament
- Posterior tibiotalar
- Tibiocalcanean

Groove for tendon of flexor hallucis longus

For bursa

Posterior tibiofibular ligament

Tibial fibers of posterior talofibular ligament

Lateral malleolus

Posterior talofibular ligament

Calcaneofibular ligament

Tendo calcaneus

B

FIGURE 32-1. *Continued.*

extremity and includes a radiolucent table that can accommodate image intensification, a sterile bolster, osteotomes, curettes, a sagittal saw, and cannulated screws. Intraoperative fluoroscopy is mandatory to confirm foot position, bony cuts, and screw placement. A secondary plan of action should be available if the bone stock is not adequate to accept stable fixation. In this case, an external fixator is usually the implant of choice and should be available (Fig. 32-3).

PATIENT POSTIONING

Patients should be positioned supine with a bolster under the ipsilateral hip (Fig. 32-4). The ipsilateral iliac crest should be prepared and draped if a need for autogenous

bone graft is contemplated. A well-padded tourniquet should be placed on the ipsilateral proximal thigh. The patient's position should take into account the need for intraoperative image intensification, with the ability to obtain anteroposterior, lateral, and mortise views. The draping of the extremity should allow for 90 degrees of knee flexion.

SURGICAL INCISION

Usually, the procedure is performed through two incisions; however, if there was no previous surgery and no internal fixation is present, a lateral incision alone may be used. Laterally, the incision parallels the fibula and begins 8 cm proximal to the tip of the lateral malleolus (Fig. 32-5).This

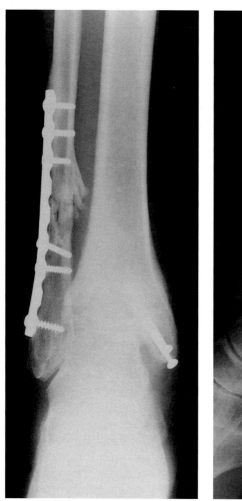
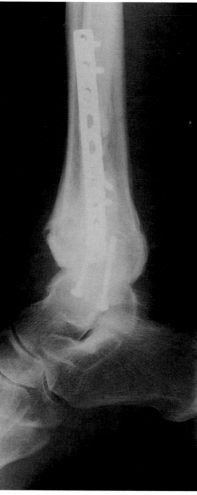
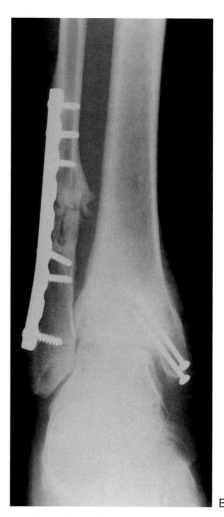

A

B, C

FIGURE 32-2. Anteroposterior **(A)**, lateral **(B)**, and mortise **(C)** preoperative radiographs.

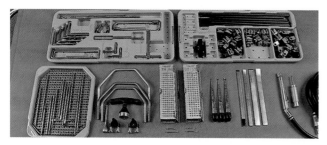

FIGURE 32-3. Equipment for ankle fusion. *Bottom row, third from left*: cannulated screws and curettes (3), osteotomes (4), and sagittal saw. *Top row and bottom left*: external fixator trays (3) and rings from a fixator set. The fixator is used when a patient's bone stock is not adequate for stable fixation.

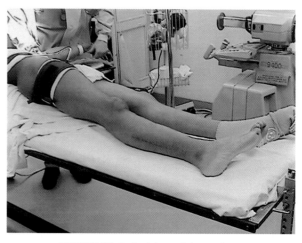

FIGURE 32-4. Position of the patient.

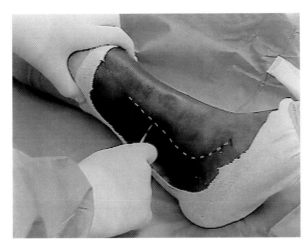

FIGURE 32-5. The lateral incision begins 8 cm from the tip of the malleolus.

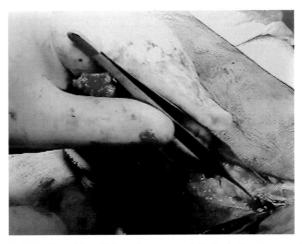

FIGURE 32-7. Identifying the external hallucis brevis muscle belly.

incision extends distally and curves toward the fourth metatarsal across the sinus tarsi. A second anteromedial incision is made over the medial malleolus (Fig. 32-6). The lengths of these incisions are altered, depending on the presence of preexisting hardware. If hardware from a previous internal fixation or attempted fusion is present, it should be removed after the exposure has been performed and before any osteotomies are performed.

PROCEDURE

Beginning on the lateral side, soft tissues, including the peroneals and flexor hallucis longus are sharply elevated from the fibula. An oblique osteotomy is performed 6 to 8 cm proximal to the tip of the fibula. ◼ The fibula is freed of all soft tissue by subperiosteal elevation. A towel clip is used to pull traction on the fibula, and the bone is released from its ligamentous attachments at the distal end. ◼ Exposure to the lateral talotibial joint is now afforded. Deep dissection

distally occurs between the extensor hallucis brevis muscle belly and the peroneal tendons (Fig. 32-7). Attention is then tuned to the medial side. Care is taken to preserve the saphenous vein and its branches. The posterior tibial tendon and posteromedial neurovascular structures are freed and protected. The medial malleolus is then osteotomized at a 45-degree angle toward the corner of the joint. ◼ Care is taken to avoid overresection of the medial tibial flare, because it serves to anchor hardware. The anterior ankle capsule is then elevated to view the articular surface from both sides (Fig. 32-8).

At this point, the articular surfaces of the tibial plafond and talar dome are denuded of remaining cartilage down to bleeding subchondral bone. ◼ If severe deformity exists, the appropriate osteotomy is performed to get the surfaces of the tibia and talus opposed. This is accomplished with the aid of an oscillating saw or osteotomes. ◼ **In either case, it is critical to avoid overresection of bone, especially on the talar side, so as not to compromise bone stock. No more than 3 to 4 mm of the bone should be resected.**

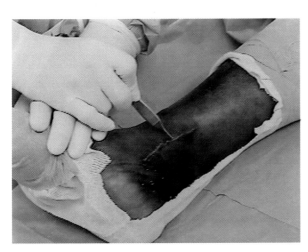

FIGURE 32-6. Anteromedial incision over the medial malleolus.

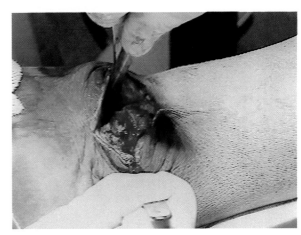

FIGURE 32-8. Elevation of the ankle joint capsule.

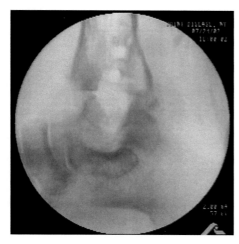

FIGURE 32-9. Angle of Gissane should line up with the mid-axis of the tibia.

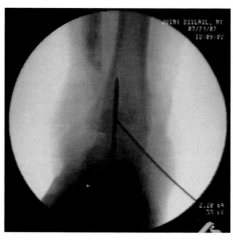

FIGURE 32-11. A second provisional Kirschner wire is placed for rotational control.

A critical point is positioning of the foot before internal fixation. The hindfoot should be placed in a plantigrade position with the ankle at 90 degrees. The hindfoot should be placed in 5 degrees of valgus and slight external rotation. The talus is translated slightly posteriorly to place the foot in line with the weight-bearing axis. This can be confirmed radiographically by aligning the angle of Gissane with the midshaft of the tibia on the lateral radiograph (Fig. 32-9). ◨

At this point, a smooth Steinman pin is placed retrograde from the calcaneus across the subtalar joint and across the ankle (Fig. 32-10). ◨ A second, smaller Kirschner wire is placed across the tibiotalar articulation for rotational control (Fig. 32-11). At this point, the position of the fusion is checked radiographically on anteroposterior, lateral, and mortise views. With acceptable alignment achieved, the guide wires for the cannulated screws are placed. These can be 6.5-, 7.3-, or 8.0-mm, cannulated, partially threaded cancellous screws, depending on the size of the patient. Two

screws are placed from proximal to distal aspects. The proximal, medial guide wire is placed approximately 2 cm above the articular surface, about 5 mm posterior to the midaxis of the tibia and angling about 60 degrees toward the anterolateral talus. ◨ The second wire is placed 2 cm proximal to the joint on the lateral side and 5 mm anterior to the midaxis of the tibia and is angled posteromedially into the talus. ◨ The third wire starts distally and enters the talus anterolaterally, and it is angled proximally into the posteromedial tibia. ◨ After the guide wires are placed and confirmed radiographically, the lengths are measured and the outer cortices overdrilled. The shorter thread screws (16 mm) should be used to avoid threads across the fusion site, allowing for maximal compression. ◨ It is critical to check screw lengths radiographically and by direct visualization if possible to avoid penetration of the subtalar joint, which may lead to subtalar joint irritability. The medial screw may need to be countersunk to avoid prominent hardware in the subcutaneous medial tibia (Fig. 32-12). In the laboratory,

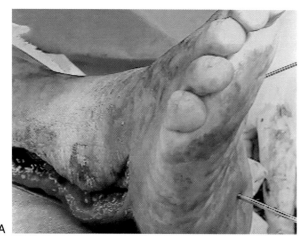

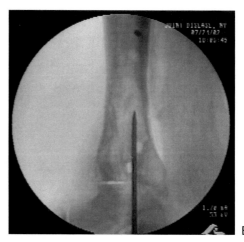

FIGURE 32-10. A and B: A Steinmann pin is placed across ankle to hold the position of the foot.

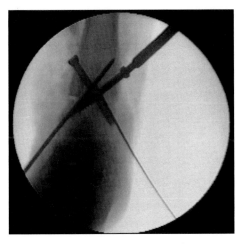

FIGURE 32-12. Medial screw placement with countersinking of the head.

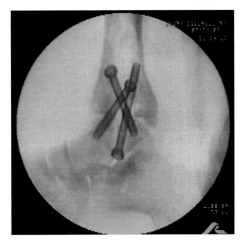

FIGURE 32-14. Final lateral view.

the cross-screw technique has been shown to be more biomechanically sound than a plate-screw construct. The final construct is confirmed on anteroposterior and lateral radiographs (Figs. 32-13 and 32-14).

If supplemental bone graft is required, it can be harvested from the distal fibula, or autogenous iliac crest bone graft can be obtained and packed around the fusion site laterally after decortication. A suction drain is placed, and the wounds are closed in layers with nylon sutures for the skin in a tension-free manner. Sterile compressive dressings are applied, and a padded posterior plaster slab with a U-shaped mold is applied to the ankle.

POSTOPERATIVE PROTOCOL

The patient's leg is strictly elevated for 24 hours. At this time, the drain can be removed. The patient is mobilized

without bearing weight on the affected site, with an emphasis on leg elevation while not ambulating. At 10 days to 2 weeks, the splint is removed, the wound checked, and the sutures discontinued. The patient is again placed in a short leg cast or a cast-brace orthosis, and weight bearing is avaoided for 3 months. The patient is followed radiographically at 6-week intervals. By 3 months, it is expected there is at least 50% bridging across the fusion site. At this point, the patient's weight-bearing status is advanced slowly to a flat foot stance, followed by full weight bearing as tolerated. At this point, physiotherapy may be initiated for lower extremity strengthening and subtalar range of motion. The patient's activity level progresses as pain-free mobility returns. A patient who has undergone ankle fusion will most likely require modifications in shoe wear. Most often, a rocker sole needs to be added to allow for easier push during gait.

COMPLICATIONS

Superficial or deep infection can complicate a well-executed ankle fusion. If recognized early, this can be treated with local wound care and intravenous antibiotics. Nerve complications may lead to suboptimal results. The superficial and deep peroneal nerves and the sural nerve are at risk laterally, as well as the posterior tibial nerve if a medial approach is used. Neuroma formation can be quite painful, and careful identification of these peripheral nerves and protection during surgery helps to avoid these complications

Malposition of the ankle is an avoidable pitfall. Excessive plantar flexion, internal rotation, or malpositioning in the varus or valgus plane can compromise the final result. Malposition can have detrimental effects on adjacent joints of the foot, with resultant progressive degenerative changes.

Nonunions, although less common with modern compression techniques, still occur with some frequency. This

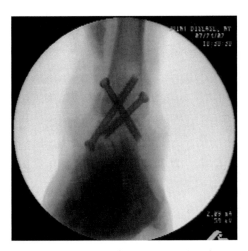

FIGURE 32-13. Final anteroposterior view.

complication leads to continued symptoms with regard to ambulatory ability. After a nonunion is established, a revision procedure should be considered.

SUGGESTED READINGS

Ahlberg A, Henricson AS. Late results of ankle fusion. *Acta Orthop Scand* 1981;52:103–105.

Hawkins BJ, Langerman RJ, Anger DM, et al. The Ilizarov technique in ankle fusion. *Clin Orthop* 1994;303:217–225.

Mann RA, Van Manen JW, Wapner K, et al. Ankle fusion. *Clin Orthop* 1991;268:49–55.

Miehlke W, Gschwend N, Rippstein P, et al. Compression arthrodesis of the rheumatoid ankle and hindfoot. *Clin Orthop* 1997;340:75–86.

Miller RA, Firoozbakhsh K, Veitch AJ. A biomechanical evaluation of internal fixation for ankle arthrodesis comparing two methods of joint surface preparation. *Orthopedics* 2000;23:457–460.

Miller SD. Late reconstruction after failed treatment for ankle fractures. *Orthop Clin North Am* 1995;26:363–373.

Morrey BF, Wiedeman GP Jr. Complications and long-term results of ankle arthrodeses following trauma. *J Bone Joint Surg Am* 1980;62:777–784.

Nasson S, Shuff C, Palmer D, et al. Biomechanical comparison of ankle arthrodesis techniques: crossed screws vs. blade plate. *Foot Ankle Int* 2001;22:575–580.

Perlman MH, Thordarson DB. Ankle fusion in a high risk population: an assessment of nonunion risk factors. *Foot Ankle Int* 1999;20:491–496.

Richter D, Hahn MP, Laun RA, et al. Arthrodesis of the infected ankle and subtalar joint: technique, indications, and results of 45 consecutive cases. *J Trauma* 1999;47:1072–1078.

Wapner KL. Salvage of failed and infected total ankle replacements with fusion. *Instruct Course Lect* 2002;51:153–157.

BIOMALLEOLAR ANKLE FRACTURES: OPEN REDUCTION AND INTERNAL FIXATION

KENNETH J. KOVAL

The ankle is a weight-bearing joint with minimal tolerance for variation from normal anatomy if good joint function is to be maintained. A congruent joint with reestablishment of normal ankle mortise relationships is necessary to prevent the long-term sequelae of painful, posttraumatic arthritis. Anatomic, stable reduction should be the goal in treatment of these intraarticular fractures. This chapter describes the operative treatment of bimalleolar ankle fractures.

ANATOMY

The ankle joint is a modified hinge joint consisting of the tibia, fibula, and talus (Fig. 33-1). The articular surface of the distal tibia is concave and broader anteriorly than posteriorly. The roof of the ankle joint (i.e., plafond) is continuous medially with the medial malleolus, which projects be-low the plafond and articulates with the medial surface of the talus. The distal aspect of the medial malleolus is divided into two prominences, the anterior and the posterior colliculi. The lateral malleolus projects about 1 cm distal and posterior to the medial malleolus. The talus is covered largely by cartilage; its body is wider anteriorly than posteriorly and is matched to the distal tibial articular surface.

Uniting these osseous structures are the medial and the lateral collateral ligaments and the ligaments of the tibiofibular syndesmosis. The deltoid ligament (i.e., medial collateral ligament) is a thick, triangular band consisting of superficial and deep fibers. The superficial fibers arise largely from the anterior colliculus of the medial malleolus and run as a continuous sheet in the sagittal plane to attach to the navicular, the sustentaculum tali, and the talus. The intraarticular and more horizontal deep fibers run from the intercollicular notch and posterior colliculus to the medial surface of the talus.

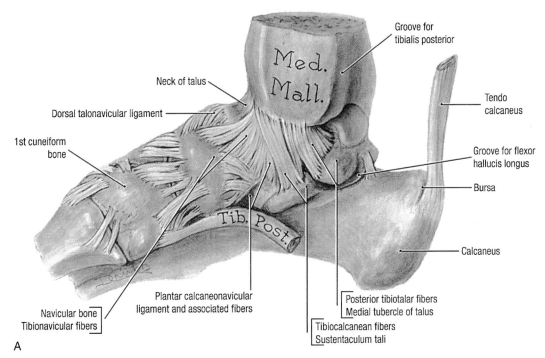

A

FIGURE 33-1. A: Medial view of the ligaments of the ankle. **B:** Lateral view of the ligaments of the ankle. **C:** Disarticulated talus. (From Agur AMR, Lee MJ. *Grant's atlas of anatomy,* 10th ed. Philadelphia: Lippincott Williams & Wilkins, 1999, with permission.) *(continued)*

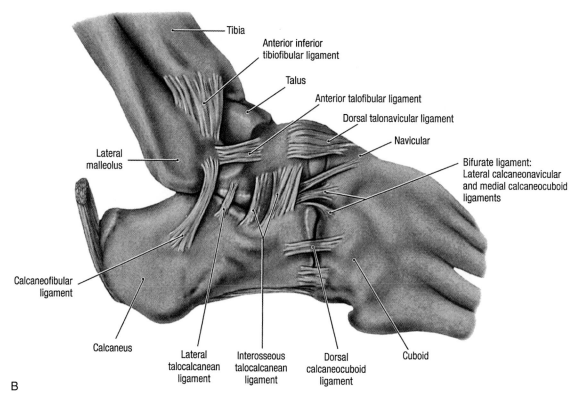

B

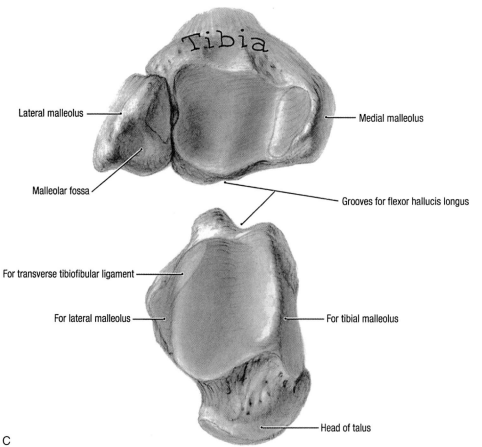

C

FIGURE 33-1. *Continued.*

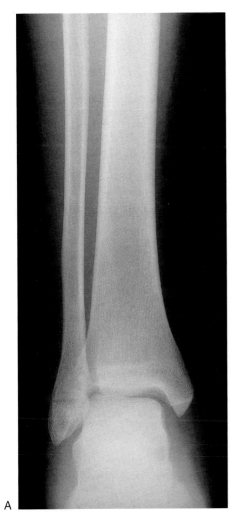
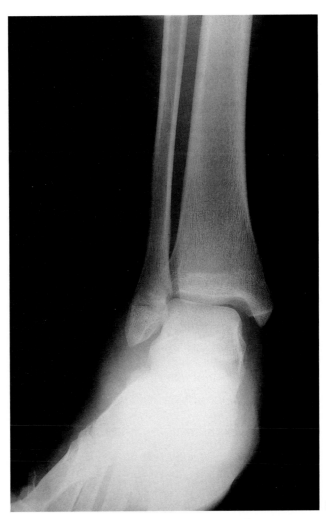

A

B

FIGURE 33-2. A: The anteroposterior radiograph demonstrates an isolated fibula fracture. **B:** A stress view, taken with external rotation of the foot with the ankle in dorsiflexion, documents medial clear space widening and talar shift.

The lateral side of the ankle has three ligaments that constitute the lateral collateral ligament: the anterior talofibular ligament, which runs from the anterior margin of the lateral malleolus to the anterior lateral facet of the talus; the calcaneofibular ligament, which extends down and posteriorly from the tip of the fibula to a tubercle on the lateral aspect of the calcaneus; and the posterior talofibular ligament, which originates on the medial surface of the lateral malleolus and inserts on the posterolateral aspect of the talus.

The most distal portions of the tibia and the fibula are joined together by four ligaments and the interosseous membrane. The ligaments are the anterior inferior tibiofibular ligament, the posterior inferior tibiofibular ligament, the inferior transverse ligament, and the posterior talofibular ligament. These ligaments stabilize the distal articulation of the tibia and fibula.

fracture patterns with an intact syndesmosis and for patients with marked osteoporosis, arterial insufficiency, limited goals for ambulation, or short life expectancy. Although it is possible to gain a satisfactory or even anatomic reduction of a displaced malleolar fracture by closed reduction, maintaining this reduction generally requires immobilization in a nonfunctional position in a long leg cast for at least 6 weeks. It is important to identify and separate patients with isolated fibular fractures from those who have obvious or occult injury to the medial side of the ankle. For patients with an isolated fibula fracture and medial pain but no talar shift, stress radiographs should be taken. If medial clear-space widening (>4 mm) with talar shift is present on stress radiographs (taken with external rotation of the foot with the ankle in dorsiflexion), the fibular fracture should be stabilized (Fig. 33-2).

INDICATIONS AND CONTRAINDICATIONS

The goal of treatment is to restore the ankle joint. Nonoperative treatment is reserved for nondisplaced, stable

CLASSIFICATION

There are several classifications for ankle fractures in clinical use. The Lauge-Hansen classification has four patterns, based on the position of the foot at the time of injury and the force direction (Fig. 33-3).

Supination-adduction accounts for 10% to 20% of malleolar fractures and is the only type associated with medial displacement of the talus:

Stage I produces a transverse avulsion-type fracture of the fibula distal to the level of the joint or a rupture of the lateral collateral ligaments.

Stage II results in a vertically oriented medial malleolus fracture.

Supination–external rotation accounts for 40% to 75% of malleolar fractures:

Stage I produces disruption of the anterior tibiofibular ligament with or without an associated avulsion fracture at its tibial or fibular attachment.

Stage II results in the typical spiral fracture of the distal fibula, which runs from anteroinferior to posterosuperior aspects.

Stage III produces a disruption of the posterior tibiofibular ligament or a fracture of the posterior malleolus.

Stage IV produces a transverse avulsion-type fracture of the medial malleolus or a rupture of the deltoid ligament.

Pronation-abduction accounts for 5% to 20% of malleolar fractures:

Stage I results in a transverse fracture of the medial malleolus or a rupture of the deltoid ligament.

Stage II produces a rupture of the syndesmotic ligaments or an avulsion fracture at their insertion sites.

Stage III produces a transverse or short oblique fracture of the distal fibula at or above the level of the syndesmosis; this results from a bending force that causes medial tension and lateral compression of the fibula, producing lateral comminution or a butterfly fragment.

Pronation–external rotation accounts for 5% to 20% of malleolus fractures:

Stage I produces a transverse fracture of the medial malleolus or a rupture of the deltoid ligament.

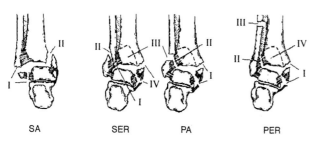

FIGURE 33-3. The Lauge-Hansen classification for ankle fractures is based on the position of the foot at the time of injury and the force direction. SA, supination-adduction; SER, supination–external rotation; PA, pronation-abduction; PER, pronation–external rotation. (From Carr JP, Trafton PG: Malleolar fractures and soft tissue injuries of the ankle. In: Browner BD, Jupiter JB, Levine AM, eds. *Skeletal trauma,* 2nd ed. Philadelphia: WB Saunders, 1998, with permission.)

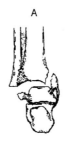
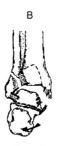
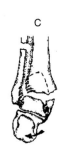

FIGURE 33-4. The Danis-Weber classification is based on the level of the fibular fracture. (From Carr JP, Trafton PG. Malleolar fractures and soft tissue injuries of the ankle. In: Browner BD, Jupiter JB, Levine AM, eds. *Skeletal trauma,* 2nd ed. Philadelphia: WB Saunders, 1998, with permission.)

Stage II results in disruption of the anterior tibiofibular ligament with or without avulsion fracture at its insertion sites.

Stage III results in a spiral fracture of the distal fibula at or above the level of the syndesmosis running from anterosuperior to posteroinferior.

Stage IV produces a rupture of the posterior tibiofibular ligament or an avulsion fracture of the posterolateral tibia.

The Danis-Weber classification is based on the level of the fibular fracture; the more proximal the fracture, the greater is the risk of syndesmotic disruption and associated instability (Fig. 33-4):

Type A involves a fracture of the fibula below the level of the tibial plafond, an avulsion injury that results from supination of the foot and that may be associated with an oblique or vertical fracture of the medial malleolus.

Type B is an oblique or spiral fracture of the fibula caused by external rotation occurring at or near the level of the syndesmosis.

Type C involves a fracture of the fibula above the level of the syndesmosis, causing disruption of the syndesmosis, and is almost always with associated medial injury.

The Orthopaedic Trauma Association (OTA) classification of ankle fractures is based primarily on fracture level in relation to syndesmosis (Fig. 33-5):

Type A is an infrasyndesmotic lesion.
    A1: infrasyndesmotic lateral malleolus, isolated
    A2: infrasyndesmotic lateral malleolus with associated medial malleolar fracture
    A3: infrasyndesmotic lateral malleolus with associated posteromedial tibial fracture

Type B is a transsyndesmotic lesion.
    B1: transsyndesmotic lateral malleolus, isolated
    B2: transsyndesmotic lateral malleolus with associated medial lesion
    B3: transsyndesmotic lateral malleolus with medial lesion and fracture of the posterolateral rim of the tibia

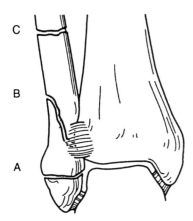

FIGURE 33-5. The Orthopaedic Trauma Association (OTA) classification of ankle fractures is based on the fracture level in relation to the syndesmosis. (From Marsh JL, Saltzman CL. Ankle fractures. In: Heckman JD, Bucholz RW, eds. *Rockwood and Green's fractures in adults,* 5th ed. Philadelphia: Lippincott Williams & Wilkins, 2001, with permission.)

Type C is a suprasyndesmotic lesion.
  C1: simple diaphyseal fibular fracture
  C2: complex (multifragment) diaphyseal fibular fracture with associated medial injury
  C3: proximal fibular fracture with associated medial injury

PREOPERATIVE PLANNING

Initial radiographs for evaluation of an ankle fracture should include anteroposterior, mortise, and lateral views of the ankle (Fig. 33-6). The surgeon should also ascertain that there

is not a proximal fibula fracture by clinical or radiographic examination.

Use the anteroposterior view to assess certain features:

- Tibiofibular overlap of less than 10 mm is abnormal and implies syndesmotic injury.
- Tibiofibular clear space of more than 5 mm is abnormal and implies syndesmotic injury.
- In a talar tilt, a difference in width of the medial and lateral aspects of the superior joint space of more than 2 mm is abnormal and indicates medial or lateral disruption.

The lateral view allows evaluation of alignment and some fractures:

- The dome of the talus should be centered under the tibia and congruous with the tibial plafond.
- Posterior tibial tuberosity fractures can be identified, as well as the direction of fibular injury.
- Avulsion fractures of the talus by the anterior capsule may be identified.

The mortise view, taken with the foot in 15 to 20 degrees of internal rotation to offset the intermalleolar axis, is used to ascertain talar positioning:

- A medial clear space of more than 4 mm is abnormal and indicates lateral talar shift.
- In assessing talar tilt, a line drawn parallel to the distal tibial articular surface and a second line drawn parallel to the talar surface should be parallel. More than 2 degrees of angulation indicates talar tilt.
- In assessing the talocrural angle, the angle subtended between the intermalleolar line and a line parallel to the dis-

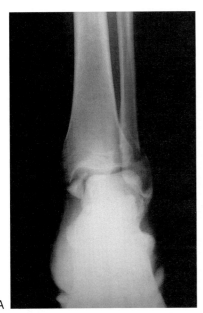

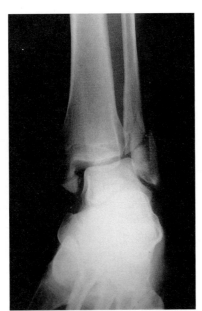

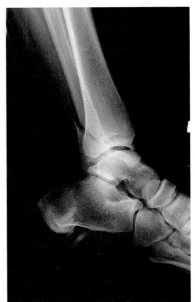

FIGURE 33-6. Anteroposterior **(A)**, mortise **(B)**, and lateral **(C)** views of the ankle demonstrate a displaced bimalleolar ankle fracture.

tal tibial articular surface should be between 8 and 15 degrees. A smaller angle indicates fibular shortening.

■ Tibiofibular overlap of less than 1 cm indicates syndesmotic disruption.

■ A talar shift of more than 1 mm is abnormal.

Computed tomography is useful in the evaluation of complex or comminuted fractures, especially of the distal tibia when plain radiographs are not able to fully delineate the fracture extent or in adolescents to demonstrate a possible triplane fracture.

EQUIPMENT

Some basic instruments are necessary for open reduction and internal fixation of the ankle (Fig. 33-7):

■ Small fragment plate and screws
■ Pelvic instrument and implant sets
■ Kirschner wires (K-wires)
■ Small-diameter, cannulated screws
■ Large and small, pointed reduction clamps
■ Cerclage wire set

SURGERY

Patient Positioning for Fracture Reduction

The patient is positioned supine, with a pad beneath the buttock on the injured side to aid access to the fibula. All pressure points are padded. A pneumatic tourniquet is applied to the upper thigh for use during surgery. The leg is prepared and draped free.

Lateral Malleolus

Approach

The fibula is approached through a straight lateral incision centered over the fracture and curving anterior distally to allow access to the anterolateral corner of the ankle joint (Fig. 33-8). The placement of this incision, however, may be adjusted, based on soft tissue conditions such as the presence of blisters or abrasions (Fig. 33-9). The deeper tissue is dissected in line with the skin incision, taking care not to injure the superficial peroneal nerve. **Division or entrapment of fixation devices the peroneal nerve in scar can lead to a symptomatic neuroma.**

Dissection is carried to the lateral border of the fibula, and the periosteum is incised over the lateral and posterior aspect of the fibula (Fig. 33-10). The full extent of the usual posterior fracture spike is exposed to allow proper fracture reduction assessment. Soft tissue stripping of butterfly fragments is kept to a minimum, particularly if there is comminution. Exposure must be sufficient to allow placement of reduction forceps, evaluation of the fracture reduction, and insertion of plate and screws.

Procedure

After fracture exposure, the fracture is mobilized and irrigated, and clot is removed from between the fracture edges (Fig. 33-11). With the usual supination–external rotation injury, external rotation of the foot opens the fracture surfaces and allows full exposure of the internal and external aspects of the fibula for irrigation and clot removal.

Fracture reduction can be accomplished by the use of clamps without strenuous manual traction. A small reduction (lion jaws) clamp from the small fragment set is placed obliquely across the fibula, perpendicular to the fracture

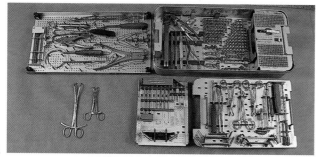
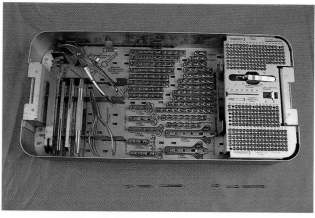

A

B

FIGURE 33-7. A: The basic instruments necessary for open reduction and internal fixation of the ankle include a cerclage wire set *(top left tray)*; small fragment plate and screw set *(top right tray)*; large and small, pointed reduction clamps (2) *(bottom left)*; drill bits, taps, Kirschner wires, and bending templates *(bottom tray, middle)*; and drill guides, screw driver, retractors, and reduction forceps *(bottom right tray)*. **B:** Small fragment plate and screw set.

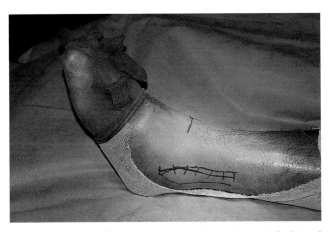

FIGURE 33-8. The fibula is approached through a straight lateral incision centered over the fracture and curving anteriorly distally to allow access to the anterolateral corner of the ankle joint.

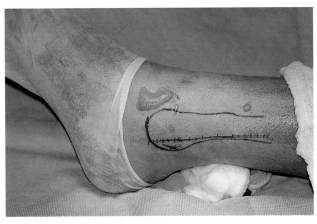

FIGURE 33-9. Modification of the lateral skin incision because of an anterolateral blister.

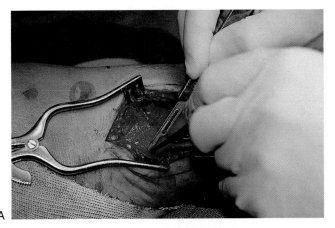

A

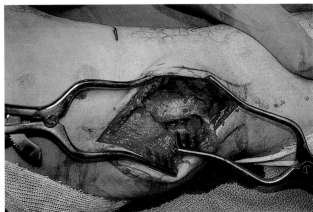

B

FIGURE 33-10. A and B: The dissection is carried to the lateral border of the fibula, and the periosteum is incised over the lateral and posterior aspects of the fibula.

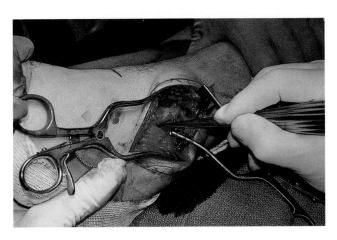

FIGURE 33-11. Removal of a clot from between the fracture edges.

plane (Fig. 33-12); this clamp is then used to obtain fracture length and rotation. ◙ A second clamp can be placed proximal or distal to the first clamp and used to fine tune the fracture reduction. **The surgeon should avoid placing the reduction clamp around the thin portion of the anterior or posterior fracture spikes to minimize the risk of iatrogenic fracture comminution.** If there is significant fracture comminution or poor bone quality, the surgeon can manually reduce the fracture and place provisional fixation with two or three 1.6-mm K-wires inserted from the tip of the fibula across the fracture.

After fracture reduction, one or two lag screws are placed across the fracture fragments from anterior to posterior aspects (Fig. 33-13). A gliding hole is made in the near cortex using a 3.5-mm drill. ◙ A 3.5/2.5 mushroom cap is then used to make a hole in the far cortex using a 2.5-mm drill. ◙ After measurement of the screw length and tapping of the screw tract, the lag screw is inserted. The surgeon must angle the drill bit laterally to capture the distal fragment. A one-third tubular plate is then contoured, placed laterally or posterolaterally, and secured to the proximal and distal fragments (Fig. 33-14). **The plate must be contoured**

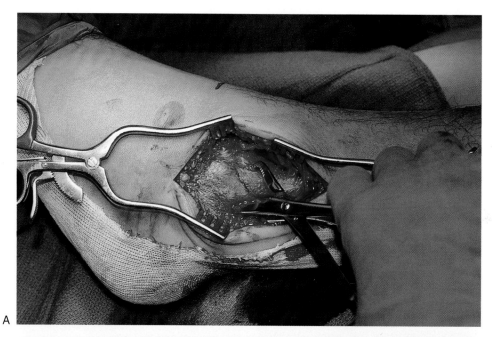

A

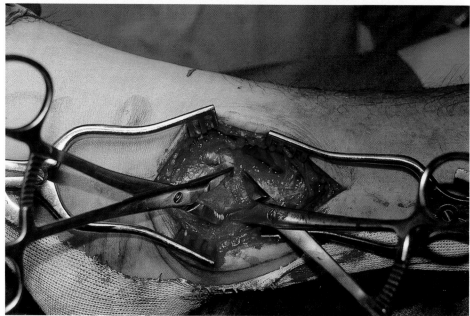

B

FIGURE 33-12. A and B: A small reduction (lion jaws) clamp from the small fragment set is placed obliquely across the fibula, perpendicular to the fracture plane, to reduce the fracture.

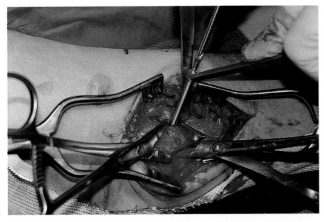

A

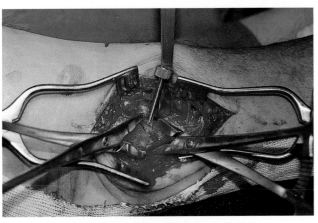

B

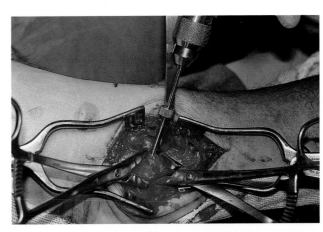

C

FIGURE 33-13. **A:** A lag screw is placed from anterior to posterior across the fracture fragments. A gliding hole is made in the near cortex using a 3.5-mm drill. **B and C:** A 3.5/2.5 mushroom cap is then used to make a hole in the far cortex using a 2.5-mm drill. **D and E:** After measurement of the screw length and tapping of the screw tract, the lag screw is inserted. **F and G:** Fluoroscopic evaluation after lag screw insertion.

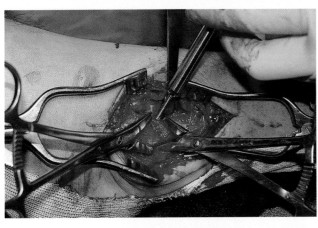

D

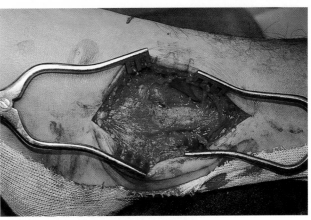

E

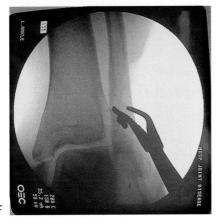

F

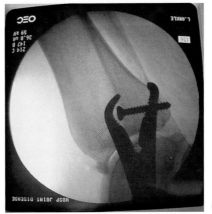

G

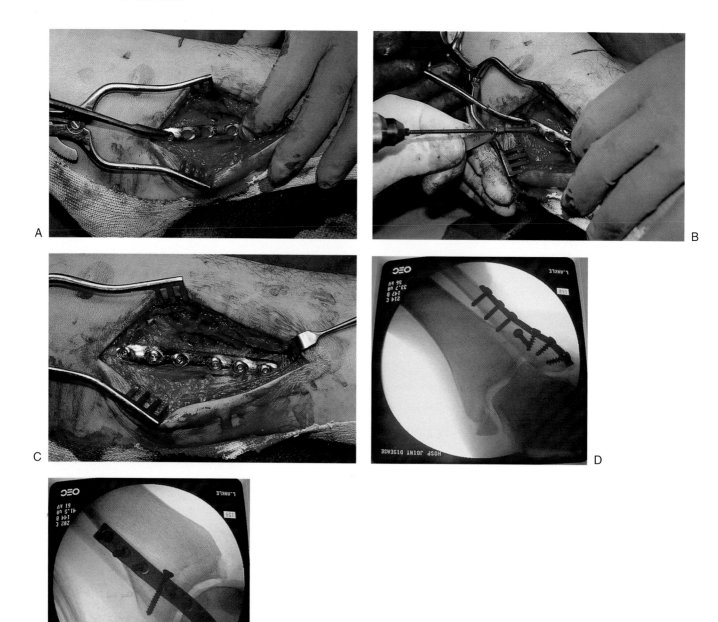

FIGURE 33-14. A to C: Lateral plate placement with screw insertion proximally and distally. The most distal screw is usually inserted first and angled proximally. **D and E:** Fluoroscopic evaluation after plate insertion.

with a bend and a twist (Fig. 33-15). ◧ The plate is bent so that it is concave just above the plafond level and gently convex over the larger lateral malleolus itself. ◧ This contouring is particularly important if fracture comminution precludes use of a lag screw, because fracture reduction can be altered by poor plate bending. I usually insert the distal screw first and then verify that the proximal aspect of the plate is centered on the fibula. After placement of a second screw, the plate position is fixed, and the plate cannot be rotated to a better position on the bone. With lateral plate placement, the distal screws must remain unicortical to

avoid intraarticular protrusion; the proximal screws are bicortical.

Medial Malleolus

Approach

The medial incision is slightly curved and centered over the medial malleolus (Fig. 33-16). It is sufficiently long to allow fracture reduction and stabilization without excessive soft tissue retraction. The saphenous vein and its accompanying saphenous nerve branches are preserved. The medial border

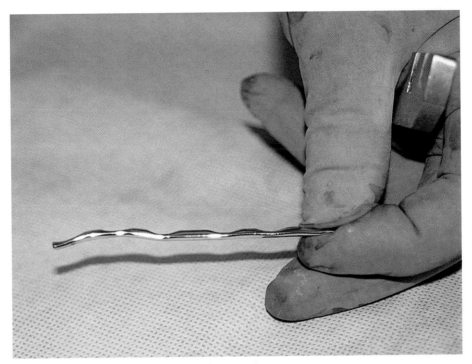

FIGURE 33-15. The plate is contoured with a bend and a twist. The plate is bent so that it is concave just above the plafond level and gently convex over the larger lateral malleolus.

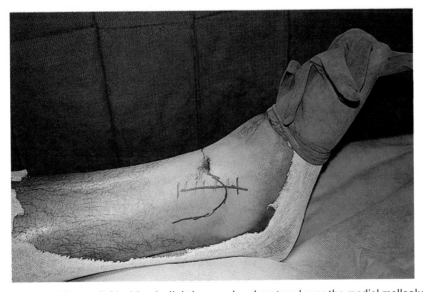

FIGURE 33-16. The medial incision is slightly curved and centered over the medial malleolus.

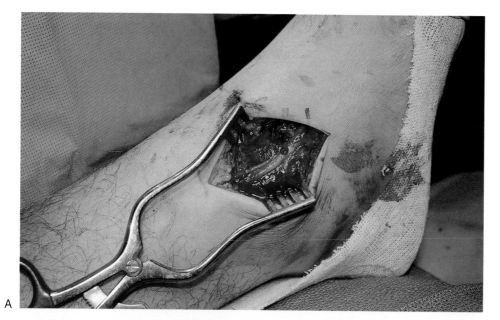

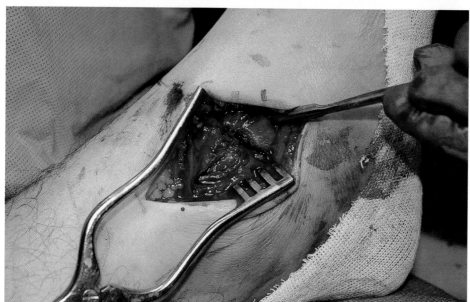

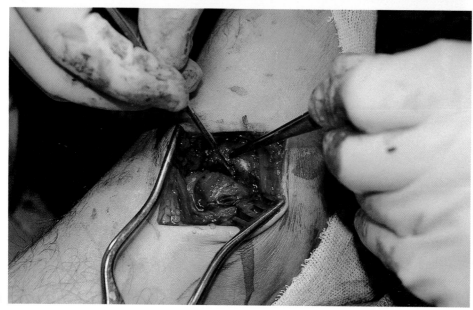

FIGURE 33-17. A and B: Soft tissues is dissected off the medial border of the medial malleolus, and the fracture is identified. **C:** The periosteum is incised on either side of the fracture.

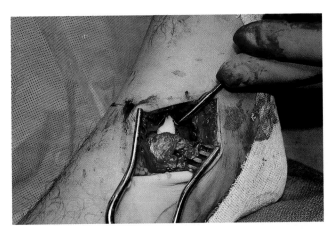

FIGURE 33-18. Visualization of the anteromedial corner of the ankle joint.

of the medial malleolus is dissected of soft tissue and the fracture identified (Fig. 33-17). ◨ The periosteum on either side of the fracture should be cleared for 2 to 3 mm to allow assessment of fracture reduction. The anteromedial corner of the ankle joint is visualized and irrigated to determine the extent of cartilage injury and remove any osteocartilaginous debris (Fig. 33-18).

Procedure

The medial malleolus can be manually reduced using a dental pick or small, pointed reduction forceps ◨ and provisionally stabilized using K-wires or reduction forceps (Fig. 33-19). ◨ Once satisfied with the fracture reduction visually and radiographically, two 4.0-mm, partially threaded, cannulated cancellous screws are inserted perpendicular to the fracture (Fig. 33-20). For most fractures, these are placed halfway between medial cortex and articular cartilage and angled proximally and laterally from the tip of the malleolus to remain entirely within the malleolus and the distal tibial metaphysis. Generally, 35- or 40-mm screw lengths are sufficient, although this depends on the patient's size and the fracture pattern. It is better to stay within the dense bone of the more distal tibial metaphysis, especially in osteoporotic patients, than to use longer screws.

Small medial malleolar fractures may be fixed with one screw, typically in the larger anterior colliculus, with a parallel K-wire in the posterior colliculus to prevent rotation. Bending the K-wire so its tip lies on the screw head aids hardware removal and minimizes the prominence. Comminuted fragments may be stabilized with K-wires and a supplementary "tension-band" suture or wire anchored around a proximal screw and washer (Fig. 33-21).

Syndesmosis Fixation

After medial and lateral malleolar reduction and stabilization, the surgeon should assess the status of the syndesmosis. Syndesmotic instability can be assessed by pulling laterally with an instrument hooked around the distal fibula or manually displacing the talus laterally with external rotation (Fig. 33-22). ◨ Displacement of more than a few millimeters, especially if there is failure or elastic recoil to the anatomic position, is an indication of soft tissue disruption and the need for syndesmotic screw fixation.

The syndesmosis is reduced with the foot in dorsiflexion to prevent narrowing of the mortise because of the trapezoidal

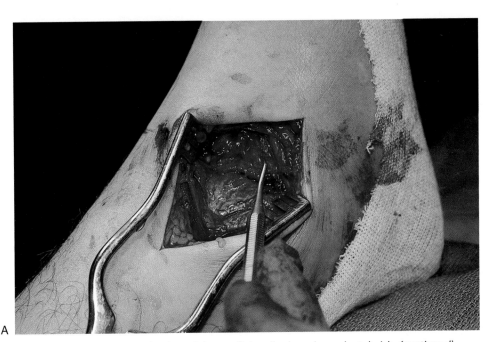

A

FIGURE 33-19. A: Reduction of the medial malleolus using a dental pick. *(continued)*

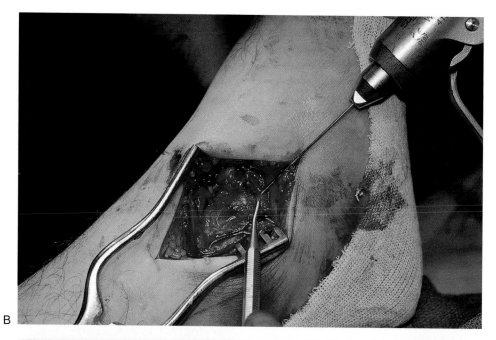

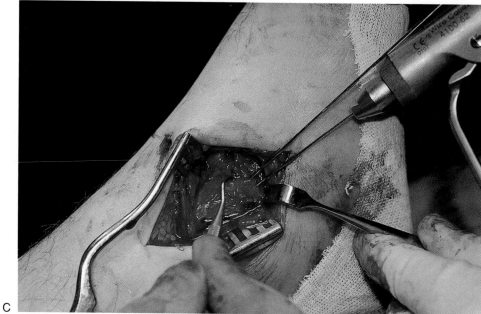

FIGURE 33-19. *Continued.* **B and C:** Provisional stabilization of the fracture using two Kirschner wires. If these wires are in a good position, they can be used for insertion of a cannulated lag screw.

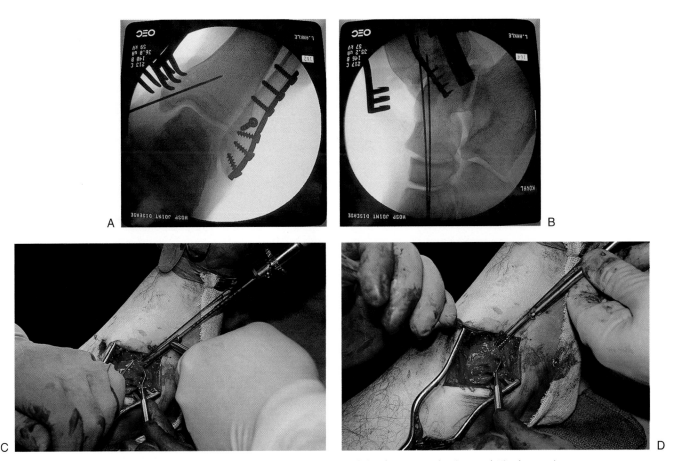

FIGURE 33-20. **A and B:** Fluoroscopic evaluation of the fracture reduction and Kirschner wire position. **C and D:** Insertion of two 4.0-mm, partially threaded, cannulated cancellous screws.

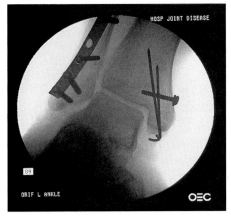

FIGURE 33-21. A small medial malleolar fragment is stabilized with Kirschner wires and a supplementary "tension-band" suture anchored around a proximal screw and washer.

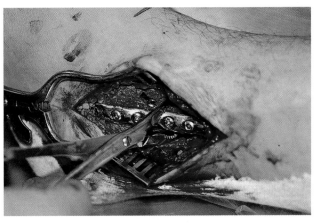

FIGURE 33-22. Assessment of syndesmotic stability by pulling laterally with a reduction clamp placed around the distal fibula.

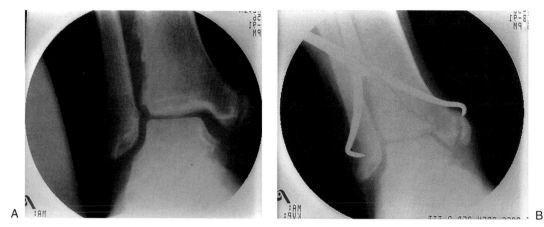

FIGURE 33-23. Reduction of a widened syndesmosis **(A)** using a tenaculum clamp placed across the distal fibula and tibia with the ankle in dorsiflexion **(B)**.

shape of the talus. A large tenaculum clamp placed across the distal tibia and fibula can be used to provisionally stabilize the syndesmosis (Fig. 33-23). After provisional fixation, radiographic confirmation of mortise alignment is obtained.

The size of the syndesmotic screw and the number of cortices of fixation remain controversial. However, I generally stabilize the syndesmosis using a fully threaded, 3.5-mm cortical screw placed through three or four cortices (Fig.

33-24). The advantage of placing the syndesmotic screw through four cortices is that, if the screw breaks, the tibial portion can be removed through a medial incision. This screw is inserted parallel to the ankle joint, from the posterolateral fibula to the anteromedial tibia, 1.5 to 2.0 cm above the plafond. If a plate was used for fibular fixation, it is often possible to place this screw through one of its holes, protruding a couple of millimeters on the medial side.

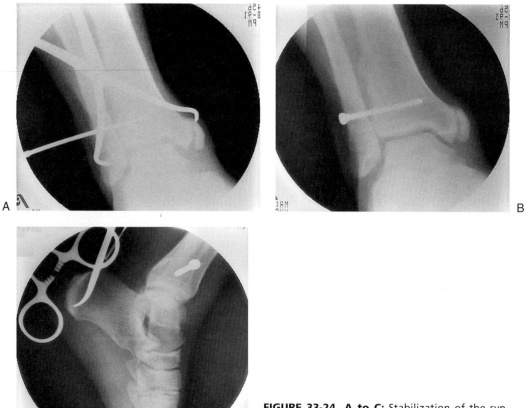

FIGURE 33-24. A to C: Stabilization of the syndesmosis using a fully threaded, 3.5-mm cortical screw placed through three cortices.

Posterior Malleolus

Small posterior malleolar fragments usually reduce with anatomic fibula reduction. Dorsiflexion of the foot may assist in reduction by a ligamentotaxis effect from the posterior capsule. If the fragment is large and involves more than 25% of the articular surface of the distal tibia, I favor fixation, particularly if associated with posterior talar subluxation or dislocation. The posterior malleolus may be stabilized using lag screws inserted in a posterior-to-anterior or anterior-to-posterior direction.

If the posterior malleolar fragment is large and requires direct reduction, exposure of this fragment and of the lateral malleolus can be performed from a posterolateral approach. The skin incision is placed posterior to the fibula. The fibula is reduced first. The approach then uses the interval between the peroneal tendons and the flexor hallucis longus muscle to expose the distal aspect of the posterior tibia (Fig. 33-25). The external edges of the fracture are used as a guide to anatomic reduction and the posterior malleolus fracture stabilized with one or two cancellous screws directed from a posterior to an anterior direction (Fig. 33-26).

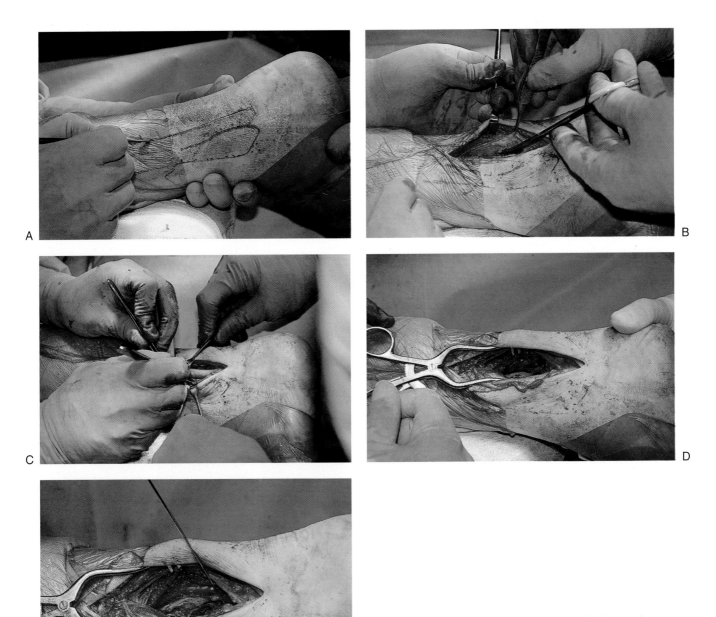

FIGURE 33-25. Exposure of the posterior malleolus can be performed from a posterolateral approach. The skin incision is placed posterior to the fibula **(A)**. The approach uses the interval between the peroneal tendons and the flexor hallucis longus muscle **(B and C)** to expose the distal aspect of the posterior tibia **(D and E)**.

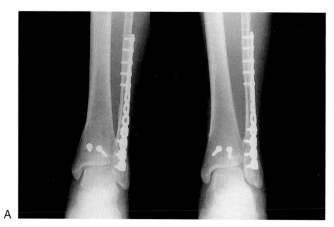

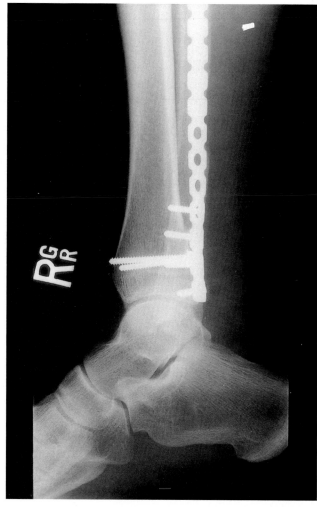

FIGURE 33-26. A and B: Stabilization of the posterior malleolus using two cancellous screws directed from posterior to anterior aspects.

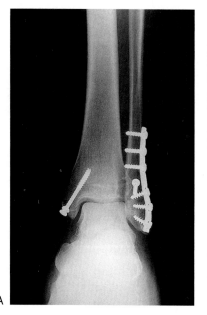

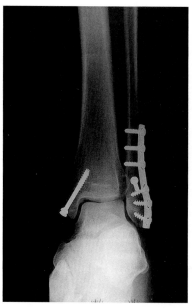

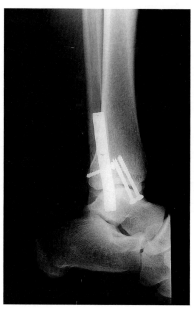

FIGURE 33-27. Final intraoperative anteroposterior **(A)**, mortise **(B)**, and lateral **(C)** radiographs.

WOUND CLOSURE

Before wound closure, the ankle is placed through a range of motion to assess fixation stability. Intraoperative radiographs are also taken to ensure that reduction and fixation are adequate (Fig. 33-27). I obtain anteroposterior, mortise, and lateral views.

The fascia is left open proximally over calf-muscle compartments but may be closed distally over the malleoli. The subcutaneous tissue is reapproximated using Vicryl sutures. The skin is closed with nylon using vertical mattress sutures to evert the wound edges. Tight closure should be avoided because of the tendency for the leg to swell in the early postoperative period. If the wound is too swollen to close without excessive tension, the wound should be left open and a delayed wound closure performed. A bulky dressing is applied with a posterior and U-shaped splints holding the ankle in a neutral position.

POSTOPERATIVE MANAGEMENT

Patients are instructed to keep the leg elevated as much as possible for the first week after surgery. They are instructed in ambulation training while not bearing weight on the injured extremity. At the first postoperative office visit, the leg is placed in a removable functional brace, and the patient is instructed on active and passive range-of-motion exercises of the ankle and subtalar joint. The brace is removed several times each day for active range-of-motion exercises. As the patient becomes more comfortable, gentle but progressive passive dorsiflexion stretching is added.

Weight bearing is allowed at 6 weeks, except for individuals in whom a syndesmosis screw had been used. These patients do not bear weight on the affected site for 8 weeks, at which time the screw is removed. Postoperative radiographs are obtained at 2 and 6 weeks. After the patient is allowed to bear weight as tolerated, resistive exercises are initiated.

SUGGESTED READINGS

Beauchamp CG, Clay NR, Tehxton PW. Displaced ankle fractures in patients over 50 years of age. *J Bone Joint Surg Br* 1983;65:329–332.

Boden SD, Labropoulos PA, McCowin P, et al. Mechanical considerations for the syndesmosis screw: a cadaver study. *J Bone Joint Surg Am* 1989;71:1548–1555.

Carr JB, Hansen ST, Benirschke SK. Surgical treatment of foot and ankle trauma: use of indirect reduction techniques. *Foot Ankle* 1989;9:176–178.

Cimino W, Ichtertz D, Slabaugh P. Early mobilization of ankle fractures after open reduction and internal fixation. *Clin Orthop* 1991;267:152–156.

Ferries JS, DeCoster TA, Firoozbakhsh KK, et al. Plain radiographic interpretation in trimalleolar ankle fractures poorly assesses posterior fragment size. *J Orthop Trauma* 1994;8:328–331.

Finsen V, Saetermo R, Kibsgaard L, et al. Early postoperative weight-bearing and muscle activity in patients who have a fracture of the ankle. *J Bone Joint Surg Am* 1989;71:23–27.

Kristensen KD, Hansen T. Closed treatment of ankle fractures: stage ii supination-eversion fractures followed for 20 years. *Acta Orthop Scand* 1985;56:107–109.

Lindsjö U. Classification of ankle fractures: the Lauge-Hansen or AO system? *Clin Orthop* 1985;199:12–16.

Mast J, Jakob R, Ganz R. *Planning and reduction techniques in fracture surgery.* New York: Springer-Verlag, 1989.

Müller ME, Allgöwer M, Schneider R, et al. *Manual of internal fixation: techniques recommended by the AO group,* 3rd ed. New York: Springer-Verlag, 1991.

Pankovich A. Fractures of the fibula proximal to the distal tibiofibular syndesmosis. *J Bone Joint Surg Am* 1978;60:221–229.

Pankovich A. Fractures of the fibula at the distal tibiofibular syndesmosis. *Clin Orthop* 1979;143:138–147.

Pankovich AM. Maisonneuve fracture of the fibula. *J Bone Joint Surg Am* 1976;58:337–342.

Pankovich AM, Shivaram MS. Anatomic basis of variability in injuries of the medial malleolus and the deltoid ligament. II. Clinical studies. *Acta Orthop Scand* 1979;50:225–236.

Pankovich AM, Shivaram MS. Anatomical basis of variability in injuries of the medial malleolus and the deltoid ligament. I. Anatomic studies. *Acta Orthop Scand* 1979;50:217–223.

Schaffer JJ, Manoli A. The antiglide plate for distal fibular fixation. *J Bone Joint Surg Am* 1987;69:596–604.

CHAPTER 34

HALLUX VALGUS CORRECTION: MODIFIED MCBRIDE AND CHEVRON OSTEOTOMY

STEVEN C. SHESKIER
PONNAVOLU D. REDDY

Hallux valgus is a radiographic diagnosis in which the angle between the first metatarsal shaft and the proximal phalanx is greater than 15 degrees. The condition represents a statistical range of normality rather than a pathologic entity in and of itself. When a patient presents complaining of a "bunion." the clinician must first determine the source of the symptoms, such as whether the chief complaint is cosmetic or there is a localized pain due to poor shoe fit, arthritis, tendonitis, neuroma, or progressive deformity of adjacent toes. The treatment should be tailored to treat the chief complaint and the inherent pathomechanics of hallux valgus. Radiographs, although useful for determining corrective procedures and their respective known limitations, are no substitute for a good history and a problem-oriented clinical examination.

ANATOMY

The first metatarsophalangeal (MTP) joint is held statically in place by medial and lateral collateral ligaments, the volar plate and the sesamoid complex on the plantar aspect, and the dorsal capsule on the dorsum of the MTP joint (Fig. 34-1). The dynamic stabilizers are the abductor hallucis medially, the adductor hallucis laterally (two heads indicate a conjoint tendon), the extensor hallucis longus (EHL) and brevis dorsally, and the flexor hallucis longus and brevis on the plantar aspect. The sesamoids sit on either side of a crista. They are also held in place by the sesamoid metatarsal retinaculum, with the lateral sesamoid tethered to the second metatarsal head by the deep transverse metatarsal ligament. As the HVA angle increases, the abductors become mechanically disadvantaged and the extensors and flexors progressively fall lateral to their neutral position and secondarily become adductors. The abductor itself can be displaced plantarward, causing pronation of the toe. Because every action has an equal and opposite reaction, the result is increasing medialization of the metatarsal head and an increase in the intermetatarsal angle. Ultimately, the static medial ligaments stretch out, and the proximal phalanx subluxates laterally, leading to an incongruous joint. Because the sesamoids are tethered by the intermetatarsal ligament,

they remain in place as the head moves medially, making them appear to have dislocated laterally.

Infrequently, there is a pure exostosis with no increase in the hallux valgus angle (HVA) or an associated bursa that thickens the area. The degenerative exostosis of hallux rigidus can be dorsomedial in location and mimic a hallux valgus but requires a different treatment.

CLASSIFICATION

Hallux valgus grading systems are devised to guide surgical decision making. **The most common cause of failure or recurrence (barring the patient returning to shoes that just do not fit) is stretching the indications for surgery.** Surgical treatment is most appropriate when it addresses the symptoms and concerns of the patient. Hence, the surgical decision-making process is "guided" by the HVA and the intermetatarsal angle (IMA) rather than being dogmatically determined by them (Fig. 34-2 and Table 34-1).

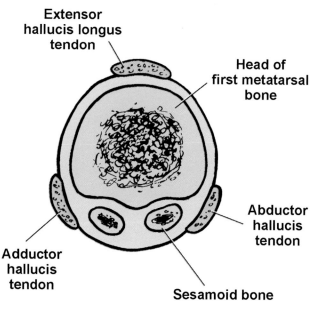

FIGURE 34-1. Anatomy of first metatarsophalangeal joint.

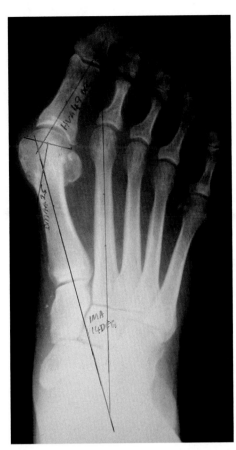

FIGURE 34-2. Weight-bearing radiograph with the hallux valgus angle (HVA), intermetatarsal angle (IMA), and distal metatarsal articular angle (DMAA) drawn.

INDICATIONS

Younger patients tend to have ligamentous laxity or a genetic predisposition, or both—hence the need for bony corrections and a subgroup of patients who have increased distal metatarsal articular angle (DMAA). For elderly patients, the surgeon should consider a simple exostectomy, Keller procedure, or a fusion. For neuromuscular conditions, the surgeon should first lean toward an MTP arthrodesis, particularly if the condition is progressive. For patients with metatarsocuneiform joint pathology (i.e., instability or degenerative arthritis), an arthrodesis of the first metatarsocuneiform joint (i.e., Lapidus procedure) should be considered. For patients with MTP arthritis (especially inflammatory joint disease), an arthrodesis should be considered. An Aiken osteotomy of the proximal phalanx is used for hallux valgus interphalangeus or to augment a procedure that does not correct the hallux valgus angle or IMA satisfactorily. It may be used in patients with asymptomatic hallux valgus associated with hammering of the second toe to make space for the second toe to be brought down into. **Clinicians should beware of younger patients with a hallux valgus and a congruent joint. They may have an increased DMAA and require a distal bony procedure that addresses this angular deformity.** In an elderly patient, remember the adage that "the punishment should fit the crime," meaning that the surgeon should perform a simple exostectomy or a Keller procedure so the foot may fit in a shoe rather than performing a complex distal soft tissue procedure with a proximal osteotomy. For patients with neuromuscular problems, arthritis, or failed hallux valgus surgery, an MTP fusion should be considered.

PREOPERATIVE PLANNING FOR BUNIONS

- Consider the symptoms (i.e., surgery should address the individuals complaints).
- Assess the angles on weight-bearing, anteroposterior radiographs (Fig. 34-2).
- Examine for instability or degenerative joint disease of the metatarsocuneiform joint.
- Consult the guide for the choice of a surgical procedure (Table 34-1).

CHEVRON OSTEOTOMY

Equipment

- Wire driver, wire cutter
- Sagittal saw
- 60-degree cutting guide (optional)

TABLE 34-1. GUIDE FOR THE CHOICE OF A SURGICAL PROCEDURE

Type	Hallux Angle	First and Second Intermetatarsal Angle	Surgical Procedure
Mild	15 to <30	9 to <15	Chevron osteotomy[a] Distal soft tissue (DST) procedure
Moderate	30 to <40	15 to <20	DST + proximal osteotomy (PO) Mitchell procedure[b]
Severe	>40	>20	DST and PO Fusion of first metatarsophalangeal joint

[a]Cannot correct pronation.
[b]A distal metatarsal step-cut osteotomy is of historical interest only because it shortens the first ray and can cause a transfer lesion under the second metatarsal head.

Patient Positioning

The patient is placed supine, with or without the use of an Esmarch tourniquet. **Sometimes, the EHL is tight and acts as a deforming force and must be lengthened. An Esmarch tourniquet may noticeably tighten the EHL tendon. If this occurs, the tourniquet is taken down so that the EHL is not Z-lengthened erroneously.** The leg can be placed on a well-padded stand to facilitate access. A hip roll can prevent external rotation of the foot.

Surgical Incision Landmarks

An incision that is approximately 6 to 8 cm long is made from the center of the middle one third of the proximal phalanx to the center of the head to the center of the first metatarsal shaft (Fig. 34-3).

Procedure

With a longitudinal incision centered over the medial eminence, the surgeon should take care to spread down to the capsule, using blunt dissection with a Stevens or Littler scissors. **Often, the dorsal digital nerve may have been displaced from its dorsomedial position to a more medial central position on the exostosis and can be inadvertently injured.** A plane should be developed over the capsule that allows a V-Y capsulotomy.

The V-Y capsulotomy is performed with the arms distal and tail proximal (Fig. 34-4). The capsule is elevated off the medial eminence with sharp dissection, and the exostosis is exposed (Fig. 34-5). ▉◗ An exostectomy is performed with a sharp osteotome or a sagittal saw at the level of the sulcus (Fig. 34-6). The cut should be made parallel to the medial margin of the foot and perpendicular to the dorsum of the foot. ▉◗ The center of the head is then determined at ap-

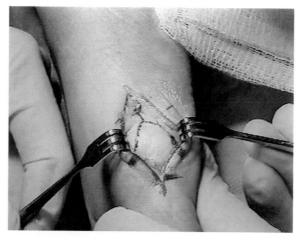

FIGURE 34-4. The V-Y capsulotomy is marked with the arms distal and the tail proximal.

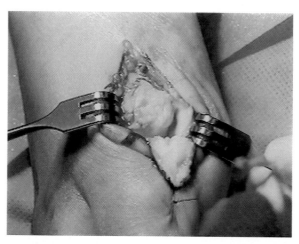

FIGURE 34-5. Exostosis exposed after sharp dissection.

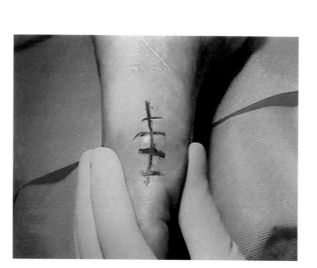

FIGURE 34-3. Incision landmarks from the center of the proximal phalanx to the center of the head to the center of the first metatarsal shaft. The incision is 6 to 8 cm long.

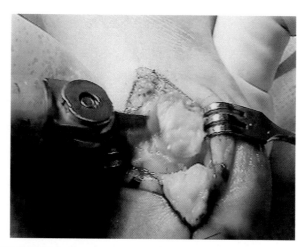

FIGURE 34-6. Exostectomy is performed with a sharp osteotome or a sagittal saw at the level of the sulcus.

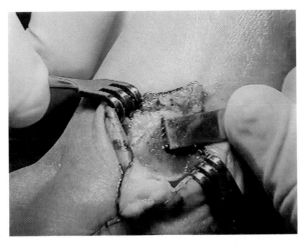

FIGURE 34-7. The center of the head is determined, and a 60-degree angled cut is marked at the center of the head so that the limbs extend proximal to the joint capsule.

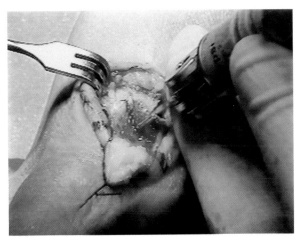

FIGURE 34-9. A saw blade is used to perform an osteotomy. A Freer elevator and a baby Hohmann retractor are used to elevate and retract the soft tissue.

proximately 1 cm from the articular margin. ◖◗ A 60-degree angled cut is marked at the center of the head in such a manner that the limbs extend proximal to the joint capsule (Fig. 34-7). ◖◗ Whether the dorsal limb is equal to the plantar limb depends on the surgeon, especially if fixation with a screw is contemplated. A 0.62-inch Kirschner wire (K-wire) is inserted at the center of the head to help in orienting the two cuts in the same plane and to help prevent cutting beyond the center of the head. ◖◗ **Divergent cuts in the mediolateral plane should be avoided, because with these type of cuts, the head may jam on the proximal shaft that then acts like a wedge and splits the head.** The wire is cut short (Fig. 34-8), and a sagittal saw blade is used to make the osteotomy (Fig. 34-9). ◖◗ Soft tissue is gently elevated with a Freer elevator and retracted with a narrow baby Hohmann retractor, taking care not to overstrip the lateral tissue and devascularize the head. After cuts are made, the blade can be removed and used as a probe to ensure a full lateral cut and further clear the soft tissue that may prevent lat-

eralization of the head. ◖◗ The head is displaced approximately 4 mm laterally ◖◗ and impacted (Fig. 34-10). ◖◗ In general, the osteotomy is stable in this position, because the normal tissue tension (e.g., tendons) provides constant impaction at the osteotomy site. ◖◗ If the osteotomy appears to be unstable, a 0.45-inch K-wire can be placed under direct visualization and left out through the skin (Fig. 34-11) ◖◗; the wire can be removed at 3 weeks after surgery . The medial eminence of the proximal shaft is shaved off and made smooth with a sagittal saw. ◖◗ The V-Y capsulotomy is advanced and closed first with a 0- Vicryl corner stitch while the toe is held in varus (Fig. 34-12). ◖◗ The capsulotomy is then closed with 0-Vicryl, taking care to identify the dorsal digital nerve that is invariably trying to be incorporated into the capsulorrhaphy. ◖◗ The skin is closed with 4-0 nylon vertical mattress sutures.

If a Chevron osteotomy is performed in a patient with an increased DMAA, a K-wire or screw stabilization is required.

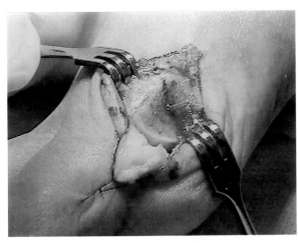

FIGURE 34-8. The Kirschner wire is cut short.

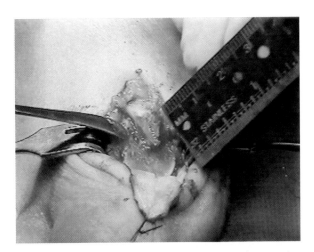

FIGURE 34-10. The head is displaced approximately 4 mm laterally and impacted.

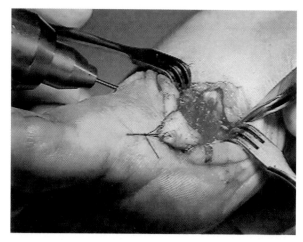

FIGURE 34-11. If the osteotomy appears to be unstable, a 0.45-inch Kirschner wire can be placed under direct visualization.

A Xeroform dressing is applied, followed by a toe spica bandage (Fig. 34-13). **If no internal fixation is used, the surgeon should exercise caution at the time of dressing; otherwise, excessive tightness of the dressing can undo the correction.**

Postoperative Protocol

The patient is in a postoperative shoe and avoids bearing weight for 2 weeks. At 2 weeks, sutures are removed, radiographs are taken, and a new toe spica is applied. The patient is then allowed to walk on the heel, bearing weight as tolerated. At 3 weeks after surgery, the pin, if present, is removed, and a toe spica is reapplied. The toe can be manipulated to break up adhesions, and the spica is reapplied. During the fourth week, if the patient is amenable, he can be placed in a Darco™ splint (Fig. 34-14), which is to be worn 24 hours each day. The splint can be removed to washing the foot. By 6 to 8 weeks, the osteotomy is healed, and the patient can go into a preapproved closed-toe shoe. Formal

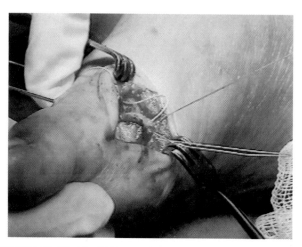

FIGURE 34-12. The V-Y capsulotomy is advanced and closed with a 0-Vicryl corner stitch while the toe is held in varus.

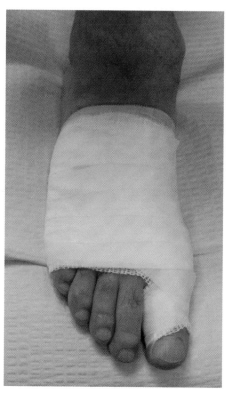

FIGURE 34-13. A xeroform dressing is applied, followed by a toe spica cast.

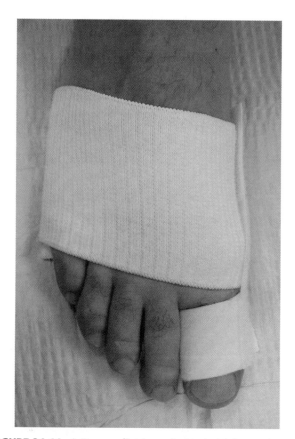

FIGURE 34-14. A Darco splint is applied to hold the toe in position.

physical therapy can be started. Three months after surgery, the patient can try to wear "dress shoes." Outlining the foot on a piece of paper and superimposing the shoe can help the clinician point out obvious sizing problems. The patient should be instructed to wear the splint at night for 6 more weeks.

MODIFIED MCBRIDE PROCEDURE

The modified McBride is the workhorse of distal soft tissue procedures. It releases the deforming force of the conjoint tendon and the lateral joint contracture. Medially, it reefs up the medial capsule after the eminence is removed. A lateral sesamoidectomy can be performed for sesamoid degenerative joint disease (i.e., component of the classic McBride procedure).

Equipment

- Standard sagittal saw
- Osteotomes

Patient Positioning

Patient positioning is the same as that for the chevron osteotomy.

Surgical Incision Landmarks

A medial eminence incision is made, as was done for the Chevron osteotomy, in addition to an incision in the 1–2 webspace (Fig. 34-15).

Procedure

The first intermetatarsal space (1–2 space) is approached dorsally. A space is developed between the metatarsal heads

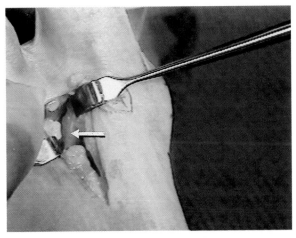

FIGURE 34-16. The conjoint tendon is identified *(arrow)* and freed inferiorly to avoid injury to the plantar digital nerve.

using blunt dissection, taking care to avoid injury to the dorsal digital nerve branches. A bursa may be encountered. The conjoint tendon is identified and freed inferiorly to avoid injury to the plantar digital nerve (Fig. 34-16). Sesamoid orientation is determined by a preoperative radiograph, which may help while performing the longitudinal capsulotomy. ◙ **Sesamoids might have become rotated and the flexor hallucis brevis inadvertently tenotomized.** The conjoint tendon is tenotomized (Fig. 34-17) at its insertion on the lateral base of the proximal phalanx, ◙ then stripped off the lateral sesamoid back to the muscle bellies, and tagged for future transfer. ◙ A lateral capsulotomy is performed ◙ with multiple stab wounds (Fig. 34-18) or a transverse capsulotomy. The toe must be stretched to at least 20 to 25 degrees of varus (Fig. 34-19). If unable to do so, consider releasing the lateral flexor hallucis brevis tendon. This should be done only when the toe cannot be stretched

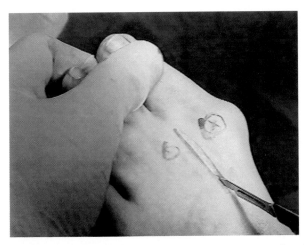

FIGURE 34-15. Incision for the modified McBride procedure is similar to that for the chevron osteotomy plus first and second intermetatarsal head incisions of 4 cm.

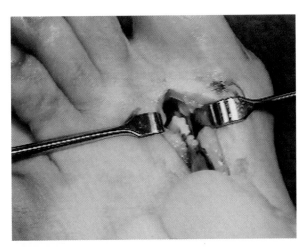

FIGURE 34-17. The conjoint tendon is tenotomized at its insertion on the lateral base of the proximal phalanx and then stripped off the lateral sesamoid back to the muscle bellies and tagged for future transfer.

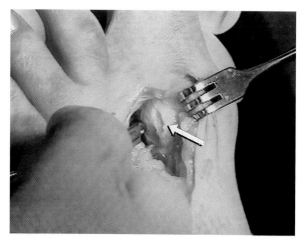

FIGURE 34-18. A lateral capsulotomy *(arrow)* is performed with multiple stab wounds.

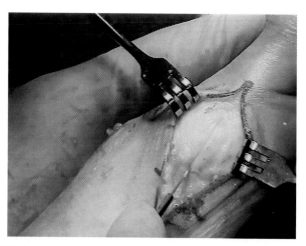

FIGURE 34-21. Longitudinal capsulotomy on the medial eminence.

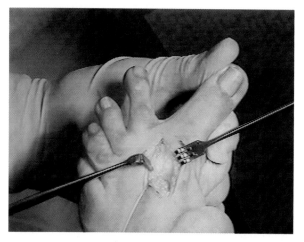

FIGURE 34-19. The toe must be brought into at least 20 to 25 degrees of varus after the capsulotomy

into adequate varus after the medial exostectomy (which may be impinging) is performed to avoid an excessive release of the lateral structures; the latter may increase the likelihood of postoperative hallux varus.

Attention is turned to the medial eminence, and a 6-cm medial incision is made (Fig. 34-20). Care is taken to avoid injuring the dorsal digital nerve, ■◄ which might have been displaced plantarward from its usual dorsomedial location. The capsulotomy can be longitudinal (Fig. 34-21) or a transverse diamond, as described by Mann. We prefer the former because it can be used to correct the valgus and pronation of the first toe. ■◄ Regardless of the method, the capsule and collateral ligament are stripped off the medial eminence to expose the exostosis. ■◄ The eminence is removed 1 mm medial to the sulcus (Fig. 34-22) ■◄ to avoid an increased likelihood of postoperative varus deformity. The sharp edges are smoothed with a rongeur and rasp (Fig. 34-23). Passive varus is rechecked to see if further lat-

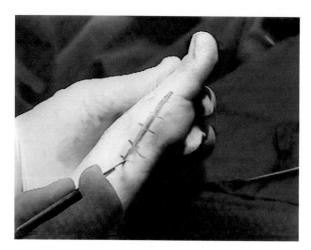

FIGURE 34-20. A 6-cm medial incision made on the medial eminence.

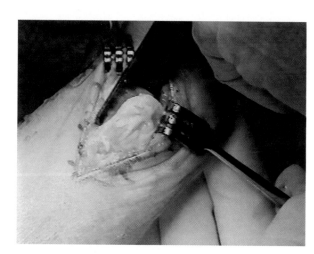

FIGURE 34-22. The eminence is removed 1 mm medial to the sulcus to avoid a postoperative varus deformity.

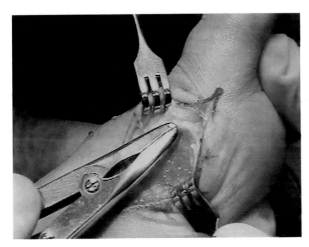

FIGURE 34-23. Edges of the exostosis are smoothed with a rongeur.

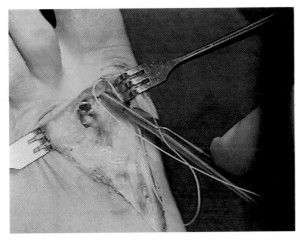

FIGURE 34-25. Suture in the dorsolateral capsule of the first metatarsal head.

eral release is indicated. **Tightness of the EHL is sometimes present, acting as a valgus deforming force, but it may be iatrogenic if an ankle Esmarch tourniquet is used.**

The conjoint tendon is transferred to the dorsal lateral capsule of the first metatarsal head with 0- Vicryl to act as a dynamic adductor of the first ray and plantar flexor (Fig. 34-24). A second 0- Vicryl suture is used to tie the capsules of the first (Fig. 34-25) and second metatarsal heads (Fig. 34-26) together to statically reduce the metatarsus primus varus if the metatarsal cuneiform joint is mobile. The heads are forced together by the assistant, who squeezes the forefoot as this suture is tied (Fig. 34-27). Patients may complain of pain in this area because of the placement of this suture. This pain resolves in time as the suture is absorbed. The medial capsulorrhaphy is closed with the toe held in slight varus. Before squaring the knot, the toe should be ranged to see if the repair of the medial capsule and ligament is isometric, akin to anterior cruciate ligament

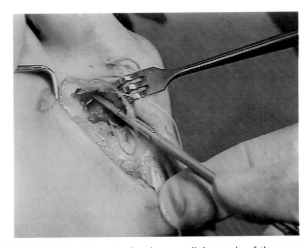

FIGURE 34-26. Suture in the dorsomedial capsule of the second metatarsal head.

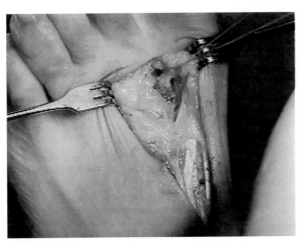

FIGURE 34-24. The conjoint tendon is transferred to the dorsal lateral capsule of the first metatarsal head with 0-Vicryl to act as a dynamic adductor of the first ray and plantar flexor.

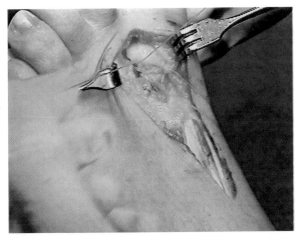

FIGURE 34-27. The capsules of the first and second heads are tied together to statically reduce metatarsus primus varus if the metatarsal cuneiform joint is mobile. The heads are forced together by the assistant, who squeezes the forefoot as the suture is tied.

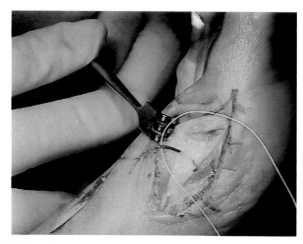

FIGURE 34-28. The first proximal knot should be tied through stable periosteum, which acts as an anchor. A drill hole is made if no stable periosteum is available.

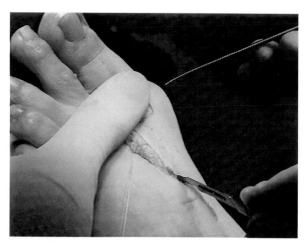

FIGURE 34-30. Surgical incision landmarks for a proximal osteotomy at the base of the first metatarsal and metatarsocuneiform joint.

isometry. The first suture of the medial capsulorrhaphy should be to periosteum (Fig. 34-28) that is stable, because it acts as an anchor, or a drill hole is made if none is available. The rest of the capsule can be closed with 2-0 Vicryl (Fig. 34-29). The skin is closed with 4-0 vertical mattress sutures. The dressing is applied as in the Chevron procedure. During toe spica application, the heads are squeezed together to augment reduction of the intermetatarsal angle.

Postoperative Protocol

The patient can bear weight during ambulation as tolerated in a stiff postoperative shoe. Sutures are removed at approximately 2 weeks, and a toe spica is reapplied on a weekly ba-

sis to assure the alignment of the toe for 4–6 weeks. During this period, undercorrection or overcorrection can be addressed. Range-of-motion exercises can be started early if stiffness is a concern.

PROXIMAL OSTEOTOMY

Proximal osteotomy is never performed alone but as an adjunct to a distal soft tissue procedure, usually in cases in which the IMA is greater than 15 degrees or when Chevron would be inappropriate (i.e., pronation of a toe or tightness of the conjoint tendon). The technique varies from a crescentic proximal osteotomy to a Chevron type or a closing

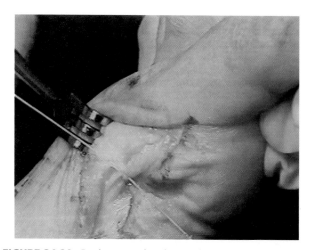

FIGURE 34-29. During capsular closure, be aware of the digital nerve.

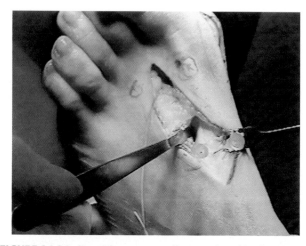

FIGURE 34-31. Two 25-gauge needles are placed in the joint to determine the plane of the metatarsal cuneiform joint. A baby Hohmann retractor is placed subperiosteally on the lateral side to protect the perforating branch of the dorsalis pedis artery and the deep peroneal nerve.

wedge. Each technique has its advantages and disadvantages. We prefer a closing wedge osteotomy similar to a high tibial osteotomy because it is stable, predictable, and adjustable.

Patient Positioning

The patient is positioned supine.

Equipment

- Micro–sagittal saw with a long blade
- Cannulated screw system with guide pins
- Over drill
- Image intensifier (optional)

Surgical Incision Landmarks

The landmarks for the incision are the bases of first metatarsal and metatarsocuneiform joints (Fig. 34-30).

Procedure

A 3-cm incision is made on the dorsum of the foot, 📹 centered over the first metatarsal cuneiform joint and taken

through the inferior bands of the extensor retinaculum. 📹 The EHL tendon is pulled medially. The metatarsocuneiform joint is delineated by placing two 25-gauge needles in it to determine the plane. The periosteum is stripped off laterally and a baby Hohmann is placed to protect the perforating branch of the dorsalis pedis artery and the deep peroneal nerve (Fig. 34-31). Preoperative radiographs determine the amount of wedge to be removed; sometimes, just the thickness of the blade is sufficient (Fig. 34-32).

Care should be taken to preserve the medial soft tissue and a bony bridge for stability. Mark the osteotomy with an osteotome (Fig. 34-33). 📹 **The thickness of the metatarsal base is deeper than initially thought, and probing with a free saw blade is recommended as is done in a Chevron. If a plantar or lateral lip is left and unrecognized, it may cause the surgeon to overcut medially or to make the wedge too large.** Place the guide wire for the screw in the proximal portion of the medial wound while carefully watching for the digital nerve. Run the guide wire up to the osteotomy site before crossing it. Saw away at the medial bone hinge until the bone can be easily bent over. Drive the wire across the osteotomy site into the proximal fragment,

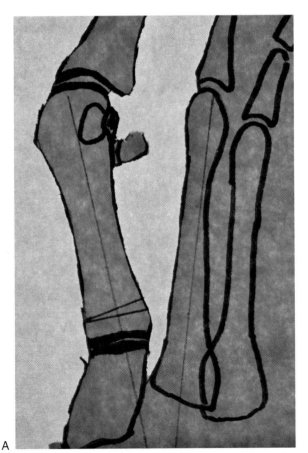
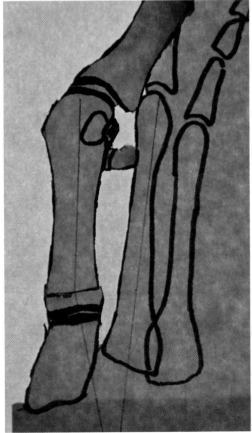

A   B

FIGURE 34-32. A: Preoperative planning tracing of a preoperative radiograph to determine the amount of wedge to be taken. **B:** Preoperative tracing for correction of the deformity with wedge removed.

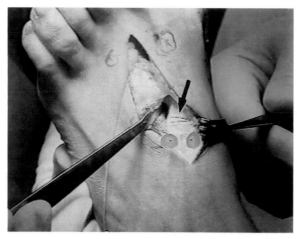

FIGURE 34-33. The osteotomy is marked *(arrow)* with an osteotome.

and continue until the wire tents the skin dorsolaterally (Fig. 34-34). ◖◼ This makes recovery of the guide wire easy if it is cut while drilling (most guide wires are very thin). Drill over the guide wire, tap the outer cortex, and insert the 4.0-mm, partially half-threaded screw. As the screw is tightened down, the metatarsal is forced into valgus as the screw head hits the cortex, allowing the surgeon to fine tune the osteotomy. ◖◼ If the medial hinge breaks, a K-wire or second screw should be placed for stability. Overcorrection of

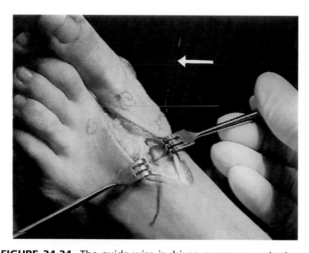

FIGURE 34-34. The guide wire is driven across one osteotomy site into the proximal fragment and continued until the wire tents the skin on the dorsolateral aspect of the foot.

metatarsus primus varus can result in hallux varus. Transfer lesion to the second metatarsal head can occur if the osteotomy is allowed to dorsiflex. Think of Newton: every action has an equal and opposite reaction. While the osteotomy is stabilized with the screw, holding the toe in varus and dorsiflexion at the MTP joint pushes the head laterally and plantarward. This maneuver can prevent dorsiflexion at the osteotomy. The sutures of the distal modified McBride (for adductor tendon transfer and approximation of first and second metatarsal heads) should be placed before the closure of the wedge osteotomy; otherwise, there will be no room to do so after the osteotomy is closed.

Postoperative Protocol

The patient does not bear weight for 2 weeks. More compliant patients can place weight on the heel, especially on stairs. The clinician should watch out for noncompliant patients. In giving patients an inch, they will often take a mile! Full weight bearing on the foot can break the screw and displace the osteotomy.

A radiograph is taken and a toe spica is applied, carefully watching for and preventing varus positioning. Follow-up evaluation is continued with the spica in place until the osteotomy is stabilized; then, a soft splint is applied. The osteotomy heals in approximately 6 to 8 weeks, at which time the screw is taken out under local anesthesia in the office or in the operating room. This is a powerful correction, and patients should be advised of the need for orthotic and physical therapy for gait training with the "new foot."

SUGGESTED READINGS

Coughlin MJ. Proximal first metatarsal osteotomy. In: Johnson KA, ed. *Master techniques in orthopaedic surgery: the foot and ankle.* Philadelphia: Lippincott-Raven Publishers, 1997:85–105.

Richardson EG. Complications after hallux valgus surgery. *Instruct Course Lect* 1999;48:331–342.

Richardson EG. Complications after hallux valgus surgery. *Instruct Course Lect* 1999;48:331–342.

Sammarco GJ, Idusuyi OB. Complications after surgery of the hallux. *Clin Orthop* 2001;391:59–71.

Thordason DB, Rudicel SA, Ebramzadeh E, et al. Outcome study of hallux valgus surgery—an AOFAS multi-center study. *Foot Ankle Int* 2001;22:956–959.

Trnka HJ, Muhlbauer M, Zembsch A, et al. Basal closing wedge osteotomy for correction of hallux valgus and metatarsus primus varus: 10–22 year follow-up. *Foot Ankle Int* 1999;20:171–177.

HAMMER TOE CORRECTION

RICHARD A. ZELL
DONNA J. ASTION

Hammer toes are a common condition of the lesser toes. They can be painful when the toe box of a shoe presses on the prominent area of the deformity, usually the flexed portion of the proximal interphalangeal joint. The deformity can be flexible or rigid and usually results from an imbalance between the extrinsic and intrinsic muscles of the foot. Often, the discomfort can be treated by shoe modifications; however, with a persistently painful hammer toe, surgery is indicated.

ANATOMY AND PATHOPHYSIOLOGY

The position of each toe depends on passive and active stabilizers of the toe. The passive stabilizers consist of the collateral ligaments, the plantar aponeurosis, the volar plate, and the capsule. The active stabilizers include the extrinsic and intrinsic muscles of the foot. Extrinsically, the flexor digitorum longus (FDL) inserts plantarly on the distal phalanx. The extensor digitorum longus (EDL) inserts dorsally on the extensor hood at the level of the proximal phalanx and then continues further to insert into the distal phalanx. The intrinsic muscles act to support and balance the extrinsic muscles. The extensor digitorum brevis (EDB) inserts onto the middle phalanx, and the lumbricals and interossei tendons course plantar to the center of rotation of the metatarsophalangeal (MTP) joint and insert into the extensor hood. The lumbricals work to plantarflex the MTP joint and extend the interphalangeal joints. There are no tendinous insertions onto the proximal phalanx (Fig. 35-1).

Lesser toe deformities result from an imbalance between the intrinsic and extrinsic muscles of the foot. The pull of the EDL and the antagonistic pull of the weaker intrinsic muscles determine the position of the proximal phalanx at the MTP joint. The pull of the long and short flexors determines the position of the middle and distal phalanges. The toe deformity is the result of an imbalance between the strong extrinsic muscles and the weaker intrinsic muscles.

Hammer toe deformities can be associated with inflammatory arthritis or with neuromuscular diseases. However, they are most commonly a result of poorly fitting shoes and are more common in women. Shoes with a narrow, pointed toe box force the proximal phalanx into extension and the proximal interphalangeal (PIP) joint into flexion. This is exacerbated by a high heel, which allows the toes to slide forward into the narrow toe box (Fig. 35-2). The second toe is most commonly affected because it is often the longest ray and therefore most affected by pressure from the toe box of the shoe.

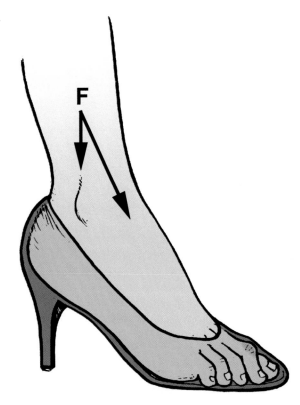

FIGURE 35-2. Poor fitting shoe with (1) a narrow toe box, which forces proximal phalanx into extension and proximal interphalangeal joint into flexion, and (2) an excessively high heel, which allows the toes to slide forward into the narrow toe box.

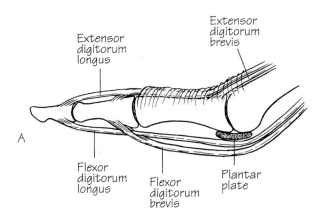

FIGURE 35-1. Normal position of the bones, joints, and extrinsic tendons of a functional lesser toe. (From Hansen ST. *Functional reconstruction of the foot and ankle.* Philadelphia: Lippincott Williams & Wilkins, 2000, with permission.)

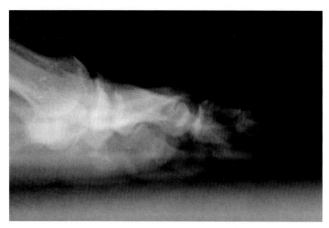

FIGURE 35-3. Weight-bearing lateral radiograph of a moderate hammer toe.

Normally, extension of the MTP joint is resisted by the plantar plate and the collateral ligaments of the MTP joint. Over time, these stabilizers become stretched, and a deformity gradually develops. As the hammer toe becomes more rigid, the toe strikes the top of the shoe at the PIP joint, and the proximal phalanx forces the metatarsal head plantarly. Eventually, the volar plate at the MTP joint stiffens, the proximal phalanx subluxates dorsally, and the plantar fat pad migrates distally. This deformity exposes the metatarsal heads plantarly, and metatarsalgia occurs. Usually, these deformities are painful at the dorsal aspect of the PIP joint, where a callous is often present. A painful callus sometimes forms at the metatarsal head plantarly.

CLASSIFICATION

Hammer toe deformities can be divided into mild, moderate, and severe forms. A mild deformity is flexible without a fixed contracture at the MTP or PIP joints. It is often caused by a contracture of the FDL. The deformity occurs with ankle dorsiflexion or with weight bearing but is absent when the patient is not bearing weight and the foot is in equinus. A moderate deformity has a fixed flexion contracture at the PIP joint but without an extension contracture at the MTP joint. (Fig. 35-3). A severe deformity has a fixed flexion contracture at the PIP joint, with a fixed extension contracture at the MTP joint (Fig. 35-4). In addition to dorsal pain at the PIP joint, patients may also complain of pain plantarly, near the corresponding metatarsal head.

INDICATIONS

Indications for surgery include difficulty with shoe wear and pain not responsive to standard conservative care. Conservative care includes properly fitting shoes, splinting devices, and doughnut cushions.

PREOPERATIVE PLANNING

A thorough physical examination allows determination of the severity of deformity (i.e., flexible or fixed). Preoperative radiographs (anteroposterior and lateral weight-bearing views of the foot) are valuable to determine the amount of contracture at the PIP and MTP joints and to rule out other pathology (Fig. 35-4).

EQUIPMENT

- Esmarch tourniquet, cast padding
- Bone cutter
- Kirschner wires (K-wires), 0.045 and 0.062 inches
- K-wire driver
- Telfa bolsters
- Postoperative shoe

PATIENT POSITIONING AND PREPARATION

Patients are positioned supine, with a bump under the ipsilateral hip to compensate for normal hip external rotation (Fig. 35-5). Surgery can be performed with use of an ankle block. A full roll of cast padding is wrapped above the malleolus. A bloodless field is obtained by exsanguinating the foot with an Esmarch and then tightly wrapping the Esmarch three times above the malleolus on the cast padding. This allows the Esmarch bandage to act as a tourniquet.

MILD DEFORMITY

Mild hammer toe deformities are managed with a flexor to extensor tendon transfer (i.e., Girdlestone-Taylor procedure). The FDL is transferred to the extensor hood, where it assumes the role of an intrinsic (i.e., plantar flexion at the MTP joint and extension of the PIP and DIP joints), thereby eliminating the deformity. Expectations for the surgery must be discussed with the patient preoperatively. A

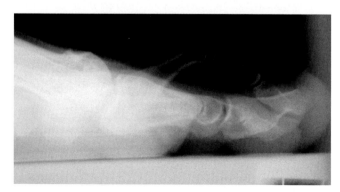

FIGURE 35-4. Weight-bearing lateral radiograph of a severe hammer toe demonstrates flexion of the proximal interphalangeal and metatarsophalangeal joints of the second toe.

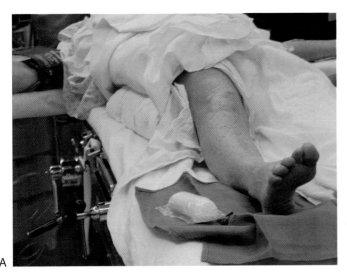

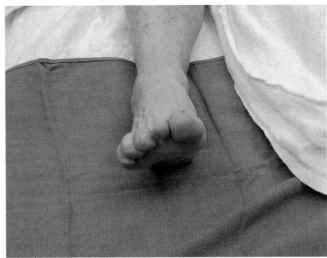

A   B

FIGURE 35-5. The patient is supine with a bump under the ipsilateral hip **(A)** to place the foot in a neutral position **(B)**.

flexor-to-extensor transfer eliminates a hammer toe deformity, but active flexion of the toe is lost.

Surgical Incision Landmarks

Three incisions are required when performing a flexor-to-extensor tendon transfer. A 1.5-cm longitudinal incision is made on the plantar surface of the toe at the level of the proximal flexion crease to harvest the FDL (Fig. 35-6). A plantar transverse stab incision is made at the distal phalanx crease to release the insertion of the FDL from the distal phalanx. A third longitudinal incision is made on the dorsal aspect of the toe over the middle phalanx to affix the FDL to the extensor hood (Fig. 35-7).

Approach and Procedure

Initially, the FDL is harvested through the longitudinal plantar incision. Dissection is carried to the level of the

flexor sheath, which is split in line with the incision. The FDL is identified as the middle of the three flexor tendons (Fig. 35-8) and held outside the skin using a hemostat. ◼ It is released from its insertion on the plantar aspect of the distal phalanx using the small plantar stab incision (Fig. 35-9). ◼ The FDL is then delivered into the proximal wound. The raphe in the midline of the FDL is split a distance of 1.5 to 2.5 cm to create two tails (Fig. 35-10). ◼

Attention is then turned to the dorsal incision. The extensor hood is exposed at the level of the proximal phalanx (Fig. 35-11). Medial and lateral tunnels are created adjacent to the extensor hood for passage of the FDL tendon slips. To create these tunnels, a hemostat is passed from dorsal to plantar aspects, deep to the neurovascular bundle, to retrieve the FDL tails ◼ and bring them to the dorsal wound (Fig. 35-12). The tails are then sutured to the extensor mechanism in the middle of the proximal phalanx using 3-0 or 4-0 absorbable suture (Fig. 35-13). ◼ The optimal position

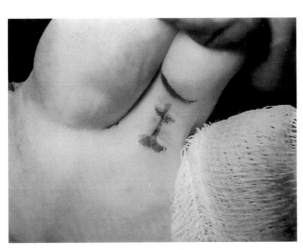

FIGURE 35-6. Plantar incision markings.

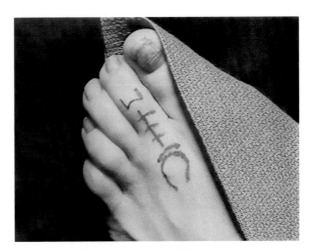

FIGURE 35-7. Dorsal incisions.

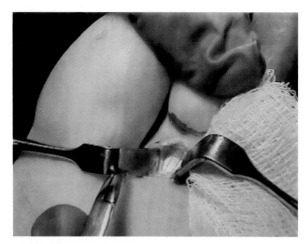

FIGURE 35-8. Flexor digitorum longus and flexor digitorum brevis tendons.

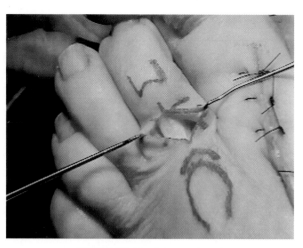

FIGURE 35-11. Extensor hood.

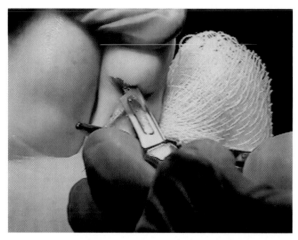

FIGURE 35-9. Release of the flexor digitorum longus tendon.

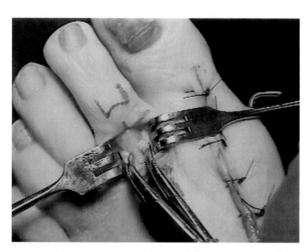

FIGURE 35-12. Retrieved flexor digitorum longus tails.

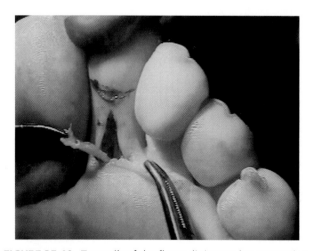

FIGURE 35-10. Two tails of the flexor digitorum longus tendon.

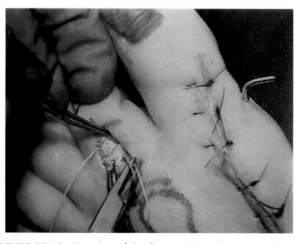

FIGURE 35-13. Suturing of the flexor tails to the extensor hood.

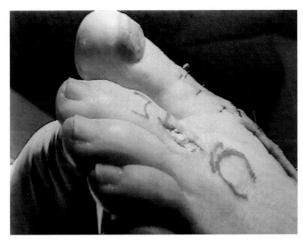

FIGURE 35-14. After the flexor tendon is sutured to the extensor tendon, the metatarsophalangeal joint should rest in neutral.

for suturing the tendon is determined with the ankle in neutral and the toe plantar flexed 20 degrees at the MTP joint. After the transfer (with the ankle in neutral), the MTP joint should rest in neutral, and the PIP joint should rest in neutral or in less than 10 degrees of flexion (Fig. 35-14). The dorsal wound is closed with nylon suture, and the plantar wound is closed with chromic suture.

Figure 35-15 shows the flexor-to-extensor tendon transfer technique using two transverse plantar incisions and one dorsal incision.

Postoperative Protocol

Weight bearing is allowed in a postoperative shoe. Sutures are removed at 3 weeks. For 6 weeks, the toe is taped to maintain PIP extension and prevent dorsiflexion at the

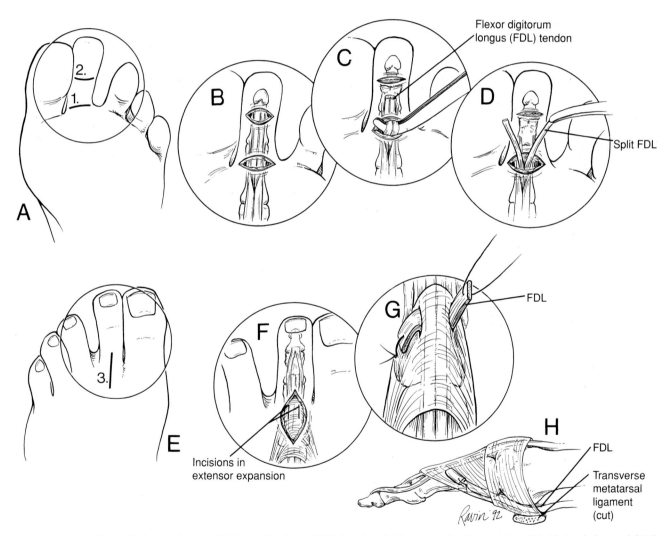

FIGURE 35-15. Flexor digitorum longus (FDL) transfer for mild deformity. **A:** Transverse incisions at the distal interphalangeal (DIP) and proximal interphalangeal joint creases. **B:** The flexor tendon is released at the DIP joint. **C:** The FDL is brought into the proximal wound with a hemostat. **D:** The FDL is split about 2 cm along natural cleavage line in its center. **E and F:** A 2-cm longitudinal incision is made over the dorsum of the proximal half of the proximal phalanx. Separate, smaller incisions are placed through the extensor expansion in the distal part of the wound for windows through which FDL slips will pass. **G:** FDL slips pass plantar to the transverse metatarsal ligament, which is essential for any flexion moment at the metatarsophalangeal joint. **H:** Tendon slips may be crossed and sutured together, but this may leave a small knot beneath skin. (From Richardson EG. Lesser toe abnormalities. In: Crenshaw AH, ed. *Campbell's operative orthopaedics,* 8th ed. St. Louis: Mosby–Year Book, 1992, with permission.)

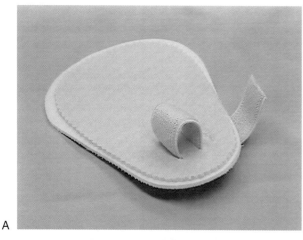

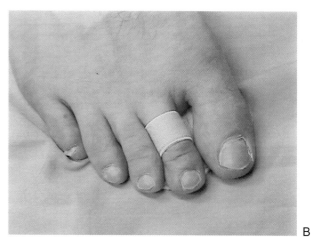

A
B

FIGURE 35-16. Budin splint **(A)** and a splint applied to the second toe to maintain proximal interphalangeal joint extension and prevent dorsiflexion at the metatarsophalangeal hammer toe **(B)**.

MTP. Alternatively, a Budin splint can be used to maintain the toe position (Fig. 35-16).

MODERATE DEFORMITY

Moderate hammer toe deformities require resection of the PIP joint (i.e., DuVries arthroplasty). The distal aspect of the middle phalanx is excised to form a fibrotic or bony union at the PIP joint with the joint in a straightened position. Expectations for the surgery must be discussed with the patient. With a DuVries arthroplasty, the deformity is eliminated, but in most cases, a stiff, shorter toe results. Rarely, a floppy toe occurs.

Surgical Incision Landmarks

The incision for a DuVries arthroplasty is an elliptical incision over the dorsal aspect of the PIP joint that includes most or all of the dorsal callus (Fig. 35-17). The extent of the transverse incision is defined by the medial and lateral aspects of the toe crease when the toe is flexed at the PIP

joint. The typical width of the ellipse is 4 to 5 mm. When operating on the fifth toe, a dorsal longitudinal incision is made over the PIP joint (Fig 35-17).

Approach and Procedure

The incision for a DuVries arthroplasty is a full-thickness incision that includes skin with the callus, the extensor tendon, and the joint capsule. After the full-thickness flap is removed, the PIP joint is flexed, and the collateral ligaments are detached from their proximal origin on the PIP joint with a no. 15 scalpel blade. To cut the medial collateral ligaments, the toe is flexed at the PIP joint, and the scalpel is passed from the plantar aspect of the proximal phalanx (parallel to the proximal phalanx) to the medial aspect of the proximal phalanx. The same is done to cut the lateral collateral ligament. Care is taken to stay close to the bone when releasing the collateral ligaments to avoid damage to the neurovascular bundles.

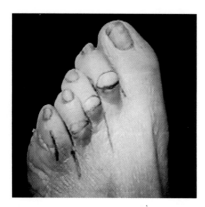

FIGURE 35-17. Incision over the dorsal aspect of the proximal interphalangeal joint.

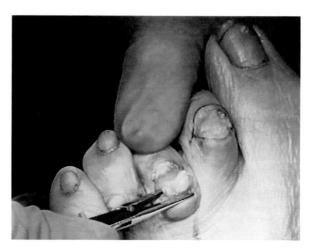

FIGURE 35-18. A straight snap is placed at the distal proximal phalanx to protect the soft tissue.

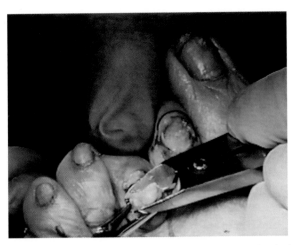

FIGURE 35-19. Cutting the distal portion of the proximal phalanx with a bone cutter.

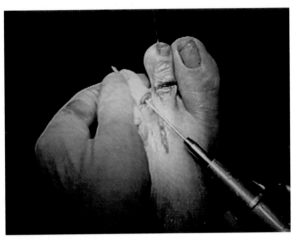

FIGURE 35-21. Kirschner wire through the middle and distal phalanx.

With the release of the collateral ligaments, the head of the proximal phalanx is delivered into the wound. Next, the soft tissue is cleared from the distal aspect of the phalanx, ◨ and a straight snap is used to define the metaphyseal-diaphyseal junction and protect the skin (Fig. 35-18). A bone cutter is used to remove the head of the proximal phalanx just proximal to the condyles of the proximal phalanx (Figs. 35-19 and 35-20). If there is continued flexion deformity at the PIP, an additional 2 to 3 mm of bone can be resected, or the FDL can be released. To release the FDL, an incision is made in the volar plate, and the FDL is cut. If an arthrodesis is desired, the articular surface of the base of the middle phalanx is roughened using a curette. <u>More bone should be resected in longer-standing deformities and in older individuals to allow adequate correction and to avoid neurovascular compromise.</u> **Removal of excessive bone from the proximal phalanx can lead to a floppy toe.**

To stabilize the arthroplasty, a K-wire (0.045 inches) is directed distally from the middle phalanx through the distal phalanx and out the tip of the toe (Fig. 35-21). The K-wire is then drilled retrograde across the resected PIP joint into the proximal phalanx (Fig. 35-22). When a K-wire is used, the wound is closed with at least two horizontal mattress sutures, incorporating the extensor tendon.

An alternative fixation technique involves use of Telfa bolsters to keep the PIP joint extended. Two Telfa bolsters are placed transversely, proximally and distally to the PIP joint. These bolsters are incorporated into the 3-0 nylon suture vertical mattress closure. When the sutures are tied over the bolsters, leverage is created that extends the PIP joint into satisfactory alignment (Fig. 35-23). <u>After a DuVries arthroplasty, the toe should be examined with the ankle in slight dorsiflexion to determine if there is an extension deformity at the MTP joint. With a mild extension deformity,</u>

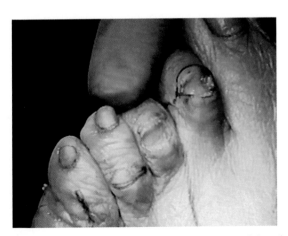

FIGURE 35-20. Appearance after removal of the condyles of the proximal phalanx.

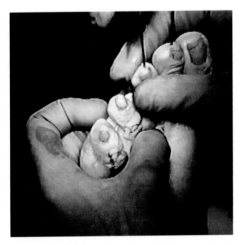

FIGURE 35-22. Kirschner wire through the proximal phalanx and metatarsophalangeal joint.

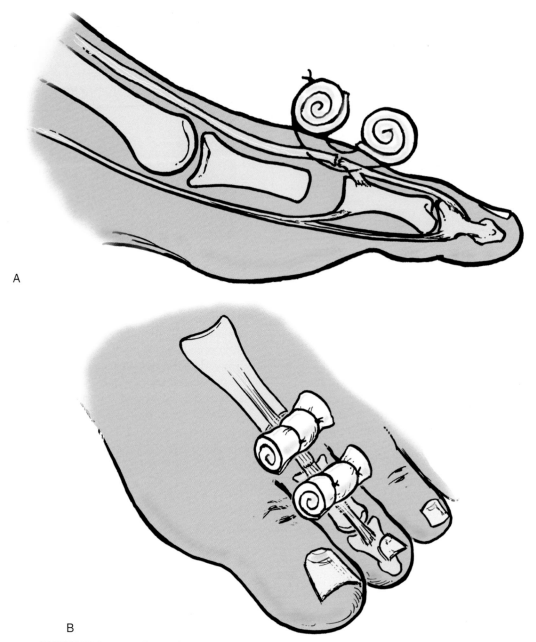

A

B

FIGURE 35-23. A and B: Telfa bolsters are used to close the proximal interphalangeal joint wound.

a percutaneous EDL tenotomy (performed at the level of the MTP) may be necessary. With a more extensive deformity, the MTP joint should be released, as discussed in the Severe Deformity procedure.

Postoperative Protocol

Patients are allowed to weight bear in a postoperative shoe. The K-wire and sutures are removed 3 weeks postoperatively. Taping (as previously described) or a Budin splint is used for 6 weeks postoperatively to keep the PIP joint extended and prevent MTP dorsiflexion.

SEVERE DEFORMITY

Severe hammer toe deformities require resection of the PIP joint (i.e., DuVries arthroplasty) with release of the extension deformity at the MTP joint (i.e., contracture, subluxation, or dislocation).

Surgical Incision Landmarks

An elliptical incision is made over the dorsal aspect of the PIP joint as described for a moderate hammer toe deformity. A second longitudinal incision (2 to 3 cm) is made over the dorsal aspect of the MTP joint.

Approach and Procedure

A PIP resection is carried out as described for a moderate hammer toe deformity. Before placement of the K-wire, attention is turned to the deformity at the MTP joint.

To address the deformity at the MTP joint, a longitudinal incision overlying the MTP joint is performed and dissection is carried down to the level of the extensor tendon (Fig. 35-17). The EDL tendon is Z-lengthened (Fig. 35-24), and a tenotomy of the EDB tendon is performed. A transverse dorsal capsulotomy of the MTP joint is executed with resection of a rectangular piece of the dorsal capsule. The joint is then manipulated out of extension. If an extension deformity persists, the collateral ligaments are released from their proximal origin on the metatarsal. The ligaments are released by making a dorsal longitudinal incision on the metatarsal neck and subperiosteally releasing the soft tissues medially and laterally. If necessary, an MTP arthroplasty (i.e., resection of the distal 2 mm of the metatarsal head) can be performed for continued extension deformity or severe arthritis.

A K-wire (0.062 inches) is then placed across the DIP and PIP joints as previously described for a moderate hammer toe deformity (Fig. 35-21). The wire is placed across the MTP joint while holding the ankle in neutral dorsiflexion and the toe in neutral alignment (Figs. 35-22 and 35-25). The foot must be held in a plantigrade position while crossing the MTP joint with the K-wire to ensure proper alignment of the joint. The EDL tendon is repaired with resorbable suture. The PIP joint wound is closed with nylon mattress sutures incorporating the extensor tendon,

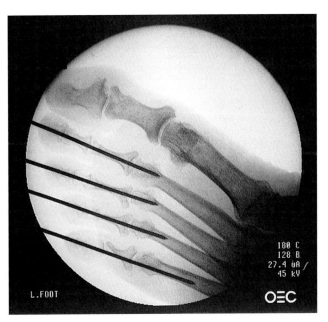

FIGURE 35-25. Kirschner wires across interphalangeal and metatarsophalangeal joints.

and the MTP joint incision is closed with interrupted nylon sutures.

Postoperative Protocol

Patients are allowed to weight bear in a postoperative shoe. The sutures and K-wire are removed 3 weeks after surgery. A Budin splint or taping is then used for 6 weeks.

In the severe deformity requiring correction at the MTP and PIP joints, reduction of the MTP and PIP joints may place tension on the neurovascular bundle. Neurovascular compromise which does not resolve several minutes after the tourniquet is removed may require removal of the K-wire to allow the toe to assume a more shortened position. After removal of a K-wire, extra care must be used with the postoperative dressing to maintain the position of the toe. The reoperated toe is particularly vulnerable to neurovascular compromise.

FOLLOW-UP

The reported rate of satisfactory results after a flexor-to-extensor transfer varies, with many studies reporting satisfactory results for more than 90% of cases. Swelling of the toe may persist for 4 to 6 months. Complications are uncommon and include transient numbness, postoperative vascular impairment, toe stiffness, hyperextension of the DIP joint, or recurrence of deformity.

The results for a DuVries arthroplasty are generally good. As with a flexor transfer, swelling of the toe commonly per-

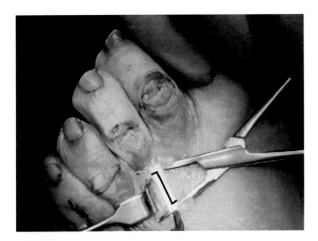

FIGURE 35-24. Z-lengthening of the extensor digitorum longus.

sists for 4 to 6 months after surgery. Complications of a DuVries arthroplasty include postoperative vascular impairment, infection, toe angulation, recurrence of deformity, flail toe, and mallet toe deformity.

SUGGESTED READINGS

Coughlin MJ, Dorris J, Polk E. Operative repair of the fixed hammer toe deformity. *Foot Ankle Int* 2000;21:94–104.

Coughlin MJ. Subluxation and dislocation of the second metatarsophalangeal joint. *Orthop Clin North Am* 1989;20:535-551.

Mann R, Coughlin MJ. Lesser toe deformities. *Instruct Course Lect* 1987;36:137–159.

Myerson MS, Shereff MJ. Th1e pathological anatomy of claw and hammer toes. *J Bone Joint Surg Am* 1989;71:45–49.

Richardson E. Lesser toe abnormalities. In *Campbell's operative orthopaedics.* St. Louis: CV Mosby, 1992:2742–2744.

Taylor RG. The treatment of claw toes by multiple transfers of flexor into extensor tendons. *J Bone Joint Surg Br* 1951;33:539–542.

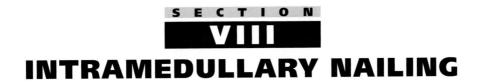

CHAPTER 36

INTRAMEDULLARY FEMORAL NAILING

KENNETH J. KOVAL

Fractures of the femoral shaft are severe injuries requiring emergent orthopaedic treatment. These fractures usually result from a directly applied, high-energy force. Important local concerns, such as limb deformity and injury to the surrounding soft tissue, can be overshadowed by associated injuries and systemic complications. However, femoral fracture management is important in the initial injury phase and in determining the patient's ultimate functional outcome. The standard of care for stabilization of femoral shaft fractures is intramedullary nailing. This chapter describes intramedullary nailing of the femoral shaft.

ANATOMY

The femur is the largest tubular bone in the body and is surrounded by the greatest mass of muscle (Fig. 36-1). The medial cortex is under compression, and the lateral cortex is under tension. The femoral shaft is subjected to major muscular forces that deform the thigh after a fracture:

Abductors (gluteus medius and minimus), which insert on the greater trochanter and abduct the proximal femur after trochanteric fractures and proximal shaft fractures

Iliopsoas, which flexes and externally rotates the proximal fragment in femoral shaft fractures by its attachment to the lesser trochanter

Adductors, which span most shaft fractures and exert a strong axial and varus load to the bone by traction on the distal fragment

Gastrocnemius, which acts on distal shaft fractures and supracondylar fractures by angulating the distal fragment into flexion

Fascia lata, which acts as a tension band by resisting the medial angulating forces of the adductors

The thigh musculature is divided into three distinct fascial compartments. The anterior compartment is composed of the quadriceps femoris, iliopsoas, sartorius, and pectineus, as well as the femoral artery, vein, and nerve and the lateral femoral cutaneous nerve. The medial compartment contains the gracilis, adductor longus, brevis, magnus,

and obturator externus muscles along with the obturator artery, vein, and nerve and the profunda femoris artery. The posterior compartment includes the biceps femoris, semitendinosus, and semimembranosus; a portion of the adductor magnus muscle; branches of the profunda femoris artery; the sciatic nerve; and the posterior femoral cutaneous nerve.

CLASSIFICATION

Many classification systems have been described for femur fractures. One such classification describes the fracture as (1) open or closed; (2) location: proximal, middle, or distal one third; supra-isthmic or infra-isthmic; (3) pattern: spiral, oblique, or transverse; (4) comminuted, segmental, or butterfly fragment; (5) angulation: varus, valgus, or rotational deformity; and (6) displacement: shortening or translation.

Winquist and Hansen developed a classification based on the amount of comminution (Fig. 36-2). Type I and II fractures have stable bone contact between the proximal and distal fragments and are considered length stable. Type III and IV comminution results in no contact between the proximal and distal fragments and requires static interlocking to maintain correct limb length and rotation.

Type I: minimal or no comminution
Type II: cortices of both fragments at least 50% intact
Type III: 50% to 100% cortical comminution
Type IV: circumferential comminution with no cortical contact at the fracture site

The Orthopaedic Trauma Association (OTA) classification of femoral shaft fractures is useful for research purposes (Fig. 36-3).

Type A: simple fracture
  A1: spiral
  A2: oblique (>30 degrees)
  A3: transverse (<30 degrees)
Type B: wedge fracture
  B1: spiral
  B2: bending
  B3: fragmented

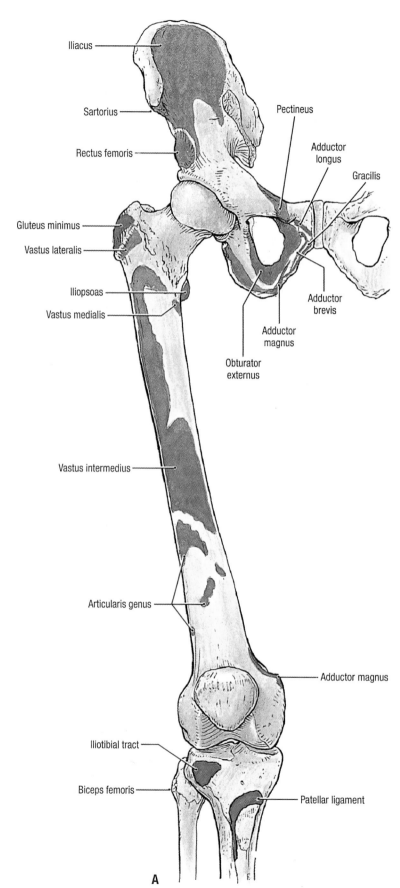

FIGURE 36-1. Bones of the lower limb showing muscle attachments. **A:** Anterior view. *(continued)*

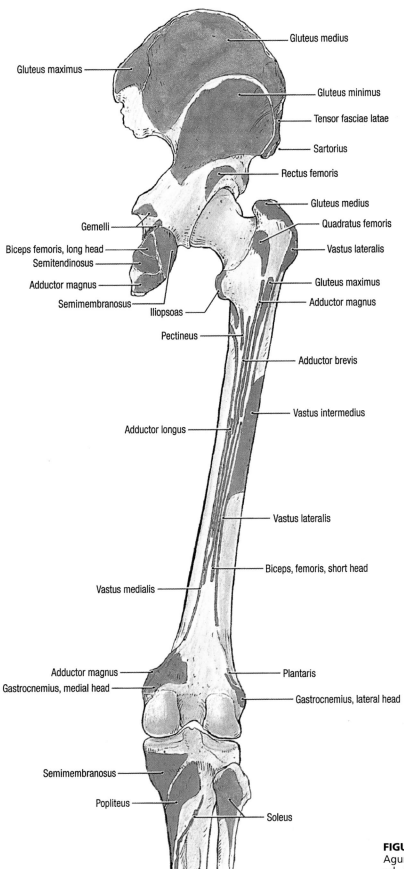

FIGURE 36-1. *Continued.* **B:** Posterior view. (From Agur AMR, Lee MJ. *Grant's atlas of anatomy,* 10th ed. Philadelphia: Lippincott Williams & Wilkins, 1999, with permission.)

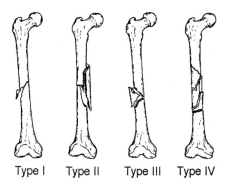

FIGURE 36-2. The Winquist and Hansen classification of femoral shaft fractures is based on the amount of comminution. (From Wolinsky PR, Johnson KD. Femoral shaft fractures. In: Browner BD, Jupiter JB, Levine AM, et al, eds. *Skeletal trauma,* 2nd ed. Philadelphia: WB Saunders, 1998, with permission.)

Type C: complex fracture
   C1: spiral
   C2: segmental
   C3: irregular

INDICATIONS AND CONTRAINDICATIONS

Intramedullary nailing is the treatment of choice for virtually all femoral shaft fractures in adults. Contraindications to intramedullary nailing include active local or systemic infection; adolescents with open growth plates in whom antegrade nailing through the piriformis fossae can damage the blood supply to the femoral head, causing osteonecrosis; a prolonged period of external fixation; patients with very narrow medullary canals; and patients with preexisting deformities that would preclude intramedullary nailing.

PREOPERATIVE PLANNING

Preoperative radiographs should visualize the entire femur, including the femoral head, femoral neck, and knee on anteroposterior and lateral views (Fig. 36-4). Radiographs should be carefully inspected for intraarticular fracture

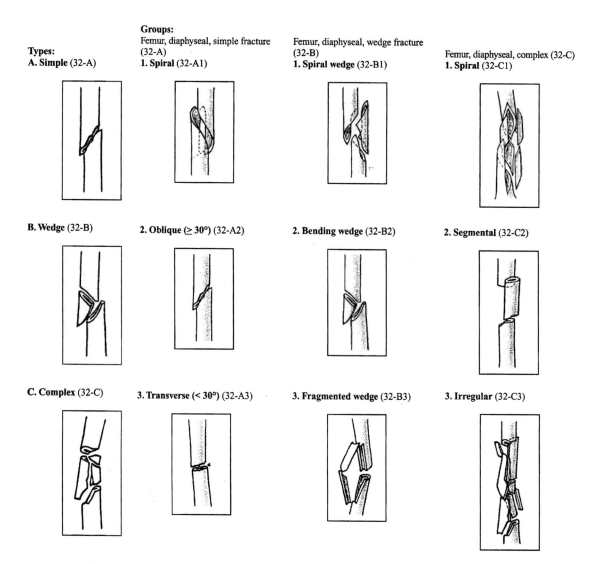

FIGURE 36-3. The Orthopaedic Trauma Association (OTA) classification of femoral shaft fractures.

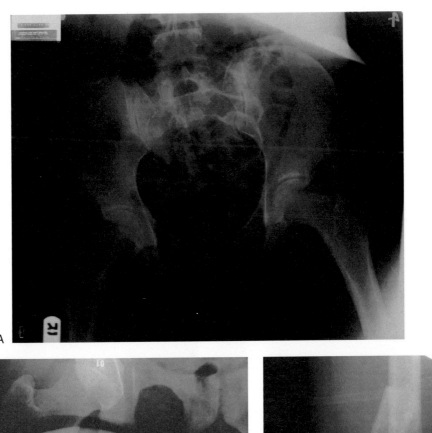

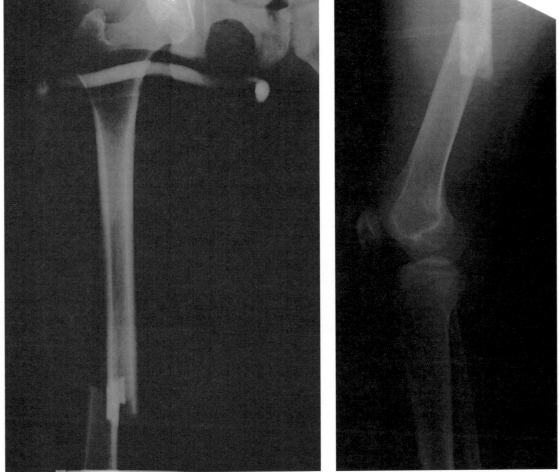

FIGURE 36-4. Preoperative anteroposterior pelvis **(A)** and anteroposterior **(B)** and lateral **(C)** femoral radiographs show a displaced femoral shaft fracture.

propagation and neoplastic disease. Preoperative radiographs of the uninjured femur may be used to estimate proper nail diameter, anticipated amount of reaming, and nail length for severely comminuted fractures (Fig. 36-5). Radiographic templates for preoperative planning are available from most nail manufacturers. In cases involving a time delay from injury to surgery, the surgeon should confirm that appropriate femoral length has been obtained with traction; excessive intraoperative traction resulting in pudendal or sciatic nerve palsy has been reported after closed antegrade intramedullary nailing.

The choice of nail size depends on the size of the patient and the extent of femoral comminution. Nevertheless, because of a small but consistently reported percentage of complications caused by nail fatigue, it is recommended that, if possible, an 11- or 12-mm-diameter nail be used.

EQUIPMENT

The equipment necessary for intramedullary femoral nailing includes the following (Fig. 36-6):

- Curved awl
- Ball-tipped and straight-tipped guide wires of identical length
- Intramedullary reamer set
- Guide wire exchange tube
- Femoral nail instrument and implant sets
- Image intensifier

PATIENT POSITIONING

When an interlocked nail is used for femoral shaft fracture fixation, the patient can be positioned supine or lateral on a fracture table or radiolucent table (Fig. 36-7). I prefer to

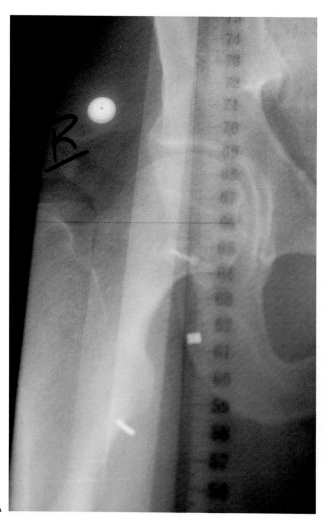

A

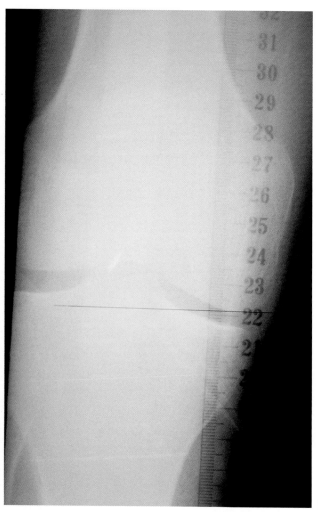

B

FIGURE 36-5. A and B: Use of preoperative radiographs of the uninjured femur to estimate proper nail length. A radiolucent ruler is placed along the femoral shaft, and the distance from the anticipated proximal to distal extent of the nail is measured.

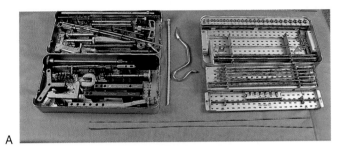

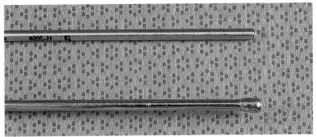

A

B

FIGURE 36-6. **A:** Selected equipment for intramedullary femoral nailing: TriGen instruments for implantation of a tibial or femoral nail *(left tray, top and bottom)*; intramedullary reamer set *(right tray, top and bottom)*; guide wire exchange tube and curved awl *(between trays)*. **B:** Intramedullary femoral nailing instruments: straight-tipped *(top)* and ball-tipped *(bottom)* guide wires of identical length.

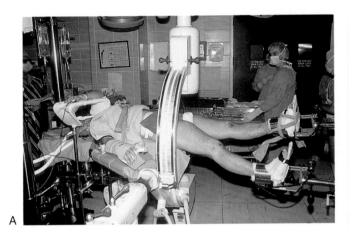

A

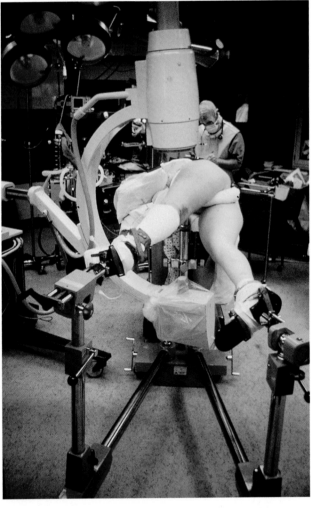

B

FIGURE 36-7. Supine **(A)** and lateral **(B)** patient positioning on a fracture table.

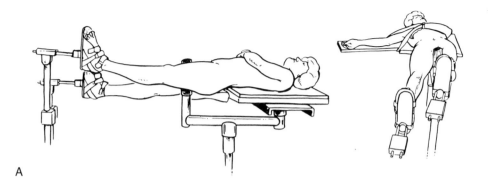

A

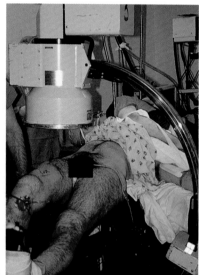

B

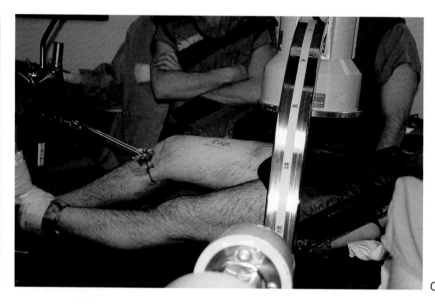

C

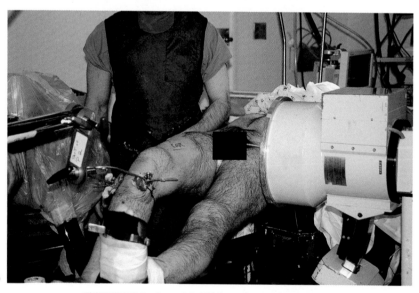

D

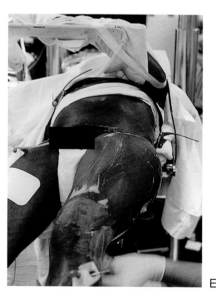

E

FIGURE 36-8. A and B: With supine patient positioning on the fracture table, the contralateral lower extremity is placed into a heel-to-toe position, adjacent but inferior to the injured extremity. **C and D:** Positioning of the image intensifier to get anteroposterior and lateral views of the proximal femur. **E:** The patient's trunk is adducted away from the operative side to facilitate access to the entry point and nail insertion.

position the patient supine on a fracture table. Supine positioning is easier to set up than the lateral decubitus and better tolerated in patients who have associated pulmonary injury or preexisting lung disease. Use of the lateral decubitus position does, however, facilitate identification and penetration of the nail entry point in the piriformis fossae, which may be the most challenging step in intramedullary nailing of a subtrochanteric fracture. Use of a fracture table allows fracture reduction through sustained longitudinal traction, with or without a skeletal pin. The design of most fracture tables allows circumferential access to the extremity for manipulation, surgical exposure, and imaging. Alternatively, intramedullary nailing can be performed on a radiolucent table. Traction can be applied manually or with the use of a femoral distractor. Set-up time is minimal, and access to the piriformis fossa is improved by abducting the limb. Disadvantages with this technique include difficulty visualizing the hip and proximal femur in lateral projection, difficulty reducing and holding the fracture alignment, and blockage of the operative field by the femoral distractor.

With supine positioning on the fracture table, the in-

jured lower extremity is adducted with the hip flexed approximately 15 degrees. The contralateral lower extremity is placed into a heel-to-toe position, adjacent but inferior to the injured extremity (Fig. 36-8). The patient's trunk is adducted away from the operative side to facilitate access to the entry point and nail insertion. Traction is applied through a skeletal pin placed in the anterior aspect of the distal femur (away from the anticipated nail position) or proximal tibia.

FRACTURE REDUCTION

Closed reduction is performed by traction through the fracture table and external manipulation. Longitudinal traction is applied through use of proximal tibial or distal femoral pin traction, and fracture alignment is checked with the image intensifier (Fig. 36-9). Occasionally, manipulation of the thigh by the surgeon or use of a crutch may help to effect fracture reduction. To minimize the risk of a pudendal nerve palsy, the traction is decreased during the preparation, draping, and proximal exposure. Frequently, a small-diameter

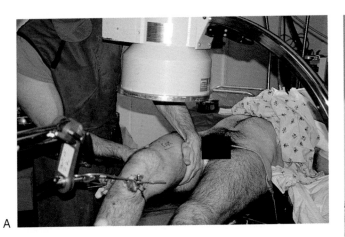

A

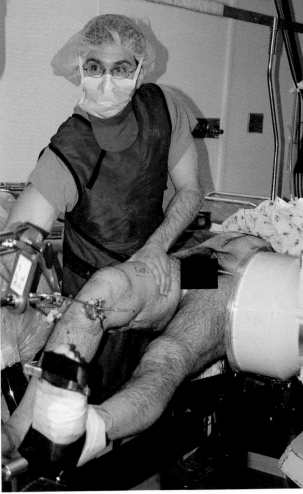

B

FIGURE 36-9. A and B: Longitudinal traction is applied by means of proximal tibial or distal femoral pin traction, and fracture alignment is checked with the image intensifier. Manipulation of the leg helps to reduce an angulated fracture.

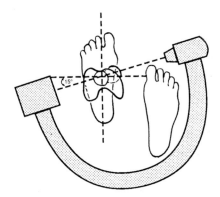

FIGURE 36-10. Determination of rotational alignment using the image intensifier. The image intensifier is rotated to obtain a perfect cross-table lateral view of the femoral head and neck. The position of the image intensifier is recorded and the unit moved to the distal femur. The image intensifier beam is rotated 15 to 20 degrees internally, and the leg is rotated until a perfect lateral view of the distal femoral condyles and knee is obtained, reestablishing the correct anteversion of the femoral neck.

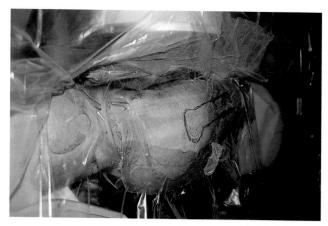

FIGURE 36-12. An oblique skin incision is made 4 to 5 cm proximal to the greater trochanter in line with the femoral shaft.

nail may be used in the proximal fragment to reduce a flexed and externally rotated proximal fragment. Alternatively, many implant manufacturers include a small-diameter rod in the nailing sets for this purpose.

Correct rotational alignment can be established using the image intensifier (Fig. 36-10). Femoral neck anteversion averages 15 degrees in most adults. The image intensifier is rotated to obtain a perfect cross-table lateral view of the femoral head and neck. The position of the image intensifier is recorded and the unit moved to the distal femur. The image intensifier beam is rotated 15 to 20 degrees internally and the leg rotated until a perfect lateral view of the distal femoral condyles and knee is obtained, reestablishing the correct anteversion of the femoral neck. Correct rotation of the distal fragment usually places the foot in 0 to 15 degrees of external rotation; with the patient placed on the fracture table, however, the proximal fragment may externally rotate as much as 45 to 50 degrees, requiring the foot to be turned out to match this external rotation.

After the fracture is reduced, the lower extremity is prepared from the rib cage to an area distal to the tibial tubercle. The operative field is draped using an isolation screen (Fig. 36-11). Alternatively, the lower extremity can be draped free, with the area from the buttocks and lateral thigh to the popliteal crease exposed and a sterile cover over the image intensifier.

APPROACH

An oblique skin incision is made 4 to 5 cm proximal to the greater trochanter, in line with the femoral shaft (Fig. 36-12). The fascia of the gluteus maximus is incised in line with its fibers, and the gluteus maximus is bluntly dissected (Fig. 36-13). The surgeon should be able to palpate the piriformis fossa posterior to the fibers of the gluteus medius. ▣

Determination of the proper entry portal is critical when using an intramedullary nail, particularly with more proximal fracture patterns. For a first-generation centromedullary nail,

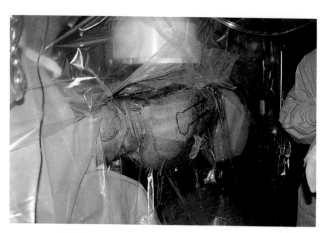

FIGURE 36-11. Use of the isolation screen.

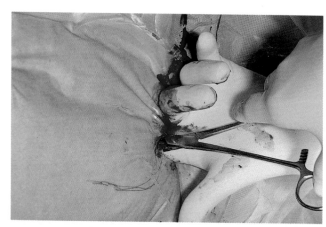

FIGURE 36-13. The fascia of the gluteus maximus is incised in line with its fibers, and the gluteus maximus is bluntly dissected.

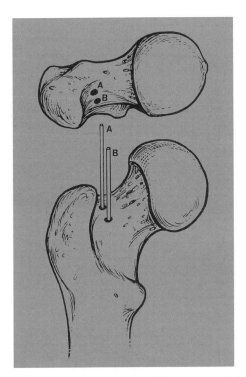

FIGURE 36-14. The entry portal should be in the middle of the piriformis fossae, in line with femoral shaft on the sagittal and coronal planes (*point B*). When using a second-generation (reconstruction) nail, the entry portal should be moved anteriorly to facilitate placement of the proximal locking screws within the femoral neck and head (*point A*).

the entry portal should be in the middle of the piriformis fossae, in line with femoral shaft in the sagittal and coronal planes (Fig. 36-14). **A lateral entry portal increases the risk of varus malalignment, and a medial entry point increases the risk of iatrogenic femoral neck fracture.** When using second-generation (reconstruction) nail, the entry portal should be moved anterior to facilitate placement of the proximal locking screws within the femoral neck and head. A curved awl or a cannulated reamer can be used to create the entry hole. I prefer a 3.2-mm tip threaded guide pin from the sliding hip screw set ◼; after its position is verified on the anteroposterior and lateral views, the entry portal is enlarged with a cannulated reamer (Fig. 36-15). ◼

PROCEDURE

After creation of the entry portal, a ball-tipped guide rod attached to a T-handled chuck is placed down the femoral canal to the fracture (Fig. 36-16). Containment of the guide wire within the femur is confirmed with anteroposterior and lateral fluoroscopic views. The fracture is reduced, and the guide wire is advanced down the center of the femoral canal to the epiphyseal scar (Fig. 36-17). ◼ **It is important to centralize the guide wire in the sagittal and coronal planes; otherwise, an angular malreduction may result when the**

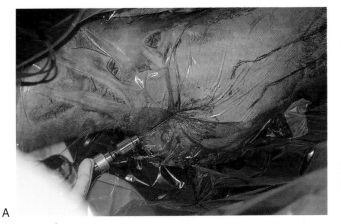
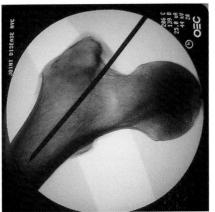
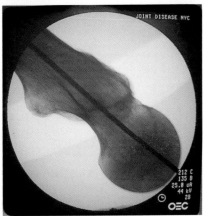

FIGURE 36-15. Use of a 3.2-mm tip-threaded guide pin from the sliding hip screw set to open the medullary canal (**A**); after its position is verified on the anteroposterior and lateral views (**B and C**), the entry portal is enlarged with a cannulated reamer (**D and E**). *(continued)*

FIGURE 36-15. *Continued.*

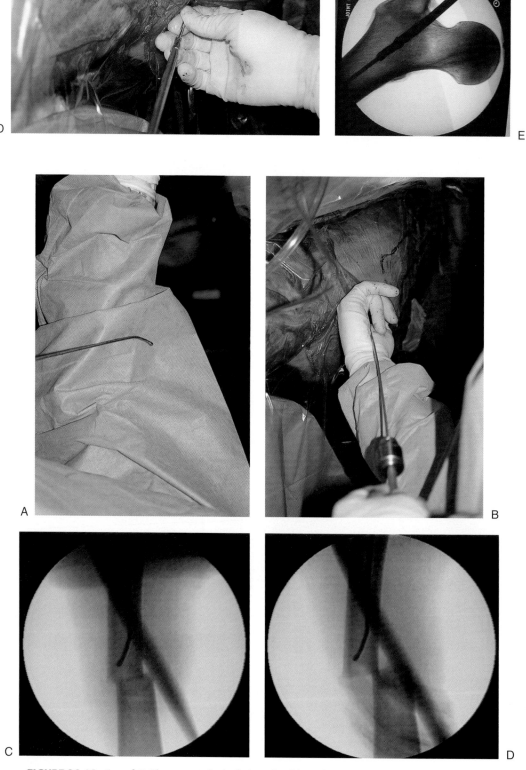

FIGURE 36-16. A and B: Placement of a ball-tipped guide rod attached down the femoral canal. **C and D:** Containment of the guide wire within the femur is confirmed with anteroposterior and lateral fluoroscopic views.

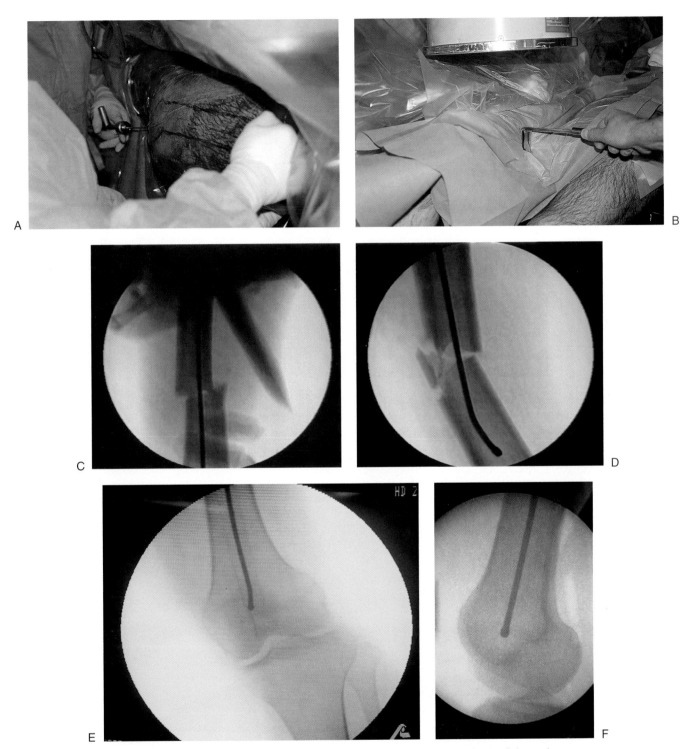

FIGURE 36-17. The fracture is reduced **(A and B)**, and the guide wire advanced down the center of the femoral canal **(C and D)** to the epiphyseal scar **(E and F)**. It is important to centralize the guide wire in the sagittal and coronal planes; otherwise, an angular malreduction may result when the nail is inserted.

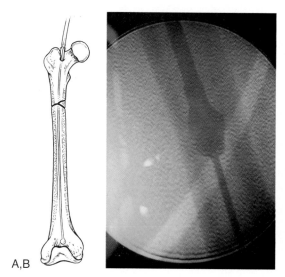
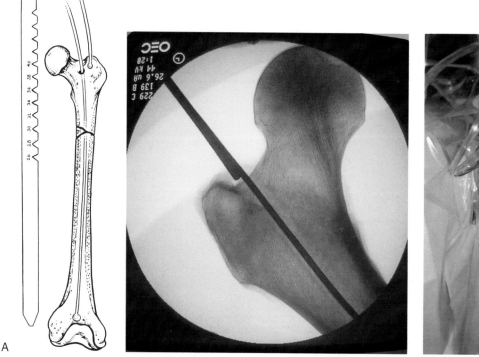
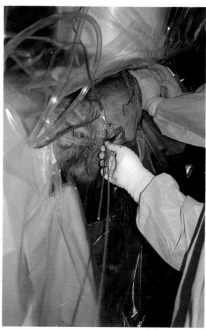

A

B,C

FIGURE 36-18. A: Determination of proper nail length using a radiolucent ruler or two identical length guide wires. **B and C:** A second guide wire is overlapped with the portion of the reduction guide wire extending proximally from the femoral entry portal; this distance is subtracted from total guide wire length to determine nail length.

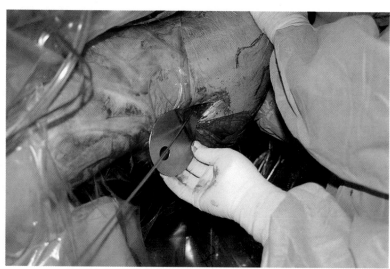

A,B

C

FIGURE 36-19. A and B: The femur is reamed over the ball-tipped guide wire in 0.5-mm increments until the desired canal diameter is achieved. **C:** A tissue protector is used at the entry portal to prevent soft tissue damage by the reamer.

nail is inserted. If the guide wire cannot be successfully advanced across the fracture site, an internal fracture alignment device can be used to reduce the fracture fragments. The proximal fragment is reamed to 10 mm and the internal fracture alignment device inserted; this cannulated device is used to directly manipulate the proximal fragment. After the fracture is reduced, the guide wire is advanced through the fracture alignment device into the distal fragment. If reducing the fracture closed proves difficult, the surgeon should not hesitate to perform a limited open reduction.

Determination of proper nail length can be made from preoperative planning and verified using two identical-length guide wires or a radiolucent ruler. In the guide wire method, a second guide wire is overlapped with the portion of the reduction guide wire extending proximally from the femoral entry portal (Fig. 36-18); this distance is subtracted from total guide wire length to determine nail length. Alternatively, the radiolucent ruler is positioned over the anterior femur, and image intensification used to make a direct reading of the distance from the entry portal to the desired distal nail tip.

The femur is reamed over the ball-tipped guide wire in 0.5-mm increments until the desired canal diameter is achieved (Fig. 36-19). I prefer to use an 11- or 12-mm-diameter nail and to overream the canal by 1 mm or, in cases of a large anterior femoral bow, 1.5 mm. If the intramedullary canal is small or if significant chatter is encountered during reaming of the femoral canal, a smaller-diameter nail should be selected.

The ball-tipped guide wire is replaced with a straight-tipped guide wire, inserted using the medullary exchange tube to maintain fracture reduction (Fig. 36-20). The se-

lected femoral nail is attached to the insertion jig; when properly assembled, the femoral nail should have an anterior bow, and the proximal guide should point laterally (Fig. 36-21). It is important to verify that the proximal targeting jig aligns with proximal nail holes before nail insertion; this can be done by assembling the drill sleeves within the insertion guide and checking that the drill bit smoothly targets the proximal nail screw holes.

The nail is advanced manually down the femoral canal over the guide wire (Fig. 36-22). The insertion handle is used to control rotation and direct nail passage. When the nail can no longer advance manually, a mallet should be used. **The mallet should only be used on the insertion driver and not on the proximal drill guide; striking the guide can alter the alignment required for proximal targeting.** As the nail is advanced down the femoral canal, correct nail rotation should be verified; the proximal insertion handle should be parallel to or pointed toward the floor to facilitate distal locking screw insertion. With the proximal handle pointed toward the ceiling, it is difficult to place the x-ray beam of many image intensifiers parallel to the distal screw holes, which complicates distal locking screw insertion. **To prevent nail incarceration, the surgeon should verify that the nail advances with each mallet blow.** During nail insertion, it may be necessary to retighten the bolts of the proximal drill guide assembly before final nail seating.

After the nail is fully seated and its position verified in the sagittal and coronal planes, the interlocking screws are inserted. For standard interlocked femoral nails, the proximal locking screws are inserted through the insertion jig and are directed obliquely or transversely from lateral to medial, depending on the nail manufacturer (Fig. 36-23). The

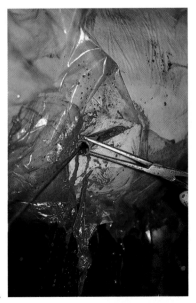
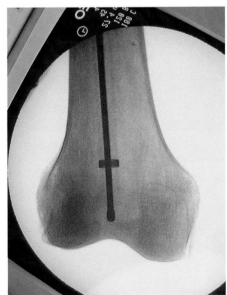
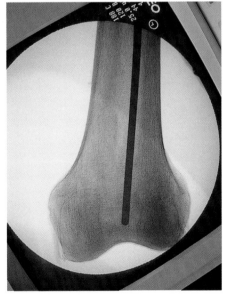

A   B,C

FIGURE 36-20. A to C: The ball-tipped guide wire is replaced with a straight-tipped guide wire, inserted using the medullary exchange tube to maintain fracture reduction.

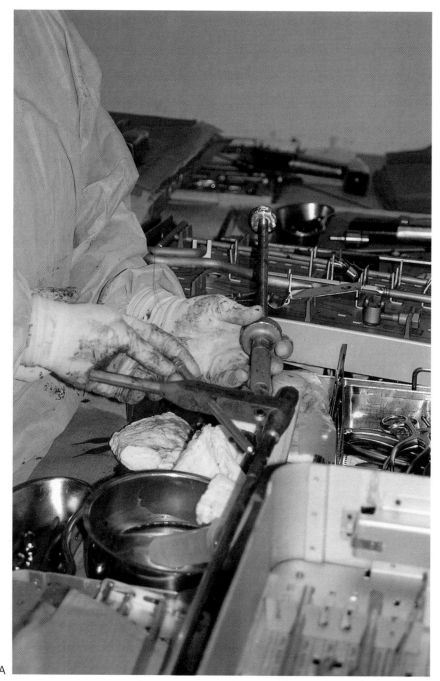

A

FIGURE 36-21. A: The selected femoral nail is attached to the insertion jig; when properly assembled, the femoral nail should have an anterior bow, and the proximal guide should point laterally. *(continued)*

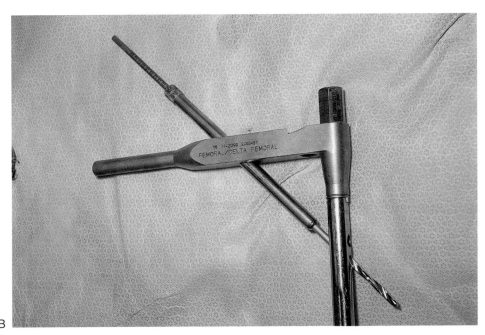

B

FIGURE 36-21. *Continued.* **B:** It is important to verify that the proximal targeting jig aligns with the proximal nail holes before nail insertion. This can be done by assembling the drill sleeves within the insertion guide and checking that the drill bit smoothly targets the proximal nail screw holes.

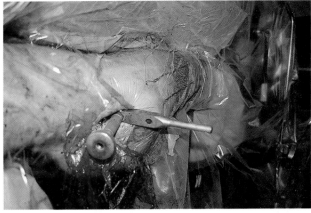

B

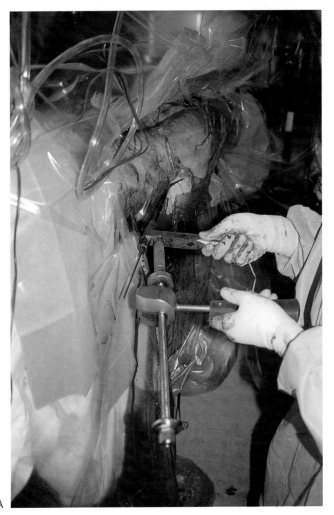

A

FIGURE 36-22. A and B: The nail is advanced manually down the femoral canal over the guide wire.

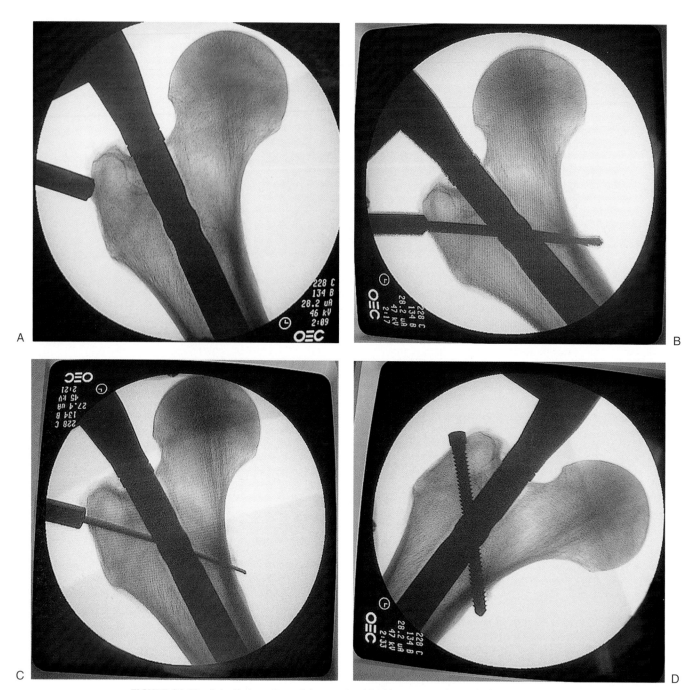

FIGURE 36-23. A to D: Insertion of the proximal locking screws through the insertion jig.

proximal locking screw is bicortical and is inserted after predrilling. The positioning of this locking screw depends on fracture geometry but is usually at the level of the lesser trochanter. **The surgeon should avoid placement of the screw in the inferior femoral neck, which could result in a stress riser effect and consequent femoral neck fracture.** The length of the locking screw can be determined directly from the drill bit. I usually measure the length of the drill bit after it contacts the inner aspect of the medial femoral cortex and add 5 mm to this measurement to determine appropriate proximal locking screw length.

Distal locking is routinely advised with the use of inter-

locked femoral nails; a static construct confers stability and is highly unlikely to lose fracture reduction in the postoperative period. **Brumback et al. reported a 10.6% loss of reduction when interlocked femoral nails were placed in a dynamically locked mode in fractures without significant fracture comminution.** Before insertion of the distal locking screw, the fracture is reassessed to verify correct fracture reduction, femoral length, and rotation. Distal locking screws are inserted using a freehand technique. There are many ways of placing the distal locking screws, but all require good image intensification (Fig. 36-24). ◼◀ The image intensifier is positioned with the beam parallel to the

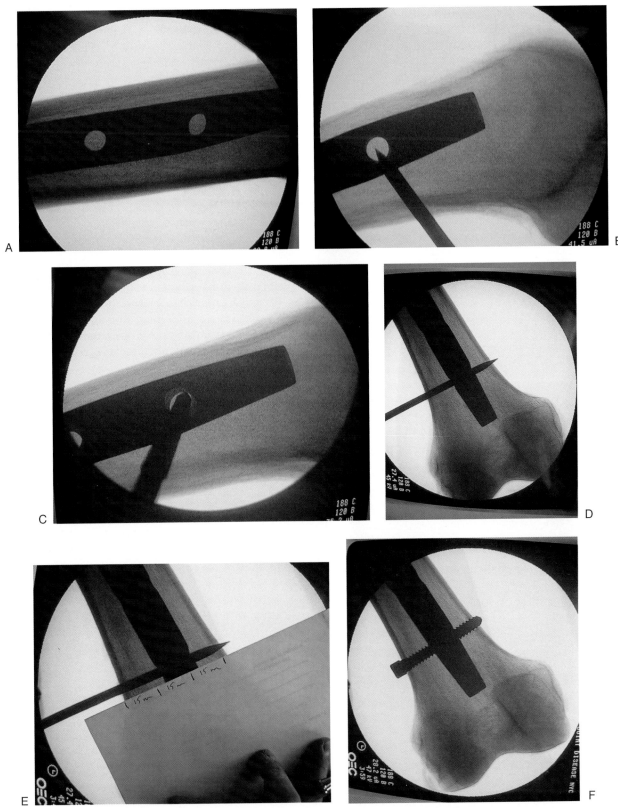

FIGURE 36-24. Insertion of the distal locking screws using a freehand technique. **A:** The image intensifier is positioned with the beam parallel to the distal locking holes; with appropriate adjustment, the holes appear perfectly round. **B:** The tip of the trocar is positioned in the middle of the locking hole, as visualized on the image intensifier. The tip of the trocar is repositioned in the middle of the locking hole and the trocar placed on end, parallel to the x-ray beam. **C:** After a halo is seen completely surrounding the trocar, it is tapped through the near cortex. **D:** The image intensifier is then positioned in an anteroposterior direction and the trocar drilled across the nail until it engages the opposite cortex. **E:** After verification of the position, the trocar is advanced through the far cortex, and the length of the locking screw is determined. **F:** Insertion of the locking screw.

distal locking holes; with appropriate adjustment, the holes appear perfectly round. I prefer to use an extra-sharp, pointed trocar to open the lateral cortex of the distal femur. The tip of the trocar is positioned in the middle of the locking hole as visualized on the image intensifier. A small skin incision is made at the tip of the trocar, and the tissue is dissected down to bone. The tip of the trocar is repositioned in the middle of the locking hole and the trocar placed on end parallel to the x-ray beam. After a halo is seen completely surrounding the trocar, it is tapped through the near cortex. Alternatively, the surgeon could use a radiolucent targeting device, which is available from various manufacturers. The image intensifier is then positioned in an anteroposterior direction and the trocar drilled across the nail until it engages the opposite cortex. Next, the image intensifier is positioned laterally to verify that the trocar has gone through the nail. After verification, the trocar is advanced through the far cortex and the length of the locking screw determined. I usually estimate the length of the locking screw based on the anteroposterior image intensifier view and the known nail diameter. Alternatively, a depth gauge or a second trocar of equal length can be used. The locking

screw is then inserted. A second distal locking screw is inserted in an identical manner. Before wound closure, fracture reduction and nail position, including all locking screws, are assessed radiographically in the sagittal and coronal planes (Fig. 36-25).

POSTOPERATIVE MANAGEMENT

Postoperative management depends on the fracture location and the amount of comminution, age of patient, preoperative mobility, and extent of coexisting injuries. Early weight bearing is encouraged for the patient with transverse or short oblique fractures when there is stable contact between two major fragments so that weight is transmitted through the bone. When comminution prevents transmission of weight through the bone, the patient is instructed to partially bear weight for 6 to 8 weeks to permit callus formation.

Patients are seen 10 to 14 days after surgery for suture removal and wound inspection. Anteroposterior and lateral radiographs are obtained to inspect the implant position, fracture alignment, and progress of union immediately after

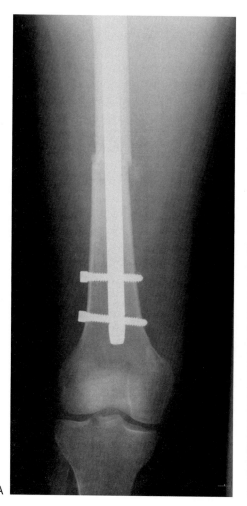
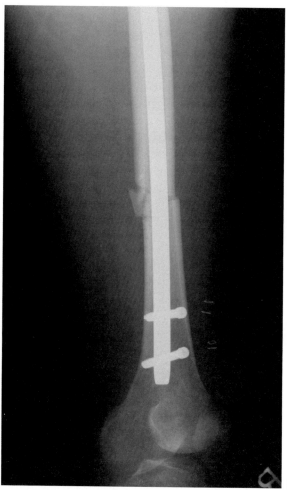

FIGURE 36-25. A and B: Final postoperative radiographs.

surgery and at 6 weeks, 12 weeks, and 20 to 24 weeks. A set of radiographs is obtained at 6 months to document adequate healing of the fracture. The average uncomplicated femoral diaphyseal fracture unites in 3 to 5 months. Several months of exercise are required to achieve the ultimate range of knee motion. The speed of recovery and degree of motion are enhanced by early physical therapy.

SUGGESTED READINGS

Benirschke SK, Melder I, Henley MB, et al. Closed interlocking nailing of femora shaft fractures: assessment of technical complications and functional outcomes of comparison of a prospective database with retrospective review. *J Orthop Trauma* 1993;7:118–122.

Bone LB, Johnson KD, Weigelt J, et al. Early versus delayed stabilization of femoral fractures: a prospective randomized study. *J Bone Joint Surg Am* 1989;71:336–340.

Braten T, Terjesen T, Rossvoll I. Femoral shaft fractures treated by intramedullary nailing: a follow-up study focusing on problems related to the method. *Injury* 1995;26:379–383.

Brumback RJ, Ellison PS Jr, Poka A, et al. Intramedullary nailing of open fractures of the femoral shaft. *J Bone Joint Surg Am* 1989;71:1324–1331.

Brumback RJ, Reilly JP, Poka A, et al. Intramedullary nailing of femoral shaft fractures. Part I. Decision-making errors with interlocking fixation. *J Bone Joint Surg Am* 1988;70:1441–1452.

Brumback RJ, Uwagie-Ero S, Lakatos RP, et al. Intramedullary nailing of femoral shaft fractures. Part II. Fracture healing with static interlocking fixation. *J Bone Joint Surg Am* 1988;70:1453–1462.

Brumback RJ, Ellison TS, Poka A, et al. Intramedullary nailing of femoral shaft fractures. Part III. Long-term effects of static interlocking fixation. *J Bone Joint Surg Am* 1992;74:106–112.

Johnson KD, Cadambi A, Seibert GB. Incidence of adult respiratory distress syndrome in patients with multiple musculoskeletal injuries: effect of early operative stabilization of fractures. *J Trauma* 1985;25:375–384.

Karpos PAG, McFerran MA, Johnson KD. Intramedullary nailing of acute femoral shaft fractures using manual traction without a fracture table. *J Orthop Trauma* 1995;9:57–62.

Kempf I, Grosse A, Beck G. Closed locked intramedullary nailing: its application to comminuted fractures of the femur. *J Bone Joint Surg Am* 1985;67:709–720.

Tornetta P III, Tiburzi D. The treatment of femoral shaft fractures using intramedullary interlocked nails with and without reaming: a preliminary report. *J Orthop Trauma* 1997;11:89–92.

Winquist RA, Hansen ST Jr, Clawson DK. Closed intramedullary nailing of femoral fractures: a report of five hundred and twenty cases. *J Bone Joint Surg Am* 1984;66:529–539.

Wiss DA, Fleming CH, Matta JM, et al. Comminuted and rotationally unstable fractures of the femur treated with an interlocking nail. *Clin Orthop* 1986;212:35–47.

CHAPTER 37

INTRAMEDULLARY TIBIAL NAILING

KENNETH J. KOVAL

Tibial shaft fractures involve the diaphysis of the tibia and can be caused by direct trauma or by torsional stress. The diagnosis is based on the presence of deformity and on anteroposterior and lateral radiographs. Associated injuries that must be excluded are arterial injuries, compartment syndrome, and injuries to the ligaments of the knee or ankle.

The goal of treatment of fractures of the lower extremity is to return the patient to his or her preinjury level of activity as soon as possible. For displaced tibial shaft fractures, this is best achieved by intramedullary nailing. This chapter discusses intramedullary nailing of the tibial shaft.

ANATOMY

The tibia is a long, tubular bone with a triangular cross section (Fig. 37-1). It has a subcutaneous anteromedial border and is bounded by four tight fascial compartments. The nutrient artery of the tibia arises from the posterior tibial artery, entering the posterolateral cortex distal to the origination of the soleus muscle, at the oblique line of the tibia. If the nutrient artery is disrupted, there is reversal of flow through the cortex, with the periosteal blood supply becoming more important. The fibula is responsible for 6% to 17% of the weight-bearing load. The common peroneal nerve courses around the neck of the fibula, where it is vulnerable to a direct blow or traction injury.

CLASSIFICATION

There is no universally accepted classification scheme. It may be best to describe the fracture in terms of (1) an open or closed injury; (2) its anatomic location (i.e., proximal, middle, or distal third); (3) the fragment number and position (e.g., comminution, butterfly fragments); (4) fracture configuration (i.e., transverse, spiral, or oblique); (5) angulation (e.g., varus or valgus, anterior or posterior); (6) shortening; and (7) displacement and percentage of cortical contact.

The Orthopaedic Trauma Association (OTA) classification of tibial fractures is useful for research purposes (Fig. 37-2):

Type A: simple
  A1: spiral
  A2: oblique (>30 degrees)
  A3: transverse (<30 degrees)
Type B: wedge (butterfly)
  B1: spiral
  B2: bending
  B3: fragmented
Type C: complex (comminuted)
  C1: spiral
  C2: segmented
  C3: irregular

INDICATIONS AND CONTRAINDICATIONS

Operative stabilization of the tibia is indicated in patients with an open fracture; multiple injuries; an ipsilateral fracture of the femur, ankle, or foot; vascular injury; compartment syndrome; and unacceptable fracture position after closed reduction and casting. An acceptable reduction includes less than 1.0 to 1.5 cm of shortening and up to 5 degrees of angulation (e.g., varus or valgus, anterior or posterior). Unstable fractures with high-grade soft tissue injury, whether closed or open, require operative stabilization.

Indications for intramedullary nailing include fractures located in the middle two thirds of the tibia. Indications for intramedullary nailing may be extended proximally or distally, but they are associated with an increased risk of fracture malreduction. Contraindications to intramedullary nailing include immature patients with open physes, patients with very small medullary canals, or a history of tibial osteomyelitis.

PREOPERATIVE PLANNING

Preoperative anteroposterior and lateral radiographs of the fractured extremity, including the knee and ankle, are critical to define the fracture and geometry of the tibial injury (Fig. 37-3). The lateral radiograph should be carefully inspected and the size of the intramedullary canal measured. An ossimeter can be used to measure the tibia and to establish the length and diameter of the nail required.

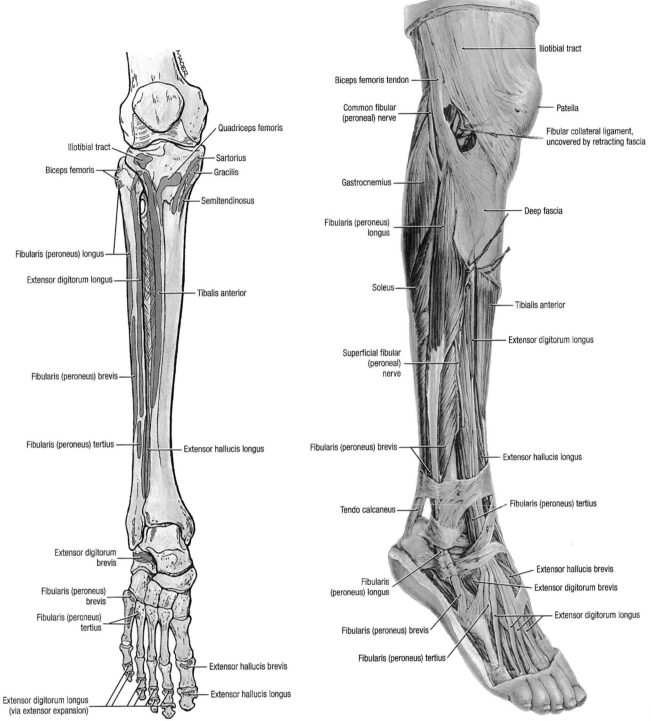

FIGURE 37-1. A: Anterior view of the tibia, fibula, and dorsum of the foot shows the muscle attachments. **B:** Anterolateral view of the muscles of the leg and foot. (From Agur AMR, Lee MJ. *Grant's atlas of anatomy,* 10th ed. Philadelphia: Lippincott Williams & Wilkins, 1999, with permission.)

A   A1   A2   A3

B   B1   B2   B3

C   C1   C2   C3

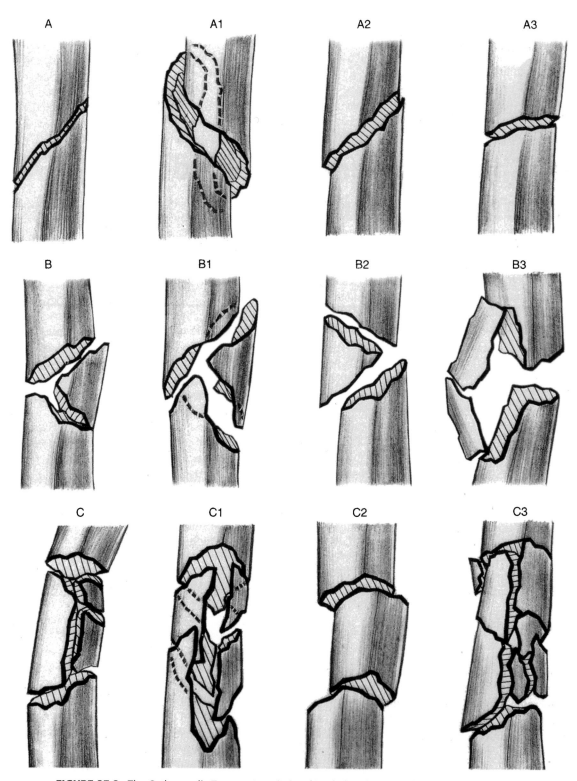

FIGURE 37-2. The Orthopaedic Trauma Association (OTA) classification of tibia fractures. (From Winquist RA. Tibial-shaft fractures: reamed intramedullary nailing. In: Wiss DA, ed. *Master techniques in orthopaedic surgery: fractures.* Philadelphia: Lippincott Williams & Wilkins, 1998:412, with permission.)

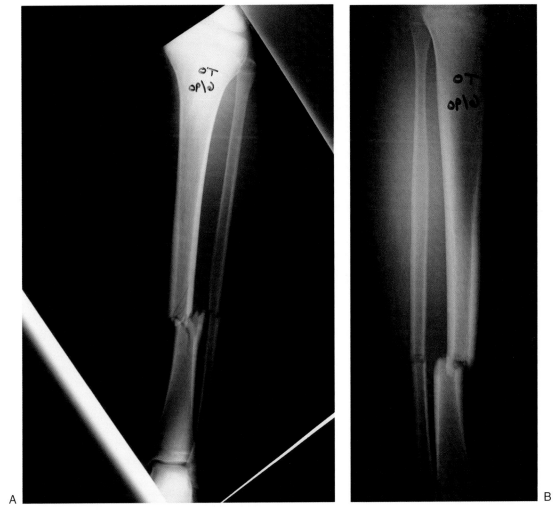

FIGURE 37-3. Anteroposterior **(A)** and lateral **(B)** radiographs demonstrating a fracture of the tibia and fibula.

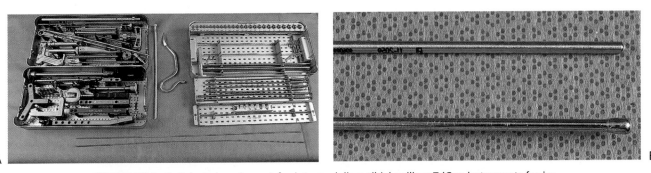

FIGURE 37-4. A: Selected equipment for intramedullary tibial nailing: TriGen instruments for implantation of a tibial or femoral nail *(left tray, top and bottom)*; Intramedullary reamer set *(right tray, top and bottom)*; guide wire exchange tube and curved awl *(between trays)*. **B:** Intramedullary tibial nailing instruments: straight-tipped *(top)* and ball-tipped *(bottom)* guide wires of identical length.

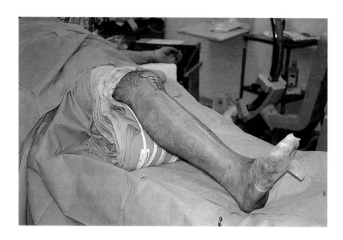

FIGURE 37-5. Supine patient positioning on a radiolucent table with a bolster under the knee. The knee is flexed to permit access to the proximal tibia.

EQUIPMENT

The equipment necessary for intramedullary tibial nailing includes the following (Fig. 37-4):

- Curved awl
- Ball-tipped and straight-tipped guide wires of identical length
- Intramedullary reamer set
- Guide wire exchange tube
- Tibial nail instrument and implant sets

PATIENT POSITIONING

Intramedullary tibial nailing can be performed with the patient positioned supine on a radiolucent table or on a fracture table. Supine positioning on a radiolucent table with a bolster under the knee is the simplest technique and is my preferred method. The knee is flexed over a radiolucent pad, which permits access to the proximal tibia and visualization of the starting point (Fig. 37-5). However, the disadvantage to this method of treatment is that it can be difficult to obtain and maintain fracture length in addition to controlling angulation and rotation.

A fracture table is more complex to set up but is more effective in maintaining length and rotation. With the fracture table, the knee is flexed 90 degrees over a post, which is placed proximal to the popliteal fossa to prevent compression of the vessels or peroneal nerve. Tape can be placed around the thigh to prevent external rotation of the extremity.

FRACTURE REDUCTION

Most tibial shaft fractures can be manually reduced using a combination of longitudinal traction and angular directed force (Fig. 37-6). Although rarely necessary, a femoral dis-

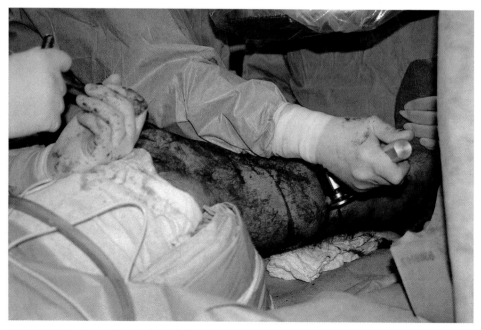

FIGURE 37-6. Manual reduction of the tibial shaft using a combination of longitudinal traction and an angularly directed force.

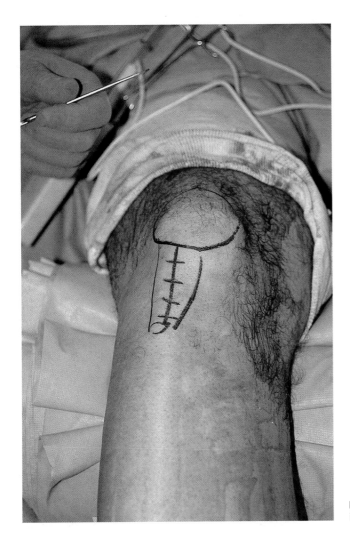

FIGURE 37-7. The incision extends from the tibial tubercle to the inferior aspect of the patella.

tractor can be used with a pin placed proximally in the posterior tibia and distally just above the ankle joint. In acute fractures, a unilateral frame is usually adequate.

INCISION AND SURGICAL APPROACH

The incision extends from the tibial tubercle to the inferior aspect of the patella (Fig. 37-7). The medial aspect of the patella tendon is identified and the patella tendon reflected laterally (Fig. 37-8). ◧ A curved awl is used to open the medullary canal at the junction of the anterior tibia and knee joint (Fig. 37-9). ◧ It is important to stay extraarticular, because backout of the nail may impinge on the femoral condyle. It is equally important not to enter at the tibia tubercle, because this leads to a more oblique anteroposterior starting angle with a greater risk for penetration of the posterior cortex with the nail. The exact starting point for the awl is determined on the anteroposterior and lateral fluoroscopic views. In midshaft and distal tibial fractures, the anteroposterior starting point should be in line with the center of the tibial shaft. On the lateral radiograph, the point of the awl should be just inferior to the joint line. In proximal fractures, the incision and starting point is just lateral to the patellar tendon; this results in the nail abutting against the lateral tibial cortex, which helps prevent translation and angulation.

OPERATIVE PROCEDURE

A bulb-tip guide wire is inserted down the canal (Fig. 37-10). It is helpful to place a small bend in the guide wire 2 cm from the tip. This often facilitates passing of the wire across the fracture site. A T-handle, which is used to control the bulb-tip guide, is placed in the midportion of the guide wire. The bulb tip is initially aimed posteriorly to enter the tibia and then immediately turned anteriorly and passed down to the fracture site, avoiding penetration of the posterior cortex proximally or exiting through the fracture site posteriorly. The guide wire is advanced to the fracture site (Fig. 37-11), the fracture is reduced, and the guide wire is

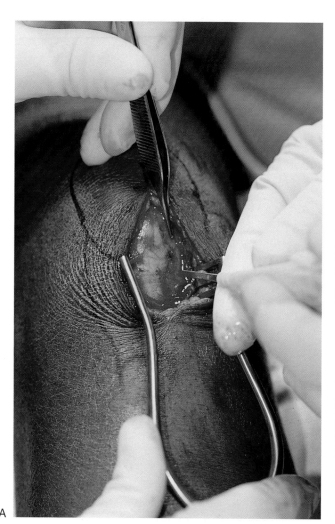

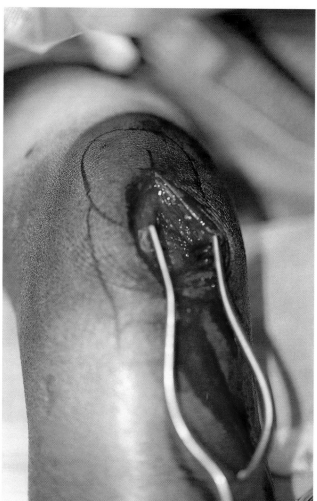

A

B

FIGURE 37-8. The medial aspect of the patella tendon is identified **(A)**, and the patella tendon is reflected laterally **(B)**.

advanced under image intensification into the distal fragment (Fig. 37-12). ◄ It is impacted into the subchondral bone above the ankle (Fig. 37-13) to stabilize the bulb tip and to aid in determining length. A second bulb tip of identical length is placed at the joint line, ◄ and a long ruler is used to determine nail length (Fig. 37-14). Another method to determine the nail length is to measure the tibia externally with a long ruler with hatch marks and confirm it with the image intensifier.

Reaming is a critical part of the surgical technique and must be done well to avoid complications (Fig. 37-15). ◄ Reaming must be done with sharp cutting reamers that dissipate heat and pressure. To prevent soft tissue damage around the incision, a skin protector should be used. **A tourniquet should be avoided because of the increased risk for thermal heat necrosis.** The surgeon starts with a small-diameter reamer and increases by 0.5-mm increments until cortical contact is reached. The fracture must be reduced as the reamer passes. The operator must take care to prevent loss of the guide wire position during each reamer introduc-

tion and removal. If the canal diameter permits, it is mechanically beneficial to place a nail that is 10 mm in diameter or larger. If necessary, an 8- or 9-mm nail may be used. However, with smaller nails, the patient's postoperative management may need to be modified.

Before nail insertion, a plastic exchange tube is passed over the bulb tip and across the fracture site (Fig. 37-16). ◄ The bulb tip is removed, a straight tip guide wire is inserted, and the plastic tube is removed. The nail is introduced down the tibial canal over this guide wire (Fig. 37-17). ◄ It is important to push posteriorly on the proximal end of the nail to minimize penetration of the posterior cortex. As the nail approaches the fracture, the fracture must be aligned in two planes. The nail should be inserted in slight external rotation. If the nail is allowed to rotate internally, interlocking occurs on the posteromedial cortex proximally and distally, which is much more difficult than if carried out on the flat surface of the tibia. To make targeting an easier process, the nail should be externally rotated approximately 10 degrees in relation to the long axis of the tibia.

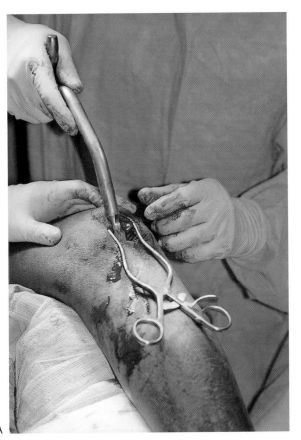
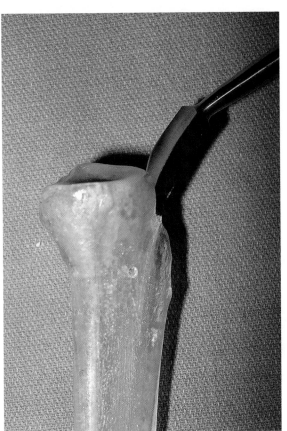

FIGURE 37-9. A and B: A curved awl is used to open the medullary canal at the junction of the anterior tibia and knee joint.

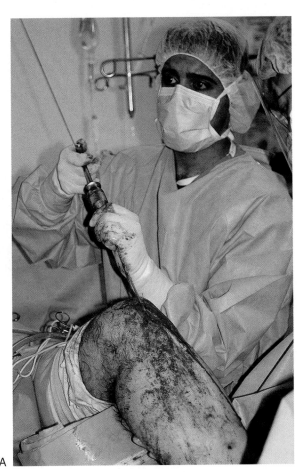
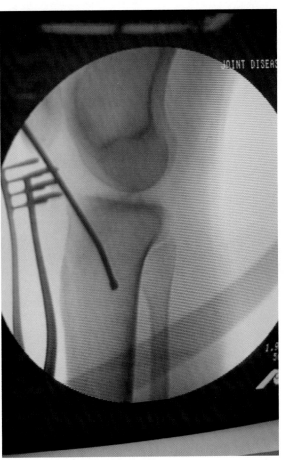

FIGURE 37-10. A and B: Insertion of a bulb-tip guide wire down the medullary canal.

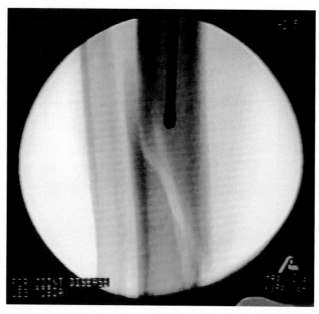

FIGURE 37-11. Advancement of the guide wire to the fracture site.

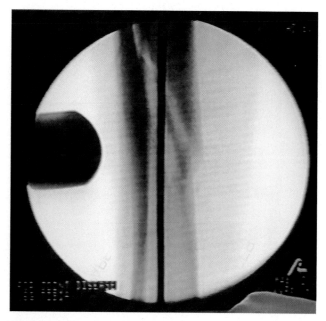

FIGURE 37-12. Fracture reduction and guide wire advancement into the distal fragment.

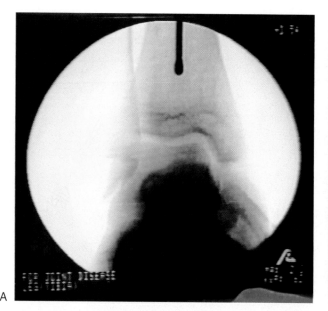

A

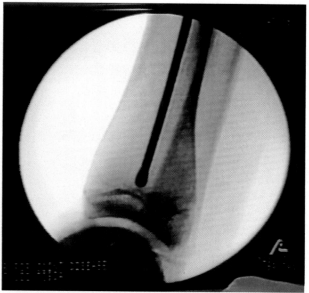

B

FIGURE 37-13. Advancement of the guide wire to the subchondral bone above the ankle. The guide wire should be centered on the anteroposterior **(A)** and lateral **(B)** radiographs.

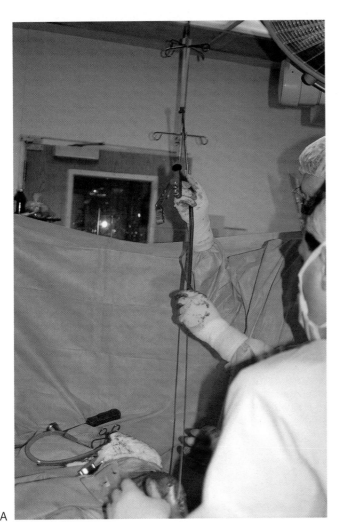

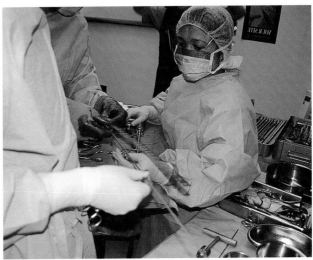

FIGURE 37-14. Determination of the tibial nail length. **A:** A second guide wire of identical length is placed at the joint line and overlapped with the external portion of the reduction guide wire. **B:** The overlapped amount is subtracted from total guide wire length to determine the nail length.

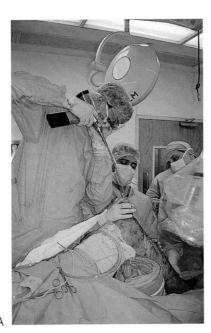

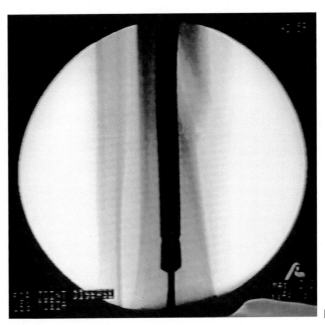

FIGURE 37-15. A and B: Reaming of the intramedullary canal.

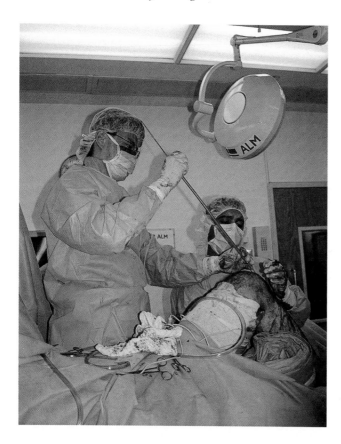

FIGURE 37-16. After intramedullary reaming, a plastic exchange tube is passed over the bulb tip and across the fracture site. The bulb tip is removed, a straight tip guide wire is inserted, and the plastic tube is removed.

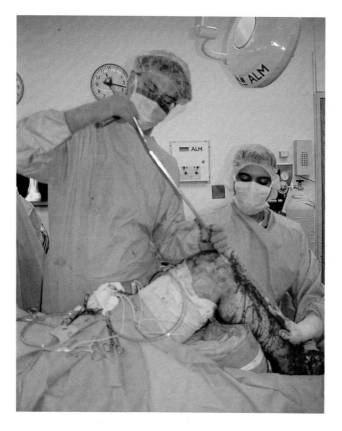

FIGURE 37-17. The nail is introduced down the tibial canal over the straight-tipped guide wire.

As the nail crosses the fracture site, it is important to avoid fracture distraction. In stable fracture patterns, traction can be released when the nail tip is 1 cm past the fracture. This allows fracture impaction and avoids distraction. Distal counterpressure can also be used as the nail crosses the fracture to prevent fracture distraction. As the nail is driven down the tibia, it is important to reassess the accuracy of its length. The tibia should be inspected proximally and distally. If the nail is too short or too long, it should be removed and replaced with another nail.

After the nail is fully seated (Fig. 37-18), proximal and distal interlocking screws are inserted. Targeting devices that attach to the intramedullary nail are very successful in placing the proximal tibial locking screws (Fig. 37-19). Only one

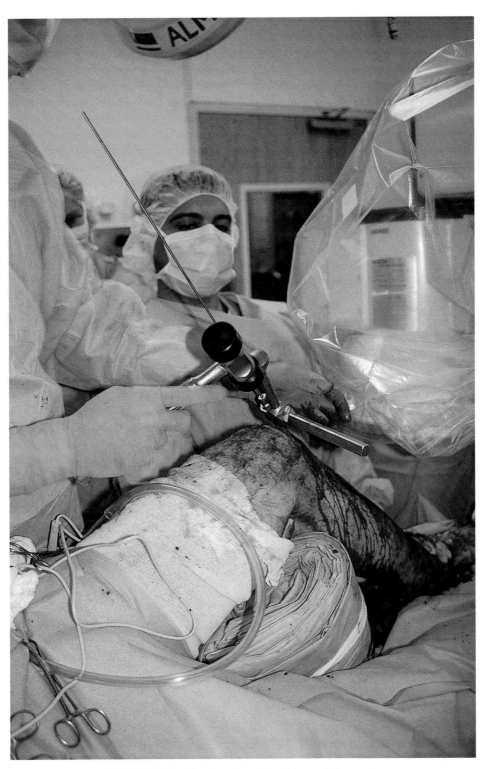

FIGURE 37-18. Final seating of the intramedullary nail.

proximal screw is necessary for fractures in the midshaft and below. For proximal fractures, two screws are necessary in the proximal end of the nail. For stable transverse or short oblique tibial fractures, the use of a dynamic slot at the proximal end of the nail is beneficial to allow impaction of the fracture. If there is any sign of comminution or a spiral component to the fracture, the nail should be statically locked.

A freehand technique is employed for distal locking screw insertion (Fig. 37-20). 🎥 Proximal and distal locking screws are inserted from medial to lateral in the subcutaneous border of the tibia. The freehand technique requires targeting of the skin incision. The image intensifier is lined up with the nail and tilted and rotated until a perfectly round hole is visualized. It is helpful to move the C-arm head away from the tibia to increase the working space and aid in magnification of the hole. The sharp point of the trocar-tipped pin is placed on the skin until it is centered in the hole. A 1-cm stab wound is made directly over the hole on the medial aspect of the tibia. The sharp, pointed pin is again placed on the bone until it is centered in the hole. It is brought into the longitudinal axis and

checked with fluoroscopy to ensure that it is centered in all planes. The pin is then passed into the tibia. Fluoroscopy is used to verify that the pin has corrected targeted the nail and the pin drilled through the far cortex. The length for the locking is determined using a second pin of the same length or a depth gauge, or it is estimated using the image intensifier. The screw is then inserted. The screw should be 5 mm too long, because this makes removal of a broken screw easier. A lateral radiograph should be checked again to be absolutely certain the screw is in the nail and has not moved anteriorly or posteriorly.

The wounds are then irrigated and closed. Before wound closure, it is important to again verify the adequacy of the fracture reduction, including rotational alignment. If necessary, the patient is checked for increased compartment pressure. Final radiographs are taken with the patient under anesthesia.

POSTOPERATIVE MANAGEMENT

The patient is placed in a well-padded posterior splint with the ankle neutral or in slight dorsiflexion to prevent an equi-

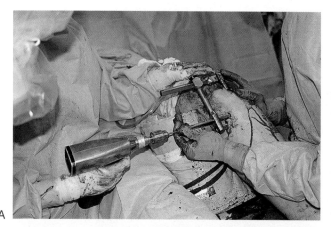

A

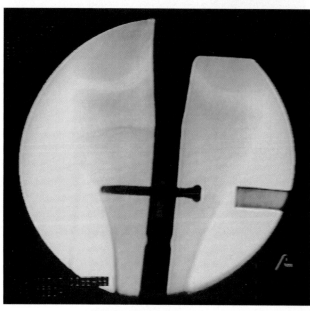

C

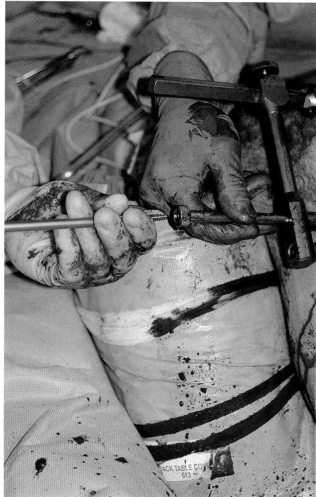

B

FIGURE 37-19. After the nail has been inserted to the appropriate depth, the proximal tibia is drilled **(A)**, the length of the locking screw measured, and the locking screw inserted **(B and C)**.

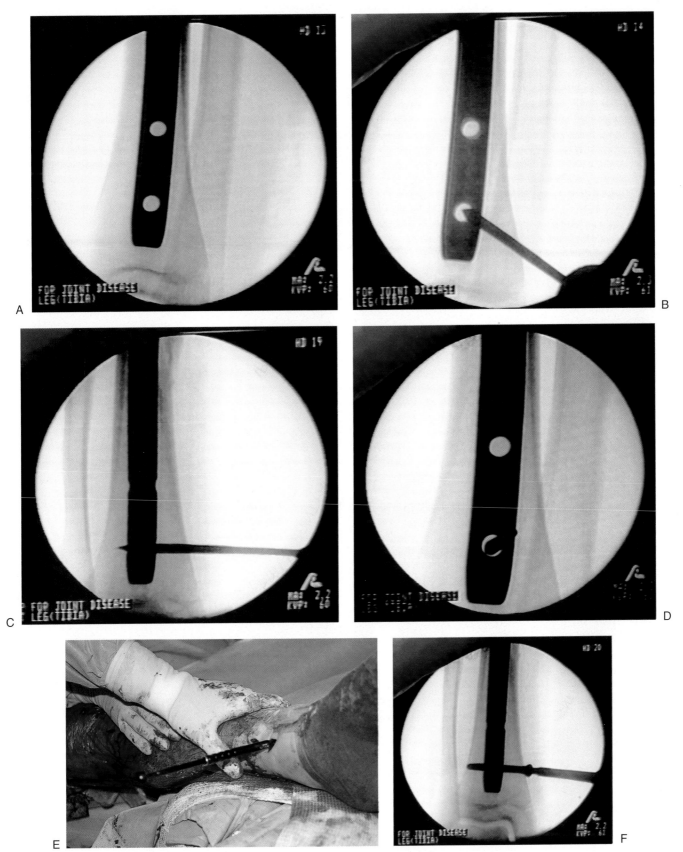

FIGURE 37-20. A freehand technique is used to insert the distal locking screws. **A:** The image intensifier is lined up with the nail and tilted and rotated until a perfectly round hole is visualized. **B:** The sharp point of the trocar-tipped pin is placed on the skin until it is centered in the hole. **C:** The pin is then brought into the longitudinal axis and passed into the tibia. **D:** Fluoroscopy is used to verify that the pin has correctly targeted the nail and that the pin drilled through the far cortex. **E:** The length for the locking screw is determined using a second pin of the same length or a depth gauge, or it is estimated using the image intensifier. **F:** The locking screw is then inserted.

nus deformity. The patient remains in a splint until the swelling decreases. In a reliable patient with a stable fracture pattern and a dynamic locking screw, toe-touch weight bearing is desirable, with progressive weight bearing over the first 4 weeks. For an unstable injury pattern or an unreliable patient, avoidance of weight bearing is recommended for the first 6 to 8 weeks.

SUGGESTED READINGS

Alho A, Benterud JG, Hogevold HE, et al. Comparison of functional bracing and locked intramedullary nailing in the treatment of displaced tibial shaft fractures. *Clin Orthop* 1992;277:243–250.

Anglen JO, Blue JM. A comparison of reamed and unreamed nailing of the tibia. *J Trauma* 1995;39:351–355.

Bone LB, Johnson KD. Treatment of tibial fractures by reaming and intramedullary nailing. *J Bone Joint Surg Am* 1986;68:877–887.

Court-Brown CM, McQueen MM, Quaba AA, et al. Locked intramedullary nailing of open tibial fractures. *J Bone Joint Surg Br* 1991;73:959–964.

Court-Brown CM, Will E, Christie J, et al. Reamed or unreamed nailing for closed tibial fractures: a prospective study in Tscherne C1 fractures. *J Bone Joint Surg Br* 1996;78:580–583.

Moed BR, Watson JT. Intramedullary nailing of aseptic tibial nonunions without the use of the fracture table. *J Orthop Trauma* 1995;9:128–134.

Tornetta P III, Collins E. Semi-extended position of intramedullary nailing of the proximal tibia. *Clin Orthop* 1996;328:185–189.

SUBJECT INDEX

Page numbers in *italics* denote figures; those followed by "t" denote tables